Comprehensive Health Insurance

Billing, Coding, and Reimbursement

Third Edition

Deborah Vines, CHAM, CRCR

Ann Braceland, NCICS

Elizabeth Stager Rollins, NCICS

Susan Miller, NCICS

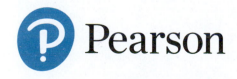 Pearson

330 Hudson Street, NY, NY 10013

Vice President, Health Science and TED: Julie Levin Alexander

Director of Portfolio Management: Marlene McHugh Pratt

Development Editor: Joan Gill

Portfolio Management Assistant: Emily Edling

Vice President, Content Production and Digital Studio: Paul DeLuca

Managing Producer, Health Science: Melissa Bashe

Content Producer: Faye Gemmellaro

Project Monitor: Meghan DeMaio

Operations Specialist: Mary Ann Gloriande

Creative Director: Blair Brown

Creative Digital Lead: Mary Siener

Managing Producer, Digital Studio, Health Science: Amy Peltier

Digital Studio Producer, REVEL and e-text 2.0: Jeff Henn

Digital Content Team Lead: Brian Prybella

Digital Content Project Lead: Lisa Rinaldi

Vice President, Product Marketing: David Gesell

Field Marketing Manager: Brittany Hammond

Full-Service Project Management and Composition: iEnergizer Aptara®, Ltd.

Full-Service Project Manager: Marianne Peters Riordan

Inventory Manager: Vatche Demirdjian

Interior and Cover Design: iEnergizer Aptara®, Ltd.

Cover Art: Frank Rohde/Shutterstock

Part and Chapter Opener Art: Frank Rohde/Shutterstock; Docent/Shutterstock; Faiz Zaki/Shutterstock

Printer/Binder: LSC Communications, Inc.

Cover Printer: Phoenix Color/Hagerstown

Credits and acknowledgments for content borrowed from other sources and reproduced, with permission, appear at the end of this textbook.

Library of Congress Cataloging-in-Publication Data

Names: Vines, Deborah, author. | Braceland, Ann, author. | Rollins, Elizabeth (NCICS) author. | Miller, Susan (Susan R.), author.

Title: Comprehensive health insurance : billing, coding, and reimbursement / Deborah Vines, Ann Braceland, Elizabeth Rollins, Susan Miller.

Description: Third edition. | Boston : Pearson, [2017] | Preceded by: Comprehensive health insurance / Deborah Vines ... [et al.]. 2nd ed. 2013. | Includes bibliographical references and index.

Identifiers: LCCN 2017001573| ISBN 013445877X (pbk.) | ISBN 9780134458779 (pbk.)

Subjects: | MESH: Forms and Records Control—methods | Insurance, Health, Reimbursement | Insurance Claim Reporting | Patient Credit and Collection—methods

Classification: LCC R728.5 | NLM W 80 | DDC 368.38/2—dc23

LC record available at https://lccn.loc.gov/2017001573

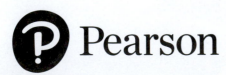

ISBN-10:   0-13-445877-X

ISBN-13: 978-0-13-445877-9

Dedication

I have had the privilege watching students of all ages dedicate time and effort to train and seek employment in the ever-changing healthcare industry. It brings great gratification to watch students complete their training, find employment, and be proud of their accomplishments. I dedicate this book to my students to express my gratitude in allowing me to share in their successes. I have benefited professionally and personally from their feedback and collaboration on the content of this textbook. Thank you.

—Deborah Vines

To My Family and Students

With special gratitude to the best caregiver, friend, and the love of my life—Norbs.

And my blessings for Lisa, Robert and Chris, each of whom have a special place in my heart.

—Ann B. Braceland

I can't think of a better field to work in than the healthcare field. Yes, things are changing constantly and there is always more to learn. There is no stagnation. This textbook gives a foundation for learning, and the students whom we have taught and who have used it have given us direction with their questions and insight. We could not have written this without them. I, too, dedicate this to all students, past and present, young or old, career changers or just starting out. Believe in yourself. You can do it!

I with to thank my fellow authors, Deborah, Ann, and Susan, who have continued to make this is a great experience.

And of course, a huge thank you to my husband and my entire family for their never-ending faith and support.

—Elizabeth Stager Rollins

To my children, Abram, Aleisha and Aaron

Their love and support assisted me through writing, and completing the third edition of this book.

—Susan Miller

Contents

Preface   xii

About the Authors   xv

Acknowledgments   xvi

Section I A Career in Healthcare   1

Chapter 1 Introduction to Professional Billing and Coding Careers   2

Employment Demand   4

Facilities   4
   Physician's Practice   4
   Multispecialty Clinic   5
   Hospital   5
   Centralized Billing Office   5

Job Titles and Responsibilities   6
   Medical Office Assistant   6
   Medical Biller   6
   Payment Poster   7
   Medical Collector   7
   Refund Specialist   7
   Insurance Verification Representative   7
   Admitting Clerk or Front Desk Representative   8

Certifications   8
   Medical Coder   10

   Privacy Compliance Officer   11

Registered Health Information Administrator (RHIA)   11
   Registered Health Information Technician (RHIT)   12
   Health Information Clerk   12
   Medical and Health Services Manager   12

Listing of Certifications   12
   Medical Office Assistant Certifications   12
   Medical Billing Certifications   13
   Medical Coding Certifications   13
   Medical Records Certification   14

Professional Memberships   14

Chapter Summary   15

Chapter Review   15

Resources   18

Section II The Relationship between the Patient, Provider, and Carrier   21

Chapter 2 Understanding Managed Care: Insurance Plans   24

The History of Healthcare in America   26

Healthcare Reform   28

Managing and Controlling Healthcare Costs   29
   Discounted Fees for Services   30
   Medically Necessary Patient Care   32
   Care Rendered by Appropriate Provider   32
   Appropriate Medical Care in Least Restrictive Setting   33

   Withholding Providers' Funds   33

Types of Managed Care Organizations   34
   Health Maintenance Organization (HMO)   34
   Preferred Provider Organization (PPO)   36
   Point-of-Service (POS) Options   36
   Exclusive Provider Organization   37
   Criticism of MCOs   37

Integrated Healthcare Delivery Systems   39
   Independent Physician Association   40
   Physician-Hospital Organization   40
   Self-Insured Plan   40

Insurance Plans   41

Commercial Health Insurance   41

Types of Insurance Coverage   42

Indemnity Plan/Fee for Service   42
Hospital Insurance   42
Hospital Indemnity Insurance   42
Medical Insurance   42
Surgical Insurance   43
Outpatient Insurance   43
Major Medical Insurance   43
Special Risk Insurance   43
Catastrophic Health Insurance   43
Short-Term Health Insurance   43
COBRA Insurance   43
Long-Term Care Insurance   44
Supplemental Insurance   44

Health Savings Accounts   44

HSA   44

HRA   45

FSA   45

Affordable Care Act   45

The Provider's View of Managed
Care   46

Patient Care   47
Facility Operations   47

Verifying Insurance Coverage   47

Collecting Insurance Payments   49

Assignment of Benefits   49

Chapter Summary   49

Chapter Review   50

Resources   53

Chapter 3 **Understanding Managed Care:
Medical Contracts and Ethics   54**

Purpose of a Contract   56

A Legal Agreement   57

Compensation and Billing Guidelines
for a MCO   57

Covered Medical Expenses   58
Payment   59

Ethics in Managed Care   60

Changes in Healthcare Delivery   60
MCO and Provider Credentialing   62
Ethics of the Medical Office Specialist   62

Contract Definitions   64

Compensation for Services   65

Patient's Bill of Rights   65

Concierge Contract   68

Chapter Summary   72

Chapter Review   73

Resources   75

Chapter 4 **Introduction to the Health
Insurance Portability and Accountability
Act (HIPAA)   76**

HIPAA Privacy Rule   78

Omnibus Rule   79
Legal Request   80

Pharmacies and Durable Medical Equipment   82

Language Barrier   82
Patient Access and Corrections   84

Transactions and Code Set Rule   84

Uniform Code Sets   85

Security Rule   85

Electronic Medical Record   85
Electronic Health Record   85

Unique Identifiers Rule   87

National Provider Identifier   88

HIPAA Enforcement Rule   88

Civil Penalties   88
Federal Criminal Penalties   88

Hitech Act   88

Meaningful Use   89

Privacy and Security Protection   91

Healthcare Reform   91

Chapter Summary   92

Chapter Review   92

Resources   95

Section III   Medical Coding   97

Chapter 5 ICD-10-CM Medical Coding   100

Definition of Diagnosis Coding   102

ICD-10-CM Guidelines   103

The Alphabetic Index   104

Neoplasm Table   104

Table of Drugs and Chemicals   104

External Causes Index   105

Structure of ICD-10-CM   105

Hyphen Usage (-)   106

√ Checkmark   106

The Tabular List   106

Placeholder   108

Laterality   108
  Coding Condition   110
  Body Mass Index   110
  Correct Coding Steps   110
  Abbreviations   114
  Surgical Coding   118
  Coding Late Effects   119
  Acute and Chronic Conditions   120
  Combination Codes: Multiple Coding   120

Chapter Summary   122

ICD-10-PCS   122

Chapter Review   124

Resources   127

Chapter 6 Introduction to CPT® and Place of Service Coding   128

Current Procedural Terminology (CPT)   130

CPT Categories   131
  CPT Category I   131
  CPT Category II   132
  CPT Category III   132

CPT Nomenclature   133
  Symbols   134
  Guidelines   134

CPT Modifiers   134
  Evaluation and Management Modifiers   135

Coding to the Place of Service   136
  Other Services Provided in the E/M Section   137

Office versus Hospital Services   137
  Emergency Department Services   138
  Preventive Medicine Services   138

Type of Patient   138
  New Patient   138
  Established Patient   138
  Referral   139
  Consultation   139

Level of E/M Service   139
  Extent of Patient's History   141
  Extent of Examination   143
  Complexity of Medical Decision Making   144
  Additional Components   145
  Assigning the Code   148

Chapter Summary   148

Chapter Review   148

Resources   151

Chapter 7 Coding Procedures and Services   152

Organization of the CPT Index   154
  Instructions for Using the CPT Index   155
  Code Range   155

Formatting and Cross-References   155
  Formatting   155
  Cross-references   157

Section Guidelines   157

Modifiers   158

Add-on Codes (+)   163

Coding Steps   164
  Coding for Anesthesia   164

Surgical Coding   166

Separate Procedure   169

Surgical Package or Global Surgery Concept   170

Supplies and Services   172

Radiology Codes   172

Pathology and Laboratory Codes   174

Medicine Codes   175

Chapter Summary　176

Chapter Review　176

Resources　181

Chapter 8　HCPCS and Coding Compliance　182

History of HCPCS　184

HCPCS Level of Codes　185
　Level I: CPT Codes　185
　Level II: HCPCS National Codes　185

HCPCS Modifiers　185
　Use of the GA Modifier　186

HCPCS Index　186

Coding Compliance　188

Code Linkage　188

Billing CPT Codes　189
　Fraudulent Claims　189
　Physician Self-Referral (Stark Law)　190
　Government Investigations and Advice　194
　Errors Relating to Code Linkage and Medical
　　Necessity　195
　Errors Relating to the Coding Process　196
　Errors Relating to the Billing Process　196

National Correct Coding Initiative　196

Fraudulent Actions　198

Federal Compliance　198
　How to Be Compliant　198

Benefits of a Compliance Program　199
Ethics for the Medical Coder　199

Chapter Summary　200

Chapter Review　200

Resources　203

Chapter 9　Auditing　204

Purpose of an Audit　206

Types of Audits　207
　External Audit　207
　Internal Audit　208
　Accreditation Audits　208

Private Payer Regulations　209

Medical Necessity for E/M Services　209

Audit Tool　212

Key Elements of Service　212
　History　213
　Examination　216
　Medical Decision Making　219

Tips for Preventing Coding Errors with Specific
　E/M Codes　227

Chapter Summary　229

Chapter Review　229

Resources　231

Section IV　Medical Claims　233

Chapter 10　Physician Medical Billing　236

Conversion to Electronic Health Records　238

Patient Information　238

Superbills　241

Types of Insurance Claims: Paper versus
　Electronic　244

Optical Character Recognition　248

CMS-1500 Provider Billing Claim Form　248

Completing the CMS-1500 Claim Form　250
　Form Locators for the CMS-1500 Form　252

Physicians' Identification Numbers　263
　Practice Exercises　264

Common Reasons for Delayed or Rejected
　CMS-1500 Claim Forms　280

HIPAA Compliance Alert　284

Filing Secondary Claims　284
　Determining Primary Coverage　285
　Practice Exercises　286

Chapter Summary　299

Chapter Review　299

Resources　302

Chapter 11 Hospital Medical Billing 304

Inpatient Billing Process 306

Charge Description Master 307

Types of Payers 308

Coding and Reimbursement Methods 308

Diagnosis Related Group System 309
    Cost Outliers 310

UB-04 Hospital Billing Claim Form 312

Instructions for Completing the UB-04
    Claim Form 315

Codes for Use on the UB-04 Claim Form 322
    Type of Bill Codes (Form Locator 4) 322
    Sex Codes (Form Locator 11) 324

Admission/Discharge Hour Codes (Form Locators 13
    and 16) 324
Admission Type Codes (Form Locator 14) 324
Source of Admission (Form Locator 15) 325
Discharge Status Codes (Form Locator 17) 325
Condition Codes (Form Locators 18–28) 326
Occurrence Code Examples (Form
    Locators 31–34) 326
Value Codes (Form Locators 39–41) 328
Revenue Codes (Form Locator 42) 328
Patient Relationship (Form Locator 59) 330
Practice Exercises 330

Chapter Summary 338

Chapter Review 339

Resources 342

Section V Government Medical Billing 343

Chapter 12 Medicare Medical Billing 346

Medicare History 348
    Medicare Administration 348

Medicare Part A Coverage and Eligibility
    Requirements 350
    Inpatient Hospital Care 351
    Skilled Nursing Facility 351
    Home Healthcare 351
    Hospice Care 351
    Blood 352
    Organ Transplants 352
    Inpatient Benefit Days 352

Medicare Part B Coverage and Eligibility
    Requirements 354

Telemedicine 354

Medicare Part C 356

Medicare Part D 356

Services Not Covered by Medicare
    Parts A and B 357

Medigap, Medicaid, and Supplemental
    Insurance 358

Requirements for Medical Necessity 359

Medicare Coverage Plans 359
    Fee-for-Service: The Original Medicare Plan 359
    Medicare Advantage Plans or Medicare Part C 359

Value-Based Payment Modifier Program 360

Medicare Providers 360
    Part A Providers 360
    Part B Providers 360
    Participating versus Nonparticipating Medicare
        Part B Providers 361

Limiting Charge 362
    Patient's Financial Responsibility 362
    Determining the Medicare Fee and Limiting
        Charge 362

Patient Registration 366
    Copying the Medicare Card 366
    Copying the Driver's License 367
    Obtaining Patient Signatures 367
    Determining Primary and Secondary Payers 367
    Plans Primary to Medicare 368
    Consolidated Omnibus Budget Reconciliation
        Act of 1985 369
    People with Disabilities 369
    People with End-Stage Renal Disease 369
    Workers' Compensation 369
    Automobile, No-Fault, and Liability Insurance 369
    Veteran Benefits 369
    Medicare Coordination 369
    Medicare as the Secondary Payer 370
    Conditional Payment 370

Medicare Documents 371

Medicare Development Letter 371

Medicare Insurance Billing Requirements 372

Completing Medicare Part B Claims 372

Filing Guidelines   374
Local Coverage Determination   374

Medicare Remittance Notice   374

Medicare Fraud and Abuse   376
Medicare Fraud   376
Medicare Abuse   377
Protecting Against Medicare Fraud and Abuse   378

Chapter Summary   380

Chapter Review   381

Resources   383

Chapter 13 Medicaid Medical Billing   384

Medicaid Guidelines   387

Eligibility Groups   387
Categorically Needy   387
Medically Needy   388
Special Groups   389

Children's Health Insurance Program Reauthorization
Act (CHIPRA)   389

Scope of Medicaid Services   390
PACE   391

Amount and Duration of Medicaid Services   391

Payment for Medicaid Services   392

Medicaid Growth Trends   393
Affordable Care Act Projections   394

The Medicaid–Medicare Relationship
(Medi-Medi)   394

Medicaid Managed Care   395

Medicaid Verification   395

Medicaid Claims Filing   396
Time Limits for Submitting Claims   396

Appeal Time Limits   396
Claims with Incomplete Information and
Zero Paid Claims   397
Newborn Claim Hints   397

Completing the CMS-1500 Form for Medicaid
(Primary)   397
Practice Exercises   398

Chapter Summary   407

Chapter Review   407

Resources   411

Chapter 14 TRICARE Medical Billing   412

TRICARE   414
TRICARE Eligibility   414
Patient's Financial Responsibilities   415
Timely Filing   415
Penalties and Interest Charges   415
Authorized Providers   415
Preauthorization   416

TRICARE Standard and TRICARE Extra   417

TRICARE Prime   418

TRICARE Prime Remote   418

TRICARE Senior Prime/TRICARE for Life   420
TRICARE Reform   420

CHAMPVA   420

Submitting Claims to TRICARE   421

Completing the CMS-1500 Form for
TRICARE (PRIMARY)   422

Confidential and Sensitive Information   424

Chapter Summary   425

Chapter Review   425

Resources   427

Section VI Accounts Receivable   429

**Chapter 15 Explanation of Benefits and
Payment Adjudication   432**

Steps for Filing a Medical Claim   434

Claims Process   437

Determining the Fees   439
Charge-Based Fee Structure   439
Resource-Based Fee Structures   439

History of the Resource-Based Relative
Value Scale   439

The RBRVS System   440

The Medicare Conversion Factor   441

Determining the Medicare Fee   441

Allowed Charges   443

Payers' Policies   444

Capitation   449

Value-based Reimbursement   450

Calculations of Patient Charges   450
   Deductible   450
   Copayments   451
   Coinsurance   451
   Excluded Services   451

Balance Billing   453

Processing an Explanation of Benefits   453
   Information on an EOB/ERA   454

Reviewing Claims Information   463

Adjustments to Patient Accounts   464
   Processing Reimbursement Information   464
   Confirming Amount Paid, Making Adjustments,
      and Determining Amount Due from Patient   464

Methods of Receiving Funds   478
   Check by Mail   478
   Electronic Funds Transfer   478
   Lockbox Services   478

Chapter Summary   479

Chapter Review   479

Resources   483

Chapter 16 Refunds, Follow-Up, and Appeals   484

Electronically Filing Claims   486

Claims Rejection Follow-Up   486

Rebilling   487

Denied or Delayed Payments   488

Answering Patients' Questions about Claims   489

Claim Rejection Appeal   490

Peer Review   492

State Insurance Commissioner   492

Carrier Audits   494

Documentation   494
   Documentation Guidelines   494
   SOAP Record-Keeping Format   495

Necessity of Appeals   495

Registering a Formal Appeal   496

The Appeals Process   496
   Reason Codes That Require a Formal Appeal   498

Employee Retirement Income Security
   Act of 1974   498
   Waiting Period for an ERISA Claim   499
   Appeal to ERISA   499

Medicare Appeals   499
   Redetermination   499
   Second Level of Appeal   500
   Third Level of Appeal and Beyond   500

Appeal Letters   500
   Closing Words   501

Appeals and Customer Service   503
   Appeals Require Perseverance and Attitude   505
   Do Not Settle for "Denial Upheld"   505

Refund Guidelines   506
   Avoid Excessive Overpayments   508
   Guidelines for Insurance Overpayments and
      Refund Requests   508
   Practice Exercises   509

Chapter Summary   514

Chapter Review   514

Resources   517

Section VII Injured Employee Medical Claims   519

Chapter 17 Workers' Compensation   522

History of Workers' Compensation   524

Federal Workers' Compensation Programs   525

State Workers' Compensation Plans   525

Overview of Covered Injuries, Illnesses,
   and Benefits   526
   Occupational Diseases and Illnesses   527
   Work-Related Injury Classifications   527

Injured Worker Responsibilities and Rights   528

Treating Doctor's Responsibilities   529
   Selecting a Designated Doctor and Scheduling an
      Appointment   530
   Communicating with the Designated Doctor   530
   What the Designated Doctor Will Do   531
   Disputing the Designated Doctor's Findings   531

Disputing Maximum Medical Improvement or
   Impairment Rating   531

Ombudsmen 531

Types of Workers' Compensation Benefits 533
Income Benefits 534
Death and Burial Benefits 535

Eligible Beneficiaries 535

Benefits and Compensation Termination 535
Types of Government Disability Policies 536

Verifying Insurance Benefits 537

Preauthorization 537
Requirements for the Preauthorization Request 537

Filing Insurance Claims 538

Completing the CMS-1500 for Workers'
Compensation Claims 538

Independent Review Organizations 539
How to Obtain an Independent Review 541
The IRO Decision 541

Medical Records 541

Fraud 542
Penalties 543
Medical Provider Fraud 543

Calculating Reimbursements 544

Chapter Summary 548
Chapter Review 549
Resources 551

Appendix A Completing the CMS-1500 Form for Physician Outpatient Billing 553

Appendix B Completing the CMS-1500 Form for Physician Outpatient Billing Plus Determining the Correct Diagnostic and Procedure Codes 616

Appendix C Completing the UB-04 Form for Hospital Billing 658

Appendix D Medical Forms 700

Appendix E Acronyms and Abbreviations 735

Appendix F Medical Terminology Word Parts 737

Glossary 750
Credits 763
Index 765

Preface

This textbook was written to provide students with the knowledge and skills necessary to work in a variety of registration (front end revenue cycle management), billing (back end revenue cycle management), and coding positions in the healthcare field. Many textbooks have been written on this subject; however, daily feedback from students has allowed the author to develop the material in this text relevant to what a medical office specialist actually experiences. The student will learn the process of billing and how to properly manage the account from the initial encounter with the patient through the resolution of the claim. In addition to submitting claims to insurance carriers, the process of billing may include reviewing medical records, verifying patient benefits, estimating patient's financial responsibility, requesting authorization, submitting a primary and/or secondary claim, posting payments, and appealing the insurance carrier's decision.

This book has been written so that it is easy to read and comprehend. It is designed for students who have not previously worked in the medical field as well as students who have worked in the field but have only been exposed to certain aspects of the registration and billing process. An ideal employee at a healthcare facility has a clear understanding of how each element in the process affects all other steps, which is the underlying concept of this textbook. Practice exercises presented throughout the text allow students to test their knowledge of the concepts presented. This hands-on practice supplements lecture content and allows for better understanding of the skills presented.

The Development of This Text

This textbook originated as a result of healthcare students and instructors expressing their concern about the complexity and flow of textbooks being used in the classroom. Students routinely expressed dismay that the required textbooks did not provide a clear understanding of the order of the steps involved in the life of the account, from the time a patient is scheduled for an appointment to the resolution of the patient's account. As a result, workbooks were developed for each course in addition to the required reading material. The workbooks ultimately became the chapters in this textbook. Students also stated that the required reading in their textbooks was outdated. Therefore, this textbook has a MyHealthProfessionsLab and a MyHealthProfessionsKit that will provide the student and instructor with updated information and URLs where they can review current changes in the healthcare industry.

Organization of the Text

A great deal of time has been spent researching the material in this text in order to address the most frequently asked student questions and to clearly illustrate the key concepts of the medical billing and coding processes. The textbook provides a unique presentation of content, exercises, examples, and professional tips within each chapter.

Features of the Text

The following special features appear in this text:

Chapter Objectives: Each chapter begins with a list of key learning objectives that students should master on completion of the chapter.

Key Terms: A list of key terms appears at the beginning of each chapter, and the terms are highlighted where they are first introduced in the text. A comprehensive glossary is provided at the end of the text.

Case Studies with Critical Thinking Questions: A thought-provoking case study is presented at the beginning of each chapter along with critical thinking questions. Students must rely on the content in the text and their own critical thinking skills to answer the questions.

Introduction: Each chapter includes introductory material that explains to readers what they will encounter within the chapter.

Examples: Numerous examples are provided throughout the text to stress the correct use of the billing and coding guidelines that are discussed.

Professional Tips: Professional Tips appear throughout the text and provide additional information related to billing and coding processes that the student might use on the job.

Practice Exercises: Practice Exercises appear in most of the chapters to allow for student practice and mastery of skills.

Chapter Summary: The chapter summary serves as a review of the chapter content.

Chapter Review: End-of-chapter questions that help reinforce learning are provided in true/false, multiple-choice, and completion formats. The review questions measure the students' understanding of the material presented in the chapter. These tools are available for use by the student or by the instructor as an outcomes assessment.

For Additional Practice: These additional case studies and billing and coding exercises allow for additional student practice and mastery of skills.

Resources: This listing provides additional information (organization contact information, websites, etc.) related to the chapter content.

New to This Edition

The healthcare industry is always a whirlwind of change, prompting government, insurance organizations, and healthcare providers to look for ways to make healthcare affordable. The Affordable Care Act is the most recent government sponsored regulation that is discussed in the text.

In Chapter 13, changes in Medicaid are discussed that were implemented by the Affordable Care Act, allowing states to opt in or opt out of the Medicaid expansion program. This will help drive consolidation, as it will add millions of new individuals and billions in new premiums to the Medicaid market.

Concierge Medicine and Telemedicine are new methods of healthcare treatment and cost-saving programs.

ICD-10 finally was implemented after many delays. All coding information and exercises in this text use 2017 codes. Chapter 5 addresses the new way to code the International Classification of Diseases using 4–7 alpha characters for more specificity of the patient's health problem.

The new CMS-1500 form is reviewed in detail and all related exercises and examples include the (02-2012) form.

Technology advances and consumer demands have increased automation of health-care, such as electronic health records (EHR), patient portals, and real time eligibility verification and claim submission.

■ New Figures and Tables have been added to this third edition to illustrate key concepts.
■ Content has been updated throughout the text to reflect current information on healthcare changes, trends, and the movement of healthcare in the future.

Ten trends for the next decade are evident:
1. more patients
2. more technology
3. more information
4. the patient as the ultimate consumer
5. development of a different delivery model
6. innovation driven by competition
7. increasing costs
8. increasing numbers of uninsured
9. less pay for providers
10. the continued need for a new healthcare system.

■ The 2017 code sets are used throughout the text.
■ ICD-9 has been eliminated.
■ ICD-10 has been added.
■ The previous chapter about completing manual claims has been eliminated, as electronic medical claims are standard practice in today's medical office.

The Learning Package

The Student Package

■ **Textbook**
■ **MyHealthProfessionsLab:** Designed to reach students in a personal way. Engaging learning and practice opportunities lead to assessments that create a personalized study plan.
■ **Student Workbook:** The *Student Workbook* contains key terms, chapter objectives, chapter outlines, critical thinking questions, practice exercises, review questions, and end-of-workbook tests/case study–type problems that test student knowledge of the key concepts presented in the core textbook.

The Instructional Package

■ **Instructor's Resource Manual:** The *Instructor's Resource Manual* contains chapter learning objectives; lesson plans for each learning objective with a customizable section for instructor notes, teaching tips, concepts for lecture; PowerPoint lecture slides that correspond to each concept for lecture; and suggestions for classroom activities.
■ **MyTest:** This electronic test generator contains more than 1,500 test questions.
■ **PowerPoint Slides:** The slides can be used during daily lectures.

About the Authors

Deborah Vines has worked extensively for more than 30 years in the healthcare industry as a practice administrator and manager in physical therapy, dermatopathology, and pediatrics. She has also held senior leadership positions in the hospital setting. As director of operations for a national healthcare staffing corporation, she has traveled across the United States, working directly with physicians and medical human resources personnel to secure jobs for individuals in the medical billing, coding, and collection fields. One of Ms. Vines's notable achievements is that in one fiscal year, through mentoring and training, she assisted 300 recruits to find employment in the medical billing industry. This achievement led her to opening Allied Career Center in Dallas, Texas, a successful vocational school specializing in medical office specialist training.

Ann Braceland has been working in the medical field since graduating from Gwynedd Mercy College with an associate's degree in nursing science. As a practice manager, her extensive work in the field of managed care and medical billing and coding have allowed her to research and find means to inform others through her teaching of the changes and challenges that arise in the medical field. Ann Braceland has established and managed satellite offices in physical and occupational medicine. She is a Medicare representative with a vast spectrum of knowledge that she uses to train staff and physicians in compliance coding and billing. As director of training for the instructors of Allied Career Center in Dallas, Texas, her presentation of the material for students led to the publication of this book. Ann Braceland is a National Certified Insurance and Coding Specialist.

Elizabeth Rollins has been in the medical billing and coding industry for 30 years, handling coding, insurance and patient billing, medical appeals, physician appeals, physician credentialing, and new employee training. She was the Vice President of Allied Career Center, where she also taught for seven years. She has been instrumental in placing hundreds of people into medical field jobs.

Susan Miller has worked in the healthcare Industry for 25 years, managing and supervising medical billing processes. She has lectured in a classroom setting, providing students with knowledge and skills on medical billing and coding. Ms. Miller continues her healthcare career in medical billing, providing support to staff members on billing and coding guidelines.

Acknowledgments

We would like to thank our publisher, Pearson, Marlene Pratt, Faye Gemmellaro, executive editor, and Joan Gill, developmental editor; and the following reviewers, who used their personal time to provide feedback for our project. Without your hard work and guidance, none of this would have been possible:

First Edition Reviewers

Vanessa Armor, RHIT
Instructor
Ivy Tech Community College, Michigan
City Campus, Indiana

Robin Berenson, Ed.D.
Spartanburg Community College,
South Carolina

Dorothy Burney
Adjunct Professor Allied Health/
Certified Coding Specialist
City College, Florida

Barbara Dahl, CMA, CPC
Medical Assisting Program Coordinator
and Department Chair
Whatcom Community College,
Washington

Susan DeGirolamo, RMA, NCPT, NCICS
Instructor
Pennsylvania Institute of Technology,
Pennsylvania

Annette Derks, CPC, CHI
Instructor
Canyon College, Florida

Shirley Jelmo, CMA, RMA
Medical Assisting Instructor
PIMA Medical Institute, Colorado

Kathy Kneifel
Instructor
Everett Community College, Washington

Tiffany Rosta, CMA
Medical Instructor
Kaplan Career Institute, Pennsylvania

Lorraine M. Smith
Instructor
Fresno City College, California

Teresa Williamson
Medical Coding and Billing Professor
Chaffey Community College, California

Second Edition Reviewers

Cindy Brassingon, MS, CMA
Professor of Allied Health
Quinebaug Valley Community College,
Connecticut

Linda H. Donahue, RHIT, CCS, CCSP, CPC
Assistant Professor, Health Information
Technology
Delgado Community College, Louisiana

Lurrean Bentley, RMA, CMRS
Instructor for Medical Assisting and
Billing/Coding Programs
Remington College, Tennessee

Michelle Edwards, CPMB, CMRS, CBCS, CCP
Medical Billing and Coding Lead
University of Antelope Valley, California

Sandra E. Fender
Instructor Southern Crescent Technical
College, Georgia

Gail High, AA
Program Coordinator, Medical Billing
and Coding Program
YTI Career Institute, Pennsylvania

Deborah McGichen, BS
Medical Billing and Coding Instructor
Allstate Career,
Allied Health Division,
Maryland

Angela Mitchell, Master of Technical Education
Instructor
Akron Institute of Herzing
University, Ohio

Julia Steff, RHIA, CCS, CCS-P
Assistant Professor, Department Chair
Palm Beach State College, Florida

Nerissa Tucker, MHA, CPC
Professor, Program Director
Allied Health Institute, Texas

Third Edition Reviewers

Lisa Mayberry
Licensed Nursing Home Administrator
Pennsylvania Institute of Technology

Grace Dimarco, CBCS, RMA
McCann School of Business
and Technology

Diana Wilcox, CPC, CPMA, CPC-I
Blue Cliff College

Deborah Malay-Hunt
The College of Healthcare Professions

Angela Campbell, RHIA, AHIMA-approved ICD-10 CM/PCS Trainer
Northwestern College

Kiyoe Irikura, CPC, CMBS
IMBC College

Rolando Russell, CPC
Ultimate Medical Academy

Robert Pezillo, CPC, CPC-I, CPPM, CPB
Community College of Rhode Island

Karlene Richardson, DHA
Mandl School

Bonnie Aspiazu, JD, FACHE, RHIA
St. Vincent Health System

Chapter Opener Features

Chapter Objectives

Each chapter opens with a list of learning objectives, which can be used to identify the material and skills the student should know upon successful completion of the chapter.

▶

Chapter Objectives

After reading this chapter, the student should be able to:

1. Understand the requirements for qualifying to receive Medicaid benefits.
2. Determine the schedule of benefits the Medicaid recipient will receive.
3. Discuss the method of verifying Medicaid benefits.
4. Submit a Medicaid claim and decipher claim status.

Key Terms

categorically needy
Children's Health Insurance Program (CHIP)
Children's Health

and Treatment (EPSDT)
Federal Medical Assistance Percentages (FMAP)

State Children's Health Insurance Program (SCHIP)
Supplemental Security Income (SSI)

◀ ## Key Terms

The Key Terms section appears at the beginning of each chapter. The terms are listed in alphabetical order, and the terminology appears in boldface on first introduction in the text. All terms are defined in the comprehensive glossary that appears at the back of the book.

Case Study with Critical Thinking Questions

Thought-provoking case studies provide scenarios that help students understand how the material presented in the chapter relates to the medical billing and coding profession. Critical thinking questions appear after each case study, and students must rely on the content in the text and their own critical thinking skills to answer the questions.

▶

Case Study
Medicaid

The office manager, Darla, had received notification from the state Medicaid program that fraudulent use of Medicaid cards was on the rise. As a result, all patients were to show a picture I.D. along with their Medicaid card. Darla had announced this new policy at the last staff meeting.

While Ginger was working as the receptionist, a patient arrived and showed her Medicaid card. Ginger explained that she needed to see a picture I.D. because of increased fraud. The patient became indignant and refused to comply because she felt she was being accused of doing something illegal. Ginger asked Darla to explain the situation to the patient.

Questions

1. Should the patient be required to comply with the new policy in order to be seen by the physician? Why?
2. Could Ginger have handled the situation differently?
3. What should Darla tell the patient in order to calm her down?

Additional Features

Professional Tips

Helpful billing and coding tips are interspersed throughout the text and provide additional information the student might use on the job.

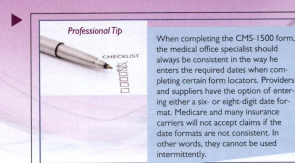

Professional Tip

CHECKLIST

When completing the CMS-1500 form, the medical office specialist should always be consistent in the way he enters the required dates when completing certain form locators. Providers and suppliers have the option of entering either a six- or eight-digit date format. Medicare and many insurance carriers will not accept claims if the date formats are not consistent. In other words, they cannot be used intermittently.

Examples

Numerous examples are provided throughout the text to stress the correct billing and coding guidelines.

Example

A patient with a headache comes in for an office visit. While being examined, the patient asks the doctor to look at his toe as long as he is there. The doctor discovers an ingrown toenail and performs minor surgery. A modifier is used to establish that a distinct and separate procedure was performed. The claims examiner disregards the modifier and denies the office visit as global. The medical office specialist should try to get the claim reconsidered by phone, requesting that the claim be paid and stating that the reason can be backed up with documentation. The medical office specialist should offer to fax the documentation.

Practice Exercises

Practice Exercises provide students with the opportunity to practice and master skills presented in the text.

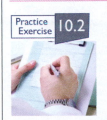

Practice Exercise 10.2

Completion of CMS-1500 (Section I)

Fill out form locators 1 through 13 on the CMS-1500 form based on the information given here. To complete this exercise, copy the CMS-1500 form provided in Appendix D or download the form from MyHealthProfessionsKit or MyHealthProfessionsLab, which accompany this text.

Liz Mary Smith is a patient in the medical office where you work. This information appears on her patient information form:

Name:	Liz Mary Smith
Gender:	Female
Birth Date:	July 1, 1996
Marital Status:	Single
Phone:	480-555-2984
Address:	4591 Explorer Drive
	Phoenix, AZ 12345
Responsible Person:	Harry L. Smith (father)
Insured's DOB:	August 5, 1950
Insured's Gender:	Male
Insured's Home Address:	5419 W. 8th Street, Apt. 306
	Norman, OK 12345
Insured's Employer Address:	Vines Lumber Co.
	6840 Judy Street
	Norman, OK 12345
Insurance Carrier:	BMA
	P.O. Box 7459
	Memphis, TN 12345
Insurance Certificate Number:	78815-080-07-000
Insurance Group Number:	G123456

Treatment and progress notes in the patient medical record indicate diagnosis of left acute otitis media ICD-10 (H66.92), on January 13, 20XX. The medical office collects only the coinsurance and waits for payment directly from the insurance carrier. Guarantor's signature on file for charges to be paid directly to provider, FORM SIGNED January 13, 20XX.

Authorization to release medical information on file.

Informational Tables and Forms

Informational tables and forms appear throughout the text and summarize pertinent information. They provide students with visuals and comparisons to reinforce the lesson.

▼

Table 16.2	Reason Codes That Require a Formal Appeal			
100	Services payable at 100%	DUP	Duplicate (previously processed)*
19	Dependent over age 19	ELIG	Pending eligibility
21	Dependent over age 21	ERR	Claim processing error or adjustment
1yr	Limited to one per year*	EXP	Experimental service not covered*
2ND	COB secondary payment	FUD	Included in surgical package*
3yr	Allowed once in 3 years*	INFO	Pending additional information
6MO	Allowed once in 6 months*	MAX	Maximum benefits paid
80%	Service(s) payable at 80%	MED	Not medically necessary*
ADD	Need additional information	N/C	Non-covered services*
ADM	Administrative adjustment	NER	Non-covered emergency services*
AOP	Approved out-of-plan	NOA	No answer to inquiry
AVE	Authorized number of visits exceeded*	NOD	No ordering doctor listed
BE	Billing error*	NPD	Nonparticipating doctor
BOI	Bill other insurance	NPP	Nonparticipating provider
CAP	Capitated services*	NREF	No referral or unauthorized*
CMC	Contractual maximum charge	PCI	Patient convenience item not covered*

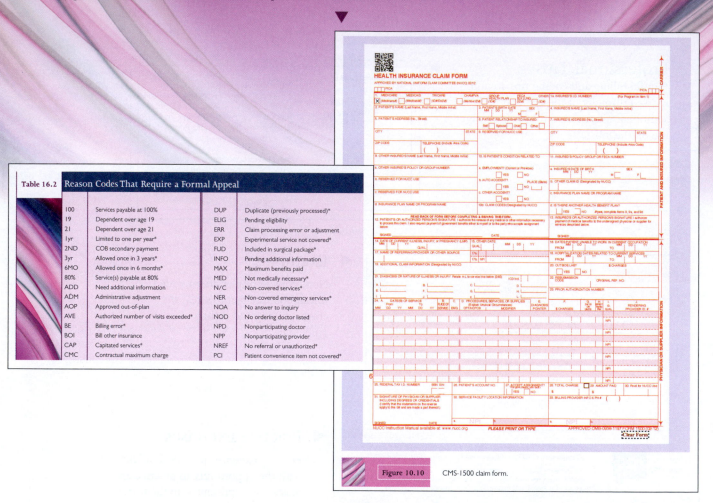

Figure 10.10   CMS-1500 claim form.

Chapter review

Chapter Summary

Each Chapter Summary is an excellent review of the chapter content.

Chapter Summary

- Changes in the way healthcare is paid for created a demand for allied health personnel trained in medical billing and coding.
- An allied health employee can find employment in a variety of medical settings.
- After completion of a course of study, the student is qualified for entry-level positions such as admitting clerk, medical biller, insurance verification representative, and medical collector.
- Certification demonstrates dedication to advancement and competency.

Chapter Review Questions

End-of-chapter questions are provided in true/false, multiple-choice, and completion formats to help reinforce learning. The review questions measure the student's understanding of the material presented in each chapter. These tools are available for use by the student or can be used by the instructor as an outcome assessment.

Chapter Review

True/False

Identify the statement as true (T) or false (F).

_____ **1.** PFS is an abbreviation for patient financial services.

_____ **2.** The medical office assistant might compile and record medical records, reports, and correspondence.

_____ **3.** HIPAA is an abbreviation for Hospital Information per American Medical Association.

_____ **4.** Certification is not required in most states.

For Additional Practice

These billing and coding exercises and case scenarios provide students with additional opportunity to practice skills and reinforce concepts presented in the chapter. These tools are available for use by the student or can be used by the instructor as an outcome assessment.

For Additional Practice

Code the following:

1. Acute bronchospasm _____

2. Herpes zoster myelitis _____

3. Smoking complicating pregnancy, childbirth, antepartum condition, or complication _____

Resources

Each end-of-chapter resources list provides additional information (organization contact information, websites, etc.) related to chapter content.

Resources

Alliance of Claims Assistance Professionals (ACAP)
873 Brentwood Drive
West Chicago, IL 60185-3743
www.claims.org; askacap@charter.net

Expert help with medical claims issues. This association works with clients and can assist with challenging denied claims and protecting clients' personal, medical, and financial information.

American Academy of Professional Coders (AAPC)
2480 South 3850 West, Suite B
Salt Lake City, UT 84120
800-626-CODE
www.aapc.com; info@aapc.com

I   Introduction to Professional Billing and Coding Careers

The content presented in this section will help the student understand the career opportunities available for the professional medical office specialist. Chapter 1 presents important information on professional billing and coding careers, including employment demands and trends, job descriptions, professional memberships, and the medical billing and coding certifications that are valuable to career advancement.

Professional Vignette

My name is Gene Simon, RHIA, my current position is Risk Manager Designee. Having gone back to college later in life, and not wanting to be in a clinical position, I decided to enter the field of health information management (HIM). It was a fascination of mine to be educated in the hugely diversified field of analyzing, abstracting, and disseminating health data. I first thought the field consisted of only reading a medical record, but I soon found out how wrong I was!

Through years of practice one becomes what the title suggests: a Registered Health Information Administrator. We work with, and must have a thorough knowledge of *every* department and *every* aspect of the medical facility. As I learned, practiced, climbed the ladder of success, and obtained positions beyond my wildest imagination, it dawned on me, "Why can't I pass on this invaluable information to the younger generation?"

I decided to become an instructor and then to become supervisor of the coding/billing and HIM departments as well as "Educator of the Year." But something was still missing from my goals: helping others to achieve their goals.

At this point in my life I have had hundreds of students in the hallways, in my classes, and especially at graduation ceremonies step up and say with big smiles on their faces and tears in their eyes, "Mr. Simon, you have changed my life, and for that I will be forever grateful." This is what being an instructor is all about: changing other people's lives for the better!

Chapter 1 / Introduction to Professional Billing and Coding Careers

Chapter Objectives

After reading this chapter, the student should be able to:

1. Recognize different types of facilities that employ allied health personnel.
2. Define job descriptions pertaining to a position.
3. Discuss options available for certification.

Key Terms

admitting clerk

centralized billing office
  (CBO)

certifications

health information clerk

insurance verification
  representative

managed care

medical and health
  services manager

medical biller

medical coder

patient financial services
  (PFS)

payer (payor)

registered health
  information
  administrator (RHIA)

registered health
  information technician
  (RHIT)

**Introduction
to Professional
Billing and
Coding
Careers**

Elizabeth had nearly completed her course on medical billing and coding. As much as she had enjoyed the class, she was now concerned that she would only have one job choice. She discussed this matter with her instructor.

The instructor explained that with the training Elizabeth had received, she would have opportunities for diverse positions in a variety of medical facilities. Continuing her education by attending seminars in order to be aware of the ever-changing aspects of medical billing would increase her marketability and potential for advancement.

Questions

1. Make a list of the pros and cons of possible career options as you currently see them. Later in the course, reevaluate the issues you listed.

2. What medical facilities in your area would be potential employers of medical coders and billers?

3. How would joining professional organizations help you advance your career?

In this textbook, the student will learn the process of submitting, coding, and resolving medical claims. There are many steps to this process. Procedures are dictated not only by the facility in which the medical office specialist works, but also by state and federal government regulations. To launch your new career, it is important that you understand the career opportunities that are available, the job titles and responsibilities for which you are qualified, and the certifications that are valuable for career advancement.

Employment Demand

Prior to the enactment of the Health Maintenance Organization Act of 1973, it was common for a physician on receipt of his or her license to open a solo/private practice. The physician would practice independently, depending on advertising and referrals for the practice to grow. The staff consisted of a receptionist, a nurse, and possibly one or two support staff. As more and more patients began to use managed care, however, physicians faced financial difficulties. Patients had previously paid for services at the time they were rendered, but with managed care contracts it became the physician's responsibility to file claims and wait 30 days or longer for payment. **Managed care** is a term used to describe a system in which healthcare delivery is monitored. Under managed care a healthcare provider will contract with a health insurance company, referred to as a **payer** (historically spelled *payor*). In this contract the provider agrees to follow guidelines and accept negotiated fees with the aim to control healthcare costs.

The delay in payment changed the way physicians' practices were managed. Physicians were forced to add additional staff to handle the processing of claims, and if claims forms were not submitted correctly or in a timely fashion, the financial health of the practice suffered because it was difficult to pay expenses with uncollected funds. The physician's increased staff needs created a demand for trained and certified medical billers, medical office assistants, and medical coders.

Physicians and nurses comprise only 40% of all healthcare providers. The other 60% are allied health employees. Allied health employees are those members of the clinical healthcare profession whose positions are distinct from the medical and nursing professions. As the name implies, they are all allies in the healthcare team, working together to make the healthcare system function.

Facilities

Physician's Practice

The size of a physician's practice is generally categorized as solo/private practice, small group (3 to 9 physicians), or large group (10 or more physicians).

Solo/Private Practice

In the solo/private practice setting, the staff may consist of a nurse, a receptionist, and a medical biller and/or office manager. The receptionist and medical biller are often cross-trained for coverage purposes.

Small-Group Practice

In a small-group practice, the physicians may have the same specialty; for instance, the group may consist of four or five general practitioners. Small-group practices frequently contract out their billing and accounts receivable. In addition to the medical receptionist, such a practice may have a staff member who verifies insurance and one who assists with scheduling and checking patients in or out. These responsibilities fall under the title of medical office assistant. Medical office assistants often compile and record medical records, reports, and correspondence. A medical records clerk or medical administrative assistant may also be employed.

Large-Group Practice

An excellent example of a large-group practice is a specialized practice, such as a back institute, which might consist of an orthopedic surgeon, neurosurgeon, internist, chiropractor, physiatrist, pain specialist, exercise physiologist, and a team of physical and occupational therapists. Large-group practices commonly handle claims and accounts receivable in house. Depending on how many physicians are in the group and what their specialties are, the large group may employ several people.

Multispecialty Clinic

A multispecialty clinic is a group of physicians with several specialties who have formed a clinic or outpatient center to provide services under each specialty. An example is an outpatient center that provides treatment for adult general internal medicine, diseases of the circulatory system and diabetes, diseases of the nervous system, gynecology, osteopathic manipulative treatment, and other services.

Hospital

Hospitals were also affected by managed care. It is very rare today to find a privately owned hospital; most are owned by corporations. In a large metropolitan area it is not uncommon for three or more hospitals with different names to actually be part of one corporation, sometimes referred to as health systems. Examples of such corporations include Hospital Corporation of America (HCA), Ascension Health, and Tenet Health Care Corporation. As an allied health employee, you may work in admissions, outpatient, inpatient, or the emergency department. You could be employed as a patient access specialist in patient services or a scheduler in the radiology department.

In the past, hospitals usually had a billing or financial department located on site that a patient could physically visit to address any billing concerns or make payments. Today there may still be a department such as this, but the staff's responsibilities are limited to answering basic questions. The actual handling and processing of data and claims are most often accomplished off site.

Many health systems centralize their billing and collections geographically. The staff responsible for processing claims will be located off site. Within the location there can be many departments: billing, revenue integrity, collections, support services, and others. These positions are part of revenue cycle or **patient financial services**. Revenue cycle is the management of healthcare reimbursement for services rendered. This includes calculating patient and payer responsibility through claims processing and collection of payment. It is the life of a patient account. In other words, it is a term that includes the entire life of a patient account from creation to payment.

Centralized Billing Office

If a hospital, physician, multi-site, or multi-physician practice chooses not to handle claims within her practice or corporation, a contract will be signed with a **centralized** billing office (CBO). CBOs contract with healthcare providers to handle their claims and/or accounts receivable. A CBO can employ just 2 or 3 people or well over 500. It is a separate entity from the healthcare provider and has different ownership, although sometimes the provider may have a financial interest.

Job Titles and Responsibilities

After completion of a course of study, the medical office specialist is qualified for entry-level positions such as patient information clerk, admitting clerk, insurance verification representative, apprentice coder, medical biller, government medical biller, payment poster, medical collector, refund specialist, medical records technician, medical receptionist, or medical secretary. Each facility will have its own specific job description and/or job title for each such position. Knowledge of medical billing and coding is imperative to performing well in all these positions because, even though medical billing may not be the primary responsibility of certain positions, every staff member influences the accuracy of information submitted on a medical claim, such as the patient data, documentation of the procedure and diagnosis, and medical coding.

Medical Office Assistant

In some facilities, this position is also referred to as a medical administrative assistant, secretary, or medical receptionist. Medical office assistants usually work in physicians' offices. They are considered front office staff and primarily handle administrative duties. Responsibilities include organization and the ability to make the office function smoothly. In this position one might perform duties such as scheduling and confirming patients' diagnostic appointments, surgeries, and medical consultations. The medical office assistant might compile and record medical records, reports, and correspondence; answer telephones; and direct calls to appropriate staff. He might also receive and route messages and documents such as laboratory results to appropriate staff as well as greet visitors, ascertain the purpose of their visit, and direct them to appropriate staff.

Education: There are no formal education or training requirements for medical office assistants. However, nearly all medical office assistant professionals hold a high school diploma or equivalent and complete a medical assisting program through a vocational school or community college. Typically, one-year programs lead to diplomas or certificates, while associate's degree programs require two years.

Medical Biller

Other job titles for a **medical biller** are billing specialist, patient account representative, claims processor, electronic claims processor, reimbursement specialist, and billing coordinator. Responsibilities may include analyzing patient data and charge information, submitting insurance claims, and contacting the insurance carrier on outstanding or incorrectly paid claims. A skillful biller helps healthcare facilities, insurance payers, and patients navigate the complexities of the many laws, regulations, and guidelines related to the business side of healthcare.

Education: A high school diploma or equivalent GED certificate is required. Many employers only look at candidates who have certification. Medical billing courses are independent of standard degree programs and may be presented in a classroom or online format. These programs usually take months rather than years to complete. The curriculum will include basic medical terminology and diagnosis, procedure, supply, and procedure and diagnostic codes. The student will also be introduced to the many and complex laws and regulations governing healthcare business, including the Health Insurance Portability and Accountability Act (HIPAA), the Affordable Care Act (ACA), Stark Laws, the False Claims Act, and the Fair Debt Collection Act.

Payment Poster

This position is sometimes called medical payment verification analyst or payment analyst. A payment poster generally reads the Explanation of Benefits documents issued by insurance carriers and posts the payments or contractual adjustments to the appropriate patient account. In a hospital billing environment, this position is also referred to as a *general* cashier. This requires excellent data entry skills, math skills, and a good working knowledge of insurance contracts.

Education: There are no formal education or training requirements for a medical payment poster. However, nearly all medical payment poster professionals hold a high school diploma or equivalent and complete a medical administrative assistant program through a vocational school or community college. Many times if the candidate does not have prior medical payment posting experience, the employer will accept previous accounting or cashiering experience with healthcare vocational training.

Medical Collector

A medical collector contacts patients and insurance carriers to collect money owed to the medical facility. This position requires a great deal of patience and tact. Most of this job is performed on the telephone; however, after contacting an insurance carrier, it may be necessary to gather and send additional information before a claim can be processed. Many of the insurance carriers have a website where the status of a claim can be checked and missing claim information can be submitted. A medical collector may also be required to send patient billing statements.

Education: A high school diploma is required for this position, though some employers prefer relevant work experience or the completion of some collegiate coursework or completing an allied healthcare vocational training program.

Refund Specialist

A refund specialist analyzes patient accounts to discern whether or not a refund is required and, if so, to whom the money should be returned. This position requires researching, analytical, and math skills.

Education: A high school diploma is required for this position, though some employers prefer relevant work experience or the completion of some collegiate coursework or completing an allied healthcare vocational training program or two years of post-secondary education.

Insurance Verification Representative

An **insurance verification representative** contacts insurance carriers by phone or via the insurance carrier's website to verify benefit information for patients. This individual may also perform precertification and/or prior authorization of services duties. Determining a patient's financial responsibility before services being rendered is often required. Many providers use web-based software programs that interface with payers to expedite benefit eligibility and provide patient balance estimates.

Education: A high school diploma is required for this position, though some employers prefer relevant work experience or the completion of some collegiate coursework or completing an allied healthcare vocational school training program or two years of post-secondary education. Training should include medical insurances, benefit verification or prior authorization, electronic health records, and basic medical terminology.

Admitting Clerk or Front Desk Representative

The **admitting clerk** or registrar, also referred to as medical admissions clerk, has face-to-face contact with patients. Registering and greeting patients, having patients complete paperwork, answering questions, data entry of patient demographic and insurance information, and requesting information and payment are the general duties of the admitting clerk position. Dealing with patients who may be upset or irritable may also be required. In some facilities, the admitting clerk is responsible for appointment scheduling; in other facilities, a scheduler is a separate position.

Education: A high school diploma or equivalent. Training or on-the-job experience as a medical secretary or a health record clerk certificate and associate's degree. Most of the education comes through job training, although there are educational programs that can assist finding employment in this role. These programs typically result in associate's degrees or in a health record clerk certificate or secretarial certificate.

Table 1.1 lists facilities, job responsibilities, and certification(s) an employee may be required to hold. The job titles and responsibilities will vary at facilities; for example, a surgeon's practice will require someone with more coding skills than a family practice will. A facility located in a rural area may need fewer employees than might a facility located in an urban area, which would require all employees to be cross-trained and able to perform varied responsibilities. There is no state or federal requirement for employees to be certified. One facility may require or encourage its employees to be certified, and another facility may train on the job.

Certifications

Medical billing and coding **certifications** are valuable to your career advancement. Medical billing and coding certificates are available at every level of expertise. Certification for medical coding and billing is not a requirement for employment in most states, but having a few billing and coding certifications will definitely help you to advance your medical billing or medical coding career and to make you more competitive in the job market. Examples of certification agencies are the American Health Information Management Association (AHIMA), American Academy of Professional Coders (AAPC), National Center for Competency Testing (NCCT), and National Healthcareer Association (NHA). General and contact information for these agencies are listed at the end of this chapter in the Resources section.

Two program accrediting agencies that are recognized by the Council for Higher Education Accreditation (CHEA) are Commission of Accreditation of Allied Health Education Programs (CAAHEP) and Accrediting Bureau of Health Education Schools (ABHES). These programs or agencies perform accrediting activities to determine if certification programs provide and maintain the highest standards. When searching for or selecting a certification program these are excellent resources.

The following vocations have been listed separately to focus on certification requirements. These job roles usually require advanced education prior to certification.

Table 1.1	Facilities, Job Titles, and Certifications	
Facilities	**Job Titles and Responsibilities**	**Certifications**
Physician's Practice		
Solo/Private Practice	Front Desk Representative	Medical Office Assistant
	Insurance Verification Representative	
	Medical Collector	Reimbursement Specialist
	Medical Office Assistant	Medical Office Assistant
	Privacy Compliance Officer	RHIT, RHIA, or CHP
Small-Group Practice	Front Desk Representative	Medical Office Assistant
	Insurance Verification Representative	
	Medical Biller	Medical Billing Specialist
		Reimbursement Specialist
	Medical Coder	Certified Coding Associate
		Certified Coding Specialist—Physician
	Medical Collector	Reimbursement Specialist
	Medical Office Assistant	Medical Office Assistant
	Privacy Compliance Officer	RHIT, RHIA, or CHP
Large-Group Practice	Front Desk Representative	Medical Office Assistant
	Insurance Verification Representative	
	Medical Biller	Medical Billing Specialist
		Reimbursement Specialist
	Medical Coder	Certified Coding Associate
		Certified Coding Specialist—Physician
		Certified Professional Coder
	Medical Collector	Reimbursement Specialist
	Medical Office Assistant	Medical Office Assistant
	Payment Poster	
	Privacy Compliance Officer	RHIT, RHIA, or CHP
Multi-specialty clinic	Admitting Clerk	Medical Office Assistant
	Health Information Clerk	Health Information Clerk
	Insurance Verification Representative	
	Medical Biller	Medical Billing Specialist
		Reimbursement Specialist
	Medical Coder	Certified Coding Associate
		Certified Coding Specialist—Physician
		Certified Professional Coder
	Medical Collector	Reimbursement Specialist
	Medical Office Assistant	Medical Office Assistant
	Payment Poster	
	Privacy Compliance Officer	RHIT, RHIA, CHP

(Continued)

Table 1.1	Facilities, Job Titles, and Certifications (Continued)		
Facilities	**Job Titles and Responsibilities**	**Certifications**	
Hospital			
Patient Financial Services	Admitting Clerk		
	Health Information Clerk	Health Information Clerk	
	Insurance Verification Representative		
	Medical Biller	Medical Billing Specialist	
		Reimbursement Specialist	
	Medical Coder	Certified Professional Coder—Hospital	
		Certified Professional Coder	
	Medical Collector	Reimbursement Specialist	
	Payment Poster		
	Privacy Compliance Officer	RHIT, RHIA, or CHP	
	Refund Specialist		
	Registered Health Information Technician (RHIT)	Registered Health Information Technician (RHIT)	
		Medical Records Certification	
Centralized Billing Office	Insurance Verification Representative	Certified Coding Specialist	
	Medical Biller	Medical Billing Specialist	
		Reimbursement Specialist	
	Medical Coder	Certified Professional Coder—Hospital	
		Certified Professional Coder	
	Medical Collector	Reimbursement Specialist	
	Payment Poster		
	Privacy Compliance Officer	RHIT, RHIA, or CHP	
	Refund Specialist		
	Registered Health Information Technician (RHIT)	Registered Health Information Technician (RHIT)	
		Medical Records Certification	

Medical Coder

Healthcare professionals who manage the coding of medical records have job titles such as **medical coder**, health information coder, medical coding specialist, coding special-ist, health information administrator or health information technician. The duties and responsibilities may include research and reference checking of medical records as well as accurately coding the primary and secondary diagnoses and procedures using the *International Classification of Diseases*, Tenth Revision, Clinical Modification (ICD-10-CM) and the American Medical Association's *Current Procedural Terminology* (CPT®) coding books.[1] Medical coders abstract and compile data from medical records regarding hospital,

---

[1]CPT® is a registered trademark of the American Medical Association.

physician, and other professional services in order to obtain appropriate optimal reimbursement. (ICD-10-CM) diagnostic codes and (CPT) procedure codes will be defined and discussed in Chapter 5 and Chapter 6.)

Education: According to the U.S. Bureau of Labor Statistics (BLS), employers typically prefer employees with certifications in this field, though this certification is not mandatory (www.bls.gov). The most common certification examination is the Certified Coding Assistant (CCA), which is administered through the American Health Information Management Association (AHIMA). This exam is typically taken after graduating from a training program. After acquiring a few years of work experience, technicians are eligible to sit for the Certified Coding Specialist (CCS) examination, which includes either a physician-based or hospital-based option.

Privacy Compliance Officer

The privacy compliance officer, also referred to as HIPAA privacy officer, is responsible for answering questions and explaining to patients and their family members about HIPAA privacy regulations, living wills, and do-not-resuscitate (DNR) orders. A privacy officer oversees all ongoing activities related to the development, implementation, and maintenance of and adherence to the organization's policies and procedures covering the privacy of, and access to, patient health information in compliance with federal and state laws and the healthcare organization's information privacy practices. In a physician setting, the privacy compliance officer is responsible for receiving and responding to requests for medical records and receiving complaints. Depending on the size of the facility, this position may also require data entry of patient demographics and/or appointment scheduling.

Education: Certification as an RHIA or RHIT with education and experience relative to the size and scope of the organization. (RHIA and RHIT certification will be defined later in this chapter). For small practices, experience and a Certified HIPAA Processional (CHP) may be acceptable.

Registered Health Information Administrator (RHIA)

The **registered health information administrator (RHIA)** performs as a critical link between care providers, payers, and patients. An RHIA is an expert in managing patient health information and medical records, administering computer information systems, collecting and analyzing patient data, and using classification systems. RHIAs possess comprehensive knowledge of medical, administrative, ethical and legal requirements, and standards related to healthcare delivery and the privacy of protected patient information. They often manage people and operational units, participate in administrative committees, and prepare budgets.

Education: Prospective RHIAs must complete a bachelor's program in health information management accredited by the Commission on Accreditation for Health Informatics and Information Management Education (CAHIIM). These programs are available in campus-based and online formats.

In many cases, students must complete two years of prerequisite coursework or an approved associate's program before applying to a health information management bachelor's program. Prerequisite topics include human anatomy, biology, psychology and computer applications. The core health information management curriculum covers medical ethics, medical law, privacy law, data analysis, and electronic records management.

Registered Health Information Technician (RHIT)

The **registered health information technician (RHIT)** position may also be referred to as coder, file clerk, health information clerk, health information systems technician, medical records analyst, medical records clerk, medical records director, medical records technician, or office manager. Job responsibilities may include compiling, processing, and maintaining medical records of physician and hospital patients in a manner consistent with the medical, administrative, ethical, legal, and regulatory requirements of the healthcare system. The job involves reviewing records for completeness, accuracy, and compliance with regulations and the release of information to persons and agencies according to regulations. As healthcare providers migrate to electronic health records mandated by the Health Insurance Portability and Accountability Act of 1996 (HIPAA) discussed in Chapter 4, registered health information technicians will evolve from the custodians of paper health records to custodians of electronic health records. This transformation will also require the registered health information technician to acquire a higher level of information technology knowledge.

Education: In order to obtain the RHIT credential, an individual will need to earn an associate's degree in health information management. This program also must be accredited by the Commission on Accreditation for Health Informatics and Information Management Education (CAHIIM). Coursework includes topics such as clinical coding and classification systems, medical terminology, data analysis, anatomy, and physiology.

Health Information Clerk

Health information clerks may work in large hospitals, clinics or for a private-practice doctor. These professionals organize and maintain health data in electronic and paper systems within various healthcare settings. They are responsible for reviewing patient records, organizing databases, tracking patient outcomes, and protecting patients' health information.

Education: An associate's degree in either of these fields will typically qualify an applicant for employment as a health information clerk; however, a growing number of employers prefer to hire health information clerks who are registered. Becoming registered requires passing a written examination overseen by the American Health Information Management Association. Only graduates of accredited 2-year programs are allowed to sit for this exam.

Medical and Health Services Manager

A **medical and health services manager**, executive, or administrator plans and directs the health services in facilities, medical practices, or specific clinical departments.

Education: A candidate will need a minimum of a bachelor's degree in health administration.

Listing of Certifications

Medical Office Assistant Certification

National Certified Medical Office Assistant

To achieve certification as a National Certified Medical Office Assistant (NCMOA), you must have a high school diploma or equivalent. You must have graduated from an approved program of study as a medical office assistant or provide documentation of 1 year of experience as a medical office assistant. The exam requires knowledge of computer literacy, business communication, medical terminology, law and ethics, patient control, insurance, office procedures, and Occupational Safety and Health Administration (OSHA) regulations. The NCMOA certification is awarded through the NCCT.

Certified Medical Administrative Assistant

To qualify as a certified medical administrative assistant (CMAA), you must be a graduate of a healthcare training program or have one or more years of full-time job experience. The CMAA certification is awarded through the NHA.

Medical Billing Certifications

Certified Medical Billing Specialist

A candidate for Certified Medical Billing Specialist (CMBS) certification is an individual who is motivated to improve her medical billing knowledge and develop new skills to assist providers in maximizing their reimbursement through proper coding and documentation. To achieve certification, an individual must successfully complete a series of six courses and provide the Medical Association of Billers (MAB) with an evaluation of billing performance from a supervisor, provider, or instructor. The CMBS certification is awarded by MAB.

Reimbursement Specialist Certification

The certified medical reimbursement specialist (CMRS) certification is a credential offered by the American Billing Association (AMBA). The CMRS designation is awarded by the Certifying Board of the American Medical Billing Association (CBAMBA) after an exam. There is no state or federal requirement for a medical billing professional to become certified; however, the goal is to provide a "professional certification."

Medical Coding Certifications

Certified Coding Associate

Coders who earn the Certified Coding Associate (CCA) certification awarded by AHIMA can immediately demonstrate their competency in the field even if they don't have much job experience. Earning a CCA demonstrates a commitment to coding even for those who are new in the field. The CCA should be viewed as a starting point for an individual beginning a new career as a coder.

Certified Professional Coder

The Certified Professional Coder (CPC) certification is designed to evaluate a medical coder's knowledge of medical terminology; human anatomy; ICD-10-CM concepts; the Health Care Procedure Coding System (HCPCS) concepts; coding concepts; surgery and coding modifiers; evaluation and management concepts; anesthesia coding; radiology, laboratory, and pathology concepts; and medicine. To receive the CPC certification, a coder must have 2 years of work experience and pass the certification exam. Those applicants who are successful in passing the certification examination, but have not met the required coding work experience, will be awarded the initial designation Certified Professional Coder–Apprentice (CPC-A). The CPC certification is awarded through the AAPC.

Certified Professional Coder–Hospital

Because there are distinct differences between CPT coding for physician services and for outpatient facility services, the AAPC has a separate examination and certification for outpatient facility coding titled Certified Professional Coder–Hospital (CPC-H). To receive the CPC-H certification, a coder must have 2 years of work experience and pass the certification exam. Those applicants who are successful in passing the certification examination, but have not met the required coding work experience, will be awarded the initial designation Certified Professional Coder–Hospital–Apprentice (CPC-H-A).

Certified Coding Specialist

Coding accuracy is very important to healthcare organizations because reimbursement cannot be received without accurate coding, and inaccurate coding results in lower productivity (due to the time needed to make corrections). Accordingly, the Certified Coding Specialist (CCS) demonstrates tested skills in medical coding. The CCS certification exam assesses mastery or proficiency in coding rather than entry-level skills. The CCS certification is awarded through AHIMA.

Certified Coding Specialist–Physician

The Certified Coding Specialist–Physician (CCS-P) certification demonstrates expertise in physician-based settings such as physicians' offices, group practices, and specialty clinics. The CCS-P certification exam assesses mastery or proficiency in coding rather than entry-level skills. If you perform coding in a doctor's office, clinic, or similar setting, you should consider obtaining the CCS-P certification to demonstrate or validate your ability. The CCS-P certification is awarded through AHIMA.

Medical Records Certification

Registered Health Information Technician

The Registered Health Information Technician is the custodian of medical records who ensures the quality of medical records by verifying their completeness, accuracy, and proper entry into computer systems. RHIT certification proves proficiency and ability in accurate patient record maintenance, management, and analysis. The RHIT certification is awarded through AHIMA. The American Health Information Management Association (AHIMA), among other organizations, provides certification programs specifically for health information technicians.

Registered Health Information Administrator

The registered Health Information Administrator acts as a critical link between care providers, payers, and patients. A RHIA candidate must have successfully completed a baccalaureate level of an HIM program accredited by the Commission on Accreditation for Health Informatics and Information Managed Education (CAHIM). The American Health Information Management Association (AHIMA), among other organizations, provides certification programs specifically for health information technicians.

Certified HIPAA Professional (CHP)

This is a two-day instructor-led HIPAA training program sponsored by the HIPAA Academy. The program covers the basics of the Administrative Simplification portion of the HIPAA legislation, which includes the HIPAA Transactions and Code Sets, Identifiers, and Privacy and Security. It is this provision of the HIPAA regulation that is the watershed legislation for healthcare information systems.

Professional Memberships

Professional memberships help you stay current in your field. They can offer information about upcoming conferences and professional development opportunities. As a member, you will be eligible to attend the group's conferences. Whether at the state, regional, or national level, professional conferences offer excellent opportunities to build your network of professionals in the field, learn the latest developments in your field, and take professional courses and seminars. Professional membership is an excellent addition to your résumé. It shows you are involved and dedicated to your particular field. Professional associations publish journals and/or newsletters that are helpful for keeping you up to date on issues and developments in your field. When you are interviewing for a position, this can be invaluable information. You can read about companies or individuals with whom you would like to work.

With your membership, you will often have access to member information. Contacting someone in your field about possible employment as a fellow member of the association may open a door. It is recommended that you join at least one professional organization, but research some beforehand to find the appropriate one for your career goals. These organizations may have a local chapter as well.

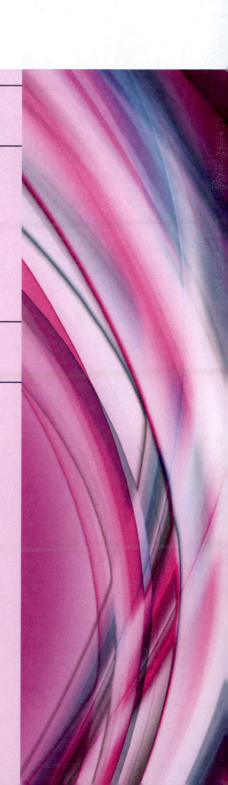

Chapter Summary

- Changes in the way healthcare is paid for created a demand for allied health personnel trained in medical billing and coding.
- An allied health employee can find employment in a variety of medical settings.
- After completion of a course of study, the student is qualified for entry-level positions such as admitting clerk, medical biller, insurance verification representative, and medical collector.
- Certification demonstrates dedication to advancement and competency.

Chapter Review

True/False

Identify the statement as true (T) or false (F).

_____ **1.** PFS is an abbreviation for patient financial services.

_____ **2.** The medical office assistant might compile and record medical records, reports, and correspondence.

_____ **3.** HIPAA is an abbreviation for Hospital Information per American Medical Association.

_____ **4.** Certification is not required in most states.

_____ **5.** Math skills are important when working with refunds and posting of payments.

_____ **6.** Coding accuracy is very important to healthcare organizations because funding cannot be received without accurate coding.

_____ 7. Registered health information technicians are health information technicians who ensure quality of medical records by verifying their completeness, accuracy, and proper entry into computer systems.

_____ 8. An admitting clerk may be responsible for appointment scheduling.

_____ 9. A collector may be required to send out patient billing statements.

_____ 10. A medical office assistant is considered front office staff and primarily handles administrative duties.

Multiple Choice

Identify the letter of the choice that best completes the statement or answers the question.

_____ 1. A business that contracts with physicians to handle its claims and/or accounts receivable is referred to as a(n):
  a. physician billing office.
  b. centralized billing office.
  c. accounts receivable corporation.
  d. billing and coding facilitator.

_____ 2. A person who is considered front office staff and primarily handles administrative duties is called a(n):
  a. medical secretary.   c. medical receptionist.
  b. medical office assistant.   d. all of the above.

_____ 3. A health information technician has the responsibility to:
  a. contact patients about their outstanding balance.
  b. assist the physician in surgery.
  c. research and code medical records.
  d. provide patients with information about their software.

_____ 4. What job description requires excellent data entry skills, math skills, and a good working knowledge of insurance contracts?
  a. Medical records technician   c. Insurance verifier
  b. Payment poster   d. Contract reviewer

_____ 5. A medical collector will contact most patients:
  a. by mail.   c. in person.
  b. during appointments.   d. by telephone.

_____ 6. A refund specialist position requires:
  a. researching, analytical, and math skills.
  b. patience and tact.
  c. data entry.
  d. organization and telephone skills.

_____ **7.** What job description routinely requires face-to-face contact with the
patient?
a. Medical biller   c. Medical collector
b. Insurance verifier   d. Admitting clerk

_____ **8.** Professional memberships help their members by:
a. providing current information in their field.
b. organizing social events.
c. providing legal services.
d. assisting with verifying benefits.

_____ **9.** An example of a certification agency is the:
a. American Health Information Management Association.
b. American Academy of Professional Workers.
c. National Center for Coding Testing.
d. National Heart Association.

_____ **10.** What abbreviation stands for a coder who specializes in hospital coding?
a. HPC-C   c. CPC-P
b. CHC-P   d. CPC-H

Completion

Complete each statement.

1. _____, _____, and _____ are the three common sizes of physician practices.

2. _____ and _____ are other job titles for a medical biller.

3. As a medical collector, it is important to have _____ and _____.

4. The knowledge of medical _____ and _____ is imperative to perform well in all medical administrative positions.

5. A medical office assistant may also be referred to as a medical _____ or
medical _____.

6. The payment poster generally reads the _____ from insurance carriers and
posts the payments or contractual adjustments to the appropriate patient account.

7. An insurance verification representative will determine the patient's financial
responsibility _____ to services being rendered.

8. Professional membership is an excellent addition to your _____.

9. To receive the CPC-H certification, you must have _____ years of work
experience and pass the certification exam.

10. The registered health information technician certification is awarded through the
_____.

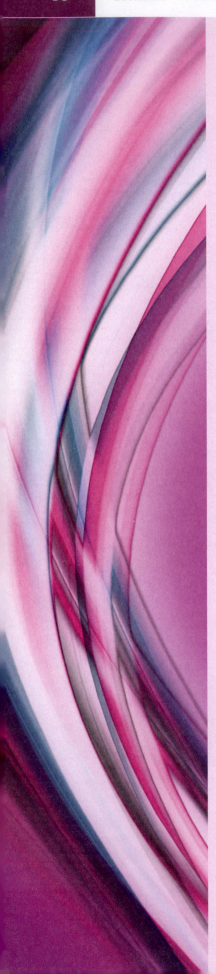

Resources

Alliance of Claims Assistance Professionals (ACAP)

873 Brentwood Drive
West Chicago, IL 60185-3743
www.claims.org; askacap@charter.net

Expert help with medical claims issues. This association works with clients and can assist with challenging denied claims and protecting clients' personal, medical, and financial information.

American Academy of Professional Coders (AAPC)

2480 South 3850 West, Suite B
Salt Lake City, UT 84120
800-626-CODE
www.aapc.com; info@aapc.com

Certification information and other extensive information for coders, office managers, claims examiners, hospital outpatient coders, experienced reimbursement specialists, and coding educators. The website job ad section lets you post your résumé and receive job alerts by email.

American Health Information Management Association (AHIMA)

233 North Michigan Avenue, 21st Floor
Chicago, IL 60601-5809
www.ahima.org

AHIMA is an association of health information management (HIM) professionals. Members are dedicated to the effective management of the personal health information needed to deliver quality healthcare to the public. Founded in 1928 to improve the quality of medical records, AHIMA is committed to advancing the HIM profession in an increasingly electronic and global environment through leadership in advocacy, education, and certification.

American Medical Billing Association (AMBA)

2465 E. Main
Davis, OK 73030
580-369-2700
www.ambanet.net/AMBA.htm

The AMBA website presents information about online courses, networking opportunities, and information on preparing for the examination to become a certified medical reimbursement specialist.

Association for Healthcare Documentation Integrity (AHDI)

4230 Kiernan Avenue
Suite 130
Modesto, CA 95356
800-982-2182
www.ahdionline.org

Provides career information, employment opportunities, networking, local association information, and approved education programs. You can post your résumé online and receive email job alerts.

Health Professions Institute (HPI)
P.O. Box 801
Modesto, CA 95355-0801
209-551-2112
www.hpisum.com

This organization publishes many books and periodicals and conducts seminars for the medical transcription community. HPI has a free student network and information on medical transcription courses. *Perspectives on the Medical Transcription Profession*, an electronic magazine, is free to medical transcription professionals.

Healthcare Financial Management Association (HFMA)
3 Westbrook Corporate Center
Suite 600
Westchester, IL 60154
800-252-4362
www.hfma.org

A nonprofit membership organization for healthcare financial leaders. The organization helps members achieve results by providing education, guidance, and tools.

Healthcare Information and Management Systems Society (HIMSS)
33 West Monroe Street, Suite 1700
Chicago, IL 60603-5616
312-664-4467
www.himss.org

The HIMSS website includes a membership directory, résumé posting, and job alerts, and it allows you to research potential employers and career development resources with résumé and interviewing advice and more. Members only.

HIPAA Academy
295 NE Venture Drive
Waukee, IA 50263
515-444-1221
www.hipaaacademy.net

The HIPAA Academy website provides current news and events plus testimonials. HIPAA Academy also provides instructor led and online training, CSCS Certification exam, training material and workshops.

Medical Association of Billers
5991 East Grant Road
Tucson, AZ 85712
www.physicianswebsites.com

Provides the AAPC Professional Medical Coding Curriculum. The organization's purpose is to provide medical billing and coding specialists with a reliable source for procedural and diagnostic coding training and information.

Medical Coding and Billing
www.medicalcodingandbilling.com

This site includes certification, education, and medical office management career information.

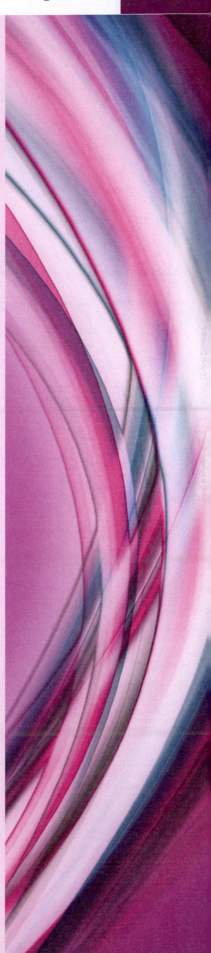

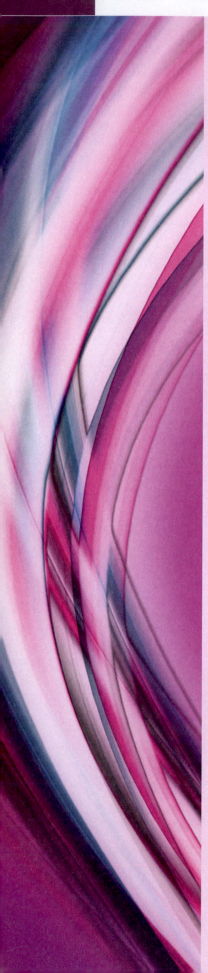

Medical Group Management Association (MGMA)
104 Inverness Terrace East
Englewood, CO 80012
303-799-1111 or 877-275-6462
www.mgma.com

This organization is designed for supervisors of medical group practices. The website lists job ads, networking and internship information, and a Core Learning Series for education. Job ads are compiled in *MGMA Connections*, a monthly publication.

MT Jobs
www.mtjobs.com

Sponsored by *MT Daily*, this website provides free job searches, résumé posting, email job alerts, and employer profiles.

MT Monthly
106 Norway Lane
Oak Ridge, TN 37830
800-951-5559 or 865-387-5555
www.mtmonthly.com

MT Monthly is a national newsletter for medical transcriptionists. *MT Monthly* currently offers the book entitled *Working as a Medical Transcriptionist at Home*. The website has links to placement services, products, and related websites.

National Center for Competency Testing (NCCT)
7007 College Boulevard, Suite 385
Overland Park, KS 66211
www.NCCTinc.com

Established in 1989, NCCT is able to work as an independent certifying agency in order to avoid any allegiance to a specific organization or association. In this way, NCCT is able to work with many organizations but can remain independent of any outside allegiance, bias, or agenda. Every applicant interested in sitting for a certification exam must meet NCCT requirements and must pass a criterion-referenced examination.

National Healthcareer Association (NHA)
7500 West 160th Street
Stilwell, KS 66085
800-499-9092
www.nhanow.com

The NHA offers education, training, and certification for many healthcare jobs, including Certified Medical Transcriptionist and Certified Billing and Coding Specialist.

Professional Association of Health Care Office Management (PAHCOM)
1576 Bella Cruz Drive, Suite 360
Lady Lake, FL 32159
800-451-9311
www.pahcom.com

The PAHCOM website contains information on education, local chapters, and the Certified Medical Manager exam. The benefits page of the website posts job openings.

Section II / The Relationship between the Patient, Provider, and Carrier

2 Understanding Managed Care: Insurance Plans

3 Understanding Managed Care: Medical Contracts and Ethics

4 Introduction to the Health Insurance Portability and Accountability Act (HIPAA)

The chapters in this section will provide the student with the knowledge of the history of healthcare in America, the different types of insurance plans and insurance plan coverage, and the types of managed care organizations and alternative healthcare plans available to patients. Because the majority of payments received in a medical facility come from health insurance carriers (also referred to as payers), it is necessary for the medical office specialist to understand the complexities of different insurance plans. This section will outline the different job responsibilities of the medical office specialist, such as contacting insurance carriers for benefits information, estimating patient financial responsibility, and filing insurance claims.

This section presents information on managed care and medical contracts and the importance of ethics in managed care, and outlines the role of the medical office specialist in reviewing and/or understanding managed care organization (MCO) contracts. It also explains the importance of the Health Insurance Portability and Accountability Act (HIPAA) and discusses the role and responsibility of the medical office specialist in protecting all patients' protected health information (PHI).

Professional Vignette

My name is Susan DeGirolamo, RMA, NCPT, NCICS. I started in this field because I needed a career in which I was able to support my two boys as a single mother. At the age of 32, I returned to school full-time. This meager leap became a major stepping stone for me. When I began my career as a medical assistant for a surgeon, I learned much more than any school could simulate. It was at this facility that I inherited the job of billing—by hand. This tedious assignment led me to continue my education and earn my certification as a biller and coder. Thanks to my experiences in the field and continued education, I went into teaching so that I can help students take that first step which may lead them anywhere. I have been presented with the opportunity to write curricula and also review medical textbooks that are used in the same type of school from which I graduated. Education is a powerful tool, and I am still learning as I write this notation. I am pursuing my associate's degree in the allied health field, not knowing the full expanse of possibilities that lie before me, but knowing that I will become even more empowered.

Chapter 2 / Understanding Managed Care: Insurance Plans

Chapter Objectives

After reading this chapter, the student should be able to:

1. Understand the history and impact of managed care.
2. Be able to discuss the organization of managed care and how it affects the provider, employee, and policyholder.
3. Calculate the financial responsibility of the patient.
4. Identify the type of managed care plan in which a patient is enrolled.
5. Recognize various types of insurance coverage.

Key Terms

Affordable Care Act (ACA)
allowed charge
assignment of benefits
carriers
case manager
coinsurance
commercial health insurance
consumer-driven healthcare (CDHC)
copay
deductible
discounted fee
Employee Retirement Income Security Act (ERISA)
enrollee
flexible spending accounts (FSA)

group insurance
health maintenance organization (HMO)
Health Reimbursement Accounts (HRAs)
health savings accounts (HSA)
high-deductible health plans (HDHP)
inpatient
insured
managed care
managed care organization (MCO)
Obamacare
outpatient
Patient Protection and Affordable Care Act (PPACA)

point-of-service (POS)
policyholder
preauthorization
pre-existing condition
preferred provider organization (PPO)
premiums
primary care physician (PCP)
providers
referral
special risk insurance
subscriber
utilization guidelines
write-off (contractual adjustment)

Upon arriving at Dr. Brown's Office, Mary was asked for her insurance card. As she handed over the card, Rebecca, the medical office specialist, noted that Mary had an HMO plan. After Mary's appointment, Rebecca was asked by Dr. Brown to schedule the patient to meet with Dr. Thomas, a general surgeon. Rebecca remembered that Mary was on an HMO plan and checked to see if the plan would allow Mary to see Dr. Thomas, who was listed as a participating provider. Rebecca scheduled the appointment and placed a referral on file with the HMO. A copy of the referral was given to Mary to take to her appointment.

Questions

1. What does it mean that Mary is on an HMO plan?

2. Why was it important that Rebecca checked to see if Mary could see Dr. Thomas?

3. What is the purpose of the referral, and why did Rebecca give the patient a copy?

Because the majority of payments received in a medical facility come from insurance **carriers**, the medical office specialist must understand the complexities of the different types of insurance plans. Understanding insurance plans and how the changes in our healthcare system came about is important for being able to explain the system to patients who have questions. Other responsibilities of the medical office specialist include contacting insurance carriers for benefits information, estimating patient financial responsibility, and filing insurance claims. The patient's benefits are also referred to as their schedule of benefits. The schedule of benefits lists what procedures will and will not be covered by the health plan. This chapter helps medical office specialists meet those responsibilities by explaining the intricacies of various types of health plans.

The History of Healthcare in America

A medical office specialist serves patients from diverse generations and ethnic groups. The medical office specialist must take this into consideration when responding to questions and remarks made by patients. Knowledge of the history of healthcare in America will assist the medical office specialist when communicating with patients.

Preceding managed care, the American healthcare system financially rewarded healthcare **providers** (individuals, group practice, or organizations providing medical or other healthcare services) for providing more care. Patients were responsible to pay directly for that care. Few controls were in place to manage costs. Patients visited a provider for illness, not for wellness and preventive services.

An employer would select a healthcare policy for its employees and pay all **premiums** (regularly scheduled payments made to purchase the insurance policy). The employee, who would be the policyholder, could accept or decline the employer's offered benefits and find insurance through his spouse or independently.

A **policyholder**, also referred to as the **subscriber**, is usually the person who contracts with an insurance company, pays the premiums, or purchases an insurance plan and is responsible for balance billing. In this case the employer pays the premium, but the employee of the company is referred to as the policyholder. A premium is the periodic payment made to the insurance company to initiate or to keep existing insurance coverage.

Usually the employee would not decline because the only expense to him would be the annual **deductible** (the amount to be paid out of pocket before insurance begins paying) that had to be met. Once the employee reached his deductible, he did not have a financial reason or concern if medical costs increased.

Medical costs continued to escalate due to an aging population and the development of high-technology procedures and pharmaceuticals. Society began excessively suing providers and, to protect themselves, providers practiced "defensive" medicine to avoid malpractice suits and jury awards. Defensive medicine resulted in tests and drugs being ordered or prescribed that might not have been necessary. Insurance companies continued to pay the providers increased fees to cover the providers' rising costs of making more services available, and the insurance companies charged higher premiums to the employers. Many employers were no longer financially able to pay the full premium for their employees and began requiring employees to contribute a percentage of the premium, such as 20% or 30%. When employees saw their take-home pay decreasing, in addition to having to meet a deductible each year, they began to protest the cost of medical care. This also happened to government-funded programs, except instead of raising premiums, the federal and state governments raised taxes. The unchecked expense of healthcare continued. The government could not ignore the outcries of the public.

The healthcare crisis meant that despite the high quality of care available to many Americans, the cost of healthcare had grown so rapidly that many people were uninsured or underinsured. Traditional ways to control costs had not proven successful. As a result employers chose not to extend health insurance to a number of employees and if necessary to hire temporary or contract employees who were not eligible for health insurance benefits to avoid the high costs of purchasing the insurance.

Likewise the federal and state governments faced a continuing budget crisis caused in large part by the rise in healthcare expenditures as a total portion of the budget. Budget cuts and deficits continued at the state and federal levels and policy makers still struggled with how to control healthcare costs. Although the answers were not easily found, the question the nation asked was "How do we lower healthcare costs without jeopardizing the quality of and access to care?"

As in most financial disputes, each party considered the other party responsible for the cost of healthcare. Employers pressured insurance companies to control premiums. Insurance companies pressured providers to control costs. Employees wanted employers to provide them with insurance options in order to feel ownership of the money spent for their care. The government felt it necessary to intervene. The government's solution was **managed care**. Managed care is a method of controlling healthcare costs and ensuring that medical care is available to everyone.

The idea of managed care was a long-standing concept, but one that was only offered to those who were employed or associated with a few visionaries, such as Henry Kaiser, an American industrialist and shipbuilder. The timeline in Table 2.1 shows the progress of managed care through its inception to today.

Table 2.1	**Managed Care Timeline**	
	1973	The Health Maintenance Organization Act (HMO Act) of 1973 is signed into law by President Richard Nixon, using federal funds and policy to promote HMOs.
	1976	Kaiser membership reaches 3 million.
	1979	Blue Cross Blue Shield collectively covers 87.4 million Americans.
	1980	Kaiser expands to the mid-Atlantic region.
	1981	Kaiser membership reaches 4 million.
	1982	California legislation is enacted that allows selective contracting for Medicaid and private insurance, paving the way for other states to enact similar laws facilitating preferred provider organizations (PPOs). The Tax Equity and Fiscal Responsibility Act (TEFRA) makes it easier and more attractive for HMOs to contract with the Medicare program.
	1985	National total HMO enrollment reaches 19.1 million.
	1990	National total HMO enrollment reaches 33.3 million. National PPO enrollment surpasses HMO enrollment with 38.1 million members. The National Committee for Quality Assurance (NCQA) is established.

(Continued)

Table 2.1	Managed Care Timeline (Continued)
1991	HEDIS is released. HEDIS is a set of standardized performance measures designed to ensure that purchasers and consumers have the information they need to reliably compare the performance of managed healthcare plans.
1994	Blue Cross Blue Shield Association eliminates requirement that all member plans must maintain not-for-profit status.
1995	National total HMO enrollment reaches 50.6 million.
1996	The Health Insurance Portability and Accountability Act of 1996 (HIPAA) includes patient privacy compliance and health plan portability provisions.
1999	NCQA initiates accreditation of PPOs, which now cover 89 million Americans.
2000	National total HMO enrollment is 80.9 million, declining for the first time from the previous year's level of 81.3 million in 1999.
2003	The Medicare Prescription Drug Improvement and Modernization Act establishes a Part D drug benefit, establishes health savings accounts (HSAs), renames the Medicare+Choice program to Medicare Advantage, and increases payment rates to Medicare Advantage plans.
2004	National total HMO enrollment is 68.8 million, and national PPO enrollment is 109 million.
2006	Medicare Part D prescription benefit becomes effective.
2010	The Affordable Care Act (ACA), officially called Patient Protection and Affordable Care Act (PPACA) and sometimes called Obamacare, is enacted by President Barack Obama, providing a comprehensive system of mandated health insurance.
2011	New healthcare reform law requires insurers to offer dependent coverage for adult children up to age 26 to be included on parents' coverage.
2012	Department of Health and Human Services found 56,257 individuals with pre-existing conditions enrolled in Pre-Existing Condition Insurance Plans (PCIPs) established under ACA.
2013	Medicare program is established for bundling to encourage doctors, hospitals and other care providers to better coordinate patient care.
2014	Employers with 50 or more workers who do not offer coverage face a fine of $2,000 for each employee if any worker receives subsidized insurance on the exchange. The first 30 employees are not counted for the fine.
	No restrictions on pre-existing conditions. Insurance companies are required to provide health insurance to any adult aged 19 to 64 who applies for coverage.
2015	Medicare creates a physician payment program aimed at rewarding quality of care rather than volume of services. This ruling will allow Medicare to reimburse physicians for having advance care planning conversations with patients.

Healthcare Reform

Healthcare reform has been ongoing for many decades. Changes to the provision of health benefits to the public affected the employer, employee, insurance companies, and healthcare providers. In reading this chapter it will become evident that since the Health Maintenance Organization Act of 1973, providers and medical facilities have been required to revamp the way they operate their businesses and provide patient care. The focus is now on extracting more value from the U.S. healthcare and aligning incentives accordingly.

In the United States, chronic diseases have caused 70% of deaths and affected 45% of all Americans. As the population ages, the likelihood of these diseases will grow rapidly. By 2023, cancer and diabetes will increase by 50%; heart disease will rise by 40%. Each year, the cost of medical treatment totals $1.7 trillion, representing 75% of all healthcare money spent. Disease prevention and wellness checkups can significantly lower the cost of being in a healthcare reform plan.

Managing and Controlling Healthcare Costs

Managed care is a specific type of healthcare system that in theory controls the cost and delivery of health services to members who are enrolled in a managed care healthcare plan. Managed care healthcare plans fall under **managed care organizations (MCO)**. A managed care organization is a health insurance organization that adheres to the principles of strong dependence on selective contracting with healthcare providers.

The goals of managed healthcare ensure that:

- Providers deliver high-quality care in a facility that manages or controls costs.
- Medical care or procedures are medically necessary and appropriate for the patient's condition or diagnosis.
- Medical care is rendered by the most appropriate provider.
- Medical care is rendered in the most appropriate, least restrictive setting.

The way in which managed care systems ensure delivery of high-quality care while managing and controlling costs is through networks and discounted fees for services.

When a managed care organization contracts with a physician or medical facility, reimbursement for each procedure is paid at a negotiated fee. Many times the negotiated fee is less than the provider's standard fee and is referred to as a **discounted fee**. The discounted fee is determined by the MCO, which views the fee as the usual and customary fee. The provider's standard fee is on the insurance claim when submitted to the MCO. The MCO will reimburse the provider according to the agreed-on discounted fee ("contract fee"), which is a component of the contract. If the provider is contracted with the MCO and the discounted fee is lower than the provider's standard fee, the provider will write off the difference between the standard fee and contract fee. The provider accepting the lower reimbursement reduces medical costs.

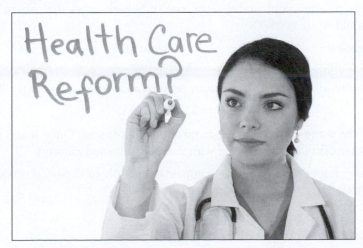

Duckman76/Fotolia LLC

Discounted Fees for Services

An insurance carrier can state in an insurance contract that it will pay "reasonable and customary fees" or "usual, customary, and reasonable fees." These may be referred to as "R and C fees" or "UCR fees," respectively.

A *usual fee* is an individual provider's average charge for a certain procedure (that is, the standard fee). For example, a general practitioner may consistently charge $65 for brief office visits. Such charges would be shown on the doctor's fee schedule and charge slip.

A *customary fee* is determined by what doctors with similar training and experience in a certain geographic location typically charge for a procedure. For example, the surgeon's charge for an appendectomy may range from $3,000 to $4,000 in a certain metropolitan area. Therefore, a surgeon's charge of $3,364 would be considered a customary fee and would be covered by insurance. Another surgeon who charges $4,200 for the same procedure would receive no more than $4,000 in payment from the insurance carrier. The $4,000 is the **"allowed" charge.**

As a medical office specialist, you may need to estimate the amount due from a patient before services are rendered. To calculate the patient's amount due you will need to adjust the balance by removing the **write-off (contractual adjustment)** dollar amount. The write-off is the difference between the provider's standard or customary fee and the allowed payment from the carrier. The following explanation and Practice Exercise 2.1 will help the medical office specialist in determining dollar amounts. To determine the amount paid by the carrier, any adjustment or write-off, and the amount due from the patient (or paid at the time of service by the patient), use the steps below.

With claims that involve unpaid deductibles and coinsurance, further math calculations are required. Determining discounted fees, write-offs, coinsurance, and copays requires knowledge of basic algebra, including addition, subtraction, and figuring of percentages.

A deductible is a specified dollar amount that the **insured** must incur and pay each policy year to a healthcare provider before the insurance company will pay toward medical care. **Coinsurance** is a specified percentage of allowed healthcare cost for each service the insured must pay the healthcare provider. Coinsurance becomes an out-of-pocket expense after the annual deductible has been met. A **copay** is a specified dollar amount the insured must pay to the provider for specific types of services such as office visits or emergency room visits. The insured is expected by contract to pay all copayments at time of service.

The carrier and the provider contract for the discounted fee, which is the allowed amount. The coinsurance is the percentage of the allowed amount for which the patient is responsible. For example, if the insurance carrier's rate of benefit is 75%, the remaining 25% is the patient's coinsurance. Total rate of benefits after the patient and carrier have paid should equal 100%.

Billed Amount	$400	No deductible
Allowed Amount	$275	$10 copay

STEP 1   *Contractual adjustment or write-off amount.* Subtract allowed amount from billed amount:

$$\$400 - \$275 = \$125$$

This will be the write-off amount or contractual adjustment. Once it has been determined, all other calculations will deal with the $275 allowed amount.

STEP 2   *Carrier's responsibility.* Subtract any unpaid deductible or copay (if no deductible or copay, go to step 3):

$$\$125 - \$10 = \$115$$

This is the portion the carrier will pay.

STEP 3   *Patient responsibility.* The patient is only responsible for the copay in this example.

Calculate the financial responsibility of the carrier and the amount the physician must write off.

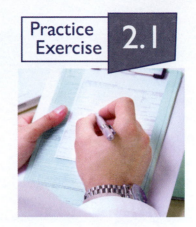

1. Ginger Smith was seen in Dr. Sampson's office today for an allergic reaction to a prescribed drug. Total charges today are $100. Allowed amount is $77.

   _____   _____

   Discount amount   Carrier pays provider

2. Wesley Camp is having outpatient surgery at the Day Surgery Center. Mr. Camp is on a PPO plan. Total charges today are $2,400.56. Allowed amount is $1,976.23.

   _____   _____

   Discount amount   Carrier pays provider

3. Scott Snyder is being seen in Dr. Eveready's office today for hypertension. Mr. Snyder is on an HMO plan. Dr. Eveready is an endocrinologist. Total charges today are $166. Allowed amount is $110.

   _____   _____

   Discount amount   Carrier pays provider

4. Andrew Payne is having outpatient surgery at the Carrollton Surgery Center. Total charges are $2,225. Allowed amount is $2,000.

   _____   _____

   Discount amount   Carrier pays provider

5. Robin Hughes is being seen in Dr. Barry's office today to have a toothpick removed from his toe. Total charges today are $125. Allowed amount is $95.

   _____   _____

   Discount amount   Carrier pays provider

6. Douglas Jackson was seen in the doctor's office today to remove a mole from his left cheek. Total charges today are $377. The allowed amount is $217.

   _____   _____

   Discount amount   Carrier pays provider

Medically Necessary Patient Care

When doctors and medical facilities sign contracts with managed care organizations, physicians and facilities must adhere to policies and guidelines regarding medically necessary procedures. These policies and guidelines are not public information. Although patients are not aware of the guidelines, they restrict a provider from ordering extensive tests or procedures to pinpoint the actual diagnosis.

Requiring the provider to justify what services are being provided to the patient emphasizes the question of medical necessity. In rendering a service to a patient, the provider must determine if the service is medically necessary. The diagnosis may be warranted; however, the treatment provided may not.

The definition of *medical necessity* is written into each contract a provider signs with an MCO. For instance, HMO contracts are stricter than preferred provider organization (PPO) contracts. Therefore, physicians have to approach the services they choose to provide to their patients based on the type of policy the patient has.

MCOs have grown, and with this growth they have developed more stringent **utilization guidelines** that providers must follow when ordering tests or surgery. Utilization guidelines are a set of methods and analyses used by healthcare carriers to manage healthcare costs by influencing patient care decision making through case-by-case assessments of the appropriateness of care. Utilization guidelines help the MCO determine if a service, whether it is a procedure or test, is medically necessary. These guidelines are used by MCOs to deny medical services to patients, so providers must determine the necessity of tests and services before providing them. They must assess the care they feel is required to accurately diagnose or treat the patient based on the MCO contract they have with the patient's insurance company.

At times, patients are forced to be discharged from hospitals when the MCO **case manager** (a person who coordinates patient care by assessing, monitoring, and evaluating options of cost-effective care) has determined that the length of hospital stay being provided is not medically necessary. For example, a physician may schedule inpatient surgery, but the MCO case manager may override an inpatient stay because according to the MCO utilization guidelines the patient's care is best suited for outpatient care.

Care Rendered by Appropriate Provider

One goal of managed care is for patient care to be delivered by the most appropriate provider. This goes hand in hand with providing cost-efficient, quality services to patients. This goal has been attained in several ways.

Managed care uses a network of providers. Each MCO provides a wide array of physicians and hospital services from which an **enrollee** (person enrolling in a contract with the insurance plan) can choose. They also contract with independent laboratory and diagnostic facilities. In doing so, each enrollee has the ability to choose his provider (depending on which managed care plan he is enrolled in) and receive services.

An MCO enrollee may be required to choose a **primary care physician (PCP)**. The PCP, also referred to as a *gatekeeper*, is the provider who coordinates a patient's care. Commonly, a general practitioner, family medicine physician, obstetrician/gynecologist (OB/GYN), or internal medicine doctor acts as the patient's PCP. If the PCP cannot provide care, the PCP will refer the patient to the appropriate specialist within the network who can provide the needed medical care. If a patient wishes to see a specialist, the patient must first schedule a visit with her primary care physician. If the PCP feels an appointment with a specialist is warranted, he will authorize the visit to the specialist. Use of a primary care physician cuts down on unnecessary visits to higher cost specialists and tests. The PCP is required to make every attempt to diagnose and treat the patient before referring her to a specialist. If a patient goes to a specialist without the PCP's referral the services may not be covered and the insured may be liable for additional charges.

Appropriate Medical Care in Least Restrictive Setting

A goal of all MCOs is for the patient to receive care in the most appropriate and least restrictive setting. These restrictive settings are important to the efficiency and delivery of healthcare in the provider's facility. The PCP or the specialist within the network has requirements to meet as to where the patient is sent for radiology, laboratory, mammography, and other types of services.

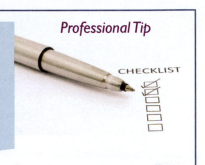

Professional Tip

CHECKLIST

The medical office specialist needs to be familiar with the patient's MCO plan with regard to where services can be obtained. In order for the insurance carrier to pay, the patient may only seek services from a facility within his plan network.

Withholding Providers' Funds

An MCO may have a *withhold program*, now known as *pay for performance*. A withhold program refers to a provision in an MCO contract that states that the MCO will withhold a percentage of the physician's revenue until year-end. This allows the MCO to evaluate the physician's medical management in terms of its cost effectiveness. If the physician has not sent the patients for numerous diagnostic tests, procedures, and so on, the amount withheld will be paid to the provider. If the physician has ordered several expensive tests, the MCO may keep the amount withheld. This type of verbiage is an incentive for the provider not to order unnecessary tests. The purpose of withholding programs is to encourage providers to use cost-effective services and procedures. The pay-for-performance program is aimed at allowing providers to give good quality care within the networks' facilities while reducing costs.

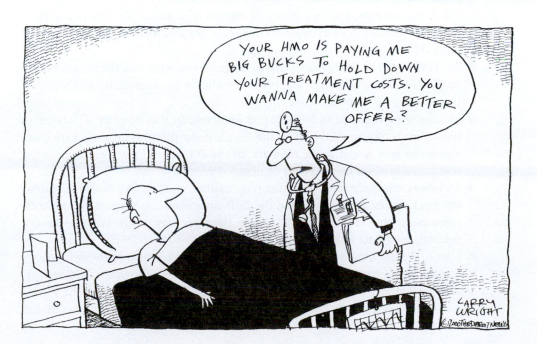

Reprinted by permission of Larry Wright.

Types of Managed Care Organizations

The major types of managed care plans are:

- Health maintenance organizations (HMOs).
- Preferred provider organizations (PPOs).
- Point-of-service plans (POSs).

Each of these plans has distinctive features or characteristics. Today it is more difficult to recognize the differences among products that bill themselves as HMOs, PPOs, or managed care.

Health Maintenance Organization (HMO)

A **health maintenance organization (HMO)** is regulated by both federal and state law. Health maintenance organizations consists of a medical center or a designated group of providers that provides medical services to subscribers (persons who are covered by an insurance policy) for a fixed monthly or annual premium. The policyholder, interchangeably called the *insured*, *subscriber*, or *member*, usually has a very small (or no) copayment when he needs services.

HMO plans have various rules for copayment, coinsurance, and deductible amounts. Remember from earlier in this chapter a copayment is a fixed dollar amount the member pays for each office visit or hospital encounter. Coinsurance is the portion of the provider's fees that the patient has to pay. A deductible is the amount a patient pays out of his own pocket before insurance begins paying any of the costs of healthcare.

The subscriber to an HMO plan is able to obtain healthcare on a regular basis with unlimited medical attention. Thus HMOs encourage subscribers to take advantage of preventive healthcare services in an attempt to make healthcare coverage more cost efficient. HMOs do tend to cover more preventive procedures, such as annual physical examinations, mammographies, and routine screening procedures.

- A distinctive feature of an HMO is that the subscriber chooses a primary care physician, who is sometimes known as a gatekeeper. The PCP arranges, provides, coordinates, and authorizes all aspects of a member's healthcare. PCPs are usually family doctors, internal medicine doctors, general practitioners, or OB/GYNs.
- An HMO enters into contractual arrangements with healthcare providers (e.g., physicians, hospitals, and other healthcare professionals) and together they form a provider network.
- Members are required to see only providers within this network if they are to have their healthcare paid for by the HMO. If the member receives care from a provider who is not in the network, the HMO will not pay for care unless it was preauthorized by the HMO or deemed an emergency.
- Members may only see a specialist (e.g., cardiologist, dermatologist, rheumatologist) if they are referred and the PCP authorizes the service. The **referral** must be approved by the HMO. If the member sees a specialist without a referral, the HMO will not pay for the service.
- HMOs are the most restrictive type of health plan because of the restrictions the members have in selecting a healthcare provider. However, HMOs typically provide members with a greater range of health benefits for the lowest out-of-pocket expenses, such as no copayment or a very low copayment and deductible.

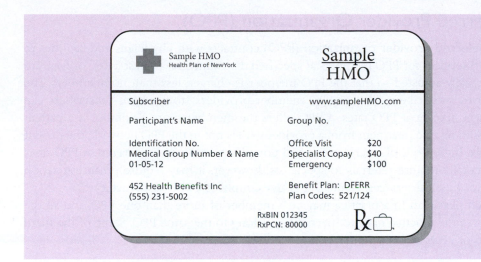

Figure 2.1

Sample HMO Insurance Card.

As mentioned, HMOs greatly restrict whom a patient may see for medical services. This restriction makes it possible to significantly reduce members' premiums. HMOs have generated considerable controversy because in many such plans doctors receive financial incentives for reducing the amount of medical services provided to patients. One method of doing this has been to pay doctors a fixed monthly fee for each patient. Another method has been to have physicians on staff. The physician works for the HMO medical center and receives an annual salary and benefits, just like any employee. Figure 2.1 is an example of an HMO insurance card.

The main types of HMOs vary in the way they link providers in order to create a healthcare delivery system.

Group Model HMO

A group model HMO is an organization that contracts with a multi-specialty physicians' group to provide physician services to an enrolled group. Physicians are employees of the group practice and generally are limited to providing care only to the HMO's members.

Individual Practice Association HMO

Individual practice association (IPA) HMOs are the most decentralized and involve contracting with individual physicians to create a healthcare delivery system. The HMO contracts with community hospitals and providers of services such as laboratories and diagnostic imaging centers. Pharmacy services are provided through a contracted network of independent and chain community pharmacies and mail order services.

Network Model HMO

Network HMOs contract with more than one community-based multi-specialty group to provide wider geographical coverage. The group practices under contract with one HMO vary from large to small, from primary care to multi-specialty practice.

Staff Model HMO

Staff model HMOs employ salaried physicians who treat members in facilities owned and operated by the HMO. Most services, including diagnostic, laboratory, and pharmacy services, are provided on site. A team of health professionals delivers the care.

Open Access HMO

Open access HMOs do not use gatekeepers. There is no requirement to obtain a referral before seeing a specialist. The copayment or coinsurance may be higher for specialist care.

Preferred Provider Organization (PPO)

The **preferred provider organization (PPO)** contracts with physicians and facilities to perform services for PPO members at specified discounted fees. These rates, or fees, are contractually adjusted so that the PPO member is charged less than nonmembers. The PPO gives subscribers a list of PPO member-providers from whom subscribers can receive healthcare at PPO rates. A PPO offers the member more flexibility. If a patient chooses to receive treatment from a provider who is not in the PPO network, the patient will have higher out-of-pocket costs, and not all services may be covered. A PPO does not generally require referrals to specialists, however, it may require preauthorization for major medical services. Figure 2.2 is an example of a PPO insurance card.

Each physician in a practice may be a member of more than one PPO, and all the doctors in the practice may not necessarily belong to the same PPO. Some of the main features of PPOs include the following:

- PPOs are similar to HMOs in that they enter into contractual arrangements with healthcare providers (e.g., physicians, hospitals, and other healthcare professionals) and together form a provider network.
- Unlike an HMO, PPO members do not have a PCP (gatekeeper) nor do they have to use an in-network provider for their care. However, PPOs offer members higher benefits as financial incentives to use network providers. The incentives may include lower deductibles, lower copayments, and higher reimbursements. For example, if the subscriber sees an in-network family physician for a routine visit, she may only have a small copayment or deductible. If she sees a non-network family physician for a routine visit, she may have to pay as much as 50% of the total bill. PPO plans customarily have an annual deductible.
- PPO members typically do not have to get a referral to see a specialist.

Point-of-Service (POS) Options

Because many patients do not wish to accept services from only their HMO providers, some HMO plans add a **point-of-service (POS)** option. Patients who choose this

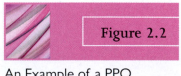

Figure 2.2

An Example of a PPO Insurance Card.

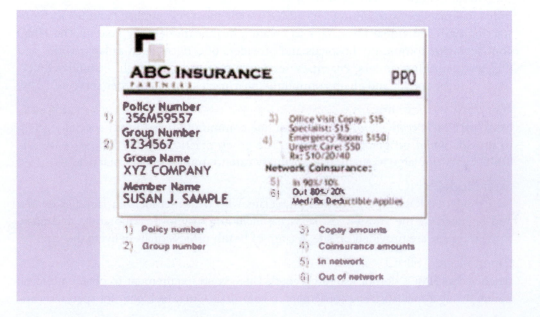

option do not have to use only the HMO's physicians. However, if they choose to see physicians outside the network, they must pay increased deductibles and coinsurance. This option makes the HMO more like a PPO in terms of choices available to the patients.

- Like an HMO and a PPO, a POS plan has a contracted provider network.
- POS plans encourage, but do not require, members to choose a primary care physician. As in a traditional HMO, the PCP acts as a gatekeeper when making referrals. POS members also may opt at their discretion to visit an out-of-network provider. If that happens, the member's copayments, coinsurance, and deductibles will be substantially higher.
- POS plans are becoming more popular because they offer more flexibility and freedom of choice than do standard HMOs.

Exclusive Provider Organization

Exclusive provider organizations (EPOs) are a type of managed care plan that combines features of HMOs (e.g., enrolled members, limited providers' network, gatekeepers, utilization management, preauthorization system) and PPOs (e.g., flexible benefit design, negotiated fees, and fee-for-service payments). Exclusive provider organizations (EPOs) are a lot like HMOs: They generally don't cover care outside the plan's provider network. However, members may not need a referral to see a specialist. An EPO is referred to as exclusive because employers agree not to contract with any other plan. Members are eligible for benefits only when they use the services of the network of providers, with certain exceptions for emergency or out-of-area services.

- If a patient decides to seek care outside the network, generally he is not reimbursed for the cost of treatment.
- Technically, many HMOs can be considered EPOs except that EPOs are regulated under insurance statutes rather than federal and state HMO regulations.
- An EPO is priced lower than a PPO to the employer, but an EPO's premiums are usually more expensive than an HMO's premiums.

Criticism of MCOs

Managed care has not been without its trouble or criticism. Some of the major issues that face HMOs, prepaid medical groups, and government-sponsored managed care plans are providing necessary care in emergency situations and providing long-term care for the chronically ill. MCOs are criticized for not offering patients the ability to appeal or hold liable the MCO with regard to procedures and even surgeries the MCO has denied on the basis of not being medically necessary. Approximately 14 states have enacted statutes that have created tort liability for patient harm caused by MCOs.

MCOs will contract with hospitals to provide care for their enrollees. When an enrollee suffers a medical emergency, she must go to an in-network hospital or emergency clinic in order for the service to be covered under the MCO's policy. In addition, policies require that the MCO be notified within 48 hours after admission; however, calling an MCO is often the last thing a patient thinks about during an emergency. An enrollee should not assume that all physicians in the hospital network are participating in the MCP.

For example, the Kaiser HMO has facilities throughout the United States that are structured as staff model HMOs. The patient must go to that one facility for all medical care, including the hospital. In an emergency this can be very risky. Consider the situation of a pregnant woman who lived 30 miles from the closest hospital in her MCO network. Her labor contractions became intense over a short period of time. She called an ambulance, and the baby was delivered while en route. If she had admitted herself, or if the ambulance had taken her to any other hospital, the medical cost would not have been covered by her Kaiser HMO policy. Many MCO contracts have been modified and addendums added to accommodate emergency situations, but sometimes it takes many phone calls and appeals to the MCO by the patient and provider to receive reimbursement. Table 2.2 outlines the advantages and disadvantages of MCOs.

Table 2.2	Advantages and Disadvantages of Managed Care Organizations
Advantages of Managed Care	**Disadvantages of Managed Care**
MCOs help to restrain the overall growth of healthcare costs by demanding discounted prices from doctors and hospitals for care.	When an enrollee suffers a medical emergency, she must go to an in-network hospital or emergency clinic in order for the service to be covered under her policy.
Hospitals and physicians are acting more efficiently in order to attract MCOs. MCOs contract with large companies and enroll a significant number of members, which forces providers to lower their own costs and to strive to improve the quality of their care. This means reducing overhead costs and the number of unnecessary tests they perform.	A managed care plan typically restricts the physician's latitude in caring for patients. The utilization guidelines of a managed care company may strongly suggest a plan of treatment different from the plan preferred by the treating physician. This situation could increase the likelihood of a malpractice suit being brought against that provider.
The MCOs collect and analyze data on how well they deliver care, such as identifying what percentage of children in an HMO are immunized. This information is combined with outcomes data to help document how well the HMO is meeting its needs. This helps consumers choose the best managed care plan for their family.	The physician runs the risk of obtaining unfavorable or undesirable evaluations collected from enrollees of the managed care company. This can have a financial impact on the physician's practice. Members can require an extraordinary amount of the physician's time because of their age group or medical conditions.
The data the managed care plan gathers is analyzed for clinical services. This tells how well a patient does when he receives a particular service, such as cataract surgery. The outcome data measures how much difference the MCO's intervention made in the consumer's health and quality of life. This data helps providers understand if a procedure or test is necessary for treatment.	Managed care companies can create an increased administrative burden on a physician's office because of incompatible claims systems, the need for authorization before providing care, required physician interaction with utilization review departments, and required quality assurance reporting.
Managed care plans are creating disease management programs and care pathways. For example, an HMO could design and implement a disease management program for patients with diabetes that combines health education, routine blood sugar testing, doctor visits, and drug therapy. HMOs develop their disease management programs with the help of experts, in particular medical specialties, and they rely heavily on the latest studies of what works best for particular types of patients.	A participating provider may experience additional financial burdens if the managed care company requires participating physicians to carry additional malpractice insurance.

Table 2.2	Advantages and Disadvantages of Managed Care Organizations (*Continued*)
Advantages of Managed Care	**Disadvantages of Managed Care**
Managed care plans make extensive use of healthcare professionals, such as physicians' assistants, nurse practitioners, and certified nurse midwives. These practitioners, who have less training than physicians, work with doctors to provide many basic healthcare services to consumers and are less costly for MCOs to employ than are physicians. They can also perform many of the primary care tasks that physicians do and provide very high-quality care for a wide range of illnesses at a lower cost.	MCOs negotiate fees with providers that are lower than the providers' usual fees. If the negotiated fees are too low this could cause the provider "to make up the difference" by seeing more patients. Seeing more patients per day may result in not enough time being spent with each patient, thus resulting in patient dissatisfaction.
Managed care plan staff members are continuously studying new medical technologies and drugs in order to keep abreast of new medical products and services and to determine what is safe and most effective for consumers and under what conditions these services or products should be made available. They are assessing everything from what prescription drugs to offer to what kinds of surgical implants MCO members should be receiving.	

Patients diagnosed with hypertension, diabetes, cancer, renal disease, or other diseases requiring ongoing treatment may run into problems with their MCO. These patients' treatments are often costly and require services from many providers. Some managed care plans' requirements, such as referrals and **preauthorization** (written approval prior to time of service) for treatment actually add a layer of bureaucracy and cost to the delivery of care and sometimes lead to delays in necessary treatment. The most progressive managed care plans identify these patients and provide case managers to ensure efficient delivery of services and patient compliance with treatment plans to provide high-quality service and to avoid the catastrophic costs associated with long and avoidable hospital stays.

Many health plans have also been criticized for not allowing patients to appeal treatment decisions other than through the MCO-governed arbitration process. A sample of a *treatment decision* would be the MCO denying a procedure or diagnostic test because it claims it is not medically necessary. For the toughest cases involving the potential use of costly, experimental treatments, progressive HMOs are adding impartial panels of medical experts to determine what care is medically appropriate. The health plans that are not addressing the concerns of their enrollees, particularly if they are for-profit plans, face an enormous backlash of public criticism for not balancing the need to control costs while preserving access to high-quality services.

Integrated Healthcare Delivery Systems

An integrated delivery system (IDS) is a network of healthcare organizations under a parent holding company. Some IDS have an HMO component, while others are a network of physicians only, or of physicians and hospitals. Thus, the term is used broadly to define an organization that provides a continuum of healthcare services. At the very least, an IDS represents providers coming together in some type of legal structure for purposes of managing healthcare and contracting with health plans such as HMOs, PPOs, or health insurance companies.

Independent Physician Association

An independent practice association (or IPA) is a U.S. term for an association of independent physicians, or other organization that contracts with independent physicians, and provides services to managed care organizations on a negotiated per capita rate, flat retainer fee, or negotiated fee-for-service basis. An HMO or other managed care plan can contract with an IPA, which in turn contracts with independent physicians to treat members at discounted fees or on a capitation basis. The typical IPA encompasses all specialties, but an IPA can be solely for primary care or could be single specialty.

IPAs are typically formed as an LLC, S Corp, C Corp, or other stock entity. Their purpose is not to generate a profit for the shareholders, although this can be done. The IPA assembles physicians in self-directed groups within a geographic region to invent and implement healthcare solutions, form collaborative efforts among physicians to implement these programs, and exert political influence upward within the medical community to effect positive change.

Despite a perception that IPAs have been formed to negotiate as a group with insurance companies in an attempt to improve rates of compensation, under the Federal Trade Commission Act, they cannot do this for the physician's other insurance reimbursement. The IPA can only negotiate for the IPA members those services which are contracted on capitated members.

Physician-Hospital Organization

A *physician-hospital organization* (PHO) is another approach to coordinating services for patients. Physicians join with hospitals to create an integrated medical care delivery system. Surgery centers, nursing homes, laboratories, and other facilities may also be connected with the PHO. This union then makes arrangements for insurance with a commercial carrier or an HMO.

Self-Insured Plan

A *self-insured plan* is one in which the payer is an employer or other group, such as a labor union. Assuming the full risk for the payment of healthcare services, the employer or labor union uses the premium it would have paid an insurance carrier to establish a fund to provide benefits for its employees or group members.

The employer may contract with an organization to manage and pay the claims for the employees' medical services. The "health plans" will be administered by an insurance company (known as a third-party administrator, or TPA).

The medical office specialist needs to know if the insured person's plan is self-insured by the patient's employer. Self-insured plans are regulated by the **Employee Retirement Income Security Act (ERISA)**. ERISA is regulated by the U.S. Department of Labor and does not abide by state insurance rules and regulations. A medical office specialist who finds it necessary to file a complaint with such a carrier on an issue such as a denied claim or an incorrect payment will be appealing to federal courts.

A medical office specialist will need to recognize the type of MCO policy a patient has and the characteristics of the policy. Table 2.3 summarizes the different MCOs and their characteristics.

Table 2.3	Various Types of MCOs and Their Characteristics			
	HMO	**PPO**	**POS**	**EPO**
	■ State licensed ■ Most stringent guidelines ■ Limited network of providers ■ Members assigned to PCPs ■ Members must use network except in emergencies or pay a penalty ■ Usually there is a financial reward to providers for managing the cost of care	■ Limited network of providers but larger than HMO ■ Members may be assigned to PCPs but restrictions on accessing other physicians not as tight as in HMO ■ Financial penalty for accessing non-network providers less severe than in an HMO ■ Usually there is no reward to providers for managing the cost of care	■ Hybrid of HMO and PPO networks ■ Members may choose from a primary or secondary network ■ Primary network is HMO-like ■ Secondary network is often a PPO network ■ Out-of-pocket expenses are lower within the primary network and higher when using the secondary network ■ Members have more choices with less expense than with a PPO	■ Doesn't have an HMO license ■ Members are eligible for benefits only when they use network providers ■ Financial penalties for members leaving the network are similar to those of HMO ■ Priced lower than a PPO but higher than an HMO
	IPA Model HMO	**Staff Model HMO**	**Network Model HMO**	**Group Model HMO**
	■ An association formed by physicians with separately owned practices (solo or small group) ■ HMO may contract with physicians separately or through the IPA	■ HMO hires the physicians and pays them salaries ■ HMO owns the network ■ HMO owns the clinic sites and health centers	■ HMO uses two or more group practices or a group practice plus a combination of staff physicians and contracted independent physicians to form a network of providers ■ Allows members to choose their providers	■ HMO contracts with multi-specialty groups. ■ May be open-panel or closed-panel

Insurance Plans

To provide protection for hospitalization and medical expenses, various prepaid medical care plans have been established. Some are private, such as Blue Cross Blue Shield, and some are government sponsored, such as Medicare, Medicaid, Tricare, and CHAMPVA. Under a written insurance contract, the policyholder pays a premium and the insurance company provides payment for medical services. If the policy is offered through employment, the employer may pay a portion of the premium.

Commercial Health Insurance

Commercial health insurance is a general term for policies offered through for-profit companies such as Aetna, Prudential, and United Healthcare. The policy can be a fee-for-service policy or a managed care one. Such policies are licensed and regulated by a state board of insurance according to the state in which the companies are located or the state in which they are incorporated.

Types of Insurance Coverage

Insurance can be classified as either **group insurance** or individual insurance. With group insurance, one master policy is issued to an organization or employer and covers the eligible members or employees and their dependents. A dependent includes same-sex and opposite-sex spouses and children. Thus, all the members or employees have similar healthcare coverage. Group insurance plans provide better benefits with lower premiums than do individual insurance plans. Individual insurance applies only to the person taking out the policy and to that person's dependents. Because it is not obtained at a group rate, the premiums are higher than for group insurance.

Descriptions of the major types of health insurance coverage follow. A basic health insurance policy might include insurance for hospital, medical, and surgical services. A comprehensive insurance package would include several of the major types of insurance listed next.

Indemnity Plan/Fee for Service

An indemnity plan provides coverage for all medically necessary services. The policyholder and/or patient may receive medically necessary services from the provider they choose. The provider is reimbursed for her services if it is the usual and customary fee. The fee for service plan typically has an annual deductible. No fee discounts are taken. The provider does not have to request preauthorization for services.

Hospital Insurance

Hospital insurance provides protection against the costs of hospital care. It generally provides a room allowance (a stated amount per day for a semiprivate room) with a maximum number of days per year. Special provisions are made for operating room charges, X-rays, laboratory work, drugs, and other medically necessary items while the insured person is an **inpatient**. (An inpatient is a person who is admitted to the hospital for a minimum of 24 hours.)

Hospital Indemnity Insurance

This insurance offers limited coverage. There are two different methods by which a patient may receive benefits. The policy may pay a per diem or fixed amount for each day the patient is in the hospital, in which case it will state a maximum number of payable days. The payment goes directly to the patient who may use it for medical services or other expenses such as prescriptions. Usually, the amount the patient receives is less than the cost of the hospital stay. The other method of payment will pay a portion of the patient's medical expenses after another policy has paid. This is considered a supplemental policy.

Medical Insurance

Medical insurance covers benefits for **outpatient** medical care, including physicians' fees for hospital visits and nonsurgical procedures. The term *medical* refers to physicians' costs. Special provisions are made for costs related to diagnostic services such as laboratory, X-ray, and pathology. (An outpatient is a person who receives medical care at a hospital or other medical facility but who is not admitted for more than 24 hours.)

Surgical Insurance

Surgical insurance provides protection for the cost of a physician's fee for surgery, whether it is performed in a hospital, in a doctor's office, or elsewhere, such as a surgical center. Charges for anesthesia generally are covered by surgical insurance.

Outpatient Insurance

Outpatient insurance usually provides protection for emergency department visits and other outpatient divisions in a hospital or medical facility, such as X-ray, pathology, and psychological services.

Major Medical Insurance

Major medical insurance offers protection for large medical expenses beyond what is established by a regular health insurance policy. There is usually an added cost for this type of insurance coverage.

Special Risk Insurance

A person can also obtain protection against a certain type of accident (e.g., an airplane crash) or illness (e.g., cancer) through **special risk insurance**.

Catastrophic Health Insurance

Catastrophic health insurance is among the least expensive forms of health insurance. Deductibles are generally large for these types of policies. There also may be caps on the amount the policy will pay in case of illness. These policies are only suitable for individuals with the financial means to handle routine illnesses and hospitalizations.

Short-Term Health Insurance

Short-term health insurance can only be purchased for a specific period of time. Coverage provided by such policies ranges from catastrophic to comprehensive, with the latter being considerably more expensive. Short-term health insurance often comes with strict qualifying procedures and may not cover preexisting medical conditions. (A **preexisting condition** is a diagnosis for which the insured has previously been treated.) In particular, pregnancy and childbirth are not usually covered by these policies.

COBRA Insurance

A federal law makes it possible for most people to continue their group health coverage for a period of time following termination of employment. Called COBRA (for the Consolidated Omnibus Budget Reconciliation Act of 1985), the law requires that if the insured works for a business of 20 or more employees and leaves his job or is laid off, he can continue to get health coverage for at least 18 months. However, the person will have to pay the entire premium, including the employer's portion, rather than just the portion of it he paid when he was working.

People are also able to get insurance under COBRA if their spouses were covered but they are now widowed or divorced. Also, if a student was covered under her parents' group plan while in school, she can continue in the plan for up to 18 months under COBRA until she finds a job that offers her health insurance.

Long-Term Care Insurance

Long-term care insurance covers both medical and custodial services. These services can range from at-home care, including assisting someone with daily personal and house-hold chores, to day care services at a facility, to assisted living residences, to nursing home care. The degree of care is based on the current requirements and condition of the person who is in need of long-term care.

Supplemental Insurance

Supplemental insurance is purchased to cover expenses, such as coinsurance, that are not covered by the primary insurance policy. An example is a Medigap policy, which is a supplemental health insurance policy sold by private insurance companies to fill the "gaps" in the original Medicare plan coverage. If a patient has a commercial policy, however, he cannot use a Medigap policy.

Health Savings Accounts

Insurance carriers may offer **high-deductible health plans (HDHP)**. The premiums on these plans are lower than other plans, but the out-of-pocket expense to the sub-scriber is much higher. The deductible on these plans can be anywhere from $3,000 to $10,000 a calendar year. Since most people cannot afford to shell out this type of money when a catastrophic medical condition requires surgery or long-term care, insurance carriers offer third-tier health insurance plans that allow members to use **health savings accounts (HSA)** and **Health Reimbursement Accounts (HRAs)**, or similar medical payment products to pay routine healthcare expenses directly. These plans fall under the concept **consumer-driven healthcare (CDHC)** which received a boost in popularity in 2003 with the passage of federal legislation providing tax incentives to those who choose such plans. Consumer-driven plans are subject to the provision of the Affordable Care Act, which mandates that routine and or health maintenance claims must be covered with no cost-sharing (copays, coinsurance, or deductibles) to the patient.

HSA

HSA is a tax savings account that helps cover additional costs not covered by a health insurance plan. Funds are placed into a savings account throughout the year to help cover deductibles and other medical expenses incurred throughout the calendar year. The amount of money deposited into the account is a tax deduction. There are limitations to what the funds can be used for without a penalty applying.

If an individual opens her own account, she must deduct the money deposited to the account yearly on her taxes. If the employer sets up the account, contributions are deducted from a paycheck before the income is taxed. If an individual takes money out of the HSA account to pay for nonmedical costs, the money withdrawn is taxed and subject to a penalty. When the individual turns 65, she can withdraw the money from the HSA for any reason without penalty. She can use the HSA to pay for medical, dental, vision, psychiatric treatments, COBRA premiums, and prescription drugs.

HRA

An employer sets the parameters regarding the HRA, meaning that any unused money is not transferred to the employee in the event the employee finds new employment. On termination of employment, participation will end automatically and expenses for services will not be eligible for reimbursement after the termination date. HRAs may allow retirees access to unused reimbursements.

Unlike the **Flexible Spending Accounts (FSA)**, which bar any amount of money not used in a single coverage period, HRAs allow any unused balance not used in a single coverage period to transfer over to the following period. When this occurs, the maximum reimbursement amount is increased for every dollar that has not been spent in the previous coverage period.

The HRA does not require that the maximum amount of reimbursement be available throughout the coverage period. Additionally, it does not require the expenses to have been incurred during the coverage period to be reimbursed. Eligible expenses that can be reimbursed by an HRA include services that are designed to diagnose, cure, or prevent illnesses as well as any service that is directly related to medical care. As of 2014, the service for which the cost is shared includes visits to the doctor's office, dental and vision care, and prescription drugs.

FSA

A **flexible spending account (FSA)**, also known as a flexible spending arrangement, is a tax-advantaged financial account that can be set up through an employer in the United States. An FSA allows an employee to set aside a portion of earnings to pay for qualified expenses as established in the plan, most commonly for medical expenses but often for dependent care or other expenses. Money deducted from an employee's pay into a FSA is not subject to taxes; therefore it is a payroll tax savings. Under the terms of the Affordable Care Act, a plan may permit an employee to carry up to $500 into the following year without losing the funds.

The most common type of flexible spending account is the medical FSA account, which is similar to a Health Saving Account (HSA) or a Health Reimbursement Account (HRA). However, while HSAs and HRAs are almost exclusively used as components of a managed care health plan, medical FSAs are commonly offered with health plans are more traditional as well. In addition, funds in an HSA are not lost when the plan year is over, unlike funds in a FSA. A FSA debit card (also known as a Flex-card) is issued to the insured person to access the account funds.

Affordable Care Act

The **Affordable Care Act (ACA)** was passed by Congress in 2010. The law is also called the **Patient Protection and Affordable Care Act**, otherwise known as **Obamacare**. The goal of the ACA is to make health insurance affordable for all Americans. Under the Affordable Care Act, insurance companies cannot deny anyone coverage because of pre-existing medical conditions. They also cannot drop an individual for simply becoming too high a liability to insure.

The federal government established the Affordable Care Act. All of these plans have the same amount of Essential Health Benefit Coverage per the Affordable Care Act. The Essential Health Benefits include preventative care, maternity and pediatric care, emergency/hospitalization care, mental health services, prescription drug coverage, lab work, and additional services.

There are five different types of Government Plans: Bronze, Silver, Gold, Platinum, and Catastrophic. All plans provide the same amount of coverage; the only difference is the cost of the premium for the policy. Bronze Plans have premiums that cost less per month or year, but an individual will pay more out-of-pocket when medical care is provided. These plans are good for normal, healthy individuals who are looking for an insurance plan for basic preventative care. Platinum Plans are the exact opposite. The individual will pay more per month or year in premiums, but less out of pocket. These plans are good for those individuals or families who have ongoing medical issues that require regular medical treatment. Catastrophic Plans are for those who need coverage in the event of a major medical issue such as a hospitalization. The individual must also be under 30 years old or undergoing some type of income hardship to qualify for this last insurance plan.

The Patient Protection and Affordable Care Act requires that all individuals have health insurance beginning in 2014. Those with low incomes who do not have access to affordable coverage through their jobs will be able to purchase a health plan with federal subsidies. Health plans cannot deny coverage for any reason, including a person's health status, race, or gender. Not having a health insurance plan will likely lead to a fine. The reason for the fine is to encourage all Americans to have health insurance. The fewer uninsured people in the United States, the lower the costs of healthcare and insurance will be for everyone.

In 2011, 26% of all U.S. citizens of working age experienced a gap in medical health insurance coverage; many lost their medical health insurance when they became unemployed or changed jobs. Medical healthcare coverage cost in 2012 was at an average of $11,204 per employee. It has also been determined that during this time period roughly two-thirds of employers increased employees' premium contributions for single coverage for 2012, and 73% increased them for employees with dependent coverage. Therefore, citizens were concerned either as an individual or as the owner of a small business that the Affordable Care Act could affect them adversely. Today, coverage under the Affordable Care Act has allowed large numbers of citizens to sign up for insurance after the deadlines in the last 2 years, destabilizing insurance markets and driving up premiums for medical health plans.

The final provision of the act prevents illegal immigrants from receiving government funds to pay for healthcare insurance. However, it does not require people to prove citizenship before getting healthcare services.

The Provider's View of Managed Care

Managed care has its pros and cons (as discussed in Table 2.2). Providers are required to follow contractual agreements with the insurance carriers in order to receive payment for services provided. Some physicians or providers see these agreements as restrictions on their way of providing medical care and managing their facilities. The standard length of a contract between an MCO and a provider is 1 year. If a physician discovers that there are too many restrictions, she has to give a written 30- or 60-day notice before she can close the practice to members of the MCO plan. (This is why a provider is sometimes listed in a directory but is no longer participating in the network.)

Patient Care

HMOs, PPOs, and fee-for-service plans often share certain features, including preauthorization, utilization review, and discharge planning.

A patient may be required to get preauthorization from his plan or insurer before admission to a hospital for certain types of surgery. If preauthorization is not obtained, then the cost of the procedure will not be covered. Utilization review is the process by which a plan determines whether a specific medical or surgical service is appropriate or medically necessary. Discharge planning is an approach that facilitates the transfer of a patient to a more cost-effective facility if the patient no longer needs to stay in the hospital. For example, if, following surgery, a patient no longer needs hospitalization but cannot be cared for at home, the person may be transferred to a skilled nursing facility.

Facility Operations

Contracting with an MCO requires that the provider implement changes in the operation of its facilities, staff, and methods of treating patients. Providers have to reduce inefficiency and waste in their own operations. As a result, physicians are joining larger groups of doctors who can provide a wide range of primary care and specialty services. This makes it easier to refer patients from one doctor to another. By joining a larger group, the doctors can share expenses by sharing office space, staff, utilities, and so forth.

Some providers are doing less testing before surgery. Hospitals are developing care pathways to help move consumers through their hospital stays as efficiently as possible. In a care pathway, the hospital studies the services the patient needs and plans the entire treatment program for the whole stay.

Verifying Insurance Coverage

The administrative staff or medical office specialist must obtain complete and accurate information on a patient who comes into the doctor's office or hospital. Not only is this information helpful in facilitating the care of the patient, but it is also necessary for the processing of insurance claims. All patient demographics and insurance information must be updated on a regular basis.

At point of service (POS), the medical office specialist should ask to see the patient's insurance card. Many practices collect the patient's insurance information before POS when they are new patients or have not been in the office for an extended length of time. The insurance card states the name of the insurance policy, the subscriber's name, and the insurance policy number. The front and back of the card should be photocopied and a current copy kept in the patient's medical record.

After receiving the insurance information, whether via phone, fax, mail, or when the patient completes information at the time of the visit, the insurance must be verified. The medical office specialist should call the insurance company and verify the information on the insurance card. The following information should be requested after establishing what type of plan the patient has: the amount of the deductible and whether it has been met or the remaining balance; coinsurance or copay amounts; any exclusions, limitations, or riders on the policy; lifetime maximum; authorizations required;

and effective coverage date. The type of facility or specialty will determine what types of information to verify. An example would be verifying a long hospital stay versus a physical examination at a family practice office. All information received should be documented. When receiving information by phone it is important to document the name and phone number of the insurance company's contact person and the date and time the medical office specialist spoke with him. The medical office specialist's name and date should also be noted. This is very important in case there is a denial of the claim or collection problems after services are provided. In addition to calling insurance companies to verify benefits, many providers verify benefits online. This can be accomplished by fax, the payer's website (portal), or through an eligibility software program. Verification of coverage is important to a practice or hospital, as it will safeguard compensation for services rendered.

When verifying benefits through the payer's website, providers enroll in the insurance company's provider online system. Many healthcare providers verify coverage through an online system designed specifically for healthcare providers. Instead of calling the insurance company, the medical office specialist can verify coverage immediately by entering patient information online through the insurance company's portal. For the most part, it will specify that the patient is still active. It will provide an effective date of coverage and show additional information such as the patient ID number, primary care physician, and deductibles, as well as copay amounts. A copy of this eligibility check should be printed or scanned and kept in the patient's medical record. In practices that are automated, the eligibility verification from the payer may automatically feed into the patient's medical record. Complete Practice Exercise 2.2 by documenting the action you would take for each situation or calculate the coinsurance.

Practice Exercise 2.2

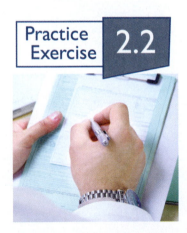

Document the action you would take for each situation or calculate the coinsurance.

1. You are the medical office specialist at the Allied Medical Clinic. Peggy Miller is being seen today. You call her insurance carrier to verify benefits. The carrier's customer services representative informs you that the patient's insurance was cancelled 2 months ago.

    What action would you take?

    _____

    _____

    _____

2. You are the medical office specialist at the Allied Medical Clinic. Your supervisor has asked you to go up to the front desk and explain to a patient what her estimated coinsurance will be for the procedure she plans to have on October 19. The total charges are $475. The allowed amount is $326. Her benefits pay at 90%.

    What is the patient's coinsurance:_____?

Collecting Insurance Payments

The medical office specialist must be well informed on managed care, including the different types of policies and methods of receiving payment, because duties will include understanding patients' health insurance coverage. Patients ask many questions about health insurance and expect the medical office specialist to know the answers. It is the medical office specialist's responsibility to see that the doctor receives compensation for services. Three conditions must be met for full payment or compensation: The insured must pay their premiums for active coverage, they must pay their deductibles and any required coinsurance, and they are also responsible for any copays due.

Assignment of Benefits

Providers may receive payment directly from the patient or accept an **assignment of benefits**. When a provider accepts an assignment of benefits, the provider and patient agree all payments will be paid directly to the provider by the patient's insurance carrier. In this case, the patient signs an assignment of benefits statement. This statement authorizes the insurance company to send payments directly to the provider.

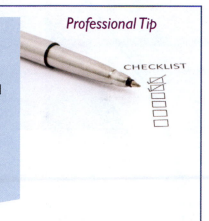

Professional Tip

The medical office specialist must be aware that some insurance carriers will not honor an Assignment of Benefits form if the provider has not contracted with the carrier (referred to as an out-of-network or nonparticipating provider). Even though the patient assigns the benefits and the provider accepts assignment, the payment for the services may be sent directly to the patient/subscriber.

When the patient does not sign the assignment of benefits, it is sometimes very difficult to receive payment in full from the patient. Providers should have a statement in their policies and procedures manual that instructs the medical office specialist not to file the claim for the patient and instead ask for payment in full at the time of service or arrange a payment agreement if the patient refuses to assign benefits. Providers have different views on handling this type of situation; be sure to check with your office manager before taking action.

Chapter Summary

- Managed care is a system that in theory controls the cost and delivery of health services to members who are enrolled in a specific type of healthcare plan.
- The goals of managed healthcare were and still are to ensure that providers deliver high-quality care in a facility that manages or controls costs, and that all medical care or procedures are medically necessary and appropriate for the patient's condition or diagnosis.
- Managed care uses a network of providers. This is true in HMOs, PPOs, POS, and EPO plans. Each MCO provides a wide array of physicians and hospital services from which enrollees can choose.
- A managed care plan typically restricts the physician's latitude in caring for patients. The utilization protocol of a managed care company may strongly suggest a plan of treatment different from the plan preferred by the treating physician.

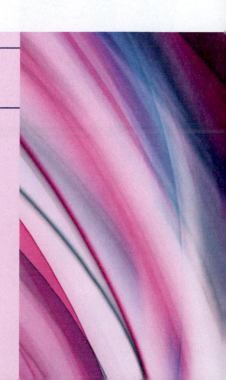

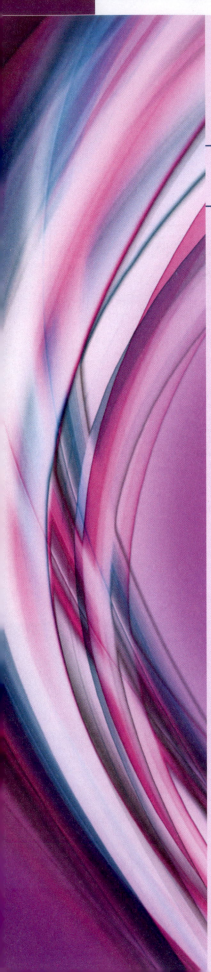

■ The administrative staff or medical office specialist must obtain complete and accurate information on a patient who comes into the doctor's office or hospital. Not only is this information helpful in facilitating the care of the patient, but it is also necessary for the processing of insurance claims.

Chapter Review

True/False

Identify the statement as true (T) or false (F).

_____ **1.** Coinsurance is paid by the provider.

_____ **2.** The deductible is the amount the insured must pay for each healthcare encounter, such as an office visit.

_____ **3.** Under a discounted fee-for-service arrangement, a provider and a payer negotiate the provider's fees.

_____ **4.** Fee-for-service contracts establish coinsurance payments for patients' charges.

_____ **5.** HMO members are usually allowed to receive medical services from any provider whom they choose without additional cost.

_____ **6.** Under an indemnity plan, an insurance company agrees to cover the financial losses of a medical practice.

_____ **7.** A managed care system combines the financing and the delivery of healthcare services.

_____ **8.** Under a POS option, HMO members can receive services from any provider, but they must pay a greater amount for encounters with non-network providers.

_____ **9.** A policyholder is a person who buys an insurance plan.

_____ **10.** Indemnity plans usually require preauthorization for many services.

_____ **11.** HDHP is abbreviation for Hitech Development Health Plans.

_____ **12.** Under a PPO, healthcare providers perform services for plan members at discounted fees.

_____ **13.** The role of a PCP is to coordinate a patient's overall care.

_____ **14.** A healthcare provider is an individual, group, or organization that provides medical or other healthcare services.

_____ **15.** A referral to a specialist by a PCP is usually required under fee-for-service plans.

_____ **16.** HMOs are usually licensed by local city or town governments.

_____ **17.** A PPO is the same as an HMO.

_____ **18.** Fee-for-service plans typically have an annual deductible.

_____ **19.** The amount of freedom offered in different managed care programs (HMO, PPO, and EPO) is basically the same.

_____ **20.** If a patient goes to a network hospital for services, she can always assume all of the physicians are in network as well.

_____ **21.** If a patient needs to receive emergency care at a hospital, he should notify his insurance company within 1 week of admission.

_____ **22.** If a provider is listed in the MCO provider directory, it can be assumed she is participating in the network.

_____ **23.** Health Reimbursement Accounts (HRAs) are part of ACA's consumer-driven plans.

_____ **24.** PPO plans do not have an annual deductible.

_____ **25.** A group model HMO contracts with multi-specialty physicians' groups to provide physician services to an enrolled group.

Multiple Choice

Identify the letter of the choice that best completes the statement or answers the question.

_____ **1.** In the United States, rising medical costs are a result of:
   a. increased spending on drugs.
   b. increased use of alternative treatments.
   c. advances in technology.
   d. all of the above.

_____ **2.** Under a written insurance contract, the policyholder pays a premium and the insurance company provides:
   a. surgery.
   b. copayments.
   c. payment for medical services.
   d. preventive medical services.

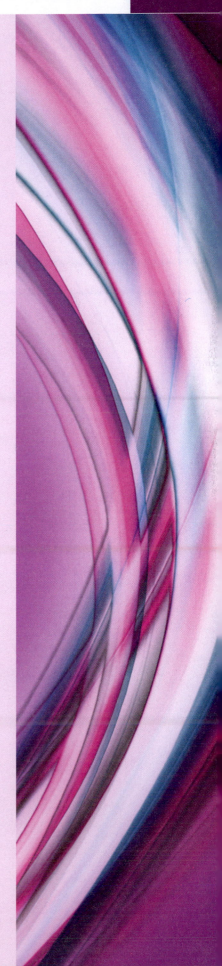

_____ **3.** An indemnity plan covers:
a. all medical services.
b. medically necessary services.
c. the episode of care.
d. all members' premiums.

_____ **4.** Which of the following conditions must be met before payment is made by the insurer?
a. Payment of premium, deductible, and coinsurance
b. Payment of the copayment
c. Payment of the premium and coinsurance
d. Payment of the deductible

_____ **5.** Under an indemnity plan a patient may use the services of:
a. only HMO network providers.
b. any provider.
c. any affiliated provider.
d. only out-of-network providers.

_____ **6.** Patients who enroll in an HMO may use the services of:
a. only HMO network providers.
b. only out-of-network providers.
c. any affiliated provider.
d. any provider.

_____ **7.** Patients who enroll in a point-of-service type of HMO may use the services of:
a. only HMO network providers.
b. only out-of-network providers.
c. any provider.
d. any affiliated provider.

_____ **8.** In a PPO plan, referrals to specialists are:
a. required.
b. more expensive.
c. not required.
d. none of the above.

_____ **9.** Four models of health maintenance organizations are:
a. staff, group, IPA, and POS.
b. staff, group, IPA, and PPO.
c. staff, group, IPA, and PCP.
d. staff, group, network, and IPA.

_____ **10.** In the staff HMO model, physicians are:
a. federal employees.
b. state employees.
c. independent contractors.
d. employees of the HMO.

_____ **11.** When a POS operation is elected under a health maintenance organization, the patient may:
a. choose providers only from the HMO's network.
b. choose providers who are not in the HMO's network.
c. choose any provider without additional expenses.
d. choose providers only from the IPA's network.

_____ **12.** Which of the following is required when an HMO patient is admitted to the hospital?

a. Referral
b. Preauthorization
c. Coinsurance
d. Utilization

_____ **13.** Health maintenance organizations are regulated:

a. only by federal law.
b. only by local law.
c. only by state law.
d. by both federal and state law.

Completion

Complete each statement.

1. Annual physical examinations and routine screening procedures are referred to as _____.

2. A policyholder's _____ includes the spouse and children.

3. _____ plans are regulated by the Employee Retirement Income Security Act (ERISA).

4. The _____ is the percentage of each claim that the insured must pay.

5. In managed care, patients often pay a specified amount called a(n) _____ for an office visit to a provider.

6. A member of an HMO must get a(n) _____ from the primary care physician before seeing a specialist.

7. The healthcare delivery system that is like an HMO but does not require the patient to get referrals from a PCP is a(n) _____.

8. The schedule of _____ lists the medical services that are covered by an insurance plan.

9. The physician who coordinates a patient's care in a health maintenance organization is called the _____.

Resources

Glossary of health management care terminology
https://www.cms.gov/apps/glossary/default.asp?Letter=A&Language=English

Managed Care Museum
www.managedcaremuseum.com

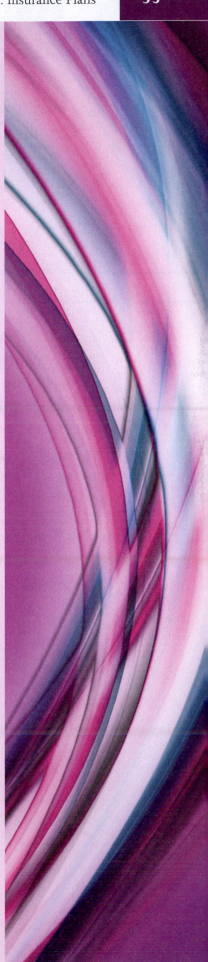

Chapter 3 | Understanding Managed Care: Medical Contracts and Ethics

Chapter Objectives

After reading this chapter, the student should be able to:

1. Understand the key elements of a managed care contract that dictates the provider's compensation for services.

2. Identify covered services for patients, which can include preventive medical services and types of office visits.

3. Recognize the obligation of a medical office specialist to uphold a standard of ethics.

4. Understand a concierge contract and an ACO contract.

5. Know definitions that are used in a managed care contract in order to understand the contract and discuss claims issues with the patient and carrier.

6. Discuss the Patient's Bill of Rights and the protections it reflects under the Affordable Care Act.

7. Conduct discussions with the patient regarding their accounts, copays, coinsurance, and deductibles.

Key Terms

accountable care organization (ACO)	National Committee for Quality Assurance (NCQA)	nonparticipating provider (non-PAR)
concierge medicine	network	participating provider (PAR)
		schedule of benefits

Case Study

**Understanding
Managed Care:
Medical
Contracts and
Ethics**

Evelyn has been going to Dr. Blake's Office for 15 years. On her most recent visit Dr. Blake requested that Shea, the front office manager, waive the copay. Shea informed Dr. Blake that it was not allowed. Dr. Blake was upset and stated that it was his office and that it was his choice if he wanted to waive a copay for a patient. Shea then allowed the patient to be seen without collecting a copay. Later the office manager came to Shea and informed her that per the doctor's contract with the insurance company, taking the copay is a requirement, and she requested that Shea call the patient and inform her of the situation.

Questions

1. Did Shea do the right thing in allowing the patient to be seen without collecting the copay?

2. Why is the physician not allowed to waive a copay for a patient?

3. What would be the best way for Shea to explain to the patient during the phone call that it is the patient's responsibility to pay the copay?

In order for a provider to be reimbursed for treatment of a patient who is a member of a managed care plan, that provider must sign a contract with the plan. The contract outlines what is expected of the provider, reimbursement amounts, time limits for submitting insurance claims, and other details. The medical office specialist may be asked to review a managed care organization (MCO) contract to determine if it would be a financially rewarding arrangement between the insurance carrier and the provider. Within a managed care contract, the medical office specialist may be required to refer to the contract to determine the compensation and billing guidelines and the covered medical expenses for the particular MCO, as discussed in this chapter. In working with patients and their insurance carriers, medical office specialists are entrusted with patients' personal information. This chapter discusses the standards of ethics that a medical office specialist is expected to uphold.

The introduction of the Affordable Care Act led to accountable care organizations (ACOs) being formed to manage care for Medicare patients. At the same time, many providers do what they always have done, caring for their patients and not participating in managed care contracts; this type of medicine is referred to as concierge medicine. The concierge physician does not participate in any plans, including Medicare and Medicaid. The medical office specialist must be aware of what is covered and not covered under a concierge contract and uphold the standards of ethics delineated in the Patient's Bill of Rights.

Purpose of a Contract

Many patients and providers are affected on a daily basis by the use of managed care. Will all of the services a physician provides be covered by the managed care contract? Will the reimbursement for services be adequate? Will the physician be able to provide the necessary services to the patients she will be treating?

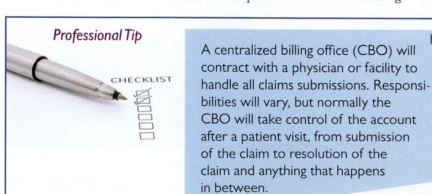

Professional Tip

CHECKLIST

A centralized billing office (CBO) will contract with a physician or facility to handle all claims submissions. Responsibilities will vary, but normally the CBO will take control of the account after a patient visit, from submission of the claim to resolution of the claim and anything that happens in between.

Contracts between the physician or a healthcare facility are generally negotiated by the physician(s) or upper management. The contract will affect all staff members. In certain facilities, especially in a medical central billing office, a medical office specialist may be responsible for posting payments received from the insurance carrier, appealing denials, or explaining nonpayment to the contracted physician.

A physician or facility may find it necessary to contract with outside services or hire additional personnel to ensure that all accounts receivable are received and paid to the fullest amount.

A Legal Agreement

A managed care contract is a legal agreement or document between a healthcare provider (physician, hospital, and clinic or outpatient center) and an insurer, health maintenance organization (HMO), or other network, whereby the provider agrees to discount the usual and customary charges in exchange for an increase in patient load. By contracting with a provider to deliver care to the policyholders (also called *members* and *enrollees*) of a managed care plan, the MCO develops a **network** for its members. The provider must contract with the managed care organization to be in the MCO's network.

MCOs contract with physicians, facilities, pharmacies, and laboratories to offer a full-service network of providers who have agreed to discount their fees for members of the managed care plan. These network providers have also agreed to use other providers in the network when the patient needs to be referred outside of their respective offices. This keeps costs down for the patient and insurance carrier, and it benefits the providers by bringing in more patients who are plan members. The provider who signs an MCO contract is classified as a **participating provider (PAR)**. When a patient is seen by a provider who is not under contract with the MCO, the provider is a **nonparticipating provider (non-PAR)**.

A concierge contract is another form of a legal agreement between the provider and the patient, under which the patient pays the provider an annual fee or retainer. The ACOs are a group of doctors, hospitals, pharmacies and other healthcare providers who voluntarily have an agreement specifically to improve delivery of care, improve health, and reduce growth in costs through improvement of care. When an ACO succeeds both in delivering high-quality care and in spending healthcare dollars more wisely, it will share in the savings it achieves for the program. The ACO shares the patient's information with their network of providers. The patient must give authorization for her medical information to be released. The medical office specialist should review these different types of ACO programs so that the information can be explained to the patient.

Compensation and Billing Guidelines for a MCO

A key element of any managed care contract is the provider's compensation for services. The contract and its related documents contain detailed requirements for claims submission and reimbursement requirements.

First, the contract should clearly state how and when the provider is to be paid. On reading the contract, the medical office specialist should clearly understand the administrative requirements of submitting claims and the timing of receiving payment. For example, the time period within which a provider must submit claims must be clearly stated on the contract. Second, the particular forms used to submit claims must be identified by name. Third, all arrangements with regard to the coordination of benefits and late payments must be carefully spelled out in the contract. Finally, because providers do not contract directly with the various payers and plans administered by the MCO, language must be added to the contract that requires the MCO to use its "best efforts" to ensure timely payments by these third-party payers and plans.

A managed care contract may offer different types of payment. Common types of payments include discounted fee-for-service, per diem, per case, percentage of premiums, and capitation arrangements. Any of these payment methods can be satisfactory, but each may pose problems as well. In today's managed care environment, the most common compensation options for licensed professionals are the discounted fee-for-service, per case charges, and capitation arrangements.

Under a discounted fee-for-service arrangement, covered services are compensated at a discount of the provider's usual and customary charges. The provider's discounted fee is negotiated by the provider and the payer. Providers are inclined to accept these discounts in return for the increased patient volume that results from an arrangement of this type with the payers. Under a per case or per visit charge arrangement, the payer compensates the provider at a predetermined rate for each episode of care provided. Because discounted fee-for-service and per case charges can arguably encourage a provider to increase the level of services provided, payers often implement strict rules or incentives to restrain any such resulting increases. Under a capitation arrangement, the provider, typically a primary care provider, is compensated for covered services based on a fixed prepaid monthly payment that is often referred to as a per-member-per-month (PMPM) amount. The PMPM amount will take into consideration the age and gender of the enrolled members. For example, the capitation rate for a member younger than 18 months of age may be $65 PMPM to reflect high utilization of services by newborns, then fall to $8 PMPM for members 2 to 18 years of age. Certain services that have a volatile usage, such as vaccinations or lab work, may be excluded from the capitation rate and paid under HMO fees. Unlike the discounted fee-for-service or per case payment methods, a capitation arrangement typically presents a heightened case management or "gatekeeper" obligation and an increased financial risk to the provider. Providers who treat patients covered by a capitation plan have an incentive to provide more preventive care, such as a mammogram, to prevent illnesses. Preventive care tends to keep patients healthy, which reduces the need to refer patients to a specialist. As a gatekeeper, the provider is expected to treat the patient as much as possible without referring to a specialist. Providers under a capitation plan receive incentives or bonuses by providing care for the patient and not referring the patient to a specialist. When the patient is referred to a specialist, the incentive or bonus may be reduced. With a capitation plan, the provider is already risking not covering his or her expenses, and by referring patients to a specialist the provider takes a greater financial risk. In reviewing any managed care contract, be alert for any provisions that allow the MCO to rebundle, or add to the covered services included in a single bundled fee, or to amend any terms of the compensation arrangement at will. To accommodate the provider's fiscal planning, all material terms of the agreement, particularly those having to do with compensation and payment, should only be modified at the time the contract is renewed, or with the prior express consent of both parties to the contract.

Managed care contracts often prohibit, or otherwise limit, the provider from seeking payment directly from members of the MCO and related plans. The medical office specialist should be aware of the applicable rules that control when, how, and under what circumstances the provider may seek particular payments from either members or the MCO when the provider is not otherwise reimbursed for services rendered. Complete Practice Exercise 3.1 to test your knowledge.

Covered Medical Expenses

All managed care contracts should contain a section that lists all services that are considered "covered" services for patients. The list of medical services covered under the insured's policy is called the **schedule of benefits**. This schedule includes preventive medical services and lists types of office visits. If a plan is capitated, this section should discuss which office procedures are covered in the capitated plan and which are not. This

In the compensation and billing section of an MCO contract, what three things will pertain to the job responsibilities of a medical office specialist?

1. _____

2. _____

3. _____

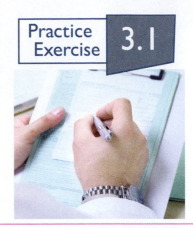

will allow the medical office specialist to determine which of the provided services should be billed to the insurer and which to the patient. This list should include the procedure code (CPT®) and the rate for each service.[1]

The type of plan that is being contracted for is also listed in this section. If it is a preferred provider organization (PPO), HMO, or exclusive provider organization (EPO), this section should list the prospective plan's guidelines.

Payment

With a fee-for-service plan, the medical office specialist should check the time limit for submitting claims. This is usually a 3- to 6-month period. The standard is 90 days. What billing requirements must be met to allow for processing and payment of claims? Does the MCO provide ongoing staff training as billing requirements change? Does the contract provide for payment to physicians within a specified period? What penalty or interest charge will be paid to the practice if payment is delayed? When are late charges paid to the practice? Some providers negotiate for language in the contract that specifies that the MCO will reimburse the practice at its usual and customary fee—not at the discounted fee-for-service rate stipulated in the contract—if payment is not made in the specified period. Also, if a plan is truly a capitated plan, does it pay at the beginning of the month? Many MCOs pay on the 15th or 30th of the month and can thus hinder a practice's cash flow. When a plan has problems paying providers on a timely basis, this may indicate inefficient claims processing, insufficient enrollees, or a lack of the required start-up funds.

Who handles the coordination of benefits? The ability to request payment from another insurer for the amount due should be specifically delegated through the managed care contract. Can the fee schedule be changed without prior notice or agreement by the practice? Are periodic reviews of charges and changes made in the fee schedule? On what are the changes based? An increasing number of managed care plans are looking at a resource-based relative value scale (RBRVS), using the Medicare RBRVS with a different conversion factor. A medical office specialist should beware of language stipulating that a fee schedule can be derived using other value scales that are generally accepted in the community.

---

[1]CPT® is a registered trademark of the American Medical Association.

Ethics in Managed Care

The healthcare reform debate in 1992–1993 during President Bill Clinton's administration demonstrated the inevitability of fundamental changes in the financing and delivery of healthcare. The demise of the Clinton proposals, which advocated a strong role for government, left the field of healthcare reform wide open to the private sector. Insurance companies and other healthcare corporations responded rapidly and aggressively, developing and marketing new models of healthcare delivery. The evolution of these models, collectively referred to as *managed care*, has changed the American healthcare system.

As transformation of this industry continues, corporate business values, such as efficiency, cost reduction, inventory management, competition, and profit, are influencing the traditional medical ethics and values of the solo practitioner: the one-on-one doctor–patient relationship and fee-for-service payment. The shift in values and structure of the healthcare system is inherently neither bad nor good. In fact, in a system where demand seems infinite and resources are finite, such shifts are both necessary and desirable.

The healthcare system can no longer accommodate unlimited demand for medical services. In 2016, the trilliondollar healthcare industry continued to experience extraordinary change spurred by the Affordable Care Act (ACA), the growth of large health systems, technological advances, and an emphasis on quality and outcomes.

Healthcare providers can no longer pretend to offer the maximum benefits of technology to all comers. It is time to accept that cost matters as much as access and quality. Managed care organizations of various sizes and types have brought the principles and values of business into the front ranks of healthcare delivery. The MCOs are trying to reduce costs by standardizing, regulating, and streamlining the supply side (providers) and by reducing demand and controlling access on the buyer's side (patients).

Medicine and business have always been somewhat uneasy partners. Most physicians have also been, to one degree or another, businesspersons who were well paid for their professional services. Now, however, business, health, and government are intertwined in new ways. Instead of the business aspects being controlled by physicians, now managers, accountants, and actuaries often control the business aspects. The values and ethical principles of business and medicine have evolved largely separately and distinctly from each other. Now that the lines of distinction are blurring, conflicts are inevitable.

Changes in Healthcare Delivery

The commingling of business and medical values is changing the types of services offered and the way in which they are delivered. The Patient Protection and Affordable Care Act, often referred to as the Affordable Care Act or Obamacare, represents the most significant overhaul of the U.S. healthcare system since the passage of Medicare and Medicaid in 1965. This act is changing the very roots of the system, including the fundamental relationships among patient, employer, provider, and third-party payer, and even the motivation for providing (or not providing) a particular service.

In many cases, the vendor of healthcare is no longer a private physician or group of providers but, rather, a large, usually for-profit corporation. In a system based on managed care, the patient's choice of provider usually is much more limited than under a traditional fee-for-service structure. In fee-for-service systems, patients could choose nearly any provider or self-refer to specialists if they wished. Now many coverage arrangements are negotiated between employers or unions and MCOs. Physicians are now becoming employees of the hospitals and MCOs. Patients must choose from a list of providers who have contracted with the new vendor (MCO) and agreed to a predetermined payment rate. In most managed care plans, if a patient needs to see a specialist, she must be referred by the primary care provider or the visit is not covered by the plan.

On March 23, 2010, President Barack Obama signed the Patient Protection and Affordable Care Act (ACA). Along with the Health Care and Education Reconciliation Act of 2010, the law put in place comprehensive health insurance reforms. The law makes preventive care—including family planning and related care—more accessible and affordable for many Americans. Employees were mandated to furnish healthcare to their employees or be fined. The Affordable Care Act required all U.S. insurance plans to cover varieties of FDA-approved contraceptives at no cost to patients. A number of organizations objected, saying that some of the approved forms of contraception are equivalent of abortifacients, or drugs that cause abortion. If they refused to provide the coverage, they would face heavy fines. The government set about making exceptions. Explicitly religious organizations, churches, and synagogues are exempt from this requirement. The Supreme Court decided in the Hobby Lobby case, regarding a for-profit business with a religious objection, that a form could be completed and submitted to the government, which then prompts a third-party organization to provide the coverage instead. The Affordable Care Act is evolving and could possibly see changes over the next several years.

Another example of a Supreme Court ruling involved the Little Sisters of the Poor, a religious institution that won a decision in 2016 which allowed them not to participate in family planning. The Supreme Court unanimously overturned the lower court rulings against the Little Sisters, ordered the government not to fine the Little Sisters, and said the lower courts should provide the government an opportunity "to arrive at an approach going forward that accommodates the petitioner's religious beliefs."

The ACA relies heavily on **accountable care organizations (ACOs)**. They were formed to provide comprehensive, coordinated, and seamless, high-quality medical care to patients. This is known as evidence-based medicine and is also cost effective. These organizations are expected to provide patients with immunizations, nutritional education, medications, and everything that guidelines from evidence-based medicine recommend for optimal patient care for disease prevention and chronic condition management. The key component is that the ACO receives a lump sum payment, from either a government insurance plan like Medicare or a commercial insurer, to divide among the various parties caring for the patient including primary care physician, specialty physician, radiology, durable medical equipment suppliers, pharmacists, the hospital, etc. If the ACO provides quality care based on metrics set by the government or insurance company and saves money on the estimated average cost for the patient's condition, the accountable care organization receives a bonus to distribute to various providers of service, including the physicians. Physicians no longer receive a fee for each service they perform, but are given some sort of basic payment per patient similar to HMO capitation or managed care. To form ACOs, hospitals have ventured into the practice of employing doctors. This has led to a loss of professionalism in medicine (unintentional). Doctors now are employees just like any other employee of the hospital, resulting in the physician's loss of control of their own office and in the physician's general dissatisfaction with all parties. Primary physicians have reacted by not going to the hospital to see their patients. The hospital employs physicians known as hospitalists to admit and care for patients during their stay, which has led to very fractionated care. Patients may see a doctor or nurse practitioner (NP) in the office, a doctor or NP in the ER, a hospitalist or hospitalist NP in the hospital, and then eventually return to their primary care doctor. During this process vital information is lost in all the handoffs, leading to patient dissatisfaction. Concierge medicine bridges this gap by doing what physicians have done for hundreds of years—caring for their patients and not participating in managed care.

MCO and Provider Credentialing

To ensure that providers are adhering to the MCO's ethics in providing patient care, the managed care organization evaluates the provider through a credentialing process designed to check the provider's medical credentials, service fees, and workplace environment. The **National Committee for Quality Assurance (NCQA)**, which is an accrediting agency for MCOs, requires that an MCO plan being reviewed for accreditation must demonstrate that it has a thorough credentialing process for its providers. The MCO's provider credentialing process must examine each physician's background for evidence of fraud, criminal activity, disciplinary actions, and malpractice history.

Although this is an admirable standard, not all managed care plans are accredited, nor have they all asked to be accredited, so not all provider credentialing processes are as good as they could be. If an MCO examines a doctor's background, it may still elect to contract with a doctor with a questionable record. Sometimes this is the only doctor in the area with a specialty that the managed care plan needs to include in its network in order to be competitive.

Also, the MCO's credentialing process does not guarantee that a doctor who is a member of an MCO is better than one who is not. Despite what the managed care plan learns about physicians during the credentialing process, the plan provides limited information to consumers about the qualifications of doctors in contracts. The amount of physician information provided to consumers varies from plan to plan.

After the provider credentialing process, the managed care organization will decide whether or not to extend an invitation, or contract, to the provider. The written contract states, among many other things, that the provider will provide medically appropriate care at a discounted rate for plan enrollees. Providers who sign these contracts are considered part of a network.

Medical management components are being focused on and the services that are being provided are being looked at more carefully today than they have been during the past decade. The physicians are often required to keep a log of when the patient arrived, when the patient was seen for the visit, and when the patient departed. MCOs want their policyholders to be satisfied with the care they are receiving from the physicians within the network but also are in the business to be financially successful. To ensure this, MCOs are grading these physicians on the services that they render to their patients.

Ethics of the Medical Office Specialist

Ethics are the rules or standards governing conduct of a person or the members of a profession. A medical office specialist has an obligation to uphold a standard of ethics. With the medical office specialist working as a liaison between the provider and patient, and between the provider and carrier, it is difficult at times to determine where the specialist's loyalty lies. As long as the medical office specialist follows the MCO contractual guidelines and is knowledgeable about the Patient's Bill of Rights (discussed later in this chapter), no ethics conflicts should arise.

Occasions have arisen when a medical office specialist has been asked to perform job assignments that do not follow legal guidelines. A medical office specialist can and will be held liable for fraudulent billing. Historically, all legal burdens fell on

Professional Tip

CHECKLIST

A medical office specialist should always document, sign, and date all conversations regarding any patient's account whether the conversation is with the provider, patient, or carrier.

the provider, but today the medical office specialist can be prosecuted. Consider these examples of fraudulent billing in Figure 3.1:

As noted in the news stories in Figure 3.1, those who break the law and steal money from these government programs will be prosecuted. If a medical office specialist is asked to conduct any services that are fraudulent, he is legally and morally obligated to say no. If it is mandatory as a condition of employment, then it is time to find another job and report the request of criminal activity to the proper authorities.

Figure 3.1

Former Owner and Operator of New York Health Clinics Sentenced for $30 Million Medicare Fraud Scheme.

On August 25, 2015, in Manhattan, NY, Oscar Huachillo was sentenced to 87 months in prison, three years of supervised release and ordered to pay $3,454,244 in restitution and $31,177,987 in forfeiture, including forfeiture of approximately $14 million of assets that were seized at or around the time of Huachillo's arrest in August 2013. Huachillo previously pleaded guilty to orchestrating a scheme to defraud Medicare out of $31 million and evading more than $3.4 million in federal income taxes by falsely underreporting his income. Huachillo set up and operated multiple healthcare clinics in NYC that purported to provide injection and infusion treatments to Medicare-eligible HIV/AIDS patients but that were, in reality, healthcare fraud mills that routinely billed Medicare for medications that were never provided or were provided at highly diluted doses, and often unnecessary because the person being "treated" did not medically need the treatments. In addition, Huachillo willfully evaded over $3.4 million in taxes owed to the IRS during the tax years 2009 through 2011 by falsely underreporting his taxable income, including income he had obtained through fraudulent Medicare claims.

Thursday, May 12, 2016

Florida Woman Sentenced for Health Care Fraud

Jenifer Engorn to Serve Two Years' Probation, Repay More than $8,000

ROANOKE, VIRGINIA – A Florida woman, who billed Medicaid for services she did not provide while living and working in the New River Valley, was sentenced today in the United States District Court for the Western District of Virginia in Roanoke on healthcare fraud charges, United States Attorney John P. Fishwick Jr. and Virginia Attorney General Mark R. Herring announced today.

Jennifer Ashlee Zenitz Engorn, 28, of Miami, Florida, who previously pled guilty to one count of healthcare fraud, was sentenced today to two years of probation, a fine of $1,100 and a $100 special assessment. Engorn was also ordered to pay $8,352 in restitution to the Department of Medical Assistance Services.

"Healthcare fraud cannot and will not be tolerated," United States Attorney John P. Fishwick Jr. said today. "Our diminishing health care dollars must be used wisely and legally. Those who break the law and steal money from these important programs will be held accountable. We are proud to work with the professional investigators in the Medicaid Fraud Control Unit to protect these important programs."

According to evidence presented at previous hearings by Assistant United States Attorney Jennie L.M. Waering, Engorn was employed to provide mental health skill building services to low income patients served by Medicaid. However, Engorn did not provide these services and provided false documentation to her employer causing the billing of Medicaid for the services that were not rendered.

Contract Definitions

The following definitions are used in MCO contracts. A medical office specialist should be familiar with these terms in order to review contracts and discuss claims issues with patients and carriers.

- *Benefit plan:* The contract issued by a payer, the plan document, or any other legally enforceable instrument under which a covered person may be entitled to covered services and which is in force with respect to such covered person.
- *Contracted services:* Those covered services provided by a physician that are consistent with the physician's training, licensure, and scope of practice.
- *Coordination of benefits (COB):* The determination of which of two or more health benefit plans will provide health benefits for a covered person as primary or secondary payers.
- *Copayment:* The charge, as determined by the benefit plan, a covered person is required to pay at the time covered services are provided.
- *Covered person:* An individual who is an insured, enrolled participant or enrolled dependent under a benefit plan.
- *Covered services:* Those healthcare services provided to covered persons under the terms of the benefit plan.
- *Emergency services:* Those services provided after the sudden onset of a medical condition manifesting itself by acute symptoms of sufficient severity, including severe pain, such that the absence of immediate medical attention reasonably could be expected to result in:
  - placing the covered person's health in serious jeopardy;
  - serious impairment to bodily functions; or
  - serious dysfunction of any bodily organ or part.
- *Fee maximum:* The maximum allowable fee payable by the corporation or payer for the provision of a given contracted service by a physician to a covered person; such fee is determined by the corporation in accordance with corporation policies and procedures.
- *Medical director:* The physician specified by the corporation as its medical director.
- *Medically necessary:* Refers to the use of services or supplies, or both, as determined by the corporation's medical director, or his designee, that:
  - are accepted by the healthcare profession as appropriate and effective for the condition being treated;
  - are based on recognized standards of the healthcare specialty involved;
  - are not experimental, investigative, or unproven;
  - are not solely for the convenience of a covered person or a healthcare provider; and
  - do not involve the use of greater resources than are required for adequate medical care.

Benefit plans may use the term *medically efficient* and other terms rather than, or in addition to, the term *medically necessary*.

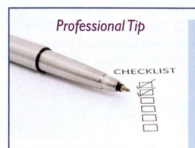

Professional Tip

CHECKLIST

The medical office specialist should always keep in mind when discussing claims issues with a patient that the patient may not be familiar with these terms, so layperson's terms may be needed.

- *Participating hospital:* A state-licensed hospital that has been designated by the corporation as a hospital to which a participating provider may authorize the admission of covered persons for covered services, provided, however, that covered persons may be admitted to any appropriate hospital for the provision of emergency services.
- *Participating provider:* A licensed healthcare professional, including the physician, a facility, or an entity that has entered into a participation agreement to provide covered services to covered persons.
- *Payer:* An insurance company, third-party administrator, or self-insured health benefit plan that is contractually obligated to indemnify or make payment on behalf of covered persons with respect to covered services and that has contracted directly or indirectly with the corporation to arrange for the provision of covered services to covered person.
- *urgent care:* A category of walk-in clinic focused on the delivery of ambulatory care in a dedicated medical facility outside of a traditional emergency room. Urgent care centers primarily treat injuries or illnesses requiring immediate care, but not serious enough to require an ER visit.

Compensation for Services

Each MCO contract has a section that addresses the compensation of the provider for services rendered to the patient. Figure 3.2 is based on an actual managed care contract. The compensation section is one that a medical office specialist will need to be familiar with for future reference.

The concierge contract between the patient and the provider is a cash only contract. The provider does not participate in any MCOs, ACOs, or Medicare. The patient cannot submit the services for their reimbursement. If the patient needs hospitalization, laboratory services, surgery, and so on, the patient's insurance is submitted. The medical office specialist needs to be able to explain this to the patient before a contract is signed.

Patient's Bill of Rights

Along with MCO contracts between the managed care plan and the provider, patients are provided with protection and should be made aware of their rights. The concierge contract is between the provider and the patient, but all providers and managed care organizations ethically must abide by the Patient's Bill of Rights. Many health plans have adopted the principles outlined in Figure 3.3.

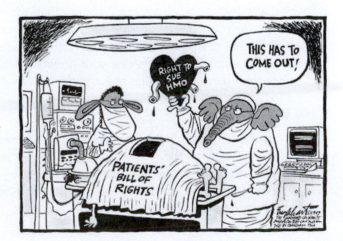

Reprinted by permission of Bob Englehart.

Billing

With respect to all Contracted Services provided by Physician to Covered Person pursuant to this Agreement, Physician shall bill Corporation or Payer, as applicable, on a form mutually agreed to, at Physician's usual and customary rate that is charged by Physician without regard to whether a particular person has health plan benefits. Billing information provided by Physician shall include Covered Person identification information and an itemization of all services and charges provided as Contracted Services hereunder.

COB Recoveries

After Physician has billed Corporation or Payer as Provided in Section IV(A) of this Agreement and has collected applicable copayments, coinsurance, and deductibles. Physician shall seek recovery from Payers having primary payment responsibility according to the COB rules of the applicable Benefit Plan. In the event that Corporation or Payer is not the initial Payer, Corporation or Payer shall pay in accordance with Section IV(D) of this Agreement and will take as credits against such payment amounts any payment Physician has received from the initial Payer(s). In the event Physician subsequently receives any payment from initial Payer(s) after Corporation or Payer has paid for such services, Physician shall promptly pay to Corporation or Payer the amount of the overpayment.

Third-Party Liability Recoveries and Subrogation

As applicable, Physician, Corporation, or Payer shall also seek payment from applicable third-party Payers who have payment responsibility other than as health benefit plan Payers. Except that Physician agrees to allow Corporation or Payer to acquire and exercise full and exclusive rights of subrogation whenever a third party, other than health benefit plan Payer, is liable for payment for services that are provided by Physician for which Corporation or Payer would otherwise be responsible hereunder.

Payment

In connection with Contracted Services provided by Physician hereunder, Corporation or Payer shall pay to Physician an amount equal to the lesser of Physician's usual and customary charge or the Fee maximum, less all coinsurance, copayments, deductibles, and recoveries described above. Payment shall be remitted to Physician generally within thirty (30) days of the later of (1) receipt of a fully completed, uncontested claim submitted in accordance with the billing procedures of Corporation, or (2) the resolution of all applicable recovery issues. Any portion of such payment that is not remitted to Physician within such period shall be subject to an interest penalty at the rate of eighteen percent (18%) per annum, with interest accruing from the first calendar day following the end of such period, and with such penalty being payable by Corporation or Payer, as applicable, to Physician. Corporation or Payer shall not make payment in an amount that, when added to the coinsurance, copayments, deductibles, and recoveries described in this Section, exceeds the amount payable under this Agreement. Corporation or Payer shall not be required to make payment under this Agreement pursuant to billings received later than ninety (90) days from the date Contracted Services were provided unless Physician notifies Corporation within such period that a claim for such services has been presented to another Payer for payment.

No Balance Bill

The combination of applicable copayments, deductibles, coinsurance, third-party recoveries described in this section, and amounts payable hereunder shall constitute payment in full for Contracted Services. Physician may not balance bill or impose any surcharge upon the Covered Person or individuals responsible for their care. Nor shall Physician seek payment from Covered Persons or such individuals for later billings denied by Corporation or Payer in accordance with paragraph D of this Section IV.

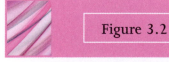

Figure 3.2   Sample Contents Based on a Managed Care Contract's Compensation Section.

Limitations Regarding Payment

To the extent that Corporation compensates Physician's services through payment to a participating Hospital for the professional component of hospital-based Physician services, Physician shall seek payment for such services solely from the Participating Hospital and shall not bill Corporation, Payer, or a Covered Person for such services.

Hold Harmless Provision for Utilization Review Decision

With respect to compensation for Contracted Services provided by Physician hereunder, Physician agrees that in no event shall Physician bill, charge, seek compensation, remuneration, or reimbursement from, or have any recourse against a Covered Person, persons, or entities other than Corporation or Payer for any benefit penalties that have been applied to such compensation subsequent to utilization review decisions over which such Covered Person has no control, provided that such covered Person has fulfilled the notification responsibilities for contacting the applicable utilization review entity as such responsibilities are set forth in the Benefit Plan. Except that, this Section shall not apply with respect to Contracted Services provided hereunder if such benefit penalties apply according to the terms of a Benefit Plan of a self-insured Payer.

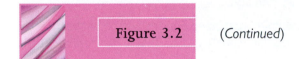

Figure 3.2   (*Continued*)

Six months after President Obama signed the Affordable Care Act into law, critical consumer protections—a "Patient's Bill of Rights"—took effect. The Patient's Bill of Rights put an end to some of the worst insurance abuses and puts consumers, not insurance companies, in control of their healthcare.

THESE NEW PROTECTIONS INCLUDE:

Ban on Discriminating against Patients with Pre-Existing Conditions. No one seeking coverage can be discriminated against, that is, denied coverage, because of a pre-existing condition.

Ban on Insurance Companies Dropping Coverage. A patient cannot be dropped from coverage due to an unintentional mistake on their application.

Ban on Insurance Companies Limiting Coverage. Insurance companies can no longer put a lifetime limit on the amount of coverage.

Ban on Insurance Companies Limiting Choice of Doctors. Before reform, insurance companies could decide which doctor you could go to. With the Patient's Bill of Rights, patients purchasing or joining a new plan the have the right to choose their own doctor in the insurer network.

Ban on Insurance Companies Restricting Emergency Room Care. Before reform, insurance companies could limit which emergency room the patient went to or charge more if the patient went out of network. Under the Patient's Bill of Rights, if the patient purchases or joins a new plan, those plans are banned from charging more for emergency services obtained out of network.

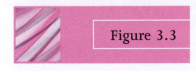

Figure 3.3   Patient's Bill of Rights.

Guarantee of the Right of Appeal. The patient has the right to appeal an insurance company decision to an independent third party.

Covering Young Adults under Their Parents' Plan. Young adults are now covered under their parents' plan until they reach their 26th birthday unless they are offered coverage at work.

Covering Preventive Care with No Cost. Services like mammograms, colonoscopies, immunizations, prenatal and new baby care will be covered and insurance companies will be prohibited from charging deductibles, copayments or coinsurance.

Information Disclosure. You have the right to accurate and easily understood information about your health plan, healthcare professionals, and healthcare facilities. If you speak another language, have a physical or mental disability, or just don't understand something, assistance will be provided so you can make informed healthcare decisions.

Choice of Providers and Plans. You have the right to a choice of healthcare providers that is sufficient to provide you with access to appropriate, high-quality healthcare.

Access to Emergency Services. If you have severe pain, an injury, or sudden illness that convinces you that your health is in serious jeopardy, you have the right to receive screening and stabilization emergency services whenever and wherever needed, without prior authorization or financial penalty.

Participation in Treatment Decisions. You have the right to know your treatment options and to participate in decisions about your care. Parents, guardians, family members, or other individuals you designate can represent you if you cannot make your own decisions.

Respect and Nondiscrimination. You have a right to considerate, respectful, and nondiscriminatory care from your doctors, health plan representatives, and other healthcare providers.

Confidentiality of Health Information. You have the right to talk in confidence with healthcare providers and to have your healthcare information protected. You also have the right to review and copy your own medical record and request that your physician change your record if it is not accurate, relevant, or complete.

Complaints and Appeals. You have the right to a fair, fast, and objective review of any complaint you have against your health plan, doctors, hospitals, or other healthcare personnel. This includes complaints about waiting times, operating hours, the conduct of healthcare personnel, and the adequacy of healthcare facilities.

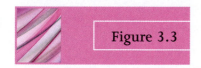

Figure 3.3   (*Continued*)

Concierge Contract

Concierge medicine is a small, personalized medical practice that takes care of a limited number of patients. This allows each patient to receive the time they need with the physician. Urgent visits are seen the same or next day. It also offers home visits and follows its patients at hospitals, nursing homes, and assisted living establishments. The patient has access to direct communication with the provider. The patient does not file insurance and the provider is non-participating. There are no deductibles, coinsurance, or copays since the physician is non-participating. The annual fee for this service is agreed upon with the patient and the provider. See Figure 3.4 for an example of a concierge contract and Figure 3.5 for an example of a list of fees for a pulmonary specialist. Figure 3.6 shows an example of an ACO contract.

This is a private contract between Dr._____ and _____ for the provision of providing the practice of medicine and payments for such services.

This Contract Agreement (the Agreement) specifies the terms and conditions under which the undersigned patient (the Patient and/or your Legal Representative) may participate in the practice of medicine offered by XYZ (the Practice).

For Medicare Beneficiaries:

1. The Patient is a Medicare beneficiary seeking services covered under Medicare.
2. Please note that the Medical Providers in XYZ have Opted-Out of Medicare on September 1, 2016 for a minimum of two (2) years.
3. Opted-Out of Medicare means the Medical Providers no longer participate in Medicare programs and that the Patient and/or the Legal Representative accepts full responsibility for payment of the provider's charge for all services furnished by the Medical Provider.
4. Please understand that Medicare limits do not apply to what the Medical Providers may charge for items or services furnished by the Medical Providers.
5. The Patient and/or their Legal Representative agree(s) not to submit a claim to Medicare or to ask the Medical Providers or the Practice to submit a claim to Medicare.
6. Medicare payment will not be made for any items or services furnished by these Medical Providers or this Practice that would have otherwise been covered by Medicare if there was no private contract and a proper Medicare claim had been submitted.
7. The Patient has the right to obtain Medicare covered items and services from providers who have not opted out of Medicare; and the Patient and/or the Legal Representative is not compelled to enter into private contracts that apply to other Medicare-covered services furnished by other providers who have not opted out of Medicare.
8. The Patient and/or the Legal Representative understand(s) that Medigap plans do not, and that other supplemental plans may elect not to, make payments for items and services not paid for by Medicare.
9. The Patient and/or the Legal Representative understand(s) that this contract cannot be entered into during a time when the Patient required emergency or urgent care services.

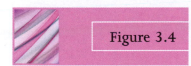

Figure 3.4   Example of a Concierge Contract.

$500.00 FIRST OFFICE VISIT (NEW PATIENT INITIAL CONSULT)

Patient initials_____

Services offered at time of office visit:

• Pulmonary care and sleep medicine
• Complete history and physical
• Medication review
• Test results review
• Medical opinion and treatment recommendations
• Presurgical pulmonary risk stratification

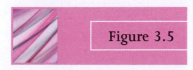

Figure 3.5   Example of a List of services and Fee Schedule for a Pulmonary Specialist.

- New medicine prescribed, if needed
- Medication refills, if needed

$1500 Annual Fee UNLIMITED OFFICE VISITS Patient Initials_____

First office visit fee is waived or, if already paid, used to offset this annual fee.

Services Offered:

- Pulmonary medicine, critical care, and sleep medicine
- Complete or interim history and physical exam
- Medication review
- Test results review
- Medical opinion and treatment recommendations
- Presurgical pulmonary risk stratification
- New medicine prescribed, if needed
- Medication refills, if needed
- Telephone medicine

$3000.00 Annual Fee UNLIMITED HOSPITAL AND OFFICE VISITS

Patient Initial_____

First office visit fee is waived or, if already paid, used to offset this annual fee.

Services Offered:

- Pulmonary medicine, critical care, and sleep medicine
- Complete or interim history and physical exam
- Medication review
- Test results review
- Medical opinion and treatment recommendations
- Presurgical pulmonary risk stratification
- New medicine prescribed, if needed
- Medication refills, if needed
- Telephone medicine

Annual Fee is for a 12-month period. The annual fee is due when the Agreement is signed by the Patient and all subsequent year's fees are due on the anniversary of the Agreement. Arrangements can be made for monthly payments.

Renewals and Termination

The Annual fee covers a period of one (1) year. The annual fee is due when the Agreement is signed. The practice is permitted to terminate this Agreement for any reason within thirty (30) days with prior written notice, in which case the Patient is entitled to a prorated refund of the Annual Fee. The patient is permitted to terminate this Agreement for any reason within thirty (30) days with prior written notice, in which case the Patient is entitled to a prorated refund of the Annual Fee.

Email Communication

Patient and or the Legal Representative understand that email communication may not be a secure medium for personal health information exchange.

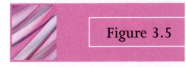

Figure 3.5   (Continued)

NOTICE TO PATIENTS:

_____is Participating in a Medicare Shared Savings Program Accountable Care Organization

Accountable Care Organizations (ACOs): Providing Better, Coordinated Care for You.

We are participating in Quality Health Alliance-ACO, LLC, a Medicare Shared Savings Program ACO. An ACO is a group of doctors, hospitals, and/or other healthcare providers working together with Medicare to give you better, more coordinated service and healthcare. Think of an ACO as a team made up of your doctors and other health-care providers. We are working together to share important information and resources about your individual needs and preferences.

Doctors and hospitals in an ACO communicate with you and with each other to make sure that you get the care you need when you're sick, and the support you need to stay healthy.

You can still choose any doctor or hospital.

Your Medicare benefits aren't changing.

ACOs are not a Medicare Advantage plan, an HMO plan, or an insurance plan of any kind. You still have the right to use any doctor or hospital that accepts Medicare, at any time. Your doctor may recommend that you see particular doctors or healthcare providers, but it's always your choice about what doctors and providers you use or hospitals you visit.

Having Your Health Information Gives Us a More Complete Picture of Your Health

To help Quality Health Alliance-ACO, LLC give you better, coordinated care, Medicare will share information with us about your care. The information will include things like dates and times you visited a doctor or hospital, your medical conditions, and a list of past and current prescriptions.

This information from other healthcare providers will give me and other healthcare providers in the ACO a more complete and up-to-date picture of your health.

If you choose to let Medicare share your healthcare information with Quality Health Alliance-ACO, LLC, it may also be shared with other ACOs in which your other doctors or healthcare providers participate. If you don't want your healthcare information shared, you can ask Medicare not to share it.

Your Privacy is Very Important to Us

Just like Medicare, ACOs must put important safeguards in place to make sure all your healthcare information is safe. ACOs respect your choice on the use of your healthcare information for care coordination and quality improvement.

Yes, share my information. If you want Medicare to share your information about care you have received from us and with other ACOs in which any of your doctors or other healthcare providers participate, **then there's nothing more you need to do.**

No, please do not share my information. If you don't want Medicare to share information with Quality Health Alliance-ACO, LLC or any other ACOs for care coordination and quality improvement purposes, you **must** do the following:

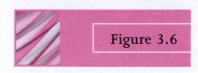

Figure 3.6   Example of an ACO Program.

- Call 1-800-MEDICARE (1-800-633-4227). Tell the representative you are calling about ACOs and you do not want Medicare to share your information with ACOs TYY users should use 1-877-486-2048.
- If you change your mind in the future, call 1-800-MEDICARE and tell the representative what you have decided. We can't communicate with Medicare on your behalf.

Even if you decline to share your health information, Medicare will still use your information for some purposes including certain financial calculations and determining the quality of care given by your healthcare providers participating in ACOs. Also, Medicare may share some of your healthcare information with ACOs when measuring the quality of care given by healthcare providers participating in ACOs.

Any Questions: any questions or concerns, call us at 800-000-0000 or contact Medicare at 1-800-MEDICARE or visit https://www.medicare.gov/manage-your-health/coordinating-your-care/accountable-care-organizations.html.

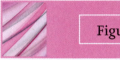

Figure 3.6   (*Continued*)

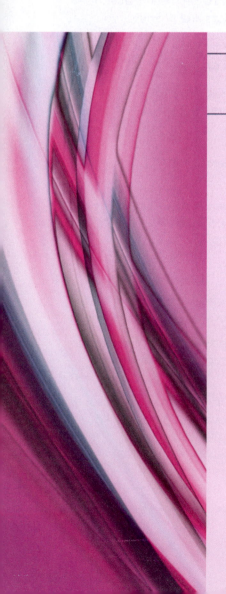

Chapter Summary

- The medical office specialist should be familiar with the billing guidelines in a contract. The contract should list all covered services and state when the provider will be paid.
- A managed care contract is a legal agreement between a healthcare provider (physician, hospital, and clinic or outpatient center) and an insurer, HMO, or other network.
- Managed care contracts often prohibit, or otherwise limit, the provider from seeking payment directly from members of the MCO and related plans.
- Managed care is undoubtedly changing how healthcare providers work. In many areas, managed care is creating fierce competition among healthcare providers for managed care plan contracts and in other areas providers are choosing not to participate with these plans.
- An ACO is a group of doctors, hospitals and other healthcare providers participating in a Medicare Shared Savings Program Accountable Care Organization.
- The medical office specialist must be able to explain the ACO to the patient before obtaining a signature.
- A concierge contract is a cash only agreement between the physician and patient. No insurance is submitted.
- A medical office specialist has the responsibility to decline if requested to act unethically.
- The patient has a bill of rights that protects his or her right to accurate and easily understood information about his or her health plan, healthcare professionals, and healthcare facilities.
- A medical office specialist should be familiar with managed care terms in order to review contracts and discuss claim issues with patients and carriers.

Chapter Review

True/False

Identify the statement as true (T) or false (F).

_____ 1. A capitated payment is prepaid to a provider to cover a plan member's health services for a specified period.

_____ 2. It is mandatory for all managed care organizations to be accredited.

_____ 3. The amount that an insured person must pay for each office visit is called the copayment.

_____ 4. Credentialing refers to the process of verifying that providers and workplaces meet certain professional standards.

_____ 5. Under a discounted fee-for-service arrangement, a provider and a payer negotiate the provider's fees.

_____ 6. Ethics are standards of behavior for licensed medical staff and other employees of medical practices.

_____ 7. Medical professional etiquette includes the respectful and courteous treatment of patients.

_____ 8. Coincerge medicine is a managed care plan.

_____ 9. A key element of any managed care contract is the provider's compensation for services.

_____ 10. A licensed healthcare professional who enters into a participation agreement with an MCO is called a nonparticipating provider.

Multiple Choice

Identify the letter of the choice that best completes the statement or answers the question.

_____ 1. Under a written insurance contract, the participating provider agrees to provide covered services to covered persons and the insurance carrier provides:
   a. payments for medical services.   c. surgery.
   b. preventive medical services.   d. copayments.

_____ 2. Payment on a capitated plan is:
   a. paid after claim is received by the carrier.
   b. paid by the patient.
   c. a retroactive payment.
   d. prepaid.

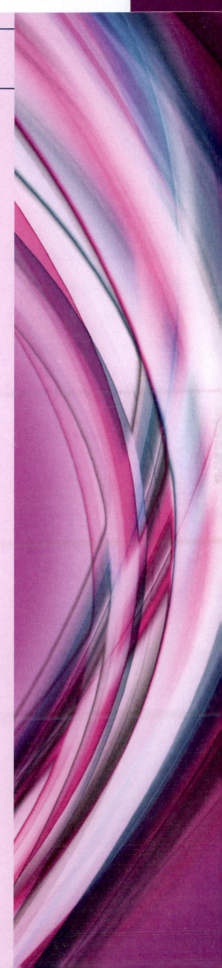

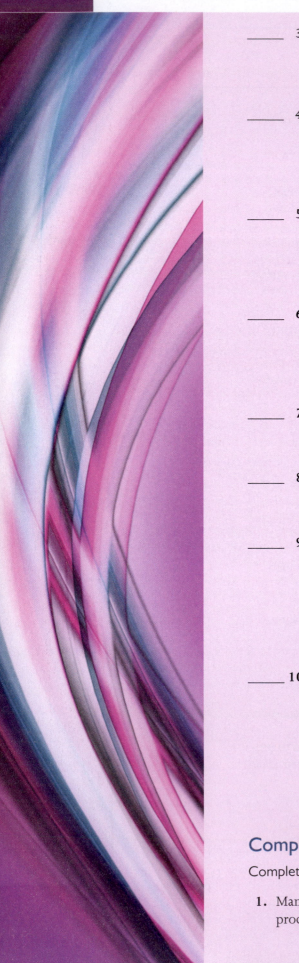

_____ 3. Under a capitated rate for each plan member, which of the following does a provider share with the third-party payer?
   a. Payments   c. Services
   b. Risk   d. The premium

_____ 4. The capitated rate per-member-per-month amount covers:
   a. all medical services.
   b. services listed on the schedule of benefits.
   c. the episode of care.
   d. all members' premiums.

_____ 5. PMPM is the abbreviation for:
   a. provider manages payments monthly.
   b. provider membership per management.
   c. per member per month.
   d. provider management by provider manual.

_____ 6. The Patient's Bill of Rights includes this principle:
   a. Respect and nondiscrimination
   b. Information disclosure
   c. Confidentiality of health information
   d. All of the above

_____ 7. COB is defined as:
   a. Contract of Benefits.   c. Contract of Business.
   b. Claim of Benefits.   d. Coordination of Benefits.

_____ 8. The list of medical services covered under the insured's policy is called the:
   a. plan of treatment.   c. fee schedule.
   b. schedule of benefits.   d. policy plan provisions.

_____ 9. The term _medically necessary_ refers to the use of services or supplies, or both, as determined by the corporation's medical director, or her designee, that:
   a. are accepted by the healthcare profession as appropriate and effective for the condition being treated.
   b. are based on unrecognized standards of the healthcare specialty involved.
   c. are experimental, investigative, or unproven.
   d. are for the convenience of a covered person.

_____ 10. When reviewing a fee-for-service plan, the medical office specialist should review:
   a. the time limit for submitting claims.
   b. what billing requirements must be met to allow for processing and payment of claims.
   c. whether the MCO provides ongoing staff training as billing requirements change.
   d. all of the above.

Completion

Complete each sentence or statement.

1. Managed care organizations evaluate the provider through a(n) _____ process.

2. Under a capitation arrangement, the provider is compensated for covered services based on a fixed prepaid monthly payment that is often referred to as a(n) _____ amount.

3. The provider must _____ with the managed care organization to be in the MCO's network.

4. The charge, as determined by the benefit plan, that a covered person is required to pay at the time covered services are provided is called a(n) _____.

5. A managed care contract is a(n) _____ agreement between a healthcare provider and an insurance carrier.

6. Network providers agree to use other providers in the _____ when the patient needs to be referred outside of their respective office.

7. The schedule of _____ lists the medical services that are covered by an insurance policy.

8. _____ refers to the use of services or suppliers, or both, as determined by the payer's or corporation's medical director, or his designee.

9. _____ is a legal agreement between the provider and patient which does not bill insurance and patient and has an annual cash fee for services.

10. An _____ is formed by providers and insurance companies. The patient must sign a contract for the provider to participate.

Resources

Advisory Commission on Consumer Protection and Quality in the Health Care Industry: **www.hcqualitycommission.gov**

American Hospital Association (AHA): **www.aha.org**

The Patient Care Partnership: Understanding Expectations, Rights, and Responsibilities is a valuable brochure that is available at the AHA website.
U.S. Department of Health and Human Services, Office of Inspector General: **http://oig.hhs.gov**

The Federal Bureau of Investigation website is a resource that can be consulted for ways to identify and prevent fraudulent billing as defined by the U.S. Attorney General: **www.fbi.gov**

This website provides information about accountable care organizations: **https://www.medicare.gov/manage-your-health/coordinating-your-care/coordinating-your-care.html**

This website provides more information about concierge medicine: **http://www.choice.md/patients-about?gclid=CIu3t5zZ7NACFUQvgQodv5wOmw**

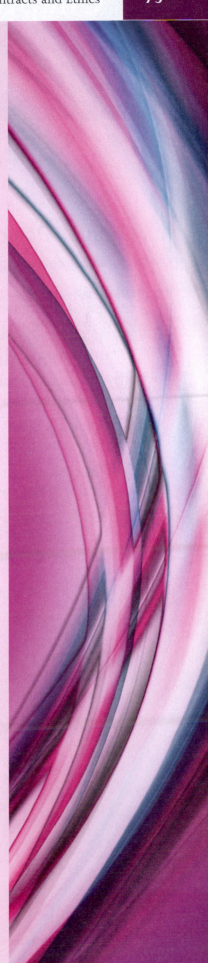

Chapter 4 | Introduction to the Health Insurance Portability and Accountability Act (HIPAA)

Chapter Objectives

After reading this chapter, the student should be able to:

1. Describe the responsibility of the medical office specialist to protect all protected health information (PHI).

2. Discuss what is required to disclose patient information to family members, friends, and when ordered by courts or government entities.

3. Understand the patient's right to request access or correction to his or her medical records.

4. Explain HIPAA security standards that require a healthcare provider to have security policies and procedures.

5. Discuss the penalties and fines involved for not being in compliance with HIPAA regulations.

6. Understand HITECH's mandatory requirements for healthcare providers to implement "meaningful use" by managing patient information and treatment through electronic health records (EHR).

Key Terms

business associates (BA)
civil money
    penalties (CMPs)
computerized provider
    order entry
    (CPOE)
covered entities (CE)
durable medical
    equipment (DME)
electronic data
    interchange (EDI)
electronic health
    records (EHR)
electronic medical
    records (EMR)

electronic protected health
    information (EPHI)
encrypted
enforcement rule
Food and Drug
    Administration (FDA)
Health and Human
    Services (HHS)
Health Information
    Technology for
    Economic and Clinical
    Health (HITECH) Act
meaningful use
National Provider
    Identifier (NPI)

Office for Civil
    Rights (OCR)
Office of the National
    Coordinator
    (ONC) for Health
    Information
Privacy Compliance
    Officer
Privacy Rule
protected health
    information (PHI)
Security Rule
transactions and code
    set rule
unique identifier rule

Audrey has worked for Dr. Jason for 6 years and has always been recognized as a model employee. While working for Dr. Jason she has also been attending college, which has prevented her from staying in touch with friends and family. In the past year she has kept in touch with friends through a social network website. When Dr. Jason's Privacy Compliance Officer brought Audrey into her office and announced Audrey's employment was being terminated for disclosing patient information, Audrey was shocked and stated she would never do such a thing. Audrey then discovered that one day at the office she had taken a picture of her desk to show where she worked, then published it on the social network. In the picture was a medical document with a patient's name.

Questions

1. Even though it was not deliberate, could Audrey or Dr. Jason be legally liable for disclosing patient information?

2. Who is responsible to train staff in regard to HIPAA rules and regulations?

3. What sections of HIPAA define the regulations to safeguard protected health information (PHI)?

The Health Insurance Portability and Accountability Act (HIPAA) was signed into law on August 21, 1996. Most healthcare insurance companies and providers were required to implement the HIPAA regulation guidelines put into place on August 21, 1996. Smaller health plans were required to implement the guidelines by October 2003. The HIPAA law is a multistep strategy that is geared to improve the health insurance system. HIPAA law provides needed information to healthcare providers for patient care and also provides patients certain rights to their personal information. HIPAA requires the Department of **Health and Human Services (HHS)** to adopt standards that **covered entities (CE)**, health plans, healthcare clearinghouses, and certain healthcare providers, employer-sponsored health plans, and health insurers must use when electronically conducting certain healthcare administrative transactions. These standards are to be applied to transactions such as claims, remittance, eligibility, and claims status requests and responses. A covered entity is any healthcare provider who transmits any health information in electronic form.

The HIPAA Administrative and Simplication Regulations: 2000–2008

HHS promulgated and modified several regulations to carry out its responsibilities and implement HIPAA Administrative Simplification provisions. These regulations are known as the Privacy Rule, the Security Rule, the Enforcement Rule, the Transactions and Code Sets Rule, and the Unique Identifier Rule.

HIPAA Privacy Rule

The HIPAA **Privacy Rule** was finalized by HHS in year 2000, in advance of the compliance deadline of April 14, 2003. The HIPAA Privacy Rule regulates the use and disclosure of protected health information held by healthcare clearinghouses, employer-sponsored health plans, health insurers, and medical service providers. By regulation, HHS extended the HIPAA Privacy Rule to independent contractors of covered entities who consider themselves as **"business associates" (BA)**. Protected health information (PHI) is any information held by a covered entity which concerns health status, provision of healthcare, or payment for healthcare that is linked to an individual. This includes any part of an individual's medical record or payment history. Covered entities may disclose protected health

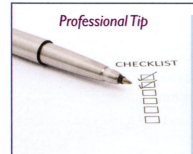

Professional Tip

CHECKLIST

The Administrative Simplification Compliance Act (ASCA) requires that as of October 16, 2003, all initial Medicare claims be submitted electronically, except in limited situations. Medicare is prohibited from payment of claims submitted on a paper claim form that do not meet the limited exception criteria. Examples of exceptions are providers that submit fewer than 10 claims per month during a calendar year and claims for dates of service that exceed Medicare timely filing guidelines.

information to law enforcement officials for law enforcement purposes as required by law, including court orders, warrants, and subpoenas and administrative requests; or to identify or locate a suspect, material witness, or missing person.

A covered entity may disclose PHI to provide treatment, payment, or healthcare without a patient's written authorization. Any other disclosures of PHI require the covered entity to obtain written authorization from the individual for the disclosure. However, when a covered entity discloses any PHI, it must make a reasonable effort to disclose only the minimum necessary information required to achieve its purpose.

Omnibus Rule

The *Omnibus Rule* is based on statutory changes under the HITECH Act. The Omnibus Rule required standards for the disclosure and use of protected health information (PHI), including established standards of enforcement for penalties and breach notification (discussed later in this chapter). The rule provides the public with increased protection and control of personal health information.

The HIPAA Privacy Rule gives individuals the right to request that a covered entity correct any inaccurate PHI. Covered entities must disclose PHI to the individual within 30 days upon request. It also requires covered entities to take reasonable steps to ensure the confidentiality of communications with individuals. For example, an individual can ask to be called on his or her cell phone instead of home or work phone numbers. An individual who believes that the Privacy Rule is not currently being upheld may file a complaint with HHS. The rule graciously enhances a patient's privacy protection by providing:

- Patients can ask for a copy of their electronic medical record in an electronic form.
- If a Medicare beneficiary requests a restriction on the disclosure of PHI to Medicare for a covered service and pays out of pocket for the service, the provider must also restrict the disclosure of PHI regarding the service to Medicare.
- The government's ability to enforce the law is strengthened, regardless of where the information is being stored.
- When patients pay out of pocket in full, they can instruct their provider to refrain from sharing information about their treatment with their health plan.
- Penalties increased for noncompliance based on the level of negligence with a maximum penalty of $1.5 million per violation.

The following are examples of when patient information may be disclosed without written consent:

- When a patient is in a treatment room and has allowed a friend or family member to remain in the room, the nurse or physician may discuss the patient's condition and treatment. The patient's action of not asking the friend or family member to leave implies permission to the physician or nurse to speak in front of the friend or family member.
- A patient's bill may be discussed when a friend or family member is with the patient at the time of service.
- Discussion may ensue when the patient has given verbal consent.
- When a patient is unconscious or incoherent after surgery, after an accident, or due to an illness, the surgeon may discuss the condition of the patient with a friend or family member.

HIPAA does not require that a healthcare provider document the patient's consent; however, a healthcare provider is advised by most legal counsel to document in writing the patient's agreement or lack of objection and to retain the document in the patient's medical file. Authority to grant authorization for use or disclosure of health information resides with:

- the patient, if the patient is a competent adult or an emancipated/mature minor; or
- a parent or legal guardian on behalf of a minor child.

Before treatment, a healthcare provider should have the patient complete a designation for release of medical information form, a document that outlines with whom the provider may share patient care information (Figure 4.1). This form should contain a method of identification such as date of birth or the last four digits of the person's Social Security number. When someone other than a friend or family member is involved, the healthcare provider must be reasonably sure that the patient asked the person to assist in her care or payment for care even though the healthcare provider may use his professional judgment.

A healthcare provider is allowed to discuss a patient's medical condition or payment with a person over the phone or in writing under the same guidelines as those that may be shared face-to-face. HIPAA does not require proof of identity in this case. However, a healthcare provider may establish his or her own rules for verifying who is on the phone.

When a patient is not present or is incapacitated, a healthcare provider is not required by HIPAA to share the patient's information with any approved friend(s) or family member(s). The provider may choose to wait until the patient has an opportunity to agree to the disclosure.

According to the U.S. Department of Health and Human Services, most privacy complaints arise because of:

1. impermissible uses and disclosures of protected health information.
2. lack of safeguards of protected health information.
3. lack of patients' access to their protected health information.
4. uses or disclosures of more than the minimum necessary protected health information.
5. lack of or invalid authorizations for uses and disclosures of protected health information.

Legal Request

The HIPAA Privacy Rule establishes guidelines for when PHI may be disclosed without a patient's authorization or objection. Each state also has laws and regulations that must be adhered to in conjunction with the HIPAA Privacy Rule. A provider must appoint a contact person or **Privacy Compliance Officer** to be responsible for receiving and responding to requests for medical records and for receiving complaints. All staff of a covered entity should be trained in rules and regulations regarding the confidentiality and release of PHI. Routine training should be provided, and the staff should be educated immediately as new rules and regulations are implemented. A covered entity's Privacy Compliance Officer must be familiar with both federal and state regulations. Some healthcare providers may contract out this service to consultants or organizations that specialize in the HIPAA Privacy Rule.

A covered entity is required to release PHI in response to a court or administrative tribunal, provided that only the PHI expressly authorized by the order is disclosed. A healthcare provider is required to release PHI to the appropriate government entity authorized by law to receive reports of child abuse or neglect.

Designation for Release of Medical Information to a Family Member, Friend, or Legal Representative

Introduction

It is the physicians' responsibility to ensure that the physician-patient relationship is confidential. The Privacy Statement of Trinity Family Medicine is the basis for how we treat your Protected Health Information. HIPAA allows physicians to use their professional judgment on disclosing certain PHI to family, friends, etc. without an authorization. This form is an aid to the physician in making a determination on disclosing such information. Trinity Family Medicine realizes that there are times when you, the patient, may want another person to be knowledgeable about your medical condition or medical needs or the status of your account. Your doctor wants you to be able, if you so desire, to name a person(s) to whom you want the office staff to speak with about your medical care and treatment. To enable that, we would ask that you complete the form listed below. Please note the following points:

- Only two people can be designated for this role
- The designation is valid until you cancel it in writing
- If you designate no one, Trinity Family Medicine may not be able to release information to any family member or friend.

Designation Statement

I, _____, designate the following person(s) to be able to speak to a physician at Trinity Family Medicine (office of Dr. David Jason, LLP), a nurse or other staff member, should it be necessary, on my behalf. I hereby give permission to Trinity Family Medicine through its physicians and staff to release to my designee any information about my medical condition or medical needs or the status of my account and I release Trinity Family Medicine, its physicians and staff, from any claim of confidentiality in connections with the release of this information.

Name of Designated Person:_____

Relationship: _____ Phone Number _____ (home/work)

Name of Designated Person:_____

Relationship: _____ Phone Number _____ (home/work)

Patient's Name: Patient's Account #: _____

Patient's Signature: _____

Date: _____ Witness: _____

I decline to designate another person to speak with my physician or clinical staff.

Patient's Signature: _____

Date: _____ Witness: _____

Figure 4.1

Designation for Release of Medical Information Form.

In regard to PHI that affects public health, a covered entity may disclose it to a public health authority that is authorized by law to collect or receive information for the purpose of preventing or controlling disease, injury, or disability. The public health authority may use this information for the reporting of disease, injury, or vital events such as birth or death. PHI must be released to a public health authority when a person may have been exposed to a communicable disease or may be at risk of contracting or spreading a disease or condition.

The U.S. **Food and Drug Administration (FDA)** may require PHI to collect or report product recalls, product defects, or product replacement. PHI may be released to an employer if the disclosed findings involve a work-related illness or injury or workplace-related medical surveillance. Only PHI related to the work-related illness or injury can be released to an employer. An employer also may have access to PHI if an employee is treated by a healthcare provider who is employed by the same company *and* the treatment was at the request of the employer. The healthcare provider must disclose to the employee that he or she will be releasing PHI to the employer by giving a copy of a notice to the individual at the time of service or posting a notice in a prominent place where services are provided. Alternatively, an employer may disclose PHI to a healthcare oversight agency for activities such as an audit, investigation, inspection, or licensure disciplinary actions.

The covered entity may disclose PHI regarding decedents to a coroner or medical examiner for the purpose of identifying the deceased, determining cause of death, or other duties as authorized by law. PHI may also be released to organ procurement organizations or other entities engaged in the procurement, banking, or transplantation of cadaveric organs, including eyes, or tissue for the purpose of facilitating the donation and transplantation.

Pharmacies and Durable Medical Equipment

Pharmacies and **durable medical equipment (DME)** have medical devices that store PHI and contain an operating system, such as Microsoft Windows. Under the new rule, companies that service medical devices and have access to the patient information they contain are considered business associates. In addition, the new rule clarifies that all BAs must comply with the HIPAA **Security Rule**. If the device manufacturer, or an intermediary, has a service contract with the provider that gives it access to electronic PHI stored within the device, then the company is a business associate under the broadened definition within the new rule. Therefore, to comply with HIPAA, medical device servicers, also known as DME servicers, will need to implement a patch management program to protect against viruses.

Manufacturers and suppliers of devices such as insulin pumps and pacemakers have resisted applying patches to the operating systems within the devices, expressing concern that modifications could affect performance.

Security for wireless implanted devices is a growing concern. For example, an "ethical hacker" recently demonstrated how an implanted wireless heart defibrillator could be hacked from 50 feet away to deliver a potentially dangerous shock.

Language Barrier

When a language barrier exists between the healthcare provider and the patient, the patient may have an interpreter or the provider may provide an interpreter. A healthcare provider may share information with an interpreter who is acting on behalf of the provider but is not a member of the provider's workforce. Providers are required under Title VI of the Civil Rights Act of 1964 to take reasonable steps to provide meaningful access to persons with limited English proficiency. A provider may contract with private companies, community-based organizations, or interpreter-service phone lines to provide language interpreter services. These arrangements must comply with the HIPAA business associate agreement requirements. The following are examples of when a provider may share patient information with an interpreter:

- When the interpreter works for the provider (e.g., a bilingual employee, a contract interpreter on staff, or a volunteer)
- When the interpreter is the patient's family member, friend, or other person identified by the patient as his or her interpreter, if the patient agrees, or does not object, or the healthcare provider determines, using his professional judgment that the patient does not object

Figure 4.2 lists HIPAA Privacy Rule disclosures to a patient's family, friends, or others involved in the patient's care or payment for care.

	Family Member or Friend	Other Persons
Patient is present and has the capacity to make healthcare decisions	Provider may disclose relevant information if the provider does one of the following: (1) obtains the patient's agreement (2) gives the patient an opportunity to object and the patient does not object (3) decides from the circumstances, based on professional judgment, that the patient does not object Disclosure may be made in person, over the phone, or in writing.	Provider may disclose relevant information if the provider does one of the following: (1) obtains the patient's agreement (2) gives the patient the opportunity to object and the patient does not object (3) decides from the circumstances, based on professional judgment, that the patient does not object Disclosure may be made in person, over the phone, or in writing.
Patient is not present or is incapacitated	Provider may disclose relevant information if, based on professional judgment, the disclosure is in the patient's best interest. Disclosure may be made in person, over the phone, or in writing. Provider may use professional judgment and experience to decide if it is in the patient's best interest to allow someone to pick up filled prescriptions, medical supplies, X-rays, or other similar forms of health information for the patient.	Provider may disclose relevant information if the provider is reasonably sure that the patient has involved the person in the patient's care and in his or her professional judgment, the provider believes the disclosure to be in the patient's best interest. Disclosure may be made in person, over the phone, or in writing. Provider may use professional judgment and experience to decide if it is in the patient's best interest to allow someone to pick up filled prescriptions, medical supplies, X-rays, or other similar forms of health information for the patient.

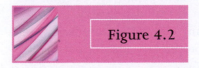

Figure 4.2   HIPAA Privacy Rule Disclosures to a Patient's Family, Friends, or Others Involved in the Patient's Care or Payment for Care.

Source: U. S. Department of Health and Human Services.

Patient Access and Corrections

The Privacy Rule covers not only the release of PHI but also the patient's access to her medical records. A patient has the right to review all of her medical records when a written request is received. The covered entity must ask for identification prior to releasing any information to protect the patient's confidentiality. The Privacy Rule also grants individuals the right to request that a covered entity correct any inaccurate PHI.

The patient has a right to contest information contained in his medical record and request that the healthcare provider correct his medical record(s) accordingly. Upon request, the covered entity must provide the information or correct the information within 30 days. It is important that a provider document any treatment or therapeutic plan as discussed in Chapter 17.

An individual, staff, or patient who believes that the Privacy Rule is not being enforced can file a complaint with the HHS **Office for Civil Rights (OCR)**. The complaint must be submitted in writing, via mail, or electronically, and must be filed within 180 days of when the complainant knew or should have known that the act had occurred. The OCR may waive this 180-day time limit if good cause is shown. Covered entities must have a written and published notice of privacy policy. After the 180-day time limit, individuals have a right to file a complaint directly with the covered entity and should refer to their privacy policy.

A provider's Privacy Compliance Officer will have the responsibility to notify OCR of any breaches of unsecured PHI. OCR requires healthcare providers and other HIPAA-covered entities to notify any individuals affected by the breach and to notify the HHS in cases where a breach affects more than 500 individuals. Breaches affecting fewer than 500 individuals will be reported to the HHS on an annual basis. The regulation also requires business associates of covered entities to notify the covered entity of breaches that are originated by the business associate.

Transactions and Code Set Rule

The HIPAA **Transactions and Code Set Rule** passed in 2005 standardizes the electronic exchange of patient-identifiable, health-related information. These transactions do contain private health information; therefore they must be sent **encrypted**, which means that the information is scrambled by rotating letters in the alphabet and/or numbers while it is being transmitted. This prevents unauthorized individuals from being able to read or decipher the information for private or monetary reasons. These transactions are based on the **electronic data interchange (EDI)** standards for the electronic transfer of information in a standard format between trading partners. EDI allows entities within the healthcare system to exchange medical, billing, and other information and to process transactions in a fast and cost-effective manner. EDI can eliminate the inefficiencies of handling paper documents, to significantly reduce administrative burden, lower operating costs, minimize risk of lost paper documents, and improve overall data quality.

Many covered entities have developed proprietary EDI formats. HIPAA

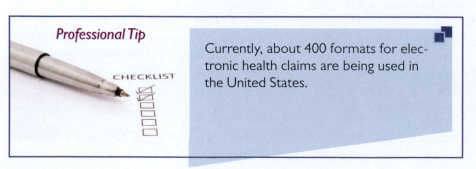

Professional Tip

CHECKLIST

Currently, about 400 formats for electronic health claims are being used in the United States.

requirements specify that all electronic data interchange formats be standardized. This includes uniform definitions of the data elements that will be exchanged in each type of electronic transaction as well as identification of the specific codes or values that are valid for each data element.

Lack of standardization makes it difficult and expensive to develop and maintain software. Moreover, the lack of standardization minimizes the ability of healthcare providers and health plans to achieve efficiency and savings.

Uniform Code Sets

HIPAA specifies that the healthcare industry use code sets when submitting healthcare claims electronically. Adopting a uniform set of medical codes is intended to simplify the process of submitting claims electronically and reduce administrative burdens on healthcare providers and health plans. Standard code sets include Healthcare Common Procedure Coding System (HCPCS), Current Procedure Terminology (CPT-4), International Classification of Diseases (ICD-10) and National Drug Codes (NDC). Finally, HHS adopted standards for unique identifiers for employers and providers in all transactions.

Security Rule

As of February 20, 2003, HHS administers and enforces the HIPAA Security Rule. The rule specifies that safeguards be implemented to protect **electronic protected health information (EPHI)**. Furthermore, covered entities and their business associates must adhere to these safeguards to protect the confidentiality, integrity, and availability of PHI. The healthcare industry relies heavily on the use of information systems to maintain **electronic medical records (EMR)**. HHS is able to protect individuals' health information by combining the authority for administration and enforcement of the federal standards for health information privacy and security called for in the HIPAA legislation. This final rule went into effect on April 21, 2006.

Electronic Medical Record

The EMR also contains health-related information about a patient that is created, gathered, managed, and consulted on by licensed clinicians and staff from a single organization who are involved in the individual's health and care. EMR are not integrated with other providers' systems.

Professional Tip

EMR is often confused with EHR (electronic health records). EMR is a legal record of what happened to a patient during an encounter with clinical services. EHR makes it possible for multiple service providers at a site (e.g., a hospital) to access or exchange information regarding patient encounters.

CHECKLIST

Electronic Health Record

The **electronic health record (EHR)** is an electronic record of patient health information that originates in a delivery setting such as a hospital, physician's practice, multi-specialty outpatient facility, or clinic. All records of patient care are retained in the EHR, including information from other systems such as X-rays, consultations, and so on. All providers who have a relationship with the patient can view the EHR. An

EHR creates and gathers information cumulatively across more than one healthcare organization. Electronic information systems have many functions that automate the covered entity's processes, such as paying claims, answering eligibility questions, and providing health information. There are three types of security safeguards required for compliance: administrative, physical, and technical.

- *Administrative Safeguards:* policies and procedures designed to demonstrate how the entity will comply with the act.
  - Covered entities must adopt a written set of privacy procedures and designate a privacy officer to be responsible for developing and implementing all required policies and procedures.
  - The policies and procedures must reference management oversight and organizational buy-in for compliance with the documented security controls.
  - Procedures should clearly identify employees or classes of employees who will have access to EPHI. Access to EPHI must be restricted to only those employees who have a need for it to complete their job function.
  - The procedures must address access authorization, establishment, modification, and termination.
  - Entities must show that an appropriate ongoing training program regarding the handling of PHI is provided to employees performing health plan administrative functions.
  - Covered entities that outsource some of their business processes to a third party must ensure that their vendors also have a framework in place to comply with HIPAA requirements. Companies typically gain this assurance through clauses in the contracts stating that the vendor will meet the same data protection requirements that apply to the covered entity. Care must be taken to determine if the vendor further outsources any data handling functions to other vendors, and to monitor whether appropriate contracts and controls are in place.
  - A contingency plan should be in place for responding to emergencies. Covered entities are responsible for backing up their data and having disaster recovery procedures in place. The plan should document data priority and failure analysis, testing activities, and change control procedures.
  - Internal audits play a key role in HIPAA compliance by reviewing operations with the goal of identifying potential security violations. Policies and procedures should specifically document the scope, frequency, and procedures of audits. Audits should be both routine and event based.
  - Procedures should document instructions for addressing and responding to security breaches that are identified either during the audit or the normal course of operations.
- *Physical Safeguards:* controlling physical access to protect against inappropriate access to protected data.
  - Controls must govern the introduction and removal of hardware and software from the network. (When equipment is retired, it must be disposed of properly to ensure that PHI is not compromised.)
  - Access to equipment containing health information should be carefully controlled and monitored.
  - Access to hardware and software must be limited to properly authorized individuals.
  - Required access controls consist of facility security plans, maintenance records, and visitor sign-in and escorts.

- Policies are required to address proper workstation use. Workstations should be removed from high-traffic areas, and monitor screens should not be in direct view of the public.
- If the covered entities use contractors or agents, they too must be fully trained on their physical access responsibilities.

■ *Technical Safeguards:* controlling access to computer systems and enabling covered entities to protect communications containing PHI transmitted electronically over open networks from being intercepted by anyone other than the intended recipient.

- Information systems housing PHI must be protected from intrusion. When information flows over open networks, some form of encryption must be used. If closed systems/networks are used, existing access controls are considered sufficient and encryption is optional.
- Each covered entity is responsible to ensure that the data within its systems has not been changed or erased in an unauthorized manner.
- Data corroboration, including the use of check sum, double-keying, message authentication, and digital signature may be used to ensure data integrity.
- Covered entities must also authenticate entities with which they communicate. Authentication consists of corroborating that an entity is what it claims to be. Examples of corroboration include password systems, two- or three-way handshakes, telephone callback, and token systems.
- Covered entities must make documentation of their HIPAA practices available to the government to determine compliance.
- In addition to policies and procedures and access records, information technology documentation should also include a written record of all configuration settings on the components of the network because these components are complex, configurable, and always changing.
- Documented risk analysis and risk management programs are required. Covered entities must carefully consider the risks of their operations as they implement systems to comply with the act. (The requirement of implementing risk analysis and risk management implies that the act's security requirements are of minimum standard and places the responsibility on covered entities to take all reasonable precautions necessary to prevent PHI from being used for non-health purposes.)

Unique Identifiers Rule

HIPAA also established uniform identifier standards which are currently being used on all claims and other data transmissions. HIPAA set the regulations to the Health Plan Identifier (HPID). On September 5, 2012, HHS published the Final Rule for Transactions and Codes Sets (the **unique identifier rule**), which adopts a unique identifier for health plans and provides a definition for health plan references code alpha and numeric definitions. This rule enforcement applies to all HIPAA-covered entities, including healthcare providers, health plans, and healthcare clearinghouses.

These standard identifiers include the following:

1. The **National Provider Identifier (NPI)** is assigned to doctors, nurses, and other healthcare providers. The use of the NPI has been in effect since May 2007 for Medicare providers.

2. The Federal Employer Identification Number (EIN) is used to identify employer-sponsored health insurance.
3. The National Health Plan Identifier is a unique identification number assigned to each insurance plan, and to the organizations that administer insurance plans, such as payers and third-party administrators.

National Provider Identifier

The NPI is the standard unique health identifier for healthcare providers, individuals, groups, or organizations that provide medical or other health services or supplies. Individuals identified in any covered electronic healthcare transaction must obtain an NPI that remains associated with the individual for life. Healthcare providers and all health plans and arm's-length clearinghouses use NPIs in the administrative and financial transactions specified by HIPAA. The NPI replaced all other identifiers used by health plans.

HIPAA Enforcement Rule

The HIPAA **Enforcement Rule** contains provisions relating to compliance and investigations, the imposition of **civil money penalties (CMPs)** for violations of the HIPAA Administrative Simplification Rules, and procedures for hearings.

Since the compliance date of the Privacy Rule in April 2003, OCR has received over 125,445 HIPAA complaints and has initiated over 854 compliance reviews. They have resolved 96% of these cases (119,964).

Civil Penalties

The American Recovery and Reinvestment Act of 2009 (ARRA) that was signed into law on February 17, 2009, established a tiered civil penalty structure for HIPAA violations. HHS has discretion in determining the amount of the penalty based on the nature and extent of the violation and the nature and extent of the harm resulting from the violation. HHS is prohibited from imposing civil penalties (except in cases of willful neglect) if the violation is corrected within 30 days (this time period may be extended).

Federal Criminal Penalties

Criminal penalties, fines, jail terms, and exclusion from the participation in the Federal healthcare programs are administrative sanctions for violating the law. Under the Civil Monetary Penalties Law (CMPL), physicians who pay or accept kickbacks also face penalties of up to $50,000 per kickback plus three times the amount of the remuneration. However, if the offense is committed with intent to sell, transfer, or use individually identifiable health information for commercial advantage, personal gain, or financial gain, they can be fined not more than $250,000, and imprisoned not more than 10 years, or both.

Hitech Act

The **Health Information Technology for Economic and Clinical Health (HITECH) Act** is contained in the American Recovery and Reinvestment Act of 2009 to strengthen HIPAA privacy and security protections, enhance enforcement efforts, and provide public education about privacy protections. The security segments of the HITECH Act were developed to help organizations that handle PHI prevent fraud, hacking, and other security threats by utilizing technology that can be used to render PHI unusable to unauthorized individuals. The act expands the privacy provisions of HIPAA to business associates of covered entities. The HITECH requirement not only expands the regulated community to include business associates but also mandates that OCR educate individuals about the potential uses of their protected health information, the effects of such uses, and the rights of individuals with respect to such uses. Finally, the HITECH Act requires OCR to conduct periodic audits to ensure that covered entities and business associates are in compliance with the law's requirements.

Meaningful Use

The HITECH Act introduced the concept of meaningful use. **Meaningful use** is a set of requirements designed to move the healthcare industry toward the implementation of standardized, certified, interoperable electronic health records and related technologies.

Under HITECH, three regulations are referred to as stages. Upon achieving the standards set by each stage, all eligible healthcare professionals and hospitals can qualify for Medicare and Medicaid incentive payments. They are eligible to receive the incentive payments once they adopt certified EHR technology and use it to achieve specified objectives.

Healthcare professionals do not achieve these benefits merely by transferring information from paper form into digital form. The EHR must deliver the information by a standardized and structured means. Therefore, the meaningful use approach requires specific standards for EHR systems. These are contained in the **Office of the National Coordinator (ONC) for Health Information**.

Similarly, EHRs cannot achieve their full potential if providers do not use the functions that deliver the most benefit: exchanging information and entering orders via computer so that the decision support functions and other automated processes are activated. Therefore, the meaningful use approach requires that providers meet specified objectives in the use of EHRs in order to qualify for the incentive payments. Basic information needs to be entered into the qualified EHR so that it exists in the structured format, information exchange begins, security checks are routinely made, and medical orders are made using **computerized provider order entry (CPOE)**. Stage 1 defines the meaningful use objectives that providers must meet to qualify for the bonus payments, and it identifies the technical capabilities required for certified EHR technology. The primary objective is to implement structure by requiring physicians and hospitals to use a CPOE system that meets certain criteria or functions. For example, the CPOE must allow the provider to maintain an up-to-date problem list of current and active diagnoses based on ICD-10-CM.

The CPOE must allow the provider to:

1. generate the list of patients by specific conditions for quality improvement.
2. have the capability to record patient information such as demographics, changes in vital signs, and smoking status for patients 13 years old or older.
3. allow the provider to check insurance eligibility and submit claims electronically from public and private payers.
4. provide patients with an electronic copy of their health information upon request and provide patients with timely electronic access to their health information.
5. provide clinical summaries for patients for each office visit.
6. exchange key clinical information among providers of care and patient-authorized entities electronically.

7. provide a summary care record for each transition of care and referral and have the capability to electronically submit reportable lab results (as required by state or local law) to public health agencies and actual submission where it can be received.

Failure to adopt a meaningful use EMR will have doctors facing penalties in the form of reductions to their Medicare fee schedule reimbursement rates. There are three stages: The penalty will equal 1% in 2015, 2% in 2016, and 3% in 2017 and each subsequent year. Under the bill, HHS can increase the penalty to 5% if fewer than 75% of eligible physicians are not utilizing an EMR by 2018.

Beyond the Stage 1 Criteria for Meaningful Use

The Centers for Medicare and Medicaid Services (CMS) intends to propose through future rulemaking two additional stages of the criteria for meaningful use.

Stage 2 Core Objectives for Meaningful Use

To secure electronic messaging to communicate with patients on relevant health information. To automatically track medication from order to administration using assistive technologies conjunction with an electronic medical administration record (eMAR) (for eligible hospitals/critical access hospitals only). Other objectives are:

Patient Access

- Provide patients the ability to view online, download, and transmit their health information within four business days of the information being availing to the eligible professionals.
- Provide patients the ability to view online, download, and transmit their health information within 36 hours after discharge from the hospital (eligible hospitals/critical access hospitals only).

Menu Objectives

- Record electronic notes in patient records.
- Access imaging results through CEHRT.
- Record patient family health history.
- Identify and report cancer cases to a state cancer registry.
- Identify and report specific cases to a specialized registry (other than a cancer registry).
- Generate and transmit permissible discharge prescriptions electronically.

Stage 3 is set to begin for physicians and hospitals as optional in 2017 and required in 2018. The rule will focus on achieving improvements in quality, safety, and efficiency while focusing on decision support for national high-priority conditions, patient access to self-management tools, access to comprehensive patient data, and improving population health outcomes. Adding uncertainty, the "final" rule for meaningful use Stage 3 includes a 60-day comment period, suggesting that there may be additional modifications or delays.

There are Medicare and Medicaid incentive payments for achieving the three successive stages of meaningful use. Healthcare professionals who are eligible for Medicare incentives under the HITECH Act are defined as, "a physician, as defined in section 1861(r)" of the Social Security Act and include the following:

- Physicians
- Dentists

- Podiatrists
- Optometrists
- Chiropractors

Privacy and Security Protection

Covered entities and business associates must uphold their responsibility to provide patients with access to their medical records, and they must adhere closely to all HIPAA requirements protecting PHI. In 2014, Dr. Lawrence Cohen shot a "selfie" while Joan Rivers was lying unconscious on an operating table at Yorkville Endoscopy in Manhattan during an outpatient surgery procedure. The anesthesiologist for the procedure, Dr. Renuka Bankulla, entered into the medical record that Dr. Cohen took a photograph of Joan Rivers while she was unconscious. As unbelievable as it seems, cases such as this one have become more frequent. In addition, it will certainly test the waters of classifications of what is a HIPAA violation. The activity of what are HIPAA violations will continue to escalate with new boundaries being set each year. The malpractice suit filed nearly a year later in January 2015 against Dr. Gwen Korovin, Ms. Rivers' private doctor; the clinic; Dr. Bankulla; and Dr. Cohen cited a number of mistakes were made that resulted in the death of Ms. Rivers a week after the August 28, 2014 procedure. The lawsuit also stated that the doctors were not sufficiently trained to handle an emergency like the one that occurred when Ms. Rivers had a laryngospasm, a spasm of the vocal cords that rendered her unable to take in enough oxygen, which resulted in her going into cardiac arrest. When Dr. Bankulla looked for Dr. Korovin to open an airway for Ms. Rivers by performing an emergency cricothyrotomy, Dr. Korovin had already left the clinic.

The Centers for Medicare and Medicaid Services issued a report of numerous errors related to a case with patient demographics similar to those of Joan Rivers, including the following violations:

- Failing to ensure that only the physicians who cared for her were granted privilege to practice medicine with the clinic's bylaws.
- Failing to get her consent for each procedure performed.
- Failing to abide by its own cell phone policy guidelines.
- Failing to identify deteriorating vital signs and provide timely intervention of lifesaving medical care.

The clinic was scheduled to lose its Medicare contract on January 31, 2015. However, the clinic was later granted an extension to correct its deficiencies and has, apparently, managed to comply.

Healthcare Reform

Healthcare reform does improve the quality of care. Disease prevention and wellness checkups can significantly lower the cost being in a healthcare reform plan. President Barack Obama campaigned to reform healthcare and make insurance more affordable to those who did not have access to employer-sponsored insurance. In 2010, the Patient Protection and Affordable Care Act became law, and started phasing in new healthcare insurance benefits that year.

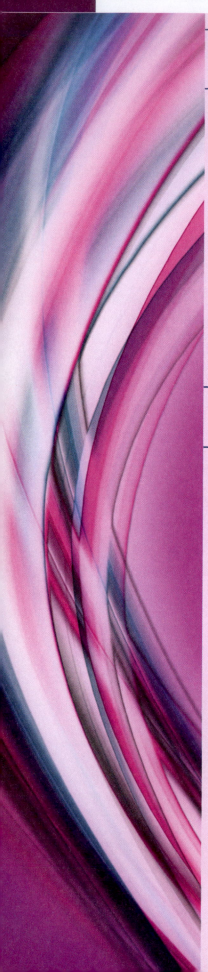

Chapter Summary

- The HIPAA Privacy Rule regulates the use and disclosure of Protected Health Information (PHI). The Privacy Rule pertains to all PHI, including paper and electronic, and about which all staff of a covered entity should be trained.
- The patient has a right to contest information contained in his medical record and to request the healthcare provider to correct his medical record(s) accordingly.
- HIPAA requires the Department of Health and Human Services (HHS) to adopt standards that covered entities, health plans, healthcare clearinghouses, and certain healthcare providers, employer-sponsored health plans, and health insurers must use when electronically conducting certain healthcare administrative transactions. These standards are applied to transactions such as claims, remittance, eligibility, and claims status requests and responses.
- The HITECH Act introduced the concept of meaningful use. Meaningful use is a set of requirements that is designed to move the healthcare industry toward the implementation of standardized, certified, interoperable electronic health records (EHRs).

Chapter Review

True/False

Identify the statement as true (T) or false (F).

_____   **1.** The HIPAA Act affects physicians and dentists in all regions.

_____   **2.** The Privacy Rule pertains to electronic PHI.

_____   **3.** A healthcare provider can make a professional judgment to decide when to discuss patient information with family and friends.

_____   **4.** When a patient is not unconscious, the healthcare provider must wait 24 hours before releasing information.

_____   **5.** A Privacy Compliance Officer must be familiar with both federal and state regulations.

_____   **6.** Pharmacies and durable medical equipment companies are more flexible with requiring a signed medical release.

_____   **7.** When a patient who does not speak the same language as the healthcare provider arrives for treatment, the provider is required by law to provide an interpreter.

_____ **8.** The Privacy Rule grants individuals the right to request that a covered entity correct any inaccurate PHI.

_____ **9.** The NPI is the standard unique health identifier for business organizations that provide medical supplies.

_____ **10.** The HIPAA Enforcement Rule sets civil money penalties for violations of the HIPAA Administrative Simplification Rules.

Multiple Choice

Identify the letter of the choice that best completes the statement or answers the question.

_____ **1.** Examples of covered entities are:
   a. health plans, healthcare clearinghouses, and certain healthcare providers.
   b. EMTs, medical supplies, and consultants.
   c. dentists, contractors, and veterinarians.
   d. healthcare providers, employers, and hospital volunteers.

_____ **2.** According to the Department of Health and Human Services, most privacy complaints arise because of:
   a. policies regarding safeguards of protected health information.
   b. providing patients access to their protected health information.
   c. a healthcare provider not providing details regarding patient care.
   d. impermissible uses and disclosures of protected health information.

_____ **3.** A covered entity is required to release PHI:
   a. in response to a court or administrative tribunal order.
   b. to a government authority authorized by law regarding reports of child abuse or neglect.
   c. to a public health authority that is authorized by law to collect or receive information for the purpose of preventing or controlling disease.
   d. All of the above

_____ **4.** PHI stands for:
   a. private healthcare identification.
   b. protected health information.
   c. physician health information.
   d. privacy health indicator.

_____ **5.** A healthcare provider may share information with an interpreter who:
   a. works in the building.
   b. is a current patient.
   c. volunteers.
   d. is a relative of an employee.

_____ **6.** An individual, staff member, or patient who believes that the Privacy Rule is not being enforced can file a complaint with the:
   a. healthcare provider.
   b. HIPAA Privacy Department.

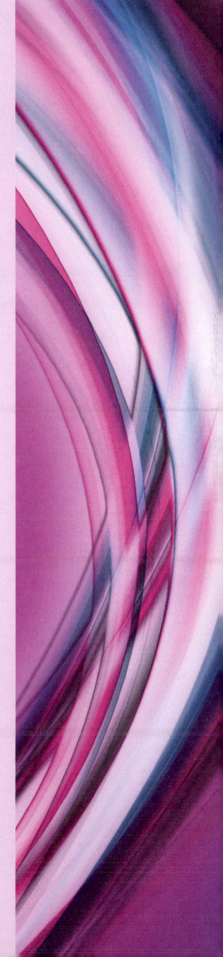

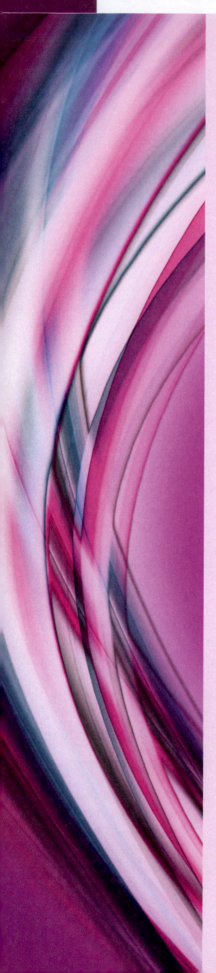

    c. HHS Office for Civil Rights.

    d. Department of Public Safety.

_____ **7.** Electronic data interchange (EDI):

    a. is the basis of HIPAA guidelines for standard coding.

    b. sets the standards for electronic transfer of information by covered entities.

    c. consists of regulations pertaining to documentation of medical records.

    d. is the coding system used to identify patient diagnosis.

_____ **8.** Electronic protected health information (EPHI) has three types of security safeguards, including:

    a. administrative, physical, and technical.

    b. vocabulary, coding, and system maintenance.

    c. procedures, support, and alarms.

    d. maintenance, regulations, and technical.

_____ **9.** The HITECH Act:

    a. strengthens privacy and security protections of health information.

    b. enhances enforcement efforts.

    c. provides public education about privacy protections.

    d. All of the above

_____ **10.** Meaningful use:

    a. sets policy standards for patient care.

    b. sets fines for illegally releasing patient information.

    c. is designed to move healthcare providers toward electronic health records.

    d. provides allied healthcare guidelines to document medical records.

Completion

Choose the best word or phrase to complete the sentence.

1. The _____ is the section of the Department of Health and Human Services where an individual, staff, or patient can file a complaint if she believes the Privacy Rule is not being enforced.

2. _____ are individuals or organizations that are regulated by the Health Insurance Portability and Accountability Act (HIPAA).

3. _____ is a system that allows various providers to access or exchange patient care information.

4. The _____ Act strengthens HIPAA privacy and security protections, enhances enforcement efforts, and provides public education about privacy protections.

5. A set of requirements designed to move the healthcare industry toward the implementation of standardized, certified, interoperable electronic health records is called _____.

6. A system referred to as _____ will allow the provider to maintain an up-to-date problem list of current and active diagnoses.

7. The primary responsibility of the designated _____ is to receive and respond to requests for medical records and to receive complaints.

8. The _____ is used to identify doctors, nurses, and other healthcare providers on medical claims.

9. Specific standards for EHR systems are maintained by _____.

Resources

UCLA Office of Compliance
http://compliance.uclahealth.org
This website provides quick guides to HIPAA guidelines which include patient privacy and security, guidance, and policies.

U.S. Department of Health and Human Services
www.hhs.gov
HIPAA government regulations and guidelines.

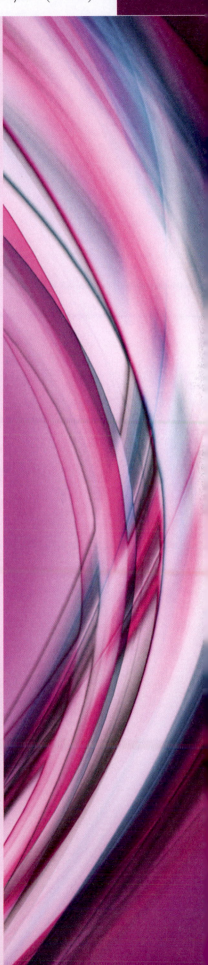

Section III / Medical Coding

5 ICD-10-CM Medical Coding

6 Introduction to CPT® and Place of Service Coding

7 Coding Procedures and Services

8 HCPCS and Coding Compliance

9 Auditing

To receive reimbursement for services provided, and prevent claim denials, diagnosis coding is a critical part of whether the physician receives payment in a timely manner. Improper medical coding can seriously affect the practice. Medical billing must be done correctly if the physician is to be successful.

Chapter 5 presents an understanding of diagnosis coding and inpatient procedure coding that begins with an understanding of the ICD-10-CM and ICD-10-PCS. The chapter provides the student with the knowledge to properly use the ICD-10-key coding guidelines, and the process to assign the correct diagnostic code(s) to the fullest extent. ICD-10-PCS will be introduced to the student for coding in-patient procedures.

Chapter 6 presents an introduction to the CPT® book and place of service coding. Understanding the use of procedure codes and the correct use of modifiers is the most important aspect of coding. This chapter discusses how evaluation and management codes are used to report office visits, hospital visits, nursing home visits, rehabilitation center visits, and home visits.

Chapter 7 presents the organization of the CPT index, instructions for using the CPT codes, the format of the terminology, and important coding steps. It presents the knowledge needed to locate the appropriate code for reporting the procedures and/or services performed.

Competent coding is part of the overall effort being made by medical practices to comply with regulations in many areas. For instance, the diagnosis code chosen must match the procedure performed. In addition, medical office specialists who work with patient records as they code must be knowledgeable about patient privacy regulations and how to keep patient data secure. Chapter 8 discusses the uniform method used by healthcare providers and medical suppliers to report professional services, procedures, and supplies.

Audits, whether performed in the office or by an external auditor, are formal examinations or reviews of documentation to determine if the documentation adequately substantiates the service billed and shows medical necessity. Chapter 9 discusses the purpose of an audit, the different types of auditing, key elements of service, the correct coding of evaluation and management (E/M) services based on medical necessity, and how to prevent coding errors with specific E/M codes.

Professional Vignette

My name is Judy Murray, and I am a Certified Medical Assistant. After my two children entered high school, I went to a local adult education school for medical assisting. I found the classes fun and exciting and discovered that I was smarter than I thought. I decided to continue on at the local community college, and received an associate's degree in Medical Assisting and then the CMA title.

I began my career doing clinical work, but soon after began to perform administrative responsibilities as well. As time passed I spent more time doing billing and less time working in the back office. Eventually, I was specializing in billing. I was able to fill in at the front desk or in the back drawing blood, performing EKGs, etc.

While I was employed in the medical office I was asked to teach bookkeeping and insurance classes at an adult education program. I found teaching at the adult level very rewarding as well as challenging. My past experience helped instill confidence that the students would be able to follow their dreams and that the profession would welcome their talents and abilities. Eventually, I taught classes at the college level, which offered me the opportunity to once again further my education and professional career. I sat for the national certification exam for Certified Professional Coders through the American Association of Professional Coders. I am now Judy Murray, CMA (AAMA), CPC.

Billing is really a team effort: Everyone in the office must do their part in order for the system to function efficiently. I love billing—it is very challenging and rewarding. It is amazing to look back to the beginning of my professional career and see how far I have grown professionally and personally in 20 years. I recently retired from teaching and am currently working 2 days a week for a plastic surgeon. The flexibility of and opportunities in this profession are numerous and very rewarding.

Chapter 5 / ICD-10-CM Medical Coding

Chapter Objectives

After reading this chapter, the student should be able to:

1 State the purpose of the ICD-10-CM and ICD-10-PCS.

2 Define abbreviations, symbols, typefaces, punctuation, and formatting conventions.

3 Use the correct Alphabetic Index and the Tabular List of ICD-10-CM to find the appropriate code.

4 Code to the highest level of certainty and specificity.

5 Assign the correct code in the proper order.

6 List the ten steps of accurate ICD-10-CM coding.[1]

7 Understand the code structure for ICD-10-PCS.

Key Terms

Alphabetic Index	ICD-10-PCS	residual effect
adverse effect	late effect	rule out
body mass index (BMI)	main term	secondary
combination code	manifestation	sign
complication code	morbidity	subterms
conventions	morphology	supplementary terms
default code	not elsewhere classified (NEC)	sequela
diagnosis		syndrome
diagnostic statement	not otherwise specified (NOS)	symptom
eponym		Tabular List
etiology	primary diagnosis	
ICD-10-CM	principal diagnosis	

[1] ICD-10-CM codes in this chapter are from the ICD-10-CM 2017 code set from the Department of Health and Human Services, Centers for Disease Control and Prevention.

Case Study

ICD-10-CM Medical Coding

Diagnostic coding is a critical part of medical billing. If the correct diagnostic code is not selected, a claim may be denied. The **diagnosis** establishes the medical necessity of the procedure or services performed for the patient. If the insurance claim is not coded to the highest level of specificity and recorded in the proper order, the claim may be reimbursed at a reduced dollar amount. Understanding diagnostic coding begins by using the *International Classification of Diseases*, Tenth Revision, Clinical Modification, known as ICD-10-CM and ICD-10-PCS correctly.

The World Health Organization (WHO) authorized the publication of the International Classification of Diseases, Tenth Revision (ICD-10), which was implemented for mortality coding and classification from death certificates in the United States in 1999. The United States developed Clinical Modification (ICD-10-CM) for medical diagnoses based on WHO's ICD-10 and CMS developed a new Procedure Coding System (ICD-10-PCS) for inpatient procedures. ICD-10-CM replaced ICD-9-CM, volumes 1 and 2, and ICD-10-PCS replaced ICD-9-CM, volume 3. This revision, which took effect on October 1, 2015, in the United States, allowed greater reporting of the descriptions of disease, morbidity, and mortality with more specificity. **Morbidity** refers to illness. The patient may have numerous comorbidities which should be coded. With this increased information of the patient, the providers will be able to attend to their patients with greater care. Did you know that the United States spends more than $150 billion annually on healthcare administration, and for the average physician, two-thirds of a full-time employee is needed to carry out billing and insurance-related tasks?

To ease these financial and administrative burdens, the Health Insurance Portability and Accountability Act (HIPAA) and the Patient Protection and Affordable Care Act established Administrative Simplification requirements. These requirements were put in place to lower costs, create uniform electronic standards, and streamline exchanges between healthcare providers and their payers. The reporting of public health statistics from this increased specific documentation of coding will improve our country's healthcare systems.

For the medical office specialist, this chapter will provide the basics of the ICD-10 CM coding and an understanding of the importance of being certified as a hospital or medical coder. The physician or any qualified healthcare practitioner who documents the patient's encounter is legally accountable for establishing the patient's diagnosis. A joint effort between the healthcare provider and the coder is essential to achieve complete and accurate documentation, code assignment, and reporting of diagnoses and procedures. The ICD-10-CM coding allows the codes to define the patient's clinical status more specifically, enabling the provider to better treat the patient's medical conditions. Please refer to www.cms.gov/ICD10 for current requirements and www.ahima.org/certification/ccs/ and www.cdc.gov/nchs/icd/icd10cm_pcs_background.htm

Definition of Diagnosis Coding

Healthcare professionals have long used coding systems to describe procedures, services, and supplies. The reason for the procedure, service, or supply must be supplied with a diagnosis for the healthcare provider to obtain reimbursement.

Proper diagnosis coding involves using the ICD-10-CM volumes to identify the appropriate codes for medical conditions that pertain to the patient's health (as recorded in the patient record) and entering those codes correctly on medical claims forms or submitting them electronically. Knowledge of medical terminology is a must for being able to read and understand the physician's documentation, which is the first step in the reimbursement process. Each service or procedure performed must be submitted with a diagnosis that will accurately link the patient's encounter to the service or procedure performed. Medical necessity must be established before the insurance carrier will make a payment to the provider of services. **Complication codes** must be coded if it is documented by the physician. ICD-10 offers an expanded selection of complication codes. A complication is an unfortunate outcome for a patient who has received medical treatment.

The ICD-10-CM codes are also used by outside agencies or organizations to forecast healthcare needs, evaluate facilities and services, review costs, and conduct studies of trends in diseases over the years. The ICD-10-PCS is used to report inpatient procedure coding.

ICD-10-CM Guidelines

Guidelines for coding and reporting the International Classification of Diseases, Tenth Revision, Clinical Modification (ICD-10-CM) were approved by the American Hospital Association, (AHA), the American Health Information Managements Association (AHIMA), Centers for Medicare and Medicaid Services (CMS), and the National Center for Health Statistics (NCHS). Adherence to these guidelines is required by HIPAA. These guidelines are organized into four sections. The medical office specialist must review all sections of these guidelines to fully understand all the rules and instructions needed to code properly. The four sections are:

1. The structure and conventions of the classification and general guidelines that apply to the entire classification. The **conventions** for the ICD-10-CM are the general rules for use of the classification independent of the guidelines. These conventions are incorporated within the Alphabetic Index and Tabular List of the ICD-10-CM as instructional notes. In section 1 there are also chapter-specific guidelines that correspond to the chapters in the classification.
2. Guidelines for selection of the principal diagnosis.
3. Guidelines for reporting additional diagnoses in a non-outpatient setting.
4. Diagnostic coding and reporting guidelines for outpatient services.

It is imperative that the provider be consistent in its documentation of the patient's medical record. Outpatient claims are paid based on medical necessity. Medical necessity can be defined in different ways by different payers to contain costs and prevent abuse of healthcare resources. The coder cannot achieve the highest code assignment of the diagnosis and procedures performed during the patient's encounter without reviewing the complete record for the specific reason for the encounter and the conditions treated. The diagnosis code can change from claim to claim or encounter to encounter. The term encounter is used for all settings, including hospital admissions. **Primary diagnosis** is used for outpatient settings and **Principal diagnosis** is used for hospital settings. A diagnosis code may be reported only once for an encounter. The ICD-10-CM is divided into two main parts, the **Alphabetic Index**, which is a list of terms and their corresponding code, and the **Tabular List**, a sequential, alphanumerical list of codes divided into chapters based on body system or condition.

The Alphabetic Index

This index consists of the Index of Diseases and Injury, which is in the main index. The Alphabetic Index to diseases is arranged in alphabetic order by disease, by specific illness, injury, eponym, abbreviation, or other descriptive term. The index also lists diagnostic terms for other reasons for encounters with healthcare professionals. Between the Alphabetic Index and the Tabular List of Diseases and Injuries, the medical office specialist will find the Neoplasm Table, the Table of Drugs and Chemicals, and the External Causes Index. To locate the correct code for the encounter, the term must be *found in the Alphabetic Index first*. The coder must verify the code in the Tabular List.

Case Study 5.1

Jacqueline is a medical coding extern in 2016. Being new to the general practitioner's practice, she is given a few medical cases to code. This first case is related to a diabetic patient. The physician has listed the following diagnoses (DX): Diabetes Mellitus with gangrene. Secondary diagnosis: BMI 41.0.

Using your ICD-10-CM book code the above diagnoses in the Alphabetic Index Only:

1. _____

2. _____

Neoplasm Table

The Neoplasm Table provides the proper code based upon the histology of the neoplasm and anatomical site. For each site there are six possible codes according to whether the neoplasm in question is:

1. Malignant Primary
2. Malignant Secondary
3. Carcinoma (Ca) in Situ
4. Benign
5. Uncertain
6. Unspecified Behavior

Example

Carcinoma of the cervix *in situ* would be coded D06.9

The coder would go to the Neoplasm Table, anatomical site, and then the type of neoplasm from the pathology report.

Table of Drugs and Chemicals

This table follows the Neoplasm Table and lists the drug and the specific codes that identify the drug and the intent. No additional external cause of injury and poisoning code is assigned in ICD-10-CM; for each drug there are six specified intents which are:

1. Poisoning, Accidental (Unintentional)
2. Poisoning, Intentional Self-harm
3. Poisoning, Assault
4. Poisoning, Undetermined
5. Adverse Effect
6. Under-dosing

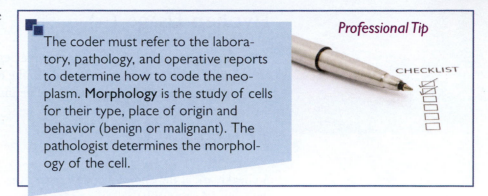

Professional Tip

The coder must refer to the laboratory, pathology, and operative reports to determine how to code the neoplasm. **Morphology** is the study of cells for their type, place of origin and behavior (benign or malignant). The pathologist determines the morphology of the cell.

CHECKLIST

Example

Self-intentional poisoning with Oxycodone, initial encounter and the code is T40.2X2A
The coder would locate the drug and then the intent of the poisoning.

External Causes Index

These codes are secondary codes for use in any healthcare setting; they provide data for injury research and evaluation of injury-prevention strategies.

In ICD-10-CM, the External Cause codes have moved to Chapter 20: External Causes of Morbidity (V01–Y99). External Cause codes capture how an injury, poisoning, or adverse effect happened (cause). An **adverse effect** is a harmful or abnormal result from a medication or an intervention such as surgery. External Cause codes also include the intent (unintentional or accidental; or intentional, such as suicide or assault), the place where the event occurred, and the activity of the patient at the time of the event.

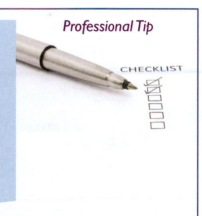

Professional Tip

Code intentional only if stated in the record, otherwise code undetermined. E codes do not have to be reported unless the provider is mandated by the payer or a state based reporting agency.

CMS streamlines ICD-10 Resources to their main new ICD-10 website. This updated website provides educational resources for coders. Go to: www.cms.gov/ICD10

CHECKLIST

Structure of ICD-10-CM

ICD-10-CM has between three and seven characters.

- Codes with three characters are included in the ICD-10-CM as the heading of a category of codes that may be further subdivided by the use of any or all of the fourth, fifth, or sixth character. Digits four to six provide greater detail of etiology, anatomical site, and severity. A code using only the first three digits is to be used if it is not further subdivided.
- A code is invalid if it has not been coded to the full number of characters required. This does not mean that all ICD-10 codes must have seven characters. The seventh character is only used in certain chapters to provide data about the characteristic of the encounters.

Hyphen Usage (-)

A hyphen at the end of the Alphabetic Index entry indicates that additional characters are required. Even if there is no hyphen in the entry, the Tabular List must be consulted to verify that no additional characters are required.

√ Checkmark

A checkmark at the end of a code √ means that an additional character is required and the Tabular List must be referred to for character selection.

Additional character required:

√4th This symbol indicates that the code requires a fourth character.
√5th This symbol indicates that the code requires a fifth character.
√6th This symbol indicates that the code requires a sixth character.
√7th This symbol indicates that the code requires a seventh character.
√×7th This symbol indicates that the code requires a seventh character following the placeholder X. Codes with fewer than six characters that require a seventh character must contain placeholder "X" to fill in the empty characters.

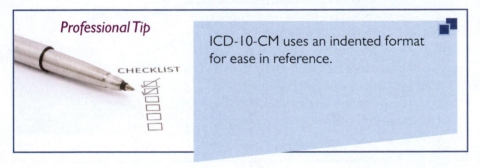

Professional Tip

CHECKLIST

ICD-10-CM uses an indented format for ease in reference.

Codes from A00.0–T88.9 and Z00–Z99.8 must be used to identify diagnoses, symptoms, conditions, problems, complaints, or other reason(s) for the encounter.

Codes that describe symptoms and signs, as opposed to diagnoses, are acceptable for reporting purposes when a related definitive diagnosis has not been established by the provider. A **symptom** is any indication of disease perceived by the patient. Chapter 18 of ICD-10-CM Symptoms, Signs, and Abnormal Clinical and Laboratory Findings, Not Elsewhere Classified (codes R00.0–R99) contain many, but not all codes for symptoms.

The Tabular List

The Tabular List is a list of codes divided into 21 separate chapters based on body system or nature of injury and disease. This list contains categories, subcategories, and valid codes which may be either a letter or a number. All categories are three characters. The first character of a three-category is a letter. The second or third characters may be numbers or alpha characters. A three-character category without further subclassification is equivalent to a valid three-character code. Subcategories are either four or five characters. Codes may be three through seven characters in length, in which each level of subdivision after a category is a subcategory. The final level of subdivision is a valid code. The final character in a code may be either a letter or a number. Codes that have applicable seventh characters are still referred to as codes, not subcategories. A code that has an applicable seventh character is considered invalid without the seventh character. When a seventh-character extension is required, a dummy placeholder "X" must be used to fill in the empty characters.

Chapter 1	Certain Infectious and Parasitic Diseases (A00–B99)
Chapter 2	Neoplasms (C00–D49)
Chapter 3	Diseases of the Blood and Blood-forming Organs and Certain Disorders involving the Immune Mechanism (D50–D89)
Chapter 4	Endocrine, Nutritional, and Metabolic Diseases (E00–E89)
Chapter 5	Mental, Behavioral, and Neurodevelopmental Disorders (F01–F99)
Chapter 6	Diseases of the Nervous System (G00–G99)
Chapter 7	Diseases of the Eye and Adnexa (H00–H59)
Chapter 8	Diseases of the Ear and Mastoid Process (H60–H95)
Chapter 9	Diseases of the Circulatory System (I00–I99)
Chapter 10	Diseases of the Respiratory System (J00–J99)
Chapter 11	Diseases of the Digestive System (K00–K95)
Chapter 12	Diseases of the Skin and Subcutaneous Tissue (L00–L99)
Chapter 13	Diseases of the Musculoskeletal System and Connective Tissue (M00–M99)
Chapter 14	Diseases of Genitourinary System (N00–N99)
Chapter 15	Pregnancy, Childbirth, and the Puerperium (O00–O9A)
Chapter 16	Certain Conditions Originating in the Perinatal Period (P00–P96)
Chapter 17	Congenital Malformations, Deformations, and Chromosomal Abnormalities (Q00–Q99)
Chapter 18	Symptoms, Signs, and Abnormal Clinical and Laboratory Findings, Not Elsewhere Classified (R00–R99)
Chapter 19	Injury, Poisoning, and Certain Other Consequences of External Causes (S00–T88)
Chapter 20	External Causes of Morbidity (V00–Y99)
Chapter 21	Factors Influencing Health Status and Contact with Health Services (Z00–Z99)

Figure 5.1

Chapters in the Tabular List.

ICD-10-CM uses an indented format for ease in reference. After verifying the code in the Tabular List, any additional instructions should be followed. Figure 5.1 shows the Tabular List.

Case Study 5.2

Jacqueline is a medical coding extern in 2016. Being new to the general practitioner's practice, she is given a few medical cases to code. This first case is related to a diabetic patient. The physician has listed the following DX: Diabetes Mellitus with gangrene. **Secondary** diagnosis BMI 41.0.

(Continued)

Using your ICD-10-CM book code the above diagnoses to the highest specificity listed.

1. _____

2. _____

1. The first section the student will use to locate the term is the Alphabetic Index. After location of the term Diabetes Mellitus, search for type 2 in the Alphabetic Index and locate the code.

2. Verify the code in the tabular as done in Case Study 5.1.

1. To code BMI (Body Mass Index) locate body in your Alphabetic Index. Find body mass index and locate the number referenced to above.

2. Again verify the code in the Tabular List.

Placeholder

The ICD-10-CM utilizes a placeholder character "X". The "X" is used as a placeholder at certain codes to allow for future expansion. A placeholder "X" is used as a fifth character placeholder at certain six-character codes to allow for further expansion, without disturbing the six-character structure.

Examples

An initial encounter for accidental poisoning by penicillin is coded:

T36.0X1A

Primary open-angle glaucoma, moderate state: H40.1192
The "X" in the fifth-character position is a placeholder, or filler character.

Z Codes
Z codes indicate a reason for an encounter.

Example

Z72 Problems related to lifestyle
  Z72.0 Tobacco use

Laterality

This also applies to bilateral conditions when there are no distinct codes identifying laterality or two different conditions. Some codes do indicate laterality, which refers to right, left, or bilateral. If the condition is bilateral and there are no distinct codes to choose, assign separate codes for the right and left side. If the side is not documented in the record, assign the code for the unspecified laterality.

Examples

C50.511—Malignant Neoplasm of lower-outer quadrant of right female breast
C50.512—Malignant Neoplasm of lower-outer quadrant of left female breast
H16.013—Central Corneal Ulcer, bilateral
L89.012—Pressure Ulcer of right elbow, stage II

Combination codes for certain conditions and common associated symptoms and manifestations

Examples

K57.21—Diverticulitis of large intestine with perforation and abscess with bleeding
E11.3419—Type 2 Diabetes Mellitus with severe nonproliferative diabetic retinopathy with macular edema
I25.110—Atherosclerotic Heart Disease of native coronary artery with unstable angina pectoris

Combination codes for poisonings and their associated external cause

Example

T42.3X2S—Poisoning by barbiturates, intentional self-harm, sequela

Obstetric codes identify trimester instead of episode of care

Example

O26.02—Excessive weight gain in pregnancy, second trimester

CHARACTER "X" is used as a fifth character placeholder in certain six-character codes to allow for future expansion and to fill in other empty characters (e.g., character five and/or six) when a code that is fewer than six characters in length requires a seventh character.

Examples

T46.1X5A—Adverse effect of calcium-channel blockers, initial encounter
T15.02XD—Foreign body in cornea, left eye, subsequent encounter

Two Types of Exclude Notes
Excludes 1 indicates that the code excluded should never be used with the code where the note is located (do not report both codes).

> ### Example
>
> Q03—Congenital Hydrocephalus
> Excludes 1: Acquired Hydrocephalus (G91.-)

Excludes 2 indicates that the condition excluded is not part of the condition represented by the code but the patient may have both conditions at the same time, in which case both codes may be assigned together (both codes can be reported to capture both conditions).

> ### Example
>
> L27.2—Dermatitis due to ingested food
> Excludes 2: Dermatitis due to food in contact with skin (L23.6, L24.6, L25.4)

Coding Condition

Code any condition described at the time of discharge as "impending" or "threatened" as follows:

- If it did occur, code as confirmed diagnosis.
- If it did not occur, refer to the Alphabetic Index to determine if the condition has a subentry term for impending or threatened and also main entries for Impending or Threatened.
- If the subterms are listed, assign the given code.
- If the subterms are not listed, code the existing underlying condition and not the condition described as impending or threatened.

Body Mass Index

If the **body mass index (BMI)** is to be documented, it must be provided by the patient's provider as a secondary diagnosis.

Chapter-Specific Guidelines

In addition to general coding guidelines, each chapter has its specific guidelines for diagnoses and/or conditions in the classifications. The coder must refer to these guidelines to accomplish coding to the highest level of certainty and specificity.

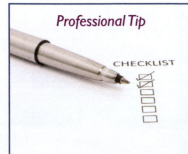

Professional Tip

CHECKLIST

Codes that describe symptoms and signs, as opposed to diagnoses, are acceptable for reporting purposes when a diagnosis has not been established (confirmed) by the provider. Chapter 18 of ICD-10-CM, Symptoms, Signs and Abnormal Clinical and Laboratory Findings Not Elsewhere Classified (codes R00–R99) contains many, but not all codes for symptoms.

Correct Coding Steps

Step 1. Identify the reason for the encounter.

The ailment, **manifestation** (**sign** or symptom of a disease), reason for the encounter, or diagnosis is looked up under the condition. Code only what is documented in the record. Oftentimes, the patient may have two or more visits before a diagnosis is determined. If *symptoms, manifestation* are documented but a definitive diagnosis has not been established, code the symptoms. *A manifestation code represents a demonstration of some aspect of an underlying disease which is separately classifiable in the Alphabetic Index. These codes are listed as secondary code in brackets. The underlying code is listed first.* For outpatient cases, do not code conditions that are referred to as "rule out," "suspected," "probable," or "questionable."

Step 2. **After selecting the reason for the encounter, always consult the Alphabetic Index before verifying the code selection in the tabular section.**

To prevent coding errors, always use both the Alphabetic Index (to identify the code) and the Tabular List to verify the code. The index does not include the important instructional notes which are found in the Tabular List and the coder can also see another more specific code in the Tabular List that wasn't in the Alphabetic Index. Many of the codes also require a fourth, fifth, sixth, or seventh character to be valid, which only will be found in the Tabular List.

Step 3. **Locate the main term entry.**

The Alphabetic Index is a listing of conditions which may be expressed as nouns or eponyms with critical use of adjectives. Reasons for encounters may be located under general terms such as admission, encounter, and examination. Other general terms could include history of, status post, or presence of, which are used to locate factors influencing health.

Examples of chart notes and the **main term** (the primary diagnosis) follow.

Example

Patient comes in for a physical examination (checkup). The *primary diagnosis* would be Physical Examination. The *main term* would be Examination, and the subterm is Physical.

Example

Patient comes in for a blood pressure check because of hypertension. The *primary diagnosis* is Hypertension. The *main term* is Hypertension.

Example (Use your ICD-10-CM to follow the coding instructions)

Patient presents with the chief complaint of right foot pain. If the physician is unable to diagnose the condition at the time of the visit/encounter, the chief complaint is used. The *main term* would be Pain, which would be located in the index:

> Pain(s) (*see also* Painful) and then the anatomic site or body part is chosen, in this case foot—see Pain, limb, lower. Search for limb, lower foot.
> M79.67

Review the Tabular List with M79.67—and locate right.
The primary diagnosis code is M79.671

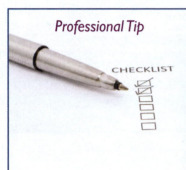

Professional Tip

CHECKLIST

At the time of their visit, patients often have more than one chief complaint or additional illnesses that may affect their present condition and/or treatment. Thus, the primary diagnosis is always listed first as the main reason for the visit/encounter, followed by any other conditions, symptoms, manifestations, or illnesses.

When researching the diagnosis, condition, or symptom, the *main term* will be in *boldface* type and followed by a code.

Example

Patient presents with the chief complaint of abdominal pain left lower quadrant. The *main term* is Pain R10.

Subterms are always indented two spaces to the right under main terms. **Subterms** may show the **etiology** (the cause or origin) of the disease or describe a particular type or body site for the main term, as shown in the following example.

Example

Pain(s) (*see also* Painful) R52   Anginoid (*see* Pain, precordial)
    abdominal R10.9   anus K62.89
    acute R52
    adnexa (uteri) R10.2   arm (*see* Pain, limb, upper
                                      axillary) (axilla) M79.62

Supplementary terms are not essential to the selection of the correct code but aid the coder in finding the correct term. Supplementary terms are in parentheses or brackets, as shown in the Example below.

Step 4. **Read cross-references listed with the main term or the subterm.**

Cross-references such as "see and "see also" are identified by italicized type and should always be checked to ensure that all alternative terms are researched.

Example

Pain(s) (*see also* Painful) R52
lower R10.30
    left quadrant R10.32

Carryover lines, or turnover lines, are always indented more than two spaces from the level of the preceding line. If the main term or subterm is too long to fit on one line, as is often the case, carryover or turnover lines are used. It is important for the coder to read carefully to distinguish between carryover lines and subterms.

Example

Pain (*see also* Painful) R52
Abdominal R10.9
  colic R10.83
  generalized R10.84
    with acute abdomen R10.0

Instructional Terms

The Alphabetic Index also includes instructional terms. These terms are discussed next.

See   The "*see*" instruction following a main term in the Alphabetic Index indicates that another term must be referenced. It is necessary to go to the main term referenced by the *see* note to locate the correct code.

Example

Infection, infected, infective (opportunistic) B99.9 locate next purulent—see condition.
Condition-see Disease

See also   A "*see also*" instruction following a main term in the Alphabetic Index indicates that another main term should be referenced. It is necessary to go to the main term referenced with the "see" note to locate the correct code. It is not necessary to follow the "*see also*" note when the original main term provides the necessary code.

> ### Example
>
> Infection, infected, infective (opportunistic) B99.9
> Sinus (chronic) (*see also* Fistula)
> Oligophrenia (*see also* Disability, intellectual)

Code also   A "code also" note instructs that two codes may be required to fully describe a condition, but this note does not provide sequencing direction.

And   The word "and" should be interpreted to mean either "and" or "or" when it appears in a title.

> ### Example
>
> Cases of "tuberculosis of bones," tuberculosis of joints," and "tuberculosis of bones and joints" are classified to subcategory A18.0, Tuberculosis of bones and joints.

With   The word "with" should be interpreted to mean "associated with" or "due to" when it appears in a code title, the Alphabetic Index, or an instructional note in the Tabular List.

The word "with" in the Alphabetic Index is sequenced immediately following the main term, not in alphabetical order.

Excludes Notes   ICD-10-CM has two types of excludes notes. Each type of note has a different definition for use but they are all similar in that they indicate that codes excluded from each other are independent of each other.

> Excludes 1: A type 1 Excludes note is a pure excludes note. It means "NOT CODED HERE!" An excludes 1 note indicates that the code excluded should never be used at the same time as the code above the Excludes 1 note. An Excludes 1 is used when two conditions cannot occur together, such as a congenital form versus an acquired form of the same condition.
>
> Excludes 2: A type 2 Excludes note represents "Not included here." An Excludes 2 note indicates that the condition excluded is not part of the condition represented by the code, but a patient may have both conditions at the same time. When an Excludes 2 note appears under a code, it is acceptable to use both the code and the excluded code together, when appropriate.

Abbreviations

Alphabetic Index abbreviations

NEC "Not elsewhere classifiable": This abbreviation in the Alphabetic Index represents "other specified." When a specific code is not available for a condition, the Alphabetic Index directs the coder to the "other specified" code in the Tabular List.

NOS "Not otherwise specified": This abbreviation is the equivalent of unspecified.

Tabular List abbreviations

NEC "Not elsewhere classifiable": This abbreviation in the Tabular Lists represents "other specified." When a specific code is not available for a condition, the Tabular List includes an NEC entry under a code to identify the code as the "other specified" code.

NOS "Not otherwise specified": This abbreviation is the equivalent of unspecified.

Step 5. Review entries for modifiers.

Nonessential modifiers are the terms in parentheses following the main term entry. These parenthetical terms are supplementary words or explanatory information that may or may not appear in the diagnostic statement and do not affect code selection. The **diagnostic statement** contains the medical term describing the condition for which a patient is receiving care. For each encounter, this medical documentation includes the main reason for the patient's visit. It may also provide description of additional conditions or symptoms that have been treated or that are related to the patient's current illness. The subterms listed under the main term are essential modifiers that do affect coding assignment. Each line of indent represents a more specific code entry.

Step 6. Interpret abbreviations, cross-references, default codes, additional characters and brackets.

The abbreviation NEC (not elsewhere classified) that follows some main terms or subterms indicates that there is no specific code for the condition even though the medical documentation may be very specific. The code next to the main term is called the **default code**.

Punctuation

The punctuations in the Alphabetic Index and Tabular List have specific meaning to the coder:

:   *Colons* are used after an incomplete phrase or term that requires one or more of the modifiers indented under it to make it assignable to a given category. The exception to this rule pertains to the abbreviation NOS, which is discussed in the next section.

[ ]   *Square brackets* are used to enclose synonyms, alternate wordings, or explanatory phrases in the Tabular List. Brackets are used in the Alphabetic Index to identify manifestation codes.

( )   *Parentheses* are used in both the Alphabetic Index and Tabular List to enclose supplementary words that may be present or absent in a statement of disease without affecting the code assignment. The terms within the parentheses are referred to as nonessential modifiers. The nonessential modifiers in the Alphabetic Index to Diseases apply to subterms following a main term, except when a nonessential modifier and a subentry are mutually exclusive, the subentry takes precedence.

Example

In the ICD-10-CM Alphabetic Index under the main term Enteritis, "acute" is a nonessential modifier and "chronic" is a subentry. In this case, the nonessential modifier "acute" does not apply to the subentry "chronic."

Example

Enteritis (acute) (diarrheal) (hemorrhagic) (noninfective) (septic) K52.9
  Chronic (noninfectious) K52.9

Practice Exercise 5.1 should be completed using your ICD10-CM.

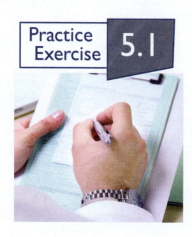

Practice Exercise 5.1

Indicate whether the following three statements are true or false about the Alphabetic Index:

1. _____ A hyphen (-) at the end of an entry indicates additional characters are required.

2. _____ The initial diagnosis search should begin in this index.

3. _____ Subcategories are either three or four characters.

Place a double underline below the main terms and a single underline below any subterms in each of the following statements. Then, using your ICD-10-CM manual, determine the correct diagnosis codes in the Alphabetic Index only:

1. Restless legs syndrome _____

2. Rheumatoid arthritis _____

3. Spasmodic asthma with status asthmaticus _____
   _____

4. Acute serous otitis media right _____

5. Congenital stenosis of the aortic valve _____

6. Occlusion and stenosis of cerebral artery without cerebral infarction
   _____

7. Bone marrow donor _____

8. Gastrointestinal disorder newborn _____

9. Tuberculin test with abnormal result _____

10. Ulcer lower limb with bone necrosis _____

11. Examination; follow-up after completed treatment for malignant neoplasm _____

12. Pneumopathy due to organic dust _____

13. Sclerosing keratitis right eye _____

14. Malocclusion due to abnormal swallowing _____

15. Obstructive (adult) (pediatric) sleep apnea _____

Etiology/manifestation ("code first," "use additional code," and "in diseases classified elsewhere" notes)

Certain conditions have both an underlying etiology and multiple body system manifestations due to the underlying etiology. For such conditions, the ICD-10-CM has a coding convention that requires the underlying condition be sequenced first followed by the manifestation (symptoms only) and never for causes. Wherever such a combination exists, there is a "use additional code" note at the etiology code, and a "code first" note at the manifestation code. These instructional notes indicate the proper sequencing order of the codes, etiology followed by manifestation.

Use Additional Code

The "Use additional code" instruction is placed in the Tabular List in those categories where the coder may wish to add further information, by means of an additional code, to give a more complete picture of the diagnosis or procedure. "*Code also*" is the same as "Use additional code."

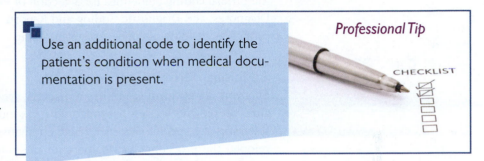

Professional Tip

Use an additional code to identify the patient's condition when medical documentation is present.

CHECKLIST

Example

An example of this would be √ 4th K25 Gastric ulcer (in the Tabular List)
Use additional code to identify:

Alcohol abuse and dependence (F10.-)

If the medical diagnosis was Acute gastric ulcer with both hemorrhage and
    perforation, alcohol abuse, uncomplicated
The coder would then code K25.2, F10.10

Step 7. Choose a potential code and locate it in the Tabular List.

The coder must follow any includes, Excludes 1, and Excludes 2 notes, and other instructional notes, such as "Code first" and "Use additional code," listed in the Tabular List for the chapter, category, subcategory, and subclassification level of code selection that directs the coder to use a different or additional code.

ICD-10-CM classifies encounters with healthcare providers for circumstances other than a disease or injury using codes in Chapter 21, "Factors Influencing Health Status and Contact with Health Services," Codes Z00–Z99.8. Circumstances other than a disease or injury are recorded as chiefly responsible for the encounter.

Step 8. Determine whether the code is at the highest level of specificity.

A code is invalid if it has not been coded to the full number of characters (greatest level of specificity) required. Codes in ICD-10-CM can contain from three up to seven alphanumeric characters. A three-character code is to be used only if the category is not further subdivided into four-, five-, or six-character codes. Placeholder character X is used both to allow for future expansion and as a placeholder for empty characters in a code that requires a seventh character but has no fourth, fifth, or sixth character. Certain categories require seventh characters that apply to all codes in that category. Always check the category level for applicable seventh characters for that category.

Step 9. Assign the code.

Having reviewed all relevant information concerning the possible choices, assign the code that most completely describes the condition.

Step 10. Sequence codes correctly.

List first the ICD-10-CM code for the diagnosis, condition, problem or other reason for the encounter which is shown in the medical record to be chiefly responsible for the services provided. List additional codes that describe any coexisting conditions. Follow the official coding guidelines for Selection of Principal Diagnosis, Reporting Additional Diagnoses, and Diagnostic Coding and Reporting guidelines for Outpatient Services on proper sequencing of codes. Assign the code.

Additional Terms

Eponyms An **eponym** is a term for diseases, syndromes, and procedures that are named after people and locales. A **syndrome** is a group of symptoms that together are characteristic of a specific disorder. Some eponyms are named after the physician who developed the procedure and some after the patient who has the disease. Examples of eponyms are Lou Gehrig's disease, Legionnaires' disease, Lyme disease, and Hodgkin's disease. The diagnostic statement may list the eponym or medical term(s) for the condition. For example, amyotrophic lateral sclerosis may be documented instead of Lou Gehrig's disease. Either the medical term or the eponym may be used to locate the main term in the Alphabetic Index.

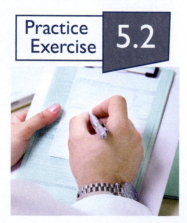

Practice Exercise 5.2

Use your ICD-10-CM manual to select the correct diagnosis codes for the following sample narrative description. Code the following:

Patient presents with severe headache; rule out brain tumor _____

Surgical Coding

For surgical procedures, use the ICD-10-CM code for the diagnosis for which the surgery was performed. If the postoperative diagnosis is known to be different from the preoperative diagnosis at the time the claim is filed, use the ICD-10-CM code for the postoperative diagnosis. Before coding, the medical office specialist should check the operative report to verify whether the postoperative diagnosis is different from the preoperative diagnosis.

Use your ICD-10-CM manual to select the correct diagnosis codes for the following sample narrative description. Code the following:

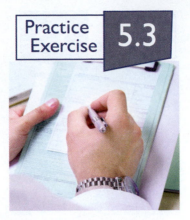

Practice Exercise 5.3

1. Outlet dysfunction constipation _____

2. Sleep disturbance _____

3. Generalized convulsive epilepsy _____

4. Chronic obstructive asthma with an acute exacerbation _____

5. Decubitus ulcer of the hip _____

Use your ICD-10-CM manual to select the correct diagnosis codes for the following sample narrative description.

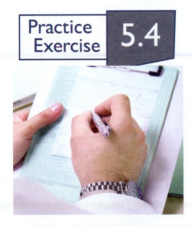

Practice Exercise 5.4

1. Code the following diagnoses:

OPERATIVE REPORT

PREOPERATIVE DIAGNOSIS: Lump in right breast _____

POSTOPERATIVE DIAGNOSIS: Malignant neoplasm primary lower_____

2. Which diagnosis is reported on the claim form? _____

Coding Late Effects

A **late effect**, also referred to as a **residual effect** or **sequela**, is a condition that remains after a patient's acute illness or injury. There is no time limit on when a late effect can be used. The residual may be apparent early, such as in stroke cases, or it may occur months or years later. The diagnostic statement may say "Late, due to an old . . ." or "Due to a previous. . . ." Thus, coding of late effects generally requires two codes sequenced in the following order:

1. The condition or nature of the late effect is sequenced first.
2. The late effect code is sequenced second.

The diagnosis will require two codes: The first code will be the late effect, followed by the code for the cause or etiology. Go to "Late effect" (sequelae) in the Alphabetic Index.

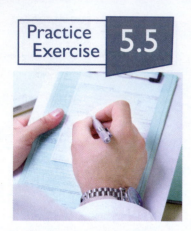

Practice Exercise 5.5

Use your ICD-10-CM manual to select the correct diagnosis codes for the following sample narrative description. Code the following:

1. Dysphagia from a CVA _____

2. Swelling due to an old fracture of the right shoulder _____

3. Nausea as a late effect of radiation sickness _____

4. Muscle weakness due to an old sprain and strain of the ankle _____

Example

Muscle weakness due to acute paralytic poliomyelitis, unspecified.

Correct Coding Order: M62.81, A80.30

Acute and Chronic Conditions

If the same condition is described as both acute (subacute) and chronic, and separate subentries exist in the Alphabetic Index at the same indentation level, code both and sequence the acute (subacute) code first. A sudden flare-up or exacerbation of a patient's chronic condition may be characterized as acute.

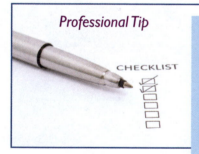

Professional Tip

CHECKLIST

If the encounter is for an illness for which the Alphabetic Index gives a choice of acute versus chronic, code the acute first.

Combination Codes: Multiple Coding

In addition to difficult coding situations, for some cases you will need to recognize the need for "multiple" or **"combination"** codes. Multiple coding means that two or more codes are used together to accurately identify a diagnosis. Multiple codes are necessary whenever you see that the ICD-10-CM notes "Use additional code" or "Code also underlying disease."

A combination code is a single code used to classify:

Two diagnoses, or
A diagnosis with an associated secondary process (manifestation)
A diagnosis with an associated complication.

Combination codes are identified by referring to subterm entries in the Alphabetic Index and by reading the inclusion and exclusion notes in the Tabular List.

Assign only the combination code when that code fully identifies the diagnostic conditions involved or when the Alphabetic Index so directs. Multiple coding should not be used when the classification code lacks necessary specificity in describing the manifestation or complication; an additional code should be used as a secondary code.

Use your ICD-10-CM manual to select the correct diagnosis codes for the following sample narrative description. Code the following:

1. Acute renal failure _____

2. Chronic renal failure _____

Practice Exercise 5.6

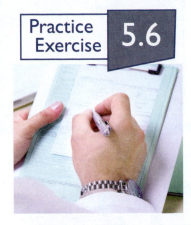

Answer the following questions, and use your ICD-10-CM manual to select the correct diagnosis code(s) for the sample narrative description:

1. What does code J01 excludes 1 mean? _____

_____

2. What does code J03 excludes 2 mean? _____

_____

3. What are the main term and cross-referenced term for "fracture"? _____

_____

4. The note under 139 instructs the coder to do what? _____

_____

5. When coding diabetic nephropathy, which code is listed first? _____

_____

Practice Exercise 5.7

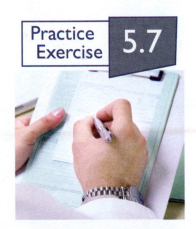

Example

Traumatic subdural hemorrhage without loss of consciousness S06.5X0

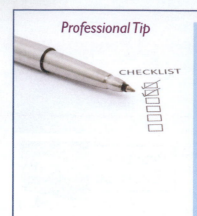

Professional Tip

CHECKLIST

Keep these important tips in mind about the ICD-10-CM manual:
- Be very familiar with the conventions of your ICD-10-CM publication.
- Use only the most current ICD-10-CM version available.
- Read all the information available in your ICD-10-CM for headings, categories, and additional characters.
- Read the Specific Guidelines to each Chapter.

Typically, the ICD-10-CM guides you to the correct codes, but you need to take the time to read through information thoroughly once you have all the facts about the patient. Oftentimes, the problem is not that coders cannot find the appropriate code in the manual, but that they have not been provided with enough information. When a treatment or diagnostic statement from a physician is too general or does not match the descriptions in the ICD-10-CM manual, the coder needs to investigate and get the information necessary to code correctly.

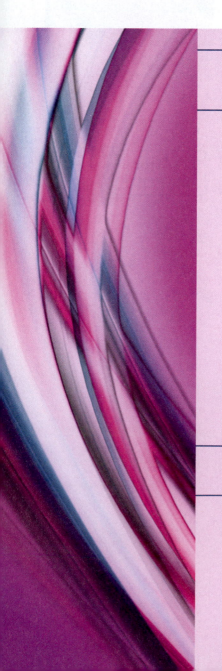

Chapter Summary

- ICD-10-CM coding is used by physicians' offices, hospitals, clinics, home healthcare agencies, and other healthcare providers to substantiate the need for patient care or treatment and to provide statistics for morbidity and mortality rates.
- The Coding Guidelines for the ICD-10-CM are as follows:

  1. Identify the reason for the encounter.
  2. After selecting the reason for the encounter, consult the Alphabetic Index.
  3. Locate the main term entry.
  4. Read cross-references listed with the main term or subterm.
  5. Review entries for modifiers.
  6. Interpret abbreviations, cross-references, default codes, additional characters, and brackets.
  7. Choose a potential code and locate it in the Tabular List.
  8. Determine whether the code is at the highest level of specificity.
  9. Assign the code.
  10. Sequence codes correctly.

ICD-10-PCS

The International Classification of Diseases, 10th Revision, Procedure Coding System was developed to replace the Volume III of the International Classification of Diseases, Ninth Revision (ICD-9-CM). ICD-10-PCS is a separate book that provides a unique code for all inpatient procedures and which also allows for new procedures, devices and technologies to be incorporated as new codes without disrupting the structure of ICD-10-PCS. The codes are seven-character alphanumeric structure.

General Characteristics of ICD-10-PCS

- Diagnostic information is not included in the procedure description and is used to report procedures only in hospital healthcare settings.
- Explicit use of NOS (not otherwise specified) options are restricted.
- Limited use of NEC (not elsewhere classified).
- Level of specificity for all procedures in ICD-10-PCS.

Code Structure

ICD-10-PCS has a seven-character alphanumeric code structure. A code is derived by choosing a specific value for each of the seven characters. The procedure performed gives value to each character. The seven characters follow the structure below:

1. Section
2. Body System
3. Root Operation
4. Body Part
5. Approach
6. Device
7. Qualifier

Because the definition of each character is also a function of its physical position in the code, the same letter or number placed in a different position in the code has a different meaning. Procedures are divided into sections that identify the general type of procedure (e.g., Medical and Surgical, Obstetrics, Imaging). The first character of the procedure code always specifies the section. The second through the seventh characters have the same meaning within each section but may mean different things in other sections. The third character specifies the general type of procedure performed (e.g., Resection, Transfusion, Transplant) while the other characters give additional information such as the body part and approach. Refer to the https://www.cms.gov/Medicare/Coding/ICD10/Downloads/2017-Official-ICD-10-PCS-Coding-Guidelines.pdf.

Example

Amputation of right elbow level.

Locate in the Index Amputation (procedure) see Detachment

Locate Detachment in the Index

Elbow Region
Right 0X6B0ZZ

Code the following:

1. Hysteroscopy with D&C, diagnostic _____
2. Excision of basal cell carcinoma of lower lip: _____
3. EGD with gastric biopsy: _____
4. Cryotherapy of wart on left hand: _____
5. Right total mastectomy, open: _____

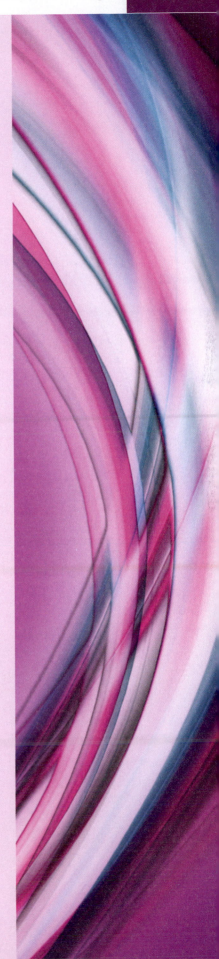

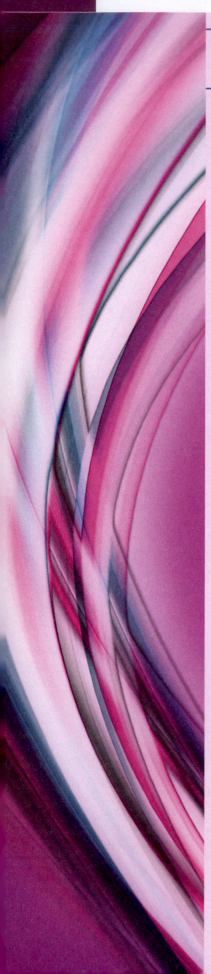

Chapter Review

True/False

Identify the statement as true (T) or false (F).

_____ 1. A sudden flare-up of a patient's chronic condition may be characterized as acute.

_____ 2. The ICD-10-CM diagnosis codes are composed of codes with three to seven characters.

_____ 3. An adverse effect is a harmful reaction caused by an overdose of a drug.

_____ 4. The Alphabetic Index of the ICD-10-CM is used first when locating a diagnostic code.

_____ 5. A coexisting condition is reported when it affects the patient's primary condition or is also treated during an encounter.

_____ 6. The etiology is the origin or cause of a disease.

_____ 7. A late effect occurs some period of time after the acute disease is resolved.

_____ 8. The manifestation is the cause or origin of an illness.

_____ 9. In the ICD-10-CM, NOS, or not otherwise specified, indicates a code to be used when too little information is available to assign another, more specific code.

_____ 10. The primary diagnosis represents the patient's most serious condition, regardless of the reason for the current encounter.

_____ 11. Subterms appear below the main term in the ICD-10-CM's Alphabetic Index.

_____ 12. Supplemental terms in the ICD-10-CM's Alphabetic Index are usually enclosed in parentheses or brackets.

_____ 13. A default code is listed next to a main term in the ICD-10-CM Alphabetic Index.

_____ 14. The ICD-10-CM diagnostic codes are made up of either three, four, or five digits and a description.

_____ 15. Codes in the Tabular List of the ICD-10-CM are organized according to anatomic system or cause.

_____ 16. In the ICD-10-CM, parentheses are used around descriptions that are not essential modifiers of the term.

_____ 17. In the ICD-10-CM, a colon used with "Includes" or "Excludes" indicates a partial term that must be completed with one of the words following the colon.

_____ 18. The Alphabetic Index of the ICD-10-CM can be used alone to correctly locate a diagnostic code.

_____ **19.** The guidelines for outpatient or physician practice diagnostic coding are the same as those that are followed to select codes for inpatients in hospitals.

_____ **20.** A late effect usually requires two diagnosis codes: first the code for the specific late effect and second the code for the cause.

_____ **21.** Signs and symptoms are reported when a patient's condition has not been diagnosed.

_____ **22.** All of the patient's conditions, including diseases or illnesses no longer active or present, must be considered when selecting the correct diagnostic code for an encounter.

_____ **23.** -Z. ICD10-PCS is used for coding outpatient procedures.

_____ **24.** A patient's chronic condition is reported each time it is treated during an encounter.

_____ **25.** ICD-10-PCS is found in ICD-10-CM.

Multiple Choice

Identify the letter of the choice that best completes the statement or answers the question.

_____ **1.** A combination code in the ICD-10-CM covers the:
   a. coexisting condition.   c. chronic and acute illness.
   b. etiology and manifestation.   d. None of the above

_____ **2.** A comparison of two coding systems that shows which codes are used for similar classifications is a:
   a. convention.   c. crosswalk.
   b. category.   d. manifestation.

_____ **3.** A disease or procedure that is named for a person is a(n):
   a. eponym.   c. etiology.
   b. E code.   d. manifestation.

_____ **4.** A placeholder must be used in the ICD-10-CM if the
   a. code requires seventh character.
   b. code requires sixth character.
   c. All of the above
   d. Where an X is noted

_____ **5.** A personal history of cancer is reported with a(n):
   a. E code.   c. combination code.
   b. Z code.   d. None of the above

_____ **6.** The cross-reference _see also_ in the ICD-10-CM means that the coder:
   a. may look up the related term(s) that follows.
   b. must refer to the term that follows.
   c. Either a or b
   d. Neither a nor b

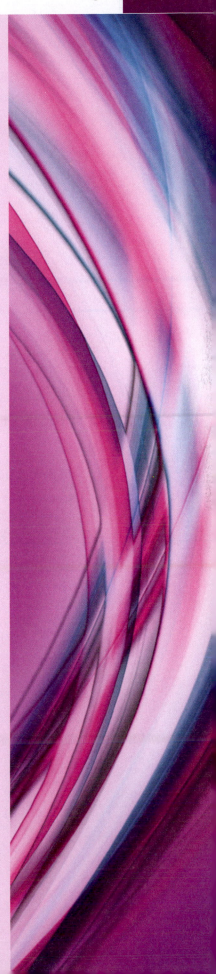

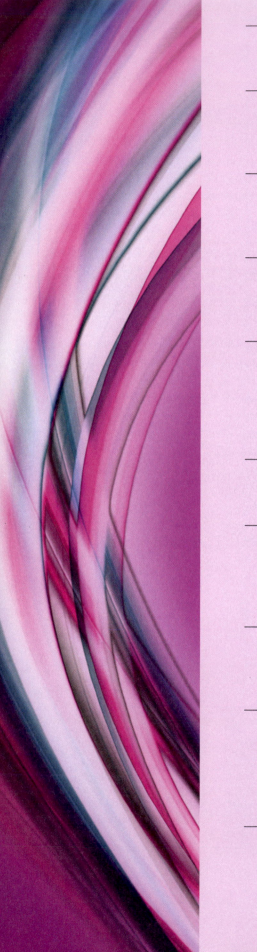

_____ **7.** An annual checkup is classified with a(n):

a. combination code.   c. H code.

b. Z code   d. five-digit code.

_____ **8.** The statement, "patient has a family history of breast cancer," requires a(n):

a. combination code.   c. Z code.

b. M code.   d. five-digit code.

_____ **9.** To find a code correctly in the ICD-10-CM, the first step is to locate the code in the:

a. Tabular List.   c. Either a or b

b. Alphabetic Index.   d. Neither a nor b

_____ **10.** A condition that arises because of an injury or illness in the patient's medical history is called a(n):

a. adverse effect.   c. comorbidity.

b. manifestation.   d. late effect.

_____ **11.** Which section of the ICD-10-CM contains the code for a diagnostic statement of "elevated blood pressure"?

a. Z Codes

b. D codes

c. Symptoms, Signs, and Ill-Defined Conditions

d. Diseases of the Circulatory System

_____ **12.** In the ICD-10-CM, M codes (morphology codes) are used by:

a. pathologists.   c. outpatient coders.

b. nutritionists.   d. radiologists.

_____ **13.** In the ICD-10-CM's Neoplasm Table, a neoplasm is categorized as either:

a. malignant, benign, uncertain, or unspecified.

b. malignant, primary, secondary, or in situ.

c. primary, secondary, uncertain, or unspecified.

d. primary, secondary, in situ, or uncertain.

_____ **14.** In the ICD-10-CM, burns are coded with the 7th character to include the : coded as to:

a. sequela.   c. subsequent encounter.

b. site initial encounter.   d. All of the above

_____ **15.** The seventh character to be added to each code from category S92 (fracture) may include:

a. initial encounter for open fracture.

b. initial encounter for closed fracture.

c. subsequent encounter for fracture with delayed healing.

d. All of the above and more

_____ **16.** Use of Z codes in any healthcare setting may be used as all of the below except:

a. principal DX in the inpatient setting.

b. as a procedure code.

c. reason for the encounter.

d. history of signs and symptoms.

Completion

Complete each sentence or statement.

1. A physician's description of the main reason for a patient's encounter is called the diagnostic _____.

2. A(n) _____ effect remains after a patient's acute illness or injury.

3. If a fracture is not recorded as either closed or open, it is coded as _____.

4. When diagnostic codes are reported, the code for the _____ diagnosis is listed first, followed by the current coexisting conditions.

5. The guideline of not assigning diagnostic codes for suspected or probable conditions is referred to as "coding to the highest level of _____."

6. After surgery, the patient's diagnosis is different from the preoperative primary diagnosis. Which diagnosis is coded? _____

For Additional Practice

Code the following:

1. Acute bronchospasm _____

2. Herpes zoster myelitis _____

3. Smoking complicating pregnancy, childbirth, antepartum condition, or complication _____

4. Epilepsy complicating pregnancy, childbirth, or the puerperium _____

5. Uterine size date discrepancy, delivered _____

6. Encounter for removal of sutures _____

7. Papanicolaou smear of cervix with cytologic evidence of malignancy _____

8. Straining on urination _____

9. Postnasal drip _____

Resources

Private Website
www.icd10data.com/ICD10CM/Codes

Free online resource of online diagnostic codes.

National Center for Health Statistics (NCHS)
www.cdc.gov/nchs/

Website for Department of Health and Human Services, Centers for Disease Control and Prevention.

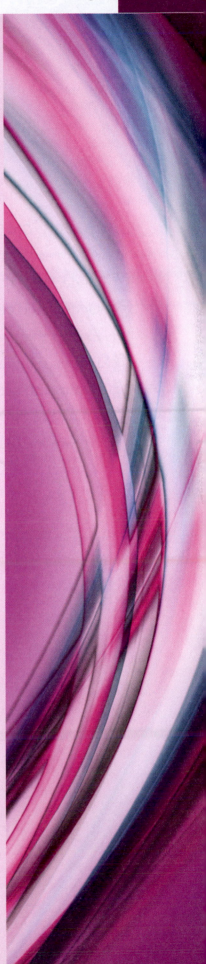

Chapter 6 / Introduction to CPT® and Place of Service Coding

Chapter Objectives

After reading this chapter, the student should be able to:

1. Understand the history of CPT.
2. Understand evaluation and management (E/M) services.
3. Explain the three types of CPT categories.
4. Distinguish the need for modifiers.
5. Distinguish between a new and established patient.
6. Know the three key elements in choosing an E/M code.
7. Determine the correct E/M code.

Key Terms

American Medical
   Association (AMA)
Centers for Medicare and
   Medicaid Services
   (CMS)
chief complaint (CC)
consultation
counseling
Current Procedural

Terminology (CPT)
E/M codes
established patient
examination
history
history of present illness
   (HPI)
medical decision making
   (MDM)

modifiers
nature of the presenting
   problem
new patient
nomenclature
past, family, and social
   history (PFSH)
review of systems (ROS)

CPT-4 codes in this chapter are from the CPT-4 2017 code set. CPT® is a registered trademark of the American Medical Association.

Introduction to CPT and Place of Service Coding

Mr. Levins previously had been a patient of Dr. Mitchell but had moved out of the area 6 years ago. He recently moved back and was seeing the doctor for the first time since he had returned. Dr. Mitchell asked the billing supervisor whether he should bill Mr. Levins as a new or established patient.

She explained that the requirement for billing as a new or established patient was determined by the date the patient had last been seen by the provider. In this case, because it had been more than 3 years since the last date of service, Mr. Levins would be considered a new patient for billing purposes.

Questions

1. Why is there a differentiation made between a new and established patient even when the patient was seen by the doctor previously?

2. Do all E/M codes contain that differentiation?

3. What would be the result of an error in coding the patient as new when he was actually established?

4. What is the rule for determining when a patient is new or established for billing purposes?

Understanding the use of procedure codes is the most important aspect of coding. If used correctly, the procedure codes determine the amount of reimbursement the provider will receive. Diagnostic codes show the reason for the procedure; the CPT codes determine whether the provider will be paid at the maximum or not.

The CPT is copyrighted and published by the American Medical Association and is updated annually. The first section of the CPT is known as Evaluation and Management (E/M) Services. These codes describe services provided by physicians to evaluate their patients and manage their care. This is the only section from which codes are used directly. The codes are widely used by physicians of all specialties and describe a very large portion of the medical care provided to patients of all ranges. This chapter discusses how the **E/M codes** are used to report office visits, hospital visits, nursing home visits, rehabilitation center visits, and home visits. The classification of E/M services is important because the nature of physician activity and practice resource costs vary by the type of service, place of service, and patient's status and age.

Current Procedural Terminology (CPT)

The **American Medical Association (AMA)** first developed and published the **Current Procedural Terminology (CPT)** in 1966. The first edition helped encourage the use of standard terms and descriptors to document procedures in the medical record, helped communicate accurate information on procedures and services to agencies concerned with insurance claims, provided the basis for a computer-oriented system to evaluate operative procedures, and contributed basic information for actuarial and statistical purposes.

This first edition of the CPT primarily contained surgical procedures, with limited sections on medicine, radiology, and laboratory procedures. When first published, CPT coding used a four-digit system. The second edition, published in 1970, presented an expanded system of terms and codes to designate diagnostic and therapeutic procedures in surgery, medicine, and specialties. It was at this time that the five-digit codes were introduced, replacing the former four-digit system. Another significant change to the book was to list procedures related to internal medicine.

In the mid to late 1970s, the third and fourth editions of the CPT were introduced. The fourth edition, published in 1977, represented significant updates in medical technology, and a system of periodic updating was introduced to keep pace with the rapidly changing medical environment.

In 1983, CPT nomenclature was adopted for use by the **Centers for Medicare and Medicaid Services (CMS)**, formerly the Health Care Financing Administration (HCFA), as part of its Healthcare Procedure Coding System (HCPCS). With this adoption, CMS mandated the use of HCPCS (CPT) to report services for Part B of the Medicare program. In October 1986, as part of the Omnibus Budget Reconciliation Act, CMS also required state Medicaid agencies to use CPT codes for reporting outpatient hospital surgical procedures. Physicians may use procedure codes from any of the sections of the CPT.

In August 2000, the CPT code set was named as a national standard under the Health Insurance Portability and Accountability Act of 1996 (HIPAA).

Procedure codes are linked with diagnostic codes to establish the medical necessity of the procedure and the fee reimbursement to the providers. Medical office specialists should be aware of the importance of correct procedure coding. With a thorough knowledge of a third-party payer's policies, definition of "medical necessity," guidelines, and reporting requirements, the medical office specialist will be able to effectively submit "clean claims" (i.e., claims with no errors).

CPT Categories

The CPT has three categories: CPT Category I, CPT Category II, and CPT Category III.

All modifications and deletions are approved by the CPT Editorial Panel. The Editorial Panel consists of staff associated with national medical specialty societies, health insurance organizations and agencies, and individual physicians and other healthcare professionals. The CPT code set is published annually in the late summer or early fall as both electronic data files and books. The release of CPT data files on the Internet typically precedes the book by several weeks. January 1 is the effective date for use of the update of the CPT code set. The exception to this schedule of release and effective dates are CPT Category II, III and vaccine product codes, which are released twice a year on January 1 or July 1 with effective dates for use 6 months later. Changes to the CPT code set are meant to be applied prospectively from the future date. The interval between the release of the update and the effective date is considered the implementation period and is intended to allow physicians and other providers, payers and vendors to incorporate CPT changes into their systems. CPT Category I is a five-digit numeric code with a descriptor. Category II is a five-digit numeric-alpha code that ends with the letter F. CPT Category III is the same as CPT Category II except the code ends with the letter T.

CPT Category I

CPT Category I codes describe a procedure or service. The descriptor in this category of CPT codes is generally based on the procedure being consistent with contemporary medical practice and widely accepted in the medical community, and thus it is being performed by many physicians in clinical settings. In a healthcare setting today, it is important for the medical office specialist to know who can bill for services. When nurse practioners and physician assistants are working with physicians, they are considered as working in exactly the same specialty and subspecialty as the physician. A physician or other qualified health care professional is an individual who is qualified by education, training, licensure/regulation (when applicable), and facility privilege (when applicable) who performs a professional service within his/her scope of practice and independently reports that professional service. These professionals are distinct from "clinical staff." A clinical staff member is a person who works under the supervision of a physician or other qualified healthcare professional and who is allowed by law, regulation, and facility policy to perform or assist in the performance of a specified professional service, but who does not individually report that professional service. In many hospital settings today, there is a team of providers for the patient. The hospital assigns a hospitalist who oversees the patient for all services. A specific modifier is used with the evaluation and management code when the hospitalist is the principal provider.

CPT Category I codes are subjected to a lengthy approval process conducted by the CPT Editorial Panel, CPT staff and the CPT/HCPAC Advisory Committee. For a procedure to be approved as a CPT Category I code, the CPT Editorial Panel requires at a minimum that many healthcare professionals perform the services across the country. In addition, FDA approval must be documented or imminent within a given CPT cycle, and the service must have proven clinical efficacy.

CPT Category I codes are restricted to clinically recognized and generally accepted services, not emerging technologies, services, and procedures (see CPT Category III discussion).

CPT Category II

CPT Category II codes are a set of optional tracking codes, developed principally for performance measurement. These codes are intended to facilitate data collection by coding certain services and/or test results that are agreed on as contributing to positive health outcomes and quality patient care. These codes may be services that are typically included in an E/M service or other component part of a service and are not appropriate for regular CPT Category I codes. Consequently, the CPT Category II codes do not have a relative value associated with them, as do CPT Category I codes.

The decision to develop CPT Category II codes for performance measures was based on a desire to standardize the collection of data for performance measurement. The current methods are based on detailed chart review or site surveys, which cost physicians time and money. By having coded data on services that are included as elements of performance measures, physicians have the option of supplying this information to plans through the administrative record. In this way, CPT Category II codes will ease the burden on physicians' offices to complete surveys and reduce the intrusion caused by chart review. Use of the administrative record for data on performance measures allows physicians to supply information without substantially adding to their paperwork because this record is currently in use. CPT Category II codes concentrate on measurements that are developed and tested by national organizations, such as the National Committee for Quality Assurance, and those that are well established and currently used by large segments of the healthcare industry. The CPT Editorial Panel does not develop any measures. As with procedures, only CPT Category II codes with standardized language for existing performance measures will be established.

CPT Category II codes are assigned a numeric-alpha identifier with the letter "F" in the last field (e.g., 1234F) to distinguish them from CPT Category I codes. These codes are located in a separate section of the CPT book, following the Medicine section. Introductory language in this code section explains the purpose of these codes. The use of these codes is optional and not required for correct coding. To expedite reporting of CPT Category II codes, once the CPT Editorial Panel has approved these codes, the newly added codes are made available on a semiannual (twice a year) basis via electronic distribution on the AMA website. These are provided for review to prepare for implementation on the effective date of January 1 of each year.

CPT Category III

CPT Category III (Emerging Technology) codes are temporary codes for emerging technologies, services, and procedures. CPT Category III codes are intended to be used for data collection purposes to substantiate widespread use of new technologies, services, and procedures or those that are in the Federal Drug Administration (FDA) approval process. Note that CPT Category III codes are *not* intended for use with services/procedures that have not been accepted by the CPT Editorial Panel because a proposal was incomplete, more information was needed, or the FDA did not support the proposal. An important part of the reasoning behind the development of CPT Category III codes was the length and requirements of the CPT approval process for CPT Category I codes, which conflicted with the needs of researchers for coded data to track emerging technology services throughout the research process.

HIPAA's Final Rule supports the elimination of these local, temporary codes and the transition to national standard code sets. Many of the local, temporary codes were used by payers until services/procedures were more fully substantiated through research and received a CPT Category I code. Thus, CPT Category III codes can take the place of local, temporary codes used for this purpose.

As with CPT Category I codes, inclusion of a descriptor and its associated code number in CPT nomenclature does not represent endorsement by the AMA of any particular diagnostic or therapeutic procedure/service. Inclusion or exclusion of a procedure/service does not imply any health insurance coverage or reimbursement policy.

CPT Category III codes are assigned a numeric-alpha identifier with the letter "T" in the last field (e.g., 1234T). These codes are located in a separate section of the CPT book, following the CPT Category II code section. Introductory language in this code section explains the purpose of these codes. Once they have been approved by the CPT Editorial Panel, the newly added CPT Category III codes are made available on a semiannual basis via electronic distribution on the AMA website. These are provided for review to prepare for implementation on the effective date of January 1 of each year. These codes will be archived after 5 years if the code has not been accepted for placement in the CPT Category I section of the CPT book, unless it is demonstrated that a CPT Category III code is still needed. These archived codes are not reused.

CPT Nomenclature

CPT **nomenclature** consists of descriptive terms, guidelines, and identifying codes for reporting medical services and procedures. Because the CPT nomenclature, a system of naming things, is not a strict classification system, some procedures may appear in sections other than those in which they might ordinarily be "classified."

There are eight sections in the CPT code book. The main body of the Category I is listed in six sections (Figure 6.1). Each section is divided into subsections with anatomic, procedural, condition, or descriptor headings. The procedures or services are presented in numeric order with one exception. The entire Evaluation and Management section appears at the beginning of the listed procedures since this section is used most often by physicians.

Evaluation and Management	99201–99499
Anesthesia	00100–01999, 99100–99140
Surgery	10021–69990
Radiology	70010–79999
Pathology and Laboratory	80048–89356
Medicine	90281–99199, 99500–99607
(except Anesthesiology)	

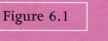

Figure 6.1

CPT Category I codes.

The seventh and eighth sections pertain to the CPT Category II and CPT Category III codes, respectively. Their section names and sequences are as follows:

- CPT Category II Performance Measurement: Codes 0001F–7025F
- CPT Category III New/Emerging Technology Codes: 0019T–0290T

Symbols

To make CPT nomenclature more user friendly, over the years a number of code symbols have been incorporated into the book. On receipt of an updated CPT book, the medical coder should review the symbols. Some of the more frequently used symbols are:

▲ *Revised code.* A triangle indicates that the code's descriptor has substantially altered the procedure descriptor.

• *New code.* This symbol indicates new to this edition.

►◄ *New or revised text.* These symbols enclose new or revised text other than the code's descriptor.

+ *Add-on code.* A plus sign describes secondary procedures only. It cannot be used as a primary code.

0 Editorial CPT Panel Actions. This symbol indicates a reinstated or recycled code.

Guidelines

Specific guidelines are found at the beginning of each of the six sections of CPT Category I. The guidelines provide information that is necessary to appropriately interpret and report procedures and services found in that section. In addition to the guidelines that appear at the beginning of each section, several of the subsections contain special instructions unique to that section, resulting in guidelines and instructional notes appearing throughout the CPT book. Note that these guidelines and notes are critical to using CPT coding correctly.

CPT Modifiers

CPT **modifiers** are two-digit numeric indicators, with the exception of the physical status modifiers found in the guidelines of the Anesthesia section. Appendix A of the CPT book has a complete listing of modifiers including the Anesthesia Physical Status Modifiers, Modifiers approved for Ambulatory Surgery Centers Outpatient Use, and Level II (HCPCS/National) Modifiers.

The two-digit modifier, with a hyphen in front of it, is placed after the five-digit CPT code to indicate that the description of the service or procedure has been altered by some specific circumstance but not changed in its definition or code. Modifiers also enable healthcare providers to effectively respond to payment policy requirements required by third-party payers. The code and modifier are reported as

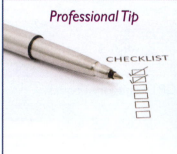

Professional Tip

CHECKLIST

Medicare and some other payers do not pay for inpatient or outpatient consults, although both consults are listed in the CPT manual. The medical office specialist should review coding guidelines provided by each payer before submitting a claim for a consultation.

a one-line entry on the claim. Some modifiers apply only to certain sections; for example, the modifier "-25" is used only for E/M coding.

Evaluation and Management Modifiers

The following modifiers are used for evaluation and management coding:

24 Unrelated Evaluation and Management Service by the Same Physician During a Postoperative Period is used when the E/M service is not related to the reason for surgery and is provided within the postoperative time period (global period) in the payer's reimbursement.

Example

An orthopedic surgeon has performed a knee replacement, and during the postop follow-up the patient presents with a sprained wrist due to a fall. The physician reports an E/M code with the 24 modifier appended to it for the management of the sprained wrist. For the normal postoperative visit, 99024 is used. The "-24" appended to the E/M code, 99024-24, informs the payer that this is separate from the visit for the knee replacement.

25 Significant, Separately Identifiable Evaluation and Management Service by the Same Physician on the Same Day of the Procedure or Other Service is used when the physician provides an E/M service in addition to another E/M service or procedure on the same day. Note: This modifier is not used to report an E/M service that resulted in a decision to perform surgery.

Example

A physician examines a patient for cervical radiculopathy. The modifier "-25" is appended to the 99214. An electromyography is reported as 95861. This shows the payer that a significant E/M service and a procedure were performed on the same day.

32 Mandated Services is used when it is requested by the third party payer, governmental, legislative, or regulatory requirement.

Example

The patient's insurance payer requests a second opinion be performed before undergoing a surgical procedure. The consult is reported with the "-32" modifier attached.

52 Reduced Service is used when an E/M service is less extensive than the descriptor indicates.

Example

The physician began an initial gynecologic exam on the patient, but due to the patient's extreme discomfort, discontinued it. The modifier "-52" is appended to the E/M code.

57 Decision for Surgery is used to indicate the visit was scheduled because a decision to have surgery was made and the patient was informed and counseled about the risks and outcomes.

Example

At the request of his primary care physician (PCP), a patient consults a surgeon about his abdominal pain. The surgeon meets the requirements to report a consultation, and the decision is made also to have surgery. The surgeon reports the consultation with the "-57" modifier attached.

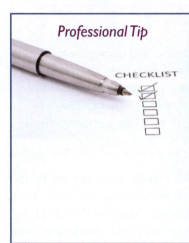

Professional Tip

CHECKLIST

The principal physician of record will append modifier "-AI" to the E/M code when billed. This modifier, which is located in Level II HCPCS, will identify the physician who oversees the patient's care from all other physicians who may be furnishing specialty care. All other physicians who perform an initial evaluation on this patient shall bill only the E/M code for the complexity level performed.

Coding to the Place of Service

The E/M section is divided into broad services such as office visits, hospital visits, assisted living facility, urgent care facility, emergency room, and consultations. Most of the categories are again divided into subcategories of services, such as new patient, established patient; initial hospital care, subsequent hospital care; initial pediatric care, subsequent pediatric care; and initial neonatal critical care, subsequent neonatal critical care.

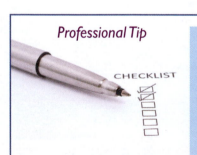

Professional Tip

CHECKLIST

Neither Medicare nor Medicaid pays for prolonged care.

The CPT coding system makes specific distinctions for place of service in the evaluation and management codes. The place of service may have a considerable impact on reimbursement. Verify the correct place of service before choosing a code. The following are some of the ranges of specific places of service:

Office (and Other Outpatient) Services	99201–99215
Observation Care Discharge	99217
Hospital Initial Observation Services	99218–99220
Subsequent Observation Care	99224–99226
Hospital (Inpatient) Services	99221–99223
Subsequent Hospital Care	99231–99233

Inpatient care with Admission & Discharge same date	99234–99236
Hospital Discharge Services	99238–99239
Consultations (Office)	99241–99245
Consultations (Inpatient)	99251–99255
Emergency Department Services	99281–99288
Critical Care Services	99291–99292
Nursing Facility Services	99304–99318
Rest Home, Custodial Care, Domiciliary	99324–99337
Oversight Services for Domiciliary, Rest Home or Home	99339–99340
Home Services	99341–99350
Prolonged Services With Direct Patient Contact	99354–99357
Prolonged Services Without Direct Patient Contact	99358–99359
Pediatric Critical Care Patient Transport	99466–99467

Other Services Provided in the E/M Section

Services found in the Evaluation and Management Section that also can be billed include the following:

Prolonged Services that are reported in addition to other physician services. For this reason these codes are add-on codes. These services can be provided either face-to-face (direct contact) with the patient or without direct contact with patient. The range of these codes is from 99354–99359.

Physician Standby Services (99360) requires prolonged physician attendance without direct patient contact. This service is requested by another physician and is coded according to time for each 30 minutes. Second and subsequent periods of standby beyond the first 30 minutes must be met to bill each unit of time. Examples of standby services include operative standby, standby for cesarean/high-risk birth, standby for frozen section, and for monitoring an EEG.

Other services found in this section that are not coded according to place of service include Case Management Services, team conferences, telephone calls, anticoagulant management, disability and life insurance evaluations, and work-related or medical disability evaluation services and Preventive Medicine Services. The Preventive Medicine Services are used to report the preventive medicine evaluation and management of infants, children, adolescents and adults. The extent and focus of the services will largely depend on the age of the patient.

Office versus Hospital Services

Office and other outpatient services are the most often reported E/M services. A patient is an *outpatient* unless admitted to a healthcare facility such as a hospital or skilled nursing facility for a 24-hour period or longer. When a patient is evaluated and then admitted to a healthcare facility, the service is reported using the codes for initial hospital care. An *inpatient* is a patient who has been admitted to the hospital and is expected to stay 24 hours or more.

Hospital observation service codes are used to report E/M services provided to patients designated as "observation status" in a hospital. These patients are there to be observed to determine whether they should be admitted to the hospital, transferred to another facility, or sent home. Not all hospitals have a specific area designated for observation patients. The patient does not have to be located in an observation area designated by the hospital, but rather designated as observation status.

The codes in this category of service are not used to report hospital observation services involving admission and discharge services provided on the same date. Hospital observation services involving admission and discharge are reported with codes 99234–99236.

Emergency Department Services

E/M services provided in the emergency department are reported with the codes in this series. These codes are not limited to use by emergency department physicians. No distinction is made between new and established patients. The reason for this is that many different physicians staff emergency departments, and the services they provide are unscheduled and episodic. Time is not a factor in selecting the E/M service code.

Preventive Medicine Services

This is a specific category of E/M codes for reporting preventive medicine services. These services include physical examination according to age, ordering of appropriate immunization(s), and laboratory/diagnostic procedures. The performance of immunizations and ancillary studies involving laboratory, radiology, and other procedures or screening tests identified with a specific CPT code is reported separately.

When reporting a preventive medicine E/M service and a problem-oriented E/M service on the same day, pay close attention to the diagnostic codes submitted on the claim. The diagnoses reported should justify the reason for reporting both services on the same day. A modifier -25 should be added to the Office/Outpatient code (99201–99215) to indicate that a significant, separately identifiable evaluation and management service was provided on the same day as the preventive medicine service. The appropriate preventive medicine service is additionally reported.

The initial preventive E/M codes are used to report the preventive medicine evaluation and management of infants, children, adolescents and adults, which include counseling/anticipatory guidance/risk factor reduction interventions which are provided at the time of the initial or periodic comprehensive preventive medicine examination. The "comprehensive" nature of the Preventive Service codes 99381–99397 reflects an age and gender appropriate history/exam and is *not* synonymous with the "comprehensive" examination required in Evaluation and Management codes 99201–99350.

Type of Patient

Once the place of service has been chosen, the type of patient must be identified. To determine if a patient is new or established, one must know the definitions of each.

New Patient

A **new patient** is one who has not received any professional services within the past 3 years from the physician or another physician of the same specialty who belongs to the same group practice.

Established Patient

An **established patient** is one who has received professional services within the past 3 years from the physician or another physician of the same specialty who belongs to the same group practice. Services that have been provided, such as telephone renewal of a prescription, if provided without a face-to-face encounter, are no longer considered when identifying patients as new or established.

Referral

A **referral** is the transfer of the total care or specific portion of care of a patient from one physician to another. A referral is not a request for consultation. If a patient is referred to the physician for total care or a portion of his care, use E/M codes and other CPT codes if appropriate to report the services provided. If a patient is sent to the physician for a consultation, use E/M consultation codes to report the services provided.

Consultation

A **consultation** occurs when a second physician, at the request of the patient's physician or another appropriate source, examines the patient and renders an opinion. The patient must present with a written request for a consultation from the requesting physician (usually the PCP) or source, which should be filled in on the chart. The consultant must document her opinion in the patient's medical record as well as any services performed. The consultant must also render her opinion in writing to the requesting physician. The patient returns to the requesting physician. The consulting physician uses the E/M codes from the Consultations section. The definition of "another appropriate source" includes a physician assistant, nurse practitioner, doctor of chiropractic, physical therapist, occupational therapist, speech language therapist, psychologist, social worker, lawyer, or insurance company.

Level of E/M Service

With each category or subcategory of E/M services, three to five levels are available for reporting purposes. The number of levels within a category varies and is dependent on the types of services that might be provided.

The various levels describe the wide variations in skill, effort, time, and medical knowledge required for the prevention or diagnosis and treatment of illness or injury, and the promotion of optimal health.

The code descriptors for the level of service identify seven components, six of which are used in defining the levels of E/M services:

1. The extent of the history documented
2. The extent of the examination documented
3. The complexity of the medical decision making documented
4. Counseling
5. Coordination of care with other providers
6. Nature of the presenting problem
7. Time

Specific steps must be taken to select the appropriate level of E/M service. Selection is based on the extent of three key components of the seven just listed:

1. The extent of the patient's history obtained
2. The extent of the examination documented
3. The complexity of the medical decision making

These three components are discussed in more detail next. Figure 6.2 is an example of the range of E/M codes that can be used for a new patient.

New Patient

99201 **Office or other outpatient visit** for the evaluation and management of a new patient, which requires these three key components:

- **a Problem Focused History;**
- **a Problem Focused Examination;**
- **straightforward medical decision making.**

Counseling and/or coordination of care with other providers or agencies are provided consistent with the nature of the problem(s) and the patient's and/or family's needs.

Usually the presenting problem(s) are self-limited or minor. Physicians typically spend 10 minutes face-to-face with the patient and/or family.

99202 **Office or other outpatient visit** for the evaluation and management of a new patient, which requires these three key components:

- **an Expanded Problem Focused History;**
- **an Expanded Problem Focused Examination;**
- **straightforward medical decision making.**

Counseling and/or coordination of care with other providers or agencies are provided consistent with the nature of the problem(s) and the patient's and/or family's needs.

Usually, the presenting problem(s) are of low to moderate severity. Physicians typically spend 20 minutes face-to-face with the patient and/or family.

99203 **Office or other outpatient visit** for the evaluation and management of a new patient, which requires these three key components:

- **a Detailed History;**
- **a Detailed Examination;**
- **medical decision making of low complexity.**

Counseling and/or coordination of care with other providers or agencies are provided consistent with the nature of the problem(s) and the patient's and/or family's needs.

Usually, the presenting problem(s) are of moderate severity. Physicians typically spend 30 minutes face-to-face with the patient and/or family.

99204 **Office or other outpatient visit** for the evaluation and management of a new patient, which requires these three key components:

- **a Comprehensive History;**
- **a Comprehensive Examination;**
- **medical decision making of moderate complexity.**

Counseling and/or coordination of care with other providers or agencies are provided consistent with the nature of the problem(s) and the patient's and/or family's needs.

Usually the presenting problem(s) are of moderate to high severity. Physicians typically spend 45 minutes face-to-face with the patient and/or family.

99205 **Office or other outpatient visit** for the evaluation and management of a new patient, which requires these three key components:

- **a Comprehensive History;**
- **a Comprehensive Examination;**
- **medical decision making of high complexity.**

Counseling and/or coordination of care with other providers or agencies are provided consistent with the nature of the problem(s) and the patient's and/or family's needs.

Usually, the presenting problem(s) are of moderate to high severity. Physicians typically spend 60 minutes face-to-face with the patient and/or family.

Figure 6.2   Example of the range of E/M codes available for use with a new patient.

Extent of Patient's History

To determine the extent of the **history** documented, the following information must be obtained from the patient. If the patient is incapacitated, the physician may obtain the history from a family member. The history is documented as follows: (1) chief complaint, (2) history of present illness, (3) review of systems, and (4) past, family, and/or social history. These are discussed in the following subsections.

Chief Complaint

The **chief complaint (CC)** is a concise statement describing the symptom, problem, condition, diagnosis, or other factor that is the reason for the visit/encounter, usually stated in the patient's or guardian's words.

History of Present Illness

The **history of present illness (HPI)** is a chronological description of the development of the patient's present illness from the first sign and/or symptom to the present. Patients usually express their problems as symptoms (e.g., pain or discomfort) or signs (e.g., lump, cut, bruise, rash), with the exception of a newborn, whose presenting complaint may be related to his mother's complaint (e.g., maternal fever during labor). The further elaboration of any symptom requires attention to some or all of the dimensions of the HPI. Signs are better described by physical findings. Problems can also be described as the status of one or more chronic conditions.

CPT guidelines recognize eight dimensions of the HPI, including a description of the following:

1. Location (where in body the CC is occurring)
2. Quality (the character of the pain)
3. Severity (the rank of the symptoms or pain on a scale, such as 1 to 10)
4. Duration (how long the symptom or pain has been present or how long it lasts when it occurs)
5. Timing (when the symptom or pain occurs)
6. Context (the situation that is associated with the pain or symptom, such as eating dairy products)
7. Modifying factors (things done to make the pain or symptom change, such as using an ice pack)
8. Associated signs and symptoms (other things that happen when the symptom or pain happens, such as "When my chest pain occurs I have shortness of breath")

Review of Systems

The **review of systems (ROS)** is an inventory of body systems obtained through a series of questions asked by the physician. The physician seeks to identify signs and/or symptoms that the patient may be experiencing or has experienced. This helps define the problem, clarify the differential diagnosis, identify testing needed, or serve as baseline data on other systems that might be affected by any possible management (treatment) options. An ROS may be highly dependent on the age of the patient and irrelevant for newborns and young infants. The following elements of a system review have been identified in the CPT code set:

- Constitutional symptoms (fever, weight loss, etc.)
- Eyes
- Ears, nose, mouth, throat
- Cardiovascular

- Respiratory
- Gastrointestinal
- Genitourinary
- Musculoskeletal
- Integumentary (skin and/or breast)
- Neurologic
- Psychiatric
- Endocrine
- Hematologic/lymphatic
- Allergic/immunologic

Past, Family, and Social History

The **past, family, and social history (PFSH)** includes a review of past medical experiences of the patient and the patient's family. Past history is dependent on the patient's age and not appropriate for a newborn infant.

The past history is a review of the patient's past experiences with illnesses, injuries, and treatments that includes significant information about the following:

- Prior major illnesses and injuries
- Prior operations
- Prior hospitalizations
- Current medications
- Allergies (e.g., drug, food)
- Age-appropriate immunization status
- Age-appropriate feeding/dietary status

The family history is a review of medical events in the patient's family including significant information about the following:

- The health status or cause of death of parents, siblings, and children
- Specific diseases related to problems identified in the CC, HPI, and/or ROS
- Diseases of family members that may be hereditary or place the patient at risk

The social history is an age-appropriate review of past and current activities that includes significant information about the following:

- Marital status and/or living arrangements
- Immunization history
- Current employment
- Developmental history
- School history
- Use of drugs, alcohol, and tobacco
- Levels of education
- Sexual history
- Other relevant social factors

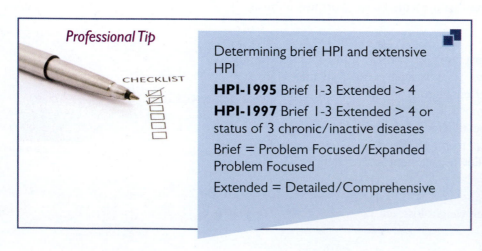

Professional Tip

CHECKLIST

Determining brief HPI and extensive HPI

HPI-1995 Brief 1-3 Extended > 4

HPI-1997 Brief 1-3 Extended > 4 or status of 3 chronic/inactive diseases

Brief = Problem Focused/Expanded Problem Focused

Extended = Detailed/Comprehensive

The levels of E/M services recognize four types of history as follows:

Problem Focused	CC; brief HPI
Expanded Problem Focused	CC; brief HPI, problem-pertinent ROS
Detailed	CC; extended HPI, problem-pertinent ROS, including review of a limited number of additional systems; pertinent PFSH (directly related to the patient's problems)
Comprehensive	CC; extended HPI; ROS directly related to problems identified in HPI plus review of all additional body systems; complete PFSH.

Extent of Examination

The extent of the **examination** performed depends on the clinical judgment of the physician and the nature of the patient's presenting problems. The levels of E/M services recognize four types of examinations:

Problem Focused	A limited exam of the affected body area or organ system
Expanded Problem Focused	A limited exam of the affected body area or organ system and other symptomatic or related organ systems(s)
Detailed	An extended exam of the affected body area(s) and other symptomatic or related organ system(s)
Comprehensive	A general multisystem exam or a complete exam of a single organ system

The following body areas are recognized:

- Head, including the face
- Neck
- Chest, including breasts and axilla
- Abdomen
- Genitalia, groin, buttocks
- Back
- Each extremity

The following organ systems are recognized:

- Eyes
- Ears, nose, mouth, and throat
- Cardiovascular
- Respiratory
- Gastrointestinal
- Genitourinary
- Musculoskeletal
- Skin
- Neurologic
- Psychiatric
- Hematologic/lymphatic/immunologic

Complexity of Medical Decision Making

To determine the complexity of the **medical decision making (MDM)**, the physician must establish a diagnosis and/or select a management option as measured by the following:

1. The number of possible diagnoses and/or the number of management options that must be considered
2. The amount and/or complexity of medical records, diagnostic tests, and/or other information that must be obtained, reviewed, and analyzed
3. The risk of significant complications, morbidity, and/or mortality, as well as comorbidities, associated with the patient's presenting problem

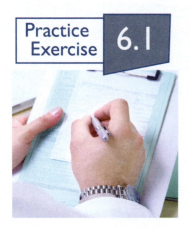

Practice Exercise 6.1

Determine in which history category—Problem Focused, Expanded Problem Focused, Detailed, or Comprehensive—you would document the following statements:

1. Patient presents with sore throat for 2 days. She has used saltwater gargle, which has not helped. She denies having any cough. Review of symptoms reveals no known allergies or family history of asthma.

2. Patient returns for follow-up visit for COPD. She states that the shortness of breath (SOB) has improved with Advair and Spiriva, which were prescribed at the last visit. Denies any chest pain. Patient takes Norvasc for hypertension. Lungs are clear to auscultation. Discussed the importance of diet and exercise. Return in 3 months.

Four types of medical decision making are recognized in the CPT nomenclature. Table 6.1 lists the types and the elements required to qualify for each type. To qualify for a given type of MDM, two of the three elements in Table 6.1 must be met or exceeded.

Table 6.1	The Four Types of Medical Decision Making		
Type of MDM	**Number of Diagnoses or Management Options**	**Amount and/or Complexity of Data to Be Reviewed**	**Risk of Complications and/or Morbidity or Mortality**
Straightforward	Minimal	Minimal or none	Minimal
Low complexity	Limited	Limited	Limited
Moderate complexity	Moderate	Moderate	Multiple
High complexity	Extensive	Extensive	Extensive

Source: Elements for Each Level of Medical Decision Making from Evaluation and Management Services. Published by Centers for Medicare and Medicaid Services (CMS).

> ### Example
>
> Low-complexity MDM is a limited number of diagnoses or management options, a moderate amount and/or complexity of data to be reviewed, and low risk of complications and/or morbidity or mortality.

After determining the three key elements, the coder should analyze the requirements to report the service level:

1. The descriptor for each E/M code explains the standards for its use. For office visits and most other services to new patients, and for initial care visits, generally all three of the key component requirements must be met.

> ### Example
>
> **99203 Office or other outpatient visit** for the evaluation and management of a new patient, which requires these three key components:
> - Detailed History
> - Detailed Examination
> - Medical decision making of low complexity

2. Most services for established patients and subsequent care require two of the three components.

> ### Example
>
> **99213 Office or other outpatient visit** for the evaluation and management of an established patient, which requires at least two of these three key components:
> - Expanded Problem Focused History
> - Expanded Problem Focused Examination
> - Medical decision making of low complexity

Additional Components

Many descriptors mention additional components, as discussed next.

Counseling

For the purpose of E/M coding, **counseling** is a discussion with a patient and/or family for one of the following reasons:

- Diagnostic results, impressions, and recommended studies
- Prognosis
- Risks and benefits of treatment options
- Instructions and/or follow-up
- Importance of compliance with chosen treatment options
- Risk factor reduction
- Patient and family education

Table 6.2	Types of Presenting Problems	
Types	**Definitions**	
Minimal	May not require the presence of a physician, but service is provided under the physician's supervision	
Self-limited or minor	Runs a definite and prescribed course and is not likely to permanently alter the health status or has a good prognosis with management and compliance	
Low severity	Low risk of morbidity without treatment; little to no risk of mortality without treatment; full recovery without functional impairment expected	
Moderate severity	Moderate risk of morbidity without treatment; uncertain prognosis or increased probability of prolonged functional impairment	
High severity	High to extreme risk of morbidity without treatment; high probability of severe, prolonged functional impairment	

The Nature of the Presenting Problem

The **nature of the presenting problem** describes how severe the patient's condition is. A presenting problem is a disease, condition, illness, injury, symptom, sign, complaint, or other reason for a visit/encounter with or without a diagnosis being established at the time of the encounter. Presenting problems can be defined as shown in Table 6.2.

Time

One element of E/M coding is how much time the physician typically spends directly treating the patient. Typical times have been included in many of the code descriptors. The specific lengths of time in the visit codes are averages and therefore represent a range of times that may be higher or lower depending on the actual visit.

Example

This statement appears after the 99214 code for an established patient E/M service:
Usually, the presenting problem(s) are of moderate to high severity. Physicians typically spend 25 minutes face-to-face with the patient and or family.

As mentioned earlier, counseling is a discussion with a patient regarding areas such as diagnostic results, instructions for follow-up treatment, and patient education. When counseling and/or coordination of care constitute more than 50% of the physician/patient and/or family encounter, then time may be considered the key or controlling factor to qualify for a particular level of E/M services. This includes time spent with those who have assumed responsibility for the care of the patient or decision making, whether or not they are family members (e.g., foster parents, person acting in locum, legal guardian). The extent of

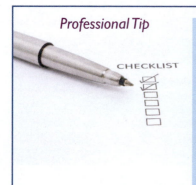

Professional Tip

CHECKLIST

When an E/M code is assigned, the patient's medical record must contain the clinical data to support it. The history, examination, and medical decision making must be sufficiently documented in the medical record so that the medical necessity and appropriateness of the service can be validated.

Read the following chart notes, and using your CPT manual, choose the appropriate code.

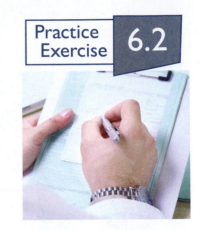

1. For several years, Dr. Bonner has been treating Mrs. Henderson for hypertension, type 2 diabetes, and obesity. Three days before this appointment, blood work was performed to determine the status of her diabetes. She presents to the physician's office, and the physician examines her for evidence of infection or circulatory problems. He then asks the patient about her compliance with the 1,200-calorie diet she has been on for the past 6 months.

   After reviewing these findings, the physician indicates to the patient that she will have to begin using insulin because her diabetes is not responding to the current treatment. Mrs. Henderson begins to sob uncontrollably. She tells Dr. Bonner that this means she is going to die because her grandmother got gangrene from this kind of diabetes and died from it.

   After calming Mrs. Henderson, Dr. Bonner explains that using insulin is not a "death sentence." He discusses diet, insulin administration, and hypoglycemic reactions as well as the symptoms of hyperglycemia. He instructs Mrs. Henderson as to proper foot and skin care and stresses the importance of seeing her ophthalmologist regularly. Mrs. Henderson is much calmer and feels that she will learn a lot from the booklets Dr. Bonner has given her.

   The total time Dr. Bonner spent with Mrs. Henderson is 25 minutes, with 20 of those minutes spent providing counseling and/or coordination of care. Because more than 50% of the encounter was spent providing counseling and/or coordination of care, the total face-to-face time between Mrs. Henderson and Dr. Bonner may be considered the key factor in selecting the level of E/M service.

   Code _____

2. Chart note for an established patient: Office visit by established patient for monthly scheduled blood test to monitor Coumadin, which is an anticoagulant; nurse spends 5 minutes, reviews the test, confirms that the patient is doing well, and states that no change in the dosage is necessary.

   Code _____

3. A patient presents to Dr. Bradley's office with complaints of fever, chills, malaise, and a cough. Dr. Bradley obtains the history, performs an examination, and orders a chest X-ray. The patient is admitted to the hospital on the same day for intravenous antibiotic therapy for treatment of pneumonia. After completion of her office hours, Dr. Bradley provides an E/M service to the patient in the hospital.

   Code _____

4. Home visit for established patient, straightforward case, problem-focused examination.

   Code _____

counseling and/or coordination of care must be documented in the medical record. When coordination of care is provided but the patient is not present, the case management and care plan oversight services subsection codes are reported. These factors, although not the key components, help ensure that the correct service level is selected.

Assigning the Code

The code that has been selected is assigned. The need for any modifiers, based on the documentation of special circumstances, is also reviewed.

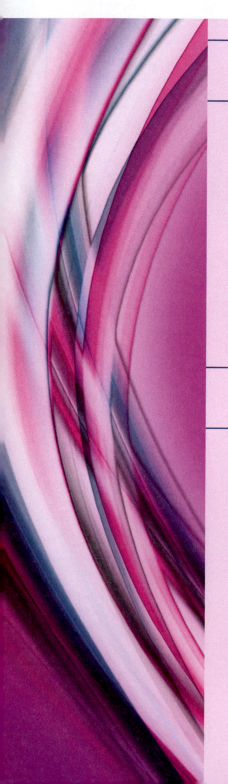

Chapter Summary

- The AMA first developed and published the CPT and updates it annually.
- The CPT has three categories: CPT Category I has six sections that refer to the CPT codes. CPT Category II contains performance measurement tracking codes. CPT Category III contains emerging technology codes.
- The CPT contains specific guidelines located at the beginning of each section.
- Modifiers are two-digit numeric indicators which indicate that the description of the service or procedure has been altered.
- The CPT coding system makes specific distinctions for place of service in the E/M codes. The place of service may have a considerable impact on reimbursement.
- Reimbursement is also related to the type of patient: new, established, or consult.
- The three key components for determining an E/M code are the extent of the history documented, the extent of the examination documented, and the complexity of the medical decision making documented.

Chapter Review

True/False

Identify the statement as true (T) or false (F).

_____ **1.** Physicians may use procedure codes from any of the sections of the CPT.

_____ **2.** In performing an E/M service, the physician often documents the HPI, which is an abbreviation for *history of previous illnesses*.

_____ **3.** In the CPT, the term *consultation* describes services that a provider performs at the request of another provider after which the patient is returned to the requesting provider's care.

_____ **4.** A new patient is one who has not received professional services within the past 2 years.

_____ **5.** An established patient is one who has received professional services from the physician or another physician of the same specialty who belongs to the same group practice within the past 3 years.

_____ **6.** Emergency department services distinguish between new and established patients.

_____ **7.** Time is a factor when choosing an emergency department service.

_____ **8.** An established patient receiving an annual exam for the first time is coded in the preventive medicine service as a new patient.

_____ **9.** Hospital observation service codes are used to code for patients admitted to the hospital.

_____ **10.** There are six categories of CPTs.

Multiple Choice

Identify the letter of the choice that best completes the statement or answers the question.

_____ **1.** Of the four types of examinations that physicians perform, which level is the most complete?
   a. Detailed
   b. Expanded Problem Focused
   c. Comprehensive
   d. Problem Focused

_____ **2.** Routine annual physical examinations are reported using CPT's:
   a. consultation codes.
   b. office services codes.
   c. preventive medicine service codes.
   d. critical care services codes.

_____ **3.** In selecting an E/M code, three components are considered: the history, the examination, and the:
   a. family background.
   b. medical decision making.
   c. diagnoses options.
   d. interval history.

_____ **4.** When choosing an E/M code, what is chosen first?
   a. Alphabetic Index
   b. Medicine section
   c. Place of service
   d. New patient

_____ **5.** A CPT code can be distinguished from an ICD-10 CM code because it contains:
   a. three digits with a decimal point.
   b. four digits.
   c. five digits with a modifier.
   d. five digits.

_____ **6.** In some billing cases it is necessary to add a two-digit modifier in order to:
   a. indicate usual charges.
   b. prevent miscoding.
   c. give a more accurate description.
   d. meet the payer's criteria.

_____ **7.** CPT codes, descriptions, and two-digit modifiers are copyrighted by the:
   a. Blue Cross and Blue Shield organization.
   b. American Medical Association.
   c. CPC coder.
   d. World Health Organization.

_____ **8.** What is the number of the modifier that is used when the physician provides an E/M service in addition to another E/M service or procedure on the same day?

    a. −25   c. −24

    b. −26   d. −32

_____ **9.** The modifier for Decision for Surgery is:

    a. −32.   c. −52.

    b. −57.   d. −21.

_____ **10.** The CPT is revised:

    a. every 2 years.   c. annually.

    b. when necessary.   d. every 6 months.

_____ **11.** In the CPT, a round bullet symbol indicates a:

    a. bundled code.   c. new code.

    b. revised code.   d. deleted code.

_____ **12.** In the CPT, a triangle symbol indicates a(n):

    a. new code.   c. decision for surgery.

    b. descriptor has changed.   d. add-on code.

_____ **13.** CPT Category I is divided into how many sections?

    a. 4   c. 5

    b. 6   d. 8

_____ **14.** Components of a medical history include all of the following except:

    a. medical decision making.   c. family history.

    b. chief complaint.   d. review of systems.

_____ **15.** A key component in coding medical decision making is the:

    a. physician's level of education.

    b. amount of time the physician spends with the patient.

    c. level of complexity.

    d. patient's childhood diseases.

Completion

Complete each sentence or statement, using your CPT manual.

1. In the CPT, E/M is the abbreviation for Evaluation and _____ Services.

2. Define the term _new patient_. _____

_____

_____

3. What subsection is used to code an annual physical examination? _____

4. What subsection is used for a consultation? _____

5. Is a patient who visits an emergency department coded as a new or an established patient? _____

6. Is critical care coded according to time? _____

7. What code is used for the annual assessment of a patient in a nursing facility whose condition could be stable, improving, or recovering? _____

8. What is the age of a neonate? _____

9. What is the age of an infant or young child? _____

10. The modifier A1 is used with an E&M code to show the _____.

For Additional Practice

Based on the description of the service, look up the appropriate CPT code in your CPT manual and write it in the space provided.

1. Complex comprehensive initial consultation, office, medical decision of high complexity: _____

2. Emergency department care, minimal care, straightforward medical decision, problem-focused history and exam: _____

3. Admission to skilled nursing facility, established patient, medical decision of low complexity, detailed history, comprehensive exam: _____

4. Subsequent hospital care for a patient in a stable condition: _____

5. Follow-up minimal consultation, office, straightforward medical decision making, Problem Focused History and Exam: _____

6. Work-related medical disability evaluation by treating physician: _____

7. Supervision of hospice patient care (25 minutes spent in 1 month): _____

8. Second opinion provided by cardiothoracic surgeon for appropriateness of a mitral valve replacement; during a 1-hour encounter, comprehensive history and exam completed; follow-up includes a written report to the PCP; MDM was moderate: _____

9. During an annual physical examination, a 45-year-old established patient complains of tiredness and shortness of breath during mild activity; physician performs a detailed cardiovascular assessment with additional detailed history; following complex MDM, the physician also schedules an immediate complete heart study: _____

10. Office visit for an established patient with a problem-focused history and examination: _____

Resources

American Medical Association
www.ama-assn.org/go/CPT

Comprehensive website devoted to Current Procedural Terminology.

American Medical Association
www.cptnetwork.com

CPT Network: a database of commonly asked questions and clinical examples (vignettes)

Chapter 7 / Coding Procedures and Services

Chapter Objectives

After reading this chapter, the student should be able to:

1. Correctly use the CPT® current procedural terminology index.
2. Understand the four primary classes of main entries in the CPT index.
3. Understand code ranges and conventions.
4. Discuss the purpose of each section and the guidelines.
5. Know how to use modifiers correctly.
6. Use add-on codes properly.
7. Review codes for accuracy.
8. Given procedural statements, apply coding guidelines to determine the correct CPT codes.

Key Terms

add-on codes
bundled code
Clinical Laboratory
    Improvement
    Amendment (CLIA)
cross-references
descriptor

fragmented billing
global period
global surgical concept
panel
physical status modifier
primary procedure
professional component

secondary procedure
separate procedure
surgical package
technical component
unbundling

CPT-4 codes in this chapter are from the CPT 2017 code set. CPT is a registered trademark of the American Medical Association.

Sandy has recently been seeing Dr. Georgio for visits pertaining to a mastectomy. In the midst of seeing Dr. Georgio for the mastectomy that was performed four weeks ago, she also saw her for a upper respiratory infection. Sandy was confused when she received a bill for the visit. Up until now she had not received any bills from the physician. Upon contacting the billing office, the biller explained that all of the visits pertaining to the mastectomy were covered under a global charge but that the most recent visit did not fall under that charge because it did not pertain to the mastectomy.

Questions

1. What does it mean that "the mastectomy visits fall under a global charge"?

2. Could there be a situation in which the upper respiratory infection could be tied to the global service?

3. Is there a universal time frame for all global services?

Current Procedural Terminology, Fourth Edition, is a listing of descriptive terms and identifying codes for reporting medical services and procedures by any qualified physician or provider. The purpose of the terminology is to provide a uniform language that will accurately describe means for reliable nationwide communication among physicians, patients, and third parties. The most recent revision is CPT 2017; the list publication was first used in 1966. This uniform language is also applicable to medical education and outcomes, health services, and quality research by providing a useful basis for local, regional, and national utilization comparisons. Each procedure or service is identified with a five-digit code. In 2000, the CPT code set was designated by the Department of Health and Human Services as the national coding standard for physician and other healthcare professional services and procedures under the Health Insurance Portability and Accountability Act (HIPAA). This means that for all financial and administrative healthcare transactions sent electronically, the CPT code set will need to be used. The subsections are divided by type of service and body system. It is important that the coder become familiar with and develop an understanding of the general layout of the CPT book. Knowledge about how to use the CPT index will assist medical coders in locating the appropriate code for reporting the procedures and/or the services performed. The CPT index is not a substitute for the main text of the CPT. Even if only one code appears in the index, the user must refer to the main text to ensure that the code selection is accurate.

Organization of the CPT Index

When using the CPT index, it is important to understand how entries to the index have been made. It cannot be stressed enough that the CPT index is not a substitute for the main text of the CPT nomenclature. As just mentioned, even if only one code appears in the index, the user must refer to the main text of the CPT book to ensure that the code selection is accurate. The CPT index is located after the appendixes. The index is organized by main terms and it contains four primary classes of main entries:

1. *Procedure or service:* Allergen Immunotherapy, Arthroscopy, Biopsy, Cardiac Catheterization, Debridement, Evaluation and Management, Laparoscopy, Osteopathic Manipulation, Physical Medicine/Therapy/Occupational Therapy, Vaccines, etc.
2. *Organ, or other anatomic site:* Abdomen, Bladder, Esophagus, Hip, Intestines, Malar Area, Olecranon Process, Prostate, etc.
3. *Condition:* Abscess, Blepharoptosis, Dislocation, Esophageal Varices, Hemorrhage, Omphalocele, Varicose Vein, etc.
4. *Synonyms, eponyms, and abbreviations:* Anderson Tibial Lengthening, CBC, Clagett Procedure, EKG, Patterson Test, etc.

Instructions for Using the CPT Index

From a historical perspective, CPT coding has always placed procedures in general sections according to where physicians will most conveniently find them. For example, the code for a diagnostic colonoscopy, although not involving an incision, is located in the Digestive System Surgery section. Keeping the endoscopies involving a biopsy, tumor removal, or other operative interventions in proximity to the diagnostic procedure was an important consideration. Similarly, cast applications are listed in the Musculoskeletal Surgery section, in proximity to the fracture and dislocation treatments, but clearly cast application is not a "surgical procedure."

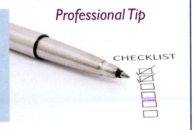

Professional Tip

In the CPT index, the CPT topics and subtopics are listed as the heading and a range of codes follows. The code(s) directs the coder to the code(s) where additional information on the topic(s) may be located. All topics referring to CPT code sections or chapter headings are listed in **BOLD UPPERCASE**.

CHECKLIST

Code Range

A range of codes is shown when more than one code applies to an entry. Two codes, either sequential or not, are separated by a comma:

Professional Tip

The CPT index provides a pointer to the correct code range in the main text. Using the CPT index makes the process of selecting procedural codes more efficient.

CHECKLIST

Biopsy
Colon...44025, 44100

More than two sequential codes are separated by a hyphen:

Biopsy
Elbow..24065–24066

Formatting and Cross-References

All CPT codes are five digits (no decimal point) followed by a **descriptor**, which is a brief description of the procedure.

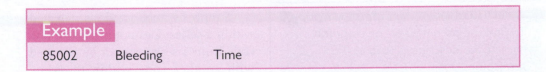

Example		
85002	Bleeding	Time

Formatting

After searching the index for the procedure, service, or condition according to the main term and any subterms, the coder searches the section in which the code or code range is located and reads all descriptors.

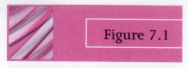

Figure 7.1

Determining the full procedure descriptor.

97010	Application of a modality to one or more areas; hot or cold packs
97012	traction, mechanical
97014	electrical stimulation (unattended)
97016	vasopneumatic devices
97018	paraffin bath

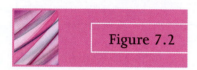

Figure 7.2

Range of procedures can be reported independently.

64400	Injection anesthetic agent; trigeminal nerve, any division or branch
64402	facial nerve
64405	greater occipital nerve
64408	vagus nerve

A main procedure descriptor may be followed by a series of up to three indented terms that modify the main descriptor. These modifying terms should be reviewed because these subterms have an effect on appropriate code selection. Note that the common descriptor begins with a capital letter, but the unique descriptors after the semicolon do not. The format of the terminology was originally developed as standalone descriptions of medical procedures.

However, to conserve space and avoid having to repeat common terminology, some of the procedure descriptors in CPT coding are not printed in their entirety but, rather, refer back to a common portion of the procedure descriptor listed in a preceding entry. Within any indented series of codes, you must refer back to the first left-justified code (the *parent code*) within that series to determine the full procedure descriptor of the indented code(s). Figure 7.1 illustrates this formatting convention.

For example, the common part of the parent code 97010—that is, the descriptor before the semicolon (in Figure 7.1, the common part descriptor is "Application of a modality to one or more areas")—should be considered part of each of the following indented codes in that series.

Thus, the full procedure descriptor represented by code 97012 is as follows:

97012 Application of a modality to one or more areas; traction, mechanical

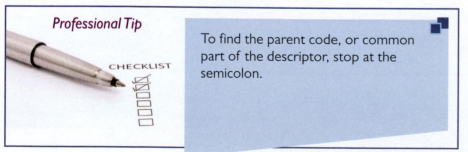

Professional Tip

CHECKLIST

To find the parent code, or common part of the descriptor, stop at the semicolon.

Simply because a code is indented within a series does not mean that one code from a series cannot be reported with another code within the same indented series. If two distinct procedures are performed then both procedures can be coded.

> ### Example
>
> The following procedures would be reported as separate codes:
>
> 64402 Injection, anesthetic agent; facial nerve
> 64408 Injection, anesthetic agent; vagus nerve
> 97014 Application of a modality to one or more areas; electrical stimulation
>   (unattended)
> 97018 Application of a modality to one or more areas; paraffin bath

Cross-references

Cross-references provide additional instructions to the user. Two types of cross-references are used in the main sections.

> ***See*** or ***Use:*** These types of entries in parentheses point to another code; (also used primarily for synonyms, eponyms, and abbreviations.)

> ### Example
>
> 82088 Aldosterone
>
> (Alkaline phosphatase, see 84075, 84080)

> ### Example
>
> 83825 Mercury, quantitative
>
> (Mercury screen, use 83015)

> ***See Also:*** These entries direct the coder to look under another main term if the procedure is not listed under the first main index entry.

> ### Example
>
> 85475 Hemolysin, acid
>
> (See also 86940, 86941)

Section Guidelines

The beginning of every section has guidelines specific to that section. The guidelines provide information that is necessary to appropriately interpret and report the procedures and services found in that section. There also may be a list of modifiers, which are specific to the section. All of the guidelines and notes are there to assist the user in appropriate interpretation and application of the codes throughout the book. These guidelines are critical to using CPT coding correctly.

Modifiers

Modifiers are used with the CPT coding system to report a service or procedure that has been modified by some specific circumstance without altering or modifying the basic definition or CPT code.

The proper use of modifiers can speed up claims processing and increase reimbursement, whereas the improper use of CPT modifiers may result in claim delays or denials. The modifiers can be readily found in the CPT book in Appendix A with their full definitions. Anesthesia has modifiers for the patient's physical status. Modifiers may be used in many instances for these reasons:

- To report a service or procedure that had both the professional component and technical component
- To report a service mandated by a third-party payer
- A service or procedure was increased or reduced
- An adjunctive service was performed
- A procedure was performed bilaterally
- A procedure or service was provided more than once
- Unusual events occurred
- To report multiple procedures performed at the same session by the same provider
- To report a portion of a service or procedure that was reduced or eliminated at the physician's discretion
- To report assistant surgeon services
- A procedure or service was performed by more than one physician or other healthcare professional and/or in more than one location

Example

A physician providing diagnostic or therapeutic radiology services, ultrasound, or nuclear medicine services in a hospital would add modifier 26 to report the professional component. 73090 with modifier 26 = Professional component only for the X-ray of the forearm.

A complete listing of modifiers is found in Appendix A of the CPT index.

22 Increased Procedural Service: When the work required to provide a service is substantially greater than typically required, it may be identified by adding -22 to the used procedure. This modifier should not be appended to an E/M service. Documentation must support the substantial work and the reason for the additional work. The report should be submitted with the claim with details including the increased intensity, time, technical difficulty of procedure, severity of patient's condition, and physical and mental effort required; it explains the patient's condition, and justifies the procedure's medical necessity.

Example

A physician excises a lesion located in a crease of the back of a very obese person. The obesity makes the excision more difficult. The physician indicates the complexity of the removal of the lesion by appending the modifier -22 to the code used to report the removal of the lesion. The operative report is included with the claim to the third-party payer.

24 Unrelated Evaluation and Management Service by the Same Physician or Other Qualified Health Care Professional During a Postoperative Period

32 Mandated Service: Services related to mandated consultation and/or related services (e.g., third-party payer, governmental, legislative, or regulatory requirement) may be identified by adding modifier -32 to the basic procedure.

47 Anesthesia by Surgeon: Regional or general anesthesia provided by the surgeon may be reported by adding modifier -47 to the basic service. This does not include local anesthesia.

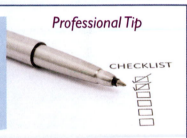

Professional Tip

This does not include local anesthesia. Modifier -47 would not be used as a modifier for the anesthesia procedure.

CHECKLIST

Example

A surgeon performs a regional nerve block before performing surgery to decompress the nerve at the carpal tunnel. To report this, the physician uses code 64721, Neuroplasty and/or transposition; median nerve at carpal tunnel. Code 64415, Injection, anesthetic agent; brachial plexus, single would also be reported to describe the regional nerve block performed. Modifier 47 is appended to the procedural code, 64721, to obtain 64721-47. The modifier alerts the third-party payer that the surgeon personally performed the anesthesia. Listing the code for the anesthesia informs the third-party payer about which nerve was blocked.

50 Bilateral Procedure: Bilateral means pertaining to two sides. Unless otherwise identified in the descriptor, bilateral procedures that are performed at the same operative session should be identified by appending modifier 50 to the procedure.

Example

A physician repairs a bilateral reducible inguinal hernia on a 2-year-old. The physician reports code 49500-50, Repair initial inguinal hernia, age 6 months to younger than 5 years, with or without hydrocelectomy; reducible. The modifier 50 is appended to the procedure code because it was performed bilaterally.

Modifier 51 should not be appended to designate add-on codes. Appendix E of the AMA's CPT summarizes the CPT codes exempt from modifier 51. Codes listed are identified in CPT with the symbol Ø.

51 Multiple Procedures: When multiple procedures are performed, other than E/M services, at the same session by the same provider, the primary procedure may be reported as listed. The additional procedures may be identified by appending modifier 51 to the additional procedure.

Modifier 51 has four applications, namely, to identify:

- Multiple medical procedures performed at the same session by the same provider
- Multiple, related operative procedures performed at the same session by the same provider
- Operative procedures performed in combination, at the same operative session, by the same provider, whether through the same or another incision or involving the same or different anatomy
- A combination of medical and operative procedures performed at the same session by the same provider

Example

A surgeon reports code 28200, Repair tendon, flexor, foot; primary or secondary, without free graft, each tendon. The second procedure performed during the same operative session by the same provider is code 28001, Incision and drainage of the bursa, foot. The modifier 51 is appended to the secondary procedure, 28001, resulting in a code of 28001-51. A **secondary procedure** is a procedure performed in addition to the primary procedure.

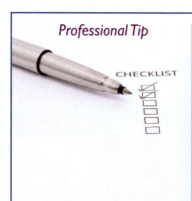

For hospital outpatient reporting of a previously scheduled procedure that is partially reduced or cancelled as a result of extenuating circumstance or threat to the well-being of the patient before or after administration of anesthesia, see modifiers 73 and 74 under Modifiers Approved for Ambulatory Surgery Center (ASC) Hospital Outpatient Use

53 Discontinued Procedure: Under certain circumstances, the physician may elect to terminate a surgical or diagnostic procedure. Due to extenuating circumstances or those that threaten the well-being of the patient, it may be necessary to indicate that a surgical or diagnostic procedure was started but discontinued. This circumstance may be reported by adding the modifier 53 to the code reported by the physician for the discontinued procedure.

Example

Following anesthesia induction, the patient experiences an arrhythmia that causes the procedure to be terminated. The physician reports the code for the planned procedure with modifier 53 appended.

54 Surgical Care Only: When one physician performs a surgical procedure and another provides preoperative and/or postoperative management, surgical services may be identified by adding modifier 54 to the usual procedure number.

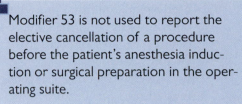
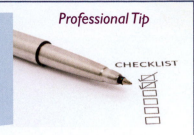

55 Postoperative Management Only: When one physician performed the postoperative management and another performed the surgical procedure, modifier 55 is appended to the usual procedure number.

56 Preoperative Management Only: When one physician performed the preoperative care and evaluation and another physician performed the surgical procedure, the preoperative component may be identified by adding modifier 56 to the usual procedure number.

Example

Example for Modifiers 54, 55, and 56: A physician may intend to perform all three components of a global service (preoperative management, surgical care, and postoperative management); however, after providing the preoperative management and performing the surgical procedure, she is unexpectedly called out of town. The surgeon in this case reports the surgical procedure with the modifiers 54 and 56 appended.

The physician who performed the postoperative management reports the operative procedure code with modifier 55 appended. Reporting the postoperative management indicates that the physician performed all of the postoperative care.

58 Staged or Related Procedure by the Same Physician During the Postoperative Period: The physician may need to indicate that the performance of a procedure or service during the postoperative period was (1) planned prospectively at the time of the original procedure (staged), (2) more extensive than the original procedure, or (3) for therapy following a diagnostic surgical procedure.

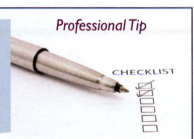

Example

A surgeon performs a mastectomy on a patient. During the postoperative global period he inserts a permanent prosthesis. The surgeon reports the code with the 58 modifier to indicate that the service was related to the mastectomy (staged to occur at a time after the initial surgery). If the physician did not append modifier 58, a third-party payer could reject the claim because the surgery occurred during the postoperative period associated with the mastectomy.

59 Distinct Procedural Service: Under certain circumstances, the physician may need to indicate that a procedure or service was distinct or independent from other services performed on the same day. Modifier 59 is used to identify procedures that are not normally reported together but are appropriate under the circumstances.

62 Two Surgeons: When two surgeons work together as primary surgeons performing a distinct part of a procedure, each surgeon should report his distinct operative work by adding modifier 62 to the procedure and any associated add-on codes for that procedure as long as both surgeons continue to work together as primary surgeons.

63 Procedure Performed on Infants less than 4 kg: Procedures performed on neonates and infants up to a present body weight of 4 kg may involve significantly increased complexity and physician work commonly associated with these patients. Appendix F in CPT Standard Edition contains a list of codes that are exempt from this modifier.

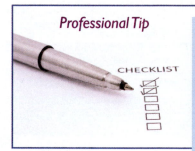

Professional Tip

CHECKLIST

Modifier 63 should not be appended to any CPT codes listed in the E/M Services, Anesthesia, Radiology, Pathology/Laboratory, or Medicine sections.

66 Surgical Team: Under some circumstances, highly complex procedures (requiring the concomitant services of several physicians, often of different specialties, plus other highly skilled, specially trained personnel, and various types of complex equipment) are carried out under the "surgical team" concept.

Example

During a heart transplant, one surgeon opens the chest and inserts the chest tubes, while another surgeon prepares the great vessels for anastomosis to the donor heart. Each surgeon reports the same code with the same modifier, in this case 33945-66.

76 Repeat Procedure by Same Physician: The physician may need to indicate that a procedure was repeated subsequent to the original procedure. Documentation should be provided to the third-party payer when reporting this modifier.

77 Repeat Procedure by Another Physician: The physician may need to indicate that a basic procedure performed by another physician had to be repeated.

78 Unplanned Return to the Operating Room by the Same Physician Following Initial Procedure for a Related Procedure During the Postoperative Period: The physician may need to indicate that another unplanned procedure was performed during the postoperative period of the initial procedure. When this subsequent procedure is related to the first and requires the use of the operating room, it may be reported by adding modifier 78 to the related procedure.

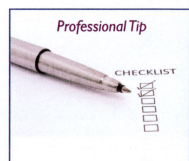

Professional Tip

CHECKLIST

It is important that all physicians on the heart transplant surgical team jointly write a description of each physician's general role on the team and send the report to each third-party payer to indicate each physician's role in the performance of the surgery.

79 Unrelated Procedure or Service by the Same Physician During the Postoperative Period: The physician may need to indicate that the performance of a procedure during the postoperative period was unrelated to the original procedure.

80 Assistant Surgeon: Surgical assistant services may be identified by adding modifier 80 to the usual procedure number.

81 Minimum Assistant Surgeon: Minimum surgical assistant services are identified by adding modifier 81 to the usual procedure number.

82 Assistant Surgeon (when qualified resident surgeon not available): The unavailability of a qualified resident surgeon is a prerequisite for appending modifier 82 to the usual procedure code.

90 Outside Laboratory: When laboratory procedures are performed by a party other than the treating or reporting physician, the procedure may be identified by adding modifier 90 to the usual procedure code.

91 Repeat Clinical Diagnostic Laboratory Test: In the course of treatment of the patient, it may be necessary to repeat the same laboratory test on the same day to obtain subsequent (multiple) test results. Under these circumstances, the test's usual procedure code and the addition of modifier 91 can identify the laboratory test performed.

92 Alternative Laboratory Platform Testing: This modifier indicates laboratory testing that is performed using a kit or transportable instrument that wholly or in part consists of a single-use, disposable analytical chamber.

99 Multiple Modifiers: Under certain circumstances two or more modifiers may be necessary to completely define a service. In such situations, modifier 99 should be added to the basic procedure, and other applicable modifiers may be listed as part of the description of service.

Add-on Codes (+)

Most of the procedures listed in the CPT can be reported by themselves because they represent the total procedure that was performed. These stand-alone codes describe the total procedure or service. Under certain circumstances, it may be necessary to report two or more stand-alone codes to completely describe the procedures performed. Add-on codes are used mainly with codes from the surgery section of the CPT book.

Some of the codes listed in the CPT code set describe procedures/services that must always be reported with a stand-alone code. These codes are referred to as add-on codes. **Add-on codes** describe procedures/services that are always performed in addition to the primary procedure; they are indicated by a plus sign (+) next to the code. The **primary procedure** is the most resource-intensive CPT procedure done during a patient's visit/encounter. The primary procedure code is listed first on the claim. Add-on codes can also be readily identified by specific language in the code descriptor, which includes phrases such as "each additional" or "List separately in addition to primary procedure."

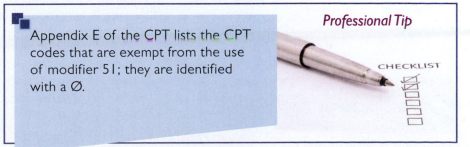

Professional Tip

Appendix E of the CPT lists the CPT codes that are exempt from the use of modifier 51; they are identified with a Ø.

CHECKLIST

The multiple modifier (51) is not appended to an add-on code. These codes are exempt from the multiple procedure concept.

Coding Steps

Perform the following steps:

1. *Determine the procedures and services to report.* The coder chooses the name and associated code of the procedure or service that most accurately identifies and describes the services performed, then chooses names and codes for additional procedures/ services. If necessary, modifiers are chosen and added to the selected procedure/ service codes. Knowledge of the payers' policies is used to decide which services can be performed in the office (or which need to be referred out of office) and can be reported and billed. All coded procedures/services must also be documented in the patient's medical record.

2. *Identify the correct codes.* The CPT index is used to locate the main term for each procedure or service. If the term is not found, the organ or body site is looked up and then the disease or injury. Further checking can be done to locate any synonyms, eponyms, or abbreviations associated with the main term. The entries under the main term are reviewed to see if any apply, and cross-references are checked. If the main term cannot be located in the index, the coder reviews the main term selection with the physician for clarification. In some cases, a better or more common term can be used.

    The main text listing, including all section guidelines and notes for particular subsections, is carefully reviewed to arrive at the final code. Items that cannot be billed separately because they are covered under another, broader code are eliminated.

    The codes to be reported for each day's service are ranked in order of highest to lowest rate of reimbursement (Figure 7.3). The actual order in which they were performed on a particular day is not important.

3. *Determine the need for modifiers.* The circumstances involved with the procedure/ service may require the use of modifiers. The patient's diagnosis may affect this determination.

Coding for Anesthesia

Anesthesia codes have their own section, which is located before the Surgery section. Basic anesthesia administration services are those services provided by or under the responsible supervision of a physician. These services include general and regional anesthesia as well as supplementation of local anesthesia. Anesthesia is reimbursed according to time. The main anesthesia codes are bundled codes. A bundled code is a

Figure 7.3

Date	Charge	Procedure
12/22/2016	$350	25500
12/22/2016	$200	99203
12/22/2016	$85	73090

The codes to be reported for each day's service are ranked in order of highest to lowest rate of reimbursement.

group of related procedures covered by a single code. These **bundled codes** include the usual services of an anesthesiologist, which are as follows:

- Routine preoperative and postoperative visits to evaluate the patient for the planned anesthesia and monitor the patient's postsurgery recovery from anesthesia
- Administration of fluids and/or blood during the period of anesthesia care
- Interpretation of noninvasive monitoring such as electrocardiography (ECG), body temperature, blood pressure, oximetry (blood oxygen concentration), capnography (blood carbon dioxide concentration), and mass spectrometry

The index is researched for the procedure under the Anesthesia section. The section's subsections are organized by body site. Under each subsection the codes are arranged by procedures. For example, under the heading "Neck," codes for procedures performed on various parts of the neck; esophagus, thyroid, larynx, trachea; lymphatic system; and major vessels are listed.

The **physical status modifier** is used only in the Anesthesia section with procedure codes to indicate the patient's health status. These modifiers, which are shown in Figure 7.4, range from P1 to P6.

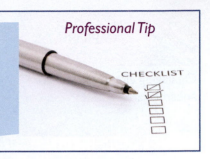

Professional Tip

CHECKLIST

In the CPT index, look for the code under Anesthesia. If you look first under the surgical procedure performed, the code will be for that surgical procedure and not the anesthesia given for the surgical procedure.

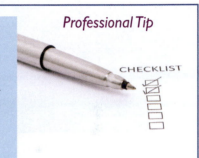

Professional Tip

CHECKLIST

The American Society of Anesthesiologists (ASA) provides a guide for the reporting of anesthesia services and procedures. The ASA publishes this billing and coding guide annually. It depicts and defines anesthesia services and modifiers. The guide assigns a relative value unit to anesthesia services, physical status modifiers, and qualifying circumstances that are added together to calculate anesthesia charges.

59 Distinct Procedural Service: Under certain circumstances, the physician may need to indicate that a procedure or service was distinct or independent from other services performed on the same day. Modifier 59 is used to identify procedures that are not normally reported together but are appropriate under the circumstances.

- P1—A normal healthy patient
- P2—A patient with mild systemic disease
- P3—A patient with severe systemic disease
- P4—A patient with severe systemic disease that is a constant threat to life
- P5—A moribund patient who is not expected to survive without the operation
- P6—A declared brain-dead patient whose organs are being removed for donor purposes

 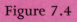

Figure 7.4

Physical status modifiers.

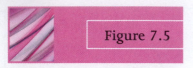

Figure 7.5

Qualifying circumstances for anesthesia.

+99100	Anesthesia for patient of extreme age; younger than 1 year and older than 70
+99116	Anesthesia complicated by utilization of total body hypothermia
+99135	Anesthesia complicated by utilization of controlled hypotension
+99140	Anesthesia complicated by emergency conditions (specify) (list separately in addition to code for primary anesthesia procedure)

Time spent providing the anesthesia service is reported separately when anesthesia services are coded. Anesthesia time begins when the anesthesia provider starts preparing the patient for anesthesia in the operating room or a similar location. Time ends when the patient is safely placed under postoperative supervision.

In the case of difficult and/or extraordinary circumstances such as extreme youth or age (under 1 year or over 70 years of age) or other unusual risk factors, it may be appropriate to report one or more of the qualifying circumstances by using an add-on code listed in Figure 7.5 in addition to the anesthesia services.

Practice Exercise 7.1

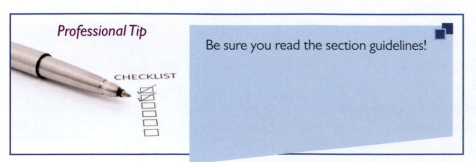

Using your CPT manual, answer the following questions:

1. What code is used to report the administration of anesthesia for a procedure on the esophagus? _____

2. Regional or general anesthesia provided by the surgeon also performing the procedure is reported with what CPT modifier? _____

3. What code is used to report repair of a ruptured Achilles tendon? _____ _____

4. Which physical status modifier is used to designate a patient with mild systemic disease? _____

5. What code is used to report anesthesia for a 72-year-old female for lens surgery of the right eye? _____

Professional Tip

CHECKLIST

Be sure you read the section guidelines!

Surgical Coding

The Surgery section is the largest section in CPT. The subsections found in the Surgery section and how they are divided according to body systems are shown in Figure 7.6.

The anatomic arrangement of each subsection is as follows:

- Head
- Neck (Soft Tissue) and Thorax
- Back and Flank
- Spine (Vertebral Column)
- Abdomen
- Shoulder
- Humerus (Upper Arm) and Elbow
- Forearm and Wrist
- Hand and Fingers
- Pelvis and Hip Joint
- Femur (Thigh Region) and Knee Joint
- Leg (Tibia and Fibula) and Ankle Joint
- Foot and Toes
- Application of Casts and Strapping
- Endoscopy/Arthroscopy

Each heading also encompasses a consistent theme of procedures described such as the following:

- Incision
- Excision
- Introduction or Removal
- Repair, Revision, and/or Reconstruction
- Fracture and/or Dislocation
- Arthrodesis/Amputation

Integumentary System	10021–19499
Musculoskeletal System	20005–29999
Respiratory System	30000–32999
Cardiovascular System	33010–39599
Digestive System	40490–49999
Urinary System	50010–53899
Male Genital System	54000–55980
Female Genital System	56405–58999
Maternity Care and Delivery	59000–59899
Endocrine System	60000–60699
Nervous System	61000–64999
Eye and Ocular Adnexa	65091–68899
Auditory System	69000–69979
Operating Microscope	69990

Figure 7.6

The subsections found in the Surgery section and how they are broken down into the body systems.

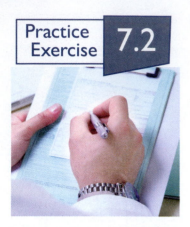

Practice Exercise 7.2

Using your CPT index, look up the following and outline how you got there:

1. Anesthetic injection of the facial nerve _____

_____

_____

_____

2. Closed treatment of the clavicle _____

_____

_____

_____

3. Excision of the gallbladder _____

_____

_____

_____

As previously discussed in this chapter, the following is an example of the use of an add-on code.

Example

Additional Lesion(s)

11100	Biopsy of skin, subcutaneous tissue and/or mucous membrane (including simple closure); unless otherwise listed (separate procedure); single lesion
+11101	Each separate/additional lesion (List separately in addition to code for primary procedure.)

Code 11100 is the primary procedure, and code 11101 is the add-on code. Code 11101 would never be reported without first reporting code 11100. As the code descriptor indicates, code 11101 is reported for each separate/additional lesion. The parenthetical note following code 11101 instructs the user regarding the code that is considered the primary procedure for that particular add-on code.

If biopsies are performed on three separate lesions of the skin, subcutaneous tissue, and/or mucous membrane, then code 11100 would be reported for the first lesion and code 11101 would be reported twice, once for the second lesion biopsy, and again for the third lesion biopsy.

Other CPT codes are also exempt from modifier 51. These codes are identified throughout the CPT book with the Ø (null) symbol placed before the code. These codes

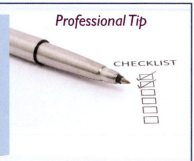

Use your CPT manual to code the following:

1. Neurorrhaphy of two digital nerves: _____

2. Xenograft, to trunk, arms and legs; 200 cm^2: _____

   _____

3. Arthrodesis, interphalangeal joint (3): _____

   _____

cannot be modified with modifier 51 multiple procedures because the add-on code is used to add increments to a primary procedure, thus the need for multiple procedures is represented by procedures that are added on.

Separate Procedure

A **separate procedure** is a descriptor used in the CPT for a procedure that is usually part of a surgical package but may also be performed separately or for a different purpose, in which case it may be reported separately.

Some of the codes listed in the CPT nomenclature have been identified by inclusion of the term *separate procedure* in the code descriptor. The separate procedure designation indicates that a certain procedure or service may be:

> *Professional Tip*
>
> The symbol ⊙ refers to the procedure that includes moderate (conscious) sedation, which is a drug-induced depression of consciousness during which the patient responds purposefully to verbal commands. The provider cannot report this as a separate procedure.
>
> CHECKLIST

1. Considered an integral component of another procedure/service.
2. Performed independently.
3. Unrelated.
4. Distinct from other procedures provided at that time.

Example

58720	Salpingo-oophorectomy, complete or partial, unilateral or bilateral (separate procedure)
58150	Total abdominal hysterectomy (corpus and cervix), with or without removal of tube(s), with or without removal of ovary(s)

When reporting a total abdominal hysterectomy with removal of the tube(s) and ovary(s), it would not be appropriate to separately report code 58720 in conjunction with code 58150. The procedure described by code 58720 is considered an integral component of the procedures described by code 58150.

However, codes designated as separate procedures should be additionally reported when performed independently, unrelated to, or distinct from other procedure(s)/service(s) provided.

Example

58720 Salpingo-oophorectomy, complete or partial, unilateral or bilateral (separate procedure)

If removal of the fallopian tubes and ovaries is the only procedure performed, then it would be appropriate to report code 58720 to describe the procedure performed.

When a procedure or service that is designated as a separate procedure is carried out independently or considered to be unrelated to or distinct from other procedures/services provided at that time, the procedure or service designated as a separate procedure may be reported by itself, or in addition to other procedures/services by appending modifier 59 to the specific separate procedure code reported. This indicates that the procedure is not considered a component of another procedure but is a distinct, independent procedure.

Surgical Package or Global Surgery Concept

A surgical CPT code is a bundled code. As mentioned, a bundled code is a single CPT code used to report a group of related procedures as in the surgical package. **Unbundling** or **fragmented billing** occurs when separate procedures are reported that should have been included under a bundled code. This practice will result in denial of a claim and can also be considered fraud.

A **surgical package** includes specific services in addition to the operation, including these:

- One related E/M encounter on the date immediately before or on the date of procedure, subsequent to the decision for surgery
- Preparing the patient for surgery including local infiltration, topical anesthesia
- Performing the operation, including normal additional procedures, such as debridement
- Immediate postoperative care, including dictating operative notes, talking with the family and other physicians
- Writing orders
- Evaluating the patient in the postanesthesia recovery area
- Typical postoperative follow-up

The typical postoperative care includes follow-up visits for normal uncomplicated care. Each third-party payer determines the number of days in which this follow-up care may take place. Therefore, it is important when certifying for surgery to ask the global period of the third-party payer. The **global period** refers to the number of days surrounding a surgical procedure during which all services relating to that procedure—preoperative, during the surgery, and postoperative—are considered part of the surgical package. This is also referred to as the **global surgical concept**. To determine global days, information from the insurance carrier or other payers may need to be obtained. Many publications and software packages on the market address global days for most carriers and unbundling.

Third-party payers have varying definitions of what constitutes a surgical package and varying policies about what is to be included in the surgical package. Because surgical package rules define what is or is not included in addition to the surgical procedure, the surgery also defines the services for which additional charges can or cannot be submitted.

The CPT code for a normal postoperative follow-up visit included in global service is 99024. This code is useful to the reporting physician for tracking the number of postoperative visits provided that are included in the "package" for the procedure performed.

Two types of services are not included in surgical package codes. These services are reported separately and reimbursed in addition to the surgical package fee:

- Complications, exacerbations, recurrence, or the presence of other diseases or injuries requiring additional services should be separately reported.
- Care for the condition for which a diagnostic surgical procedure was performed or for other coexisting conditions is not included and may be reported separately.

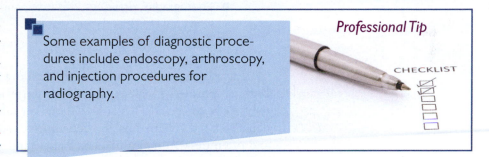

Professional Tip

Some examples of diagnostic procedures include endoscopy, arthroscopy, and injection procedures for radiography.

CHECKLIST

Example

A patient undergoes a diagnostic upper gastrointestinal endoscopy for suspected gastric ulcer disease. The findings of the endoscopy are positive for an acute gastric ulcer. At that time, the physician prescribes medication for treatment of the ulcer disease. The patient is instructed to return to the physician's office in 1 week for follow-up care related to the effectiveness of the medication prescribed.

In the preceding example, the follow-up visit is reported separately with the appropriate level of E/M code based on key components that have been met during the encounter. Care of the condition for which the diagnostic procedure was performed is not included and may be reported separately.

The following are some examples of what is included in a surgical procedure and cannot be billed separately:

- Positioning the patient
- Insertion of intravenous access for medication (IV)
- Administration of sedative by the physician performing the procedure
- Local infiltration of medication—topical, or regional anesthetic administered by the physician performing the procedure
- Surgical approach, including identification of landmarks, incisions, and evaluation of the surgical field
- Exploration of operative area

- Fulguration of bleeding points
- Simple debridement of traumatized tissue
- Lysis of a moderate amount of adhesions
- Isolation of neurovascular tissue or muscular, bony, or other structures limiting access to the surgical field
- Surgical cultures
- Wound irrigation
- Insertion and removal of drains, suction devices, dressings, pumps into or out of same site
- Surgical closure
- Application and removal of postoperative dressings, including analgesic devices
- Application of splints with musculoskeletal procedures
- Institution of patient-controlled analgesia
- Photographs, drawings, dictation, and transcription to document the services provided
- Surgical supplies

An area of great concern in medical billing is inaccurately billing separately for procedures considered incidental to the major procedure. Many CPT surgical narratives in the CPT book include "with or without" or other language to include or exclude incidental services. Numerous procedures are done in conjunction with other procedures, and often the CPT code subsection notes and guidelines will indicate that a particular code includes a variety of the supporting procedures.

The CPT book further states that follow-up care for complications, exacerbations, recurrence, and the presence of other diseases that require additional services is not included in the surgery package. General anesthesia for surgical procedures is not part of the surgical package, and the anesthesiologist bills general anesthesia services separately.

Supplies and Services

Supplies and materials provided by the physician (e.g., sterile trays/drugs) "over and above" those usually included with procedures rendered are listed separately. The guideline indicates that you should list the drugs, trays, supplies, and materials provided, and identify them as code 99070 or use the specific supply code, which can be found in Healthcare Common Procedure Coding System (HCPCS). According to the CPT nomenclature, supplies and materials provided by the physician are reported only if they are "over and above" those usually included with the office visit or other services rendered, such as drugs, special dressings used to pack a wound, wound irrigation equipment, or a pair of crutches.

Radiology Codes

The codes in the Radiology section are used to report radiological services performed by or supervised by a physician. Radiology codes may have two parts:

1. *Results are the technical component of a service. Testing leads to results.* The **technical component** is the part of the relative value associated with the procedure that reflects the test, technologist, equipment, and processing, including preinjection and postinjection

services such as local anesthesia, placement of a needle or catheter, and injection of contrast material. The technical component of taking the X-ray would be reported with the procedure code and the modifier -TC attached to the procedure.

2. *Results lead to interpretation. Reports are the work product of the interpretation of numerous test results.* The **professional component** is the part of the relative value associated with a procedure that represents a physician's skill, time, and expertise used in performing it, as opposed to the technical component. The reading, interpretation, and written report of the radiological examination by the physician would be the professional component and the modifier -26 would be attached to the procedure.

These modifiers are to be used only when the physician's office states that only part of the radiological procedure was done. Otherwise, the descriptor remains as stated with no modifier.

Note that the supervision and interpretation (S&I) descriptor means that the radiology code is only for the professional component. Modifier 26 does not need to be attached. When the word(s) *supervision and interpretation* or the acronym S&I appear, the code for the technical component is selected from another section.

Radiology codes follow the same type of guidelines noted in the Surgery section. For example, some radiology codes are identified as separate procedure codes. These codes are usually part of a larger, more complex procedure and should not be reported as separate codes unless the procedure was done independently. Also, some codes are add-on codes, such as those covering additional vessels that are studied after the basic examination. These codes are used with the primary codes and do not stand alone.

Contrast material is commonly used for imaging enhancement. Contrast material improves visualization and evaluation of the body structure or organ studied. Some of the procedures listed in the Radiology section of the CPT book may be performed with or without the use of contrast material for imaging enhancement. The phrase *with contrast* used in the codes for procedures using contrast for imaging enhancement represents contrast material administered intravascularly, intra-articularly, or intrathecally.

Use your CPT manual to the following situation:

An orthopedic surgeon sends his patient to the radiologist for an X-ray of the leg (73590) but asks that the patient return with the X-ray for his interpretation (professional component).

1. The radiologist would code 73590 with modifier _____

2. The orthopedist would code 73590 with modifier _____

3. How would it be coded if the orthopedist sent the patient to the radiologist to take the X-ray and send the report? _____

4. Complete study, cardiac MRI for function (professional component only) _____

5. Computed tomography, lumbar spine; with contrast material (technical component only) _____

Practice Exercise 7.4

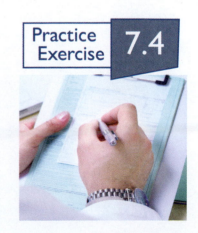

When contrast materials are only administered orally and/or rectally, the study does not qualify as "with contrast" and should be coded "without contrast."

Pathology and Laboratory Codes

The codes in the Pathology/Laboratory section cover services provided by physicians or by technicians under the supervision of a physician. A complete procedure includes the following:

- Ordering the test
- Taking and handling the sample
- Performing the actual test
- Analyzing and reporting on the test results

The 8000 series codes are used to report the performance of specific laboratory tests only and do not include the collection of the specimen via venipuncture (or finger/heel/ear stick), arterial puncture, or other collection methodology (e.g., lumbar puncture). The collection of the specimen by venipuncture or by arterial puncture is not considered an integral part of the laboratory procedure(s) performed. Codes in the 36400–36425 series are used to report venipuncture for obtaining blood samples for diagnostic purposes or to monitor levels of blood components.

A **panel** is a group of tests ordered together to detect particular diseases or malfunctioning organs. Organ or disease-oriented panels are reported with the codes from the 80047–80076 series. These panels were developed for coding purposes and should not be interpreted as clinical standards for testing. When a panel is reported, all of the listed tests must have been performed with no substitution. If fewer tests are performed than those listed in the panel code (unbundling), then the individual code number(s) for each test should be listed rather than the panel code.

Example

80051 Electrolyte Panel
This panel must include the following:

Carbon dioxide	(82374)
Chloride	(82435)
Potassium	(84132)
Sodium	(84295)

Procedures and services are listed in the index under the following types of main terms:

- Name of the test, such as urinalysis, drug test
- Procedure such as hormone assay
- Abbreviations such as CBC, RBS, TLC
- Panel of tests, under Blood Tests

Some medical practices have laboratory equipment and perform their own testing. In-office labs must be certified by the **Clinical Laboratory Improvement**

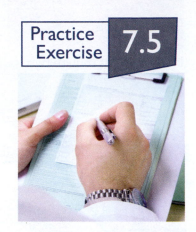
Amendment (**CLIA**) of 1988, which awards three levels of certification. The lowest level for an in-office certified lab can perform dipstick urinalysis and urine pregnancy. If the medical practice does not have a lab but obtains the specimen for the lab, the venipuncture code 36415 may be billed for obtaining the blood sample. As in every medical setting, the Occupational and Safety and Health Administration (OSHA) regulates safety.

Medicine Codes

The Medicine section of the CPT book contains a variety of listings for reporting procedures and services provided by many different types of healthcare providers. In addition, many services and procedures provided by nonphysician practitioners can be found in the Medicine section. For example, codes in the Physical Medicine and Rehabilitation subsection are often used to report the services and procedures provided by physical and occupational therapists. Audiologists and speech therapists find listings in the special Otorhinolaryngologic Services subsection that describes some of the technical procedures and services they provide.

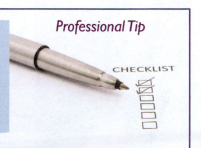

Professional Tip

Immunoglobulins use a different administration code. Always read the notes provided in the section before choosing the correct codes.

CHECKLIST

Codes from the Medicine section may be used with codes from any other section. Add-on codes and separate procedure codes are included in the Medicine section.

The descriptors for injections require two codes: one for administering the immunization and the other for the particular vaccine or toxoid that is given (Figure 7.7).

Cardiac catheterizations are the most commonly performed surgical procedure, with more than 1 million performed each year. Complete coding of cardiac catheterization requires at least three codes: a code for the catheterization procedure itself, a code for the injection procedure, and a code for the imaging supervision and interpretation.

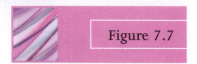

Figure 7.7

Immunizations require two codes.

| 90471 | Immunization administration |
| 90710 | Measles, mumps, rubella, and varicella vaccine (MMRV), live, for subcutaneous use |

Each of these has a professional and a technical component. Unless the physician owns the laboratory, those codes are billed using modifier 26.

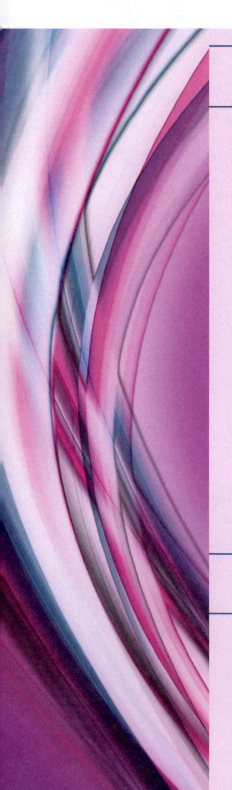

Chapter Summary

- Reimbursement is the key to a medical practice's success. Medical office specialists should be aware of the importance of correct procedure coding.
- When using the CPT index, it is important to understand how entries to the index have been made. It cannot be stressed enough that the CPT index is not a substitute for the main text of the CPT nomenclature.
- Guidelines can be found at the beginning of each of the six sections of the CPT book. These guidelines provide information that is necessary to appropriately interpret and report procedures and services found in that section.
- Modifiers more fully describe procedures that were changed in some way, and they affect the reimbursement by increasing or decreasing the amount.
- Add-on codes describe procedures/services that are always performed in addition to the primary procedure; they are indicated by a plus sign (+) next to the code.
- A bundled code is used to report a group of related procedures, as in a surgical package. Each surgical package has included in its reimbursement a certain number of days during which procedures associated with a surgery are reimbursed, as determined by third-party payers.
- Anesthesia coding requires a physical status modifier. The reimbursement is based on measurement of time.
- With 14 subsections, the Surgery section is the largest CPT section.
- Radiology codes contain two components: technical and professional.
- A panel is a group of tests ordered together to detect particular diseases or malfunctioning organs; panels are found in the Laboratory section.
- The Medicine section contains a variety of listings for reporting procedures and services provided by many different types of healthcare providers.

Chapter Review

True/False

Identify the statement as true (T) or false (F).

_____   **1.** CPT add-on codes are never used as primary procedure codes.

_____   **2.** In the CPT, a bundled code is used to report a group of related procedures.

_____ **3.** If a CPT code is not bilateral, a modifier is used with the code to report a bilateral service.

_____ **4.** The terms *unbundling* and *fragmented billing* in procedural coding have the same meaning.

_____ **5.** A CPT modifier is used to show that only part of a procedure has been done.

_____ **6.** An incomplete CPT code does not have a modifier attached.

_____ **7.** When a physician treats complications or recurrences that arise after surgery, these services are reported separately.

_____ **8.** All third-party payers use the same definitions for surgical package codes.

_____ **9.** A global surgical concept for a diagnostic procedure includes follow-up care related only to recovery from the procedure itself, not for care of the patient's underlying condition.

_____ **10.** Add-on codes that describe qualifying circumstances are available for use with codes from the Surgery section of the CPT.

_____ **11.** Codes from the Surgery section of the CPT cover only the operation itself, not postoperative care.

_____ **12.** To report a bilateral procedure, the modifier 50 (Bilateral Procedure) is attached to the CPT code for the unilateral procedure.

_____ **13.** S&I is the abbreviation for supervision and interpretation.

_____ **14.** The injection of local anesthesia or the application of topical anesthesia by the surgeon can be billed in addition to the operation itself.

Multiple Choice

Identify the letter of the choice that best completes the statement or answers the question.

_____ **1.** In the CPT, what procedure is bundled with the arthroscopy in the following entry? 23515 *Open treatment of clavicular fracture, with or without internal or external fixation*
   a. Open treatment
   b. Clavicular fracture
   c. With or without internal or external fixation
   d. None of the above

_____ **2.** The divisions of the CPT, such as Anesthesia and Radiology, are referred to as:
   a. parts.   c. sections.
   b. chapters.   d. components.

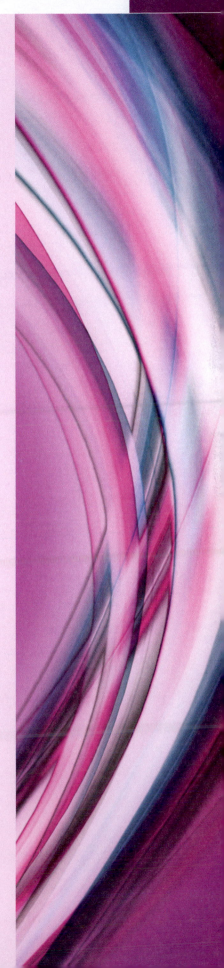

_____ **3.** If fewer tests are performed than those listed in the panel code (unbundling), then the individual code number(s) for each test should be listed rather than the panel code as:

a. unbundled. c. listed separately.

b. bundled. d. none of the above.

_____ **4.** The primary CPT code that is listed first for a claim is the procedure that:

a. is performed first.

b. is the most resource intensive.

c. appears first in the CPT-4.

d. is none of the above.

_____ **5.** Which is the correct process for selecting CPT codes?

a. Locate the probable code, determine the procedures and services it covers, and determine the need for modifiers.

b. Determine the procedures and services to report, identify the correct codes, and determine the need for modifiers.

c. Determine the correct codes and modifiers, and then place them in the proper order from primary to secondary procedures.

d. None of the above

_____ **6.** The largest section in CPT is:

a. Surgery. c. Radiology.

b. Anesthesia. d. Medicine.

_____ **7.** The bundle codes in the CPT's Anesthesia section generally cover:

a. preoperative evaluation and planning.

b. care during the procedure.

c. routine postoperative care.

d. all of the above.

_____ **8.** What is required of the physician in order to report the professional component of a CPT code from the Radiology section?

a. Reading the radiological examination

b. Writing a report of interpretation

c. Both a and b

d. Neither a nor b

_____ **9.** How many CPT codes are required to report an immunization?

a. One c. Three

b. Two d. Four

_____ **10.** A patient has an office encounter for removal of five skin tags on her hand. During the visit, she asks the physician to evaluate swelling and heat in her left knee. The physician performs an expanded history and examination with low medical decision making. What codes should be reported?

a. 11200, 99214 c. 11100, 99213-25

b. 11200, 99213-25 d. 11200, 99213-51

_____ **11.** A patient had a surgery 15 days ago to treat a dislocated ankle. Today, the same surgeon repairs the patient's flexor tendon muscle on the other foot. What code should be reported for today's service?

    a. 28200-79   c. 28200-58

    b. 28200   d. 28200-51

_____ **12.** Radiology codes may have two parts:

    a. Unlisted or guided.

    b. Supervision or interpretation.

    c. Professional or technical.

    d. Complete or partial.

_____ **13.** Under CPT guidelines, all services related to a surgical procedure are not additionally reimbursed:

    a. before the global period.   c. during the global period.

    b. after the global period.   d. during the E/M period.

_____ **14.** CPT codes from the Anesthesia section may use:

    a. standard CPT modifiers and physical status modifiers.

    b. physical status modifiers and duration modifiers.

    c. either a or b.

    d. neither a nor b.

_____ **15.** How many subsections are in the surgery section?

    a. 11   c. 14

    b. 9   d. 15

_____ **16.** In CPT, a plus sign (+) next to a code indicates a(n):

    a. add-on code.   c. revised code

    b. new code.   d. new/revised/text.

Completion

Complete each sentence or statement.

1. In CPT, some codes have both a technical component and a(n) _____ component that represents the physician's skill, time, and expertise.

2. A(n) _____ procedure can be performed in addition to the primary procedure.

3. Codes in the Anesthesia section of the CPT are reimbursed according to _____.

4. Codes for many procedures and services provided by family practice physicians, such as immunizations, are located in the CPT's _____ section.

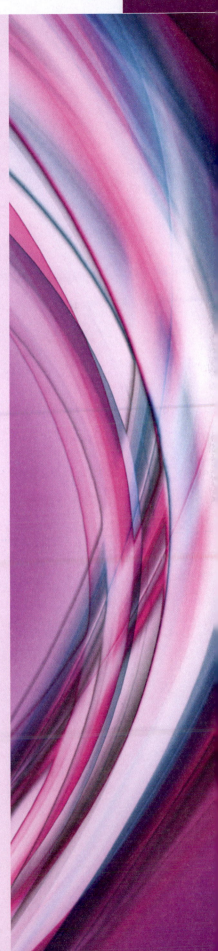

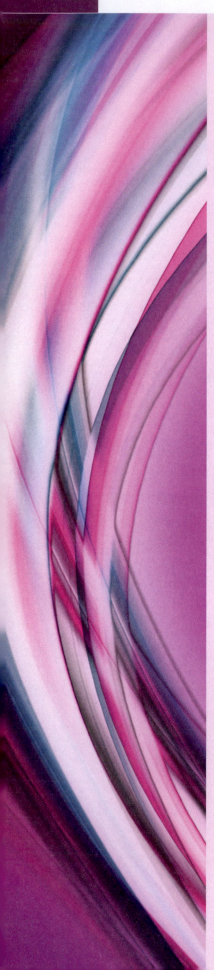

For Additional Practice

Provide the correct modifier for each of the following descriptions.

1. Distinct procedural service _____

2. Mandated service _____

3. Multiple modifiers _____

4. Discontinued procedure _____

5. Radiologist provides a report on a lateral chest X-ray _____

6. Multiple procedures _____

7. Bilateral procedure _____

8. Referenced outside laboratory _____

9. Postoperative management only _____

10. Unrelated procedure by the same physician during the postoperative period _____

Code the following using your CPT manual:

1. Debridement of 10 nails by any method _____

2. Chemical peel, facial; dermal _____

3. Preoperative placement of needle localization wire, breast _____

4. Mastectomy, subcutaneous _____

5. Incision and drainage (I&D) of hematoma, soft tissue of neck _____

6. Manipulation, elbow, under anesthesia _____

7. Endoscopy, surgical; operative tissue ablation and reconstruction of atria, without cardiopulmonary bypass _____

8. Repair atrial septal defect, secundum, with cardiopulmonary bypass, with or without patch _____

9. Laparoscopy, surgical, appendectomy _____

10. Nephrolithotomy; secondary surgical operation for calculus _____

11. Vaginal birth only, including postpartum care _____

12. Removal of lens material; intracapsular, for dislocated lens _____

13. Radiological supervision and interpretation, percutaneous vertebroplasty or vertebral augmentation including cavity creation, per vertebral body under CT guidance _____

14. Mammary ductogram, single duct, radiological supervision and interpretation _____

15. Mammography; bilateral _____

16. Therapeutic radiology treatment, intermediate _____

17. Lipase _____

18. General health panel _____

19. Triglycerides _____

20. PSA total _____

21. Tissue culture for non-neoplastic disorders; lymphocyte _____

22. Pathology consultation during surgery _____

23. Intravenous infusion, hydration 2 hours _____

24. End-stage renal disease (ESRD) related services per full month; for patient 58 years old for home dialysis _____

25. Spirometry, including graphic record, total and timed vital capacity, expiratory flow rate measurement with or without maximal voluntary ventilation _____

26. Application of a modality to one or more areas; diathermy _____

27. Hospital-mandated on-call service; in-hospital (1 hour) _____

28. Ventilation assist and management, initiation of pressure or volume preset ventilators for assisted or controlled breathing; hospital inpatient, initial day _____

29. Tobacco use assessed (CAD, CAP, COPD, PV) _____

30. Dyspnea assessed, present (COPD) _____

Resources

American Society of Anesthesiologists
www.asahq.org
2017 CPT Standard Edition
www.cptnetwork.com

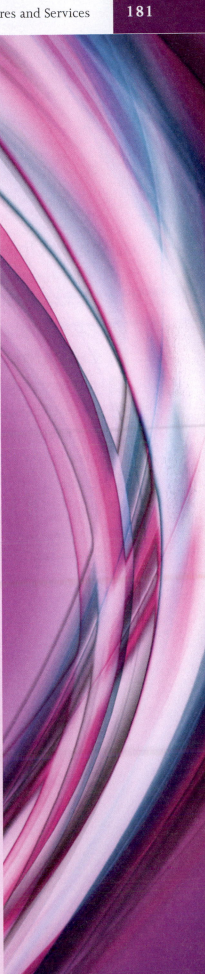

Chapter 8 / HCPCS and Coding Compliance

Chapter Objectives

After reading this chapter, the student should be able to:

1. Understand the two levels of HCPCS.
2. Recognize the need for HCPCS coding and when to report HCPCS codes.
3. Learn how to use HCPCS modifiers.
4. Interpret and identify correct code linkages.
5. Review the coding for accuracy.
6. Understand federal laws, regulations, and penalties that pertain to coding compliance.
7. Understand the responsibilities of coding and coding compliance.
8. Explain the National Correct Coding Initiative.
9. Understand medical ethics for the medical coder.

Key Terms

abuse
advance beneficiary
    notice (ABN)
advisory opinion
assumption coding
code linkage

durable medical
    equipment
    (DME)
fraud
HCPCS
Level I HCPCS

Level II HCPCS
National Correct
    Coding Initiative
    (NCCI)
OIG fraud alerts
OIG Work Plan

CPT codes in this chapter are from the CPT 2017 code set. CPT® is a registered trademark of the American Medical Association.

The physician ordered a blood test to be completed for Mrs. Rhoades, who has Medicare. The medical assistant performed the venipuncture and marked the patient encounter form with the HCPCS code G0001. The billing specialist who was to post the charges noticed that an outdated code had been used. G0001 had been deleted and the correct way to code for a venipuncture is with code 36415. She corrected the error and sent an email memo emphasizing to staff that they must review their coding manuals and use only current codes.

Questions

1. Why is it important to use only current codes and coding books?
2. How could this error have been prevented?
3. Would this claim have been denied? What are some of the effects of a denied claim?

Introduction

HCPCS (pronounced "hick-picks") is the acronym for the Healthcare Common Procedure Coding System. This system is a uniform method used by healthcare providers and medical suppliers to report professional services, procedures, and supplies. Each year in the United States, over 5 billion claims are processed by healthcare insurers for reimbursement. To insure that these claims are processed in an orderly and consistent manner, a standardized coding system is essential. HCPCS has two principal subsections, which are Level I HCPCS and Level II HCPCS. Current Procedural Terminology, referred to as CPT, is Level I HCPCS. Level II HCPCS is used to identify products, supplies, drugs, and services which are not included in the CPT coding set.

It is of the utmost importance that the medical office specialist, who may also do the coding, ensures the codes are applied correctly during the medical billing process. This includes abstracting the information from the medical documentation, assigning the appropriate codes, and creating a clean claim to be paid by the insurance carriers.

History of HCPCS

The Health Insurance Portability and Accountability Act of 1996 (HIPAA) required CMS to adopt standards for coding systems that are used for reporting healthcare transactions. The regulation that CMS published on August 17, 2000 (45 CFR 162.10002), to implement the HIPAA requirement for standardized coding systems established the HCPCS level II codes as the standardized coding system. This system described and identified healthcare equipment and supplies in healthcare transactions that are not CPT code set (HCPCS I) jurisdiction. The HCPCS Level II coding system was selected as the standardized coding system because of its wide acceptance among both public and private insurers. Public and private insurers were required to be in compliance with the August 2000 regulation by October 1, 2002.

HCPCS I and II has maintained the following:

- Meet the operational needs of Medicare/Medicaid
- Coordinate government programs by uniform application of CMS policies
- Allow providers and suppliers to communicate their services in a consistent manner
- Ensure the validity of profiles and fee schedules through standardized coding
- Enhance medical education and research by providing a vehicle for local, regional, and national utilization comparisons

The permanent national codes serve the important function of providing a standardized coding system that is managed jointly by private and public insurers. It supplies a predictable set of uniform codes that provide a stable environment for claims submission and processing.

HCPCS Level of Codes

HCPCS has two levels of coding, each of which is a unique coding system, as discussed in the following subsections. The HCPCS codes used must be valid at the time the service is rendered.

Level I: CPT Codes

The terms **Level I HCPCS** and CPT codes are synonymous. The coder will know that this refers to the CPT book.

Level II: HCPCS National Codes

The CPT book does not contain all of the codes a medical coder might need to report certain medical services, ambulance services, or use of durable medical equipment, drugs and supplies. **Durable medical equipment (DME)** is an appliance, apparatus, or product intended for use in assisting or treating a patient. The CMS developed the second level of HCPCS codes. In contrast to the five-digit codes found in Level I, Level II HCPCS are alphanumeric. These national codes consist of one alphabetic character (a letter between A and V), followed by four digits. The codes are grouped by the type of service or supply they represent and are updated annually by the CMS with input from private insurance companies.

Example

A HCPCS code from injections that may be covered by Medicare is reported from the J series of the Level II codes used for material (drug) that is injected, rather than a CPT code.

Ampicillin up to 500 mg; IM or IV   J0290

Level II codes are required for reporting most medical services and supplies provided to Medicare and Medicaid patients and by most private payers.

Each of the 22 sections covers a related group of items. Review Table 8.1 on page 186 to become familiar with the different types of procedures covered. Codes are provided for a wide range of medical services, dental services, rehabilitative services, drugs, intravenous and chemotherapy treatments, and supplies. For proper reimbursement, this book must be used for the specific supplies used.

National permanent HCPCS Level II codes are maintained by the HCPCS National Panel. The panel is comprised of representatives from the Blue Cross/Blue Shield Association (BCBSA), the Health Insurance Association of America (HIAA), and the CMS. The panel is responsible for making decisions about additions, revisions, and deletions to the permanent national alphanumeric codes. These codes are for the use of all private and public health insurers. The medical office specialist may also refer to the specific website: www.cms.gov/Medicare/Coding/MedHCPCSGenInfo/index.html?redirect=/medhcpcsgeninfo

HCPCS Modifiers

HCPCS modifiers are two-digit codes, which may be either alpha (all letters) or alphanumeric (letters plus numbers). They range from AA to VP. National modifiers can be used with all levels of HCPCS codes.

Table 8.1	Level II HCPCS Codes	
Transportation services	A0021–A0999
Medical and surgical supplies	A4206–A8004
Miscellaneous and experimental	A9150–A9999
Enteral and parenteral therapy	B4034–B9999
Temporary hospital outpatient PPS	C1300–C9899
Durable medical equipment (DME)	E0100–E8002
Procedures and services, temporary	G0008–G9156
Rehabilitative services	H0001–H2037
Drugs administered other than oral method	J0120–J9999
Temporary codes for DMERCS	K0001–K0899
Orthotic procedures	L0112–L4631
Prosthetic procedures	L5000–L9900
Medical services	M0064–M0301
Pathology and laboratory	P2028–P9615
Temporary codes	Q0035–Q9968
Diagnostic radiology services	R0070–R0076
Private payer codes	S0012–S9999
State Medicaid agency codes	T1000–T5999
Vision	V2020–V2799
Hearing services	V5008–V5364

HCPCS modifiers are used to modify procedures and services on health insurance forms filed for Medicare patients. The list of modifiers is shown in Table 8.2.

Use of the GA Modifier

An **advance beneficiary notice (ABN),** according to the CMS, is a written notification that must be signed by the patient or guardian before the provider may render a service to a Medicare beneficiary that could potentially be denied or deemed "not medically necessary." When an ABN is on file, an HCPCS GA modifier must be appended to the code for the service in question on the CMS-1500 form. Once a Medicare beneficiary signs the ABN, he is legally responsible for the charges if Medicare denies payment for the service as "not medically necessary."

HCPCS Index

Because the HCPCS is organized by code number rather than by service or supply name, the index allows you to locate any code without looking through the individual range of codes. To find a code, in the index look up the medical or surgical supply, service, orthotic, prosthetic, or generic drug you need, and you will be directed to the appropriate codes. This index also references many of the brand names by which these items are known.

Table 8.2	HCPCS Modifiers

LT	Left side (used to identify procedures performed on the left side of the body)
RT	Right side (used to determine procedures performed on the right side of the body)
A1	Principal physician of record
BL	Special acquisition of blood and blood products
CA	Procedure payable only in the inpatient setting when performed emergently on an outpatient who expires before admission
CR	Catastrophe/disaster related
E1	Upper left, eyelid
E2	Lower left, eyelid
E3	Upper right, eyelid
E4	Lower right, eyelid
FA	Left hand, thumb
F1	Left hand, second digit
F2	Left hand, third digit
F3	Left hand, fourth digit
F4	Left hand, fifth digit
F5	Right hand, thumb
F6	Right hand, second digit
F7	Right hand, third digit
F8	Right hand, fourth digit
F9	Right hand, fifth digit
FB	Item provided without cost to provider (e.g., sample or replacement of a defective device)
FC	Partial credit received for replaced device
GA	Waiver of liability statement on file
GG	Performance and payment of a screening mammogram and diagnostic mammogram on the same patient, same day
GH	Diagnostic mammogram converted from screening mammogram on same day
LC	Left circumflex, coronary artery (Hospitals use with codes 92980–92984, 92995, 92996.)
LD	Left anterior descending coronary artery (Hospitals use with codes 92980–92984, 92995, 92996.)
LM	Left main coronary artery
QM	Ambulance service provided under arrangement by a provider of services
QN	Ambulance service furnished directly by a provider of services
RC	Right coronary artery (Hospitals use with codes 92980–92984, 92995, 92996.)
TA	Left foot, great toe
T1	Left foot, second digit
T2	Left foot, third digit
T3	Left foot, fourth digit
T4	Left foot, fifth digit
T5	Right foot, great toe
T6	Right foot, second digit
T7	Right foot, third digit
T8	Right foot, fourth digit
T9	Right foot, fifth digit

Source: From HCPCS Level II Coding. Published by U. S. Department of Health and Human Services.

Coding Compliance

One of the most important documents in the medical record is the progress note, which updates the patient's clinical course of treatment and summarizes the assessment and plan of care. If a patient's condition, examination, and treatment plan are not documented in the chart, "It did not happen."

Providers have the ultimate responsibility for proper documentation and correct coding, as well as for compliance with regulations. Medical office specialists help to ensure that maximum reimbursement is received promptly for reported services by submitting correct claims.

Coding compliance is part of the overall effort of medical practices to comply with regulations in many areas, such as patient privacy and the security of patient data. In this sense, compliant claims are an indication of a compliant medical practice. On the other hand, claims that contain errors raise the question of whether the practice is generally acting in a fraudulent manner. To reduce the chances of being targeted for an investigation or an audit, and to reduce the risk of liability if there is an audit, medical practice staff as well as physicians must be aware of, understand, and comply with all applicable regulations and laws.

These claims, as well as the process used to create them, must comply with the rules imposed by federal and state law and by government and private payer healthcare program requirements. Correct claims reduce the chance of an investigation and the risk of liability if an audit occurs. Consequences of inaccurate coding and incorrect billing include the following:

- Denied claims
- Delays in processing claims and receiving payments
- Reduced payments
- Fines and other sanctions
- Exclusion from payers' programs
- Prison sentences
- Loss of the provider's license to practice medicine

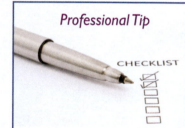

Professional Tip

CHECKLIST

Medicare has placed a cap on the number of physical, respiratory, and cardiac rehabilitation treatments that Medicare patients are allowed. If a provider exceeds that amount and cannot prove that additional therapy was medically necessary, reimbursement for the treatment will be denied. The medical office specialist must be aware of the rules and regulations issued by Medicare and have the patient sign an ABN in advance of treatment received if treatment may exceed the allowed amount and reimbursement may be denied. The Medicare Guidelines for ABNs state that the physician should have the patient sign the ABN. The physician and staff need to work as a team. The medical office specialist, medical assistant, and physician should work together to ensure that patients complete waivers as appropriate. Hospitals would require a Hospital-Issued Notice of Noncoverage (HINNs) which may be required before admission, after admission, and at any point required during an inpatient stay.

The GA modifier must be attached to the CPT code for the provider to be able to bill the patient for the denial.

Code Linkage

On a clean claim, each reported service is connected to a diagnosis that supports the procedure as necessary to investigate or treat the patient's condition. Payers analyze this connection between the diagnostic and the procedural information, called **code linkage**, to evaluate the medical necessity of the reported charges. Correct claims also comply with many other requirements issued by government and private payers. Some regulations involve the place, frequency, or level of services. Some services are always denied as not reasonable, not medically necessary, or experimental. Payers also often deny claims because of certain frequency limitations on services.

The ultimate goal of submitting claims is to be paid and not be audited after payment. If a provider is audited, it takes up time and disrupts the practice of everyday "work."

To increase the chances of submitting a clean claim and having it accepted without an audit, a medical office specialist should ask herself these questions before submitting the claim:

1. Is the coded service billable?
2. Are the codes appropriate to the patient's profile (age, gender, condition)?
3. Is there a clear and correct link between each diagnosis and procedure?
4. Is the documentation in the patient's medical record adequate to support the reported services?
5. Do the reported services comply with all regulations?

Billing CPT Codes

When entering CPT and ICD-10-PCS codes on a claim form, the most resource-intensive procedure or service should be listed first. The third-party payer or Medicare may pay the first listed code at the approved rate but reduce any following procedures by 50% or deny it as being part of the primary procedure.

Fraudulent Claims

The Federal Civil False Claims Act (31 U.S.C. §3729 False Claims) prohibits submitting a fraudulent claim or making a false statement or representation in connection with a claim. The act includes liability for certain acts. Any person who engages in an action listed in Figure 8.1 is submitting fraudulent claims.

Any person who engages in one of the following actions is submitting fraudulent claims:

- Knowingly presents, or causes to be presented to an officer or employee of the U.S. Government a false or fraudulent claim for payment or approval
- Knowingly makes, uses, or causes to be made or used, a false record or statement to get a false or fraudulent claim paid or approved by the Government
- Conspires to defraud the Government by getting a false or fraudulent claim allowed or paid
- Has possession, custody, or control of property or money used, or to be used, by the Government and intending to defraud the Government or willfully to conceal the property
- Knowingly makes, uses, or causes to be made or used, a false record or statement to conceal, avoid, or decrease an obligation to pay or transmit money or property to the Government

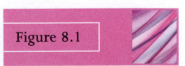

Figure 8.1

A list of fraudulent actions from Civil False Claims Act.

Since 2010, the U.S. Department of Health and Human Services (HHS), Office of Inspector General (HHS OIG), the Centers for Medicare and Medicaid Services (CMS), and the U.S. Department of Justice (DOJ) have been using powerful, new anti-fraud tools to protect Medicare and Medicaid by shifting beyond a "pay and chase" approach toward fraud prevention. Through the groundbreaking Healthcare Fraud Prevention Partnership, stronger relationships have been built between the government and private sector to help protect all consumers.

These focused efforts are successful. In Fiscal Year (FY) 2014, the government recovered $3.3 billion as a result of healthcare fraud judgments, settlements, and additional administrative impositions in healthcare fraud cases and proceedings. Since its inception in 1997, the Health Care Fraud and Abuse Control (HCFAC) Program has returned more than $27.8 billion to the Medicare Trust Funds. The HCFAC program has returned $7.70 for each dollar invested.

The Health Care Fraud Prevention and Enforcement Action Team (HEAT), a joint initiative between HHS, OIG, and DOJ, has played a critical role in the fight against healthcare fraud. A key component of HEAT is the Medicare Fraud Strike Force— interagency task force teams comprised of OIG and DOJ analysts, investigators, and prosecutors who target emerging or migrating fraud schemes, including fraud by criminals masquerading as healthcare providers or suppliers. The federal government encourages reporting of suspected fraud and abuse against the government by protecting and rewarding people involved in qui tam, or whistleblower, cases.

The whistleblower, known as the "relator," files a lawsuit on behalf of the federal government. If the government recovers money from the suit, the whistleblower is entitled to 15–30% of the government's recovery. Unlike other types of lawsuits, a False Claims Act suit cannot be filed without an attorney or "pro se." The whistleblower must find an experienced False Claims attorney to pursue this type of suit.

The Affordable Care Act required CMS to revalidate all existing 1.5 million Medicare suppliers and providers under new risk-based screening requirements. As a result of revalidation and other proactive initiatives, CMS deactivated more than 470,000 enrollments and revoked nearly 28,000 enrollments to prevent certain providers from re-enrolling and billing the Medicare program. Both of these actions immediately stop billing. A provider with deactivated billing privileges can reactivate at any time, and a revoked provider is barred from re-entry into Medicare for a period ranging from 1 to 3 years. Figure 8.2 illustrates False Claims Act judgments and settlements against individuals, groups, or corporations who are guilty of fraud.

Figure 8.3 provides settlement amounts recovered by HHS and the OIG. Note that some of these recoveries were made because the professional provider did not actually administer the service and the modalities given were not one-on-one with the patient as indicated. Although this would be the responsibility of the provider of the service, the coder must be aware of the differences in the procedures when coding.

Physician Self-Referral (Stark Law)

Physician self-referral is the practice of a physician referring a patient to a medical facility in which she has a financial interest, be it ownership, investment, or a structured compensation arrangement. Critics of the practice allege an inherent conflict of interest, given the physician's position to benefit from the referral. They suggest that such arrangements may encourage overutilization of services, in turn driving up healthcare costs. In addition, they believe that it would create a captive referral system, which limits competition from other providers. An example of federal legislation of this situation is the Stark Law (kickbacks), which governs physician self-referral for

June 1, 2016; U.S. Attorney; District of Columbia
Owners of Home Health Care Agency Sentenced to Prison For Taking Part in $80 Million Medicaid Fraud

WASHINGTON – Florence Bikundi and her husband, Michael D. Bikundi, Sr., the owners of Global Healthcare, Inc., a home care agency, were sentenced today to prison terms for health care fraud, money laundering, and other charges stemming from a scheme in which they and others defrauded the District of Columbia Medicaid program of over $80 million.

May 31, 2016; District of New Jersey
Newark Hospital To Pay $450,000 For Allegedly Billing Health Care Programs For Unnecessary Procedures

NEWARK, N.J. – Saint Michael's Medical Center Inc., located in Newark, New Jersey, has agreed to pay $450,000 to resolve allegations that it falsely billed Medicare and Medicaid for medically unnecessary cardiac procedures, U.S. Attorney Paul J. Fishman announced today.

May 20, 2016; U.S. Attorney; Northern District of Illinois
Local Physician Pleads Guilty to Health Care Fraud

ROCKFORD – A suspended physician pleaded guilty today in federal court to charges of health care fraud. CHARLES S. DEHANN, 61, of Belvidere, Ill., pleaded guilty before Judge Frederick J. Kapala to two counts of health care fraud in a scheme to defraud Medicare that included overbilling and billing Medicare for treatment of patients that were already deceased.

May 6, 2016; U.S. Attorney; Eastern District of Pennsylvania
Settlement Reached Over University's Home Health Care Billing

PHILADELPHIA – The United States has reached a settlement agreement with the Trustees of the University of Pennsylvania, on behalf of its operating divisions, including the University of Pennsylvania Health System (UPHS), for the alleged submission of false home health care billings to the Medicare program. The settlement includes $75,787 to resolve allegations that Penn Care at Home violated the False Claims Act by submitting claims to Medicare for services not rendered and for services that were not reasonable or necessary. As part of the settlement agreement, UPHS has also agreed to implement new compliance oversight measures for its home health entities and will annually submit certified compliance reports pertaining to its home health entities to the United States Attorney's Office through 2019. The settlement releases UPHS from liability for conduct pertaining to a specific limited number of episodes of patient care.

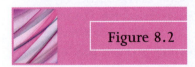

Figure 8.2   False Claims Act Legal Center.

Source: http://oig.hhs.gov/fraud/enforcement/criminal/

Medicare and Medicaid patients. The law is named for U.S. Congressman Pete Stark, who sponsored the initial bill.

The Stark Law prohibits physicians from referring Medicare patients for "designated health services" to entities with which the physician or the physician's immediate family members have a financial relationship, unless the relationship meets one of the detailed exceptions set forth in the law and accompanying regulations. Likewise, the Stark Law prohibits an entity from submitting Medicare claims based upon such prohibited referrals and requires entities to refund amounts received for items or services provided pursuant to prohibited referrals. Sanctions for violating the Stark Law include denial of payment, civil monetary penalties of up to $15,000 per claim submitted, and exclusion from the federal healthcare programs. Knowingly submitting claims based upon prohibited referrals, and retaining sums paid on such claims, constitute violations

Health Care Fraud

Including this past year's $1.9 billion, the department has recovered nearly $16.5 billion in health care fraud since January 2009 to the end of fiscal year 2015 – more than half the health care fraud dollars recovered since the 1986 amendments to the False Claims Act. These recoveries restore valuable assets to federally funded programs such as Medicare, Medicaid, and TRICARE – the health care program for the military. But just as important, the department's vigorous pursuit of health care fraud prevents billions more in losses by deterring others who might otherwise try to cheat the system for their own gain. The department's success is a direct result of the high priority the Obama Administration has placed on fighting health care fraud. In 2009, the Attorney General and the Secretary of the Department of Health and Human Services, the department that administers Medicare and Medicaid, announced the creation of an interagency task force called the Health Care Fraud Prevention and En-forcement Action Team (HEAT), to increase coordination and optimize criminal and civil enforcement. Additional information on the government's efforts in this area is available at StopMedicareFraud.gov, a webpage jointly established by the Departments of Justice and Health and Human Services.

Two of the largest health care recoveries this past year were from DaVita Healthcare Partners, Inc., the leading provider of dialysis services in the United States. DaVita paid $450 million to resolve allegations that it knowingly generated unnecessary waste in administering the drugs Zemplar and Venofer to dialysis patients, and then billed the government for costs that could have been avoided. DaVita paid an additional $350 million to resolve claims that it violated the False Claims Act by paying kickbacks to physicians to induce patient referrals to its clinics. DaVita is headquartered in Denver, Colorado, and has dialysis clinics in 46 states and the District of Columbia.

Hospitals were involved in nearly $330 million in settlements and judgments this past year. A cardiac nurse and a health care reimbursement consultant filed a *qui tam* suit against hundreds of hospitals that were allegedly implanting cardiac devices in Medicare patients contrary to criteria established by the Centers for Medicare and Medicaid Services in consultation with cardiologists, professional cardiology societies, cardiac device manufactur-ers, and patient advocates. The department settled with nearly 500 of these hospitals for a total of $250 million, including $216 million recovered in the past fiscal year. For details, see 500 Hospitals.

Several settlements involved violations of the Stark Law. The Stark Statute prohibits certain financial relationships between hospitals and doctors that could improperly influence patient referrals. Services provided in violation of the Stark Statute are not reimbursable by Medicare or Medicaid. Hospitals settling false claims involving Stark violations include Adventist Health System for $115 million, an organization that operates hospitals and other health care facilities in 10 states; North Broward Hospital District for $69.5 million, a special taxing district of Florida that operates hospitals and other health care facilities in Broward County, Florida; and Georgia hospital system Columbus Regional Healthcare System and Dr. Andrew Pippas for $25 million plus contingent payments up to an additional $10 million. The Adventist settlement also involved allegations of miscoding claims to obtain higher reimbursements for services than allowed by Medicare and Medicaid.

Claims involving the pharmaceutical industry accounted for $96 million in settlements and judgments. Daiichi Sankyo Inc., a global pharmaceutical company with its U.S. headquarters in New Jersey, paid $39 million to resolve allegations of false claims against the United States and state Medicaid programs. Daiichi allegedly paid kickbacks to physicians to induce them to prescribe Daiichi drugs, including Azor, Benicar, Tribenzor and Welchol. Medicare and Medicaid prohibit reimbursement for drugs involved in kickback schemes. AstraZeneca LP and Cephalon Inc. paid the United States $26.7 million and $4.3 million, respectively, in separate settlements for allegedly underpaying rebates owed under the Medicaid Drug Rebate Program. As part of those settlements, the two drug manufactur-ers agreed to pay an additional $23 million to state Medicaid programs for their losses. And in another settle-ment, PharMerica Corp., the nation's second largest nursing home pharmacy, agreed to pay the United States

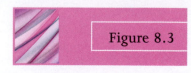

Figure 8.3   Settlement amounts recovered by the HHS and the OIG.

$9.25 million to resolve allegations that it solicited and received kickbacks from pharmaceutical manufacturer Abbott Laboratories in exchange for promoting the drug Depakote for nursing home patients. PharMerica is headquartered in Louisville, Kentucky.

Skilled nursing homes and rehabilitation facilities have also been fertile ground for civil fraud and false claims actions. In the largest failure of care settlement with a skilled nursing home chain in the department's history, Extendicare Health Services Inc. and its subsidiary, Progressive Step Corporation, agreed to pay the United States $32.3 million to resolve allegations that Extendicare billed Medicare and Medicaid for deficient nursing services and billed Medicare for medically unreasonable and unnecessary rehabilitation therapy services. Extendicare and Pro-Step paid an additional $5.7 million to eight states for their Medicaid losses. The department has ongoing litigation against additional nursing home chains and rehabilitation centers based on similar allegations of false claims for medically unreasonable or unnecessary rehabilitation therapy. For example, see HCR ManorCare.

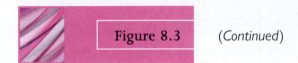

Figure 8.3   *(Continued)*

of the FCA. The FCA provides for treble damages and civil penalties between $5,500 and $11,000 per claim.

An example of a violation of this is the case, *United States ex rel. Baklid-Kunz v. Halifax Hospital Medical Center and Halifax Staffing, Inc.*, which was filed in June 2009 by a whistleblower who had served as Halifax's director of physician services. The government intervened in the case in September 2011. The case alleged, among other things, that Halifax's arrangements with medical oncologists and neurosurgeons violated the Stark Law, and that Medicare claims submitted by Halifax based upon referrals from these physicians violated the FCA.

The government alleged that the prohibited referrals in this case resulted in the submission of 74,838 claims and an overpayment of $105,366,000. Given the possibility of treble damages and civil penalties, Halifax faced a possible damage award in excess of $1.1 billion.

The case involved many important legal questions arising under the Stark Law and FCA. The parties and the court focused on two key elements common to many frequently used Stark Law exceptions—that compensation cannot take into account the volume or value of referrals and that compensation must be within fair market value. The case was set for trial in 2014 but the case was settled before trial.

The government argued that Halifax's arrangements with the medical oncologists failed to comply with a Stark Law exception because those arrangements took into account the volume or value of the physicians' referrals. The arrangements with the medical oncologists provided for a base salary and participation in a bonus pool equal to 15% of the operating margin of the medical oncology program at Halifax. The bonus pool was allocated among the physicians in proportion to their personally performed services. Because the bonus pool included revenues for designated health services referred by the physicians (i.e., services not personally performed by the physicians), the government argued that the arrangement took into account the volume or value of the physicians' referrals, regardless of how the bonus pool was allocated among the individual physicians. In a ruling prior to trial, the court agreed with the plaintiffs and found that as a matter of law these arrangements violated the Stark Law. This ruling meant that the only issue at trial related to the medical oncologist arrangements was the amount of damages to be awarded to the government.

According to the government's expert witness, these arrangements resulted in compensation to the neurosurgeons in amounts over twice the compensation paid to neurosurgeons at the 90th percentile of their specialty, despite producing below the 90th percentile. Halifax argued that a number of factors justified the levels of compensation paid to the neurosurgeons. In a pretrial ruling, the trial court found that whether the arrangements resulted in compensation that fell within fair market value was a disputed issue of fact to be resolved by the jury at trial.

The settlement of 85 million dollars brings to an end a case that demonstrates the high stakes involved in FCA cases arising out of alleged violations of the Stark Law, and the many difficult and unsettled legal issues that healthcare providers face.

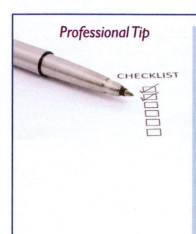

Professional Tip

CHECKLIST

Knowing the difference between a supervised modality and a constant attendance modality for physical therapy is required for proper coding. In the case of HealthSouth (see Figure 8.3), if the physical therapist was not in constant attendance with the patient the claim would be fraudulent. By contrast, supervised attendance does not require direct (one-on-one) contact by the provider.

Government Investigations and Advice

Civil Law

Under civil law the maximum penalty for medical fraud is $10,000 for each item or service for which fraudulent payment has been received. An amount up to three times the amount of the claim can also be fined.

Criminal Law

Because medical fraud can have criminal aspects, those found guilty can receive jail sentences of up to 10 years as well as fines. If a patient is seriously injured or dies, longer jail sentences—up to life imprisonment—are probable.

Administrative Law

Physicians can also be subject to administrative remedies, such as exclusion from participation as providers in all government health programs.

Most billing-related accusations are based on the Civil False Claims Act and on Section 231 of HIPAA, which broadened the definition of fraud to state that providers who knew or should have known that a claim for service was false can be held liable.

Fraud is an act of deception used to take advantage of another person or entity. If a person pretends to be a physician and treats patients without a valid medical license, these actions constitute fraud. Fraudulent acts are intentional because the person knows that the act is illegal and is trying to obtain a profit. In federal law, **abuse** is an action that misuses the money that the government has allocated, such as Medicare funds. Abuse is illegal because the taxpayers' dollars are misspent. A healthcare claim fraud occurs when healthcare providers or others falsely represent their services or charges to payers. A provider may bill for services that were not performed, code at a higher level to increase payment, or fail to provide complete services under a contract. The key difference between fraud and abuse is as follows: To bill when the procedure was not done is fraud; to bill when it was not necessary is abuse.

Each year the OIG announces the **OIG Work Plan**. This plan lists the year's planned projects for sampling types of billing to see if there are any problems. Each year a specific area of billing will be audited.

In 2016, the OIG reviewed Medicare incentive payments to eligible healthcare professionals and hospitals for adopting EHRs (electronic health records) and CMS safeguards to prevent erroneous incentive payments. The work plan also reviewed Medicare incentive payment data to identify payments to providers that should not have received incentive payments (e.g., those not meeting selected meaningful use criteria). It also assessed CMS's plans to oversee incentive payments for the duration of the program and corrective actions taken regarding erroneous incentive payments.

Medicare incentive payments are authorized over a 5-year period to physicians and hospitals that demonstrate meaningful use of certified EHR technology. (Recovery Act, §§ 4101 and 4102.) Incentive payments were scheduled to begin in 2011 and continue through 2016, with payment reductions to healthcare professionals who fail to become meaningful users of EHRs beginning in 2015. (§ 4101(b).) As of July 2015, Medicare EHR incentive payments totaled more than $20 billion. (OAS; W-00-14-31352; expected issue date: FY 2016; Recovery Act.)

Medicaid incentive payments were also reviewed to Medicaid providers and hospitals for adopting EHRs and CMS safeguards to prevent erroneous incentive payments. It also determined whether incentive payments to Medicaid providers to purchase, implement, and operate EHR technology were claimed in accordance with Medicaid requirements; assess CMS's actions to remedy erroneous incentive payments and its plans for securing the payments for the duration of the incentive program; and HHS OIG Work Plan Mid-Year Update | FY 2016 Appendix B—Recovery Act Reviews Page 76 determine whether payments to states for related administrative expenses were appropriate.

The law authorizes 100% federal financial participation for allowable expenses for eligible Medicaid providers to purchase, implement, and operate certified EHR technology. (Recovery Act, § 4201.) The section also provides a 90% federal match for state administrative expenses for the adoption of certified EHR technology by Medicaid providers. As of July 2015, Medicaid EHR incentive payments totaled more than $9 billion. Incentive payments will continue through 2021. (OAS; W-00-14-31351; W-00-15-31351; various reviews; expected issue date: FY 2016; Recovery Act.)

The OIG performed audits of various covered entities receiving EHR incentive payments from CMS to determine whether they adequately protect electronic health information created or maintained by certified EHR technology. A core meaningful-use objective for eligible providers and hospitals is to protect electronic health information created or maintained by certified EHR technology by implementing appropriate technical capabilities. To meet and measure this objective, eligible hospitals must conduct a security risk analysis of certified EHR technology as defined in Federal regulations and use the capabilities and standards of Certified Electronic Health Record Technology. (45 CFR § 164.308(a)(1) and 45 CFR §§ 170.314(d)(1)–(d)(9).) (OAS; W-00-14-42002). The OIG chooses a specific region of the country in which to conduct such audits. If the OIG finds problems with billing the targeted codes, then it will expand the investigation nationally.

OIG fraud alerts are issued periodically by the OIG and are posted on the CMS website to advise providers of problematic actions that have come to the OIG's attention. The OIG also issues CMS advisory bulletins that alert providers and government-sponsored program beneficiaries of potential problems. Providers are responsible for knowing the contents of the advisories and can be prosecuted for "not knowing." The medical office specialist must read the bulletins to be knowledgeable of any changes or updates in billing and coding procedures.

Errors Relating to Code Linkage and Medical Necessity

Three common types of errors are associated with the code linkage process and the question of medical necessity:

1. The CPT procedure codes must match the *International Classification of Diseases, Tenth Revision, Clinical Modification* (ICD-10-CM) diagnosis codes. For example, billing for

drainage of a pilonidal cyst would need a diagnosis of pilonidal cyst with or without mention of abscess.

2. The procedures must not be elective, experimental, or nonessential. For example, billing for a cosmetic surgery for an eyelift when the procedure was done for appearance only and not medically necessary is not allowed. If, however, the patient had blepharoptosis, then the eyelift would be medically necessary and would not be considered an elective surgery.

3. The procedures must be furnished at an appropriate level. Coding of the E/M codes must be done at the appropriate level that meets the reason for the encounter, history, examination, and the medical decision making.

Errors Relating to the Coding Process

Other common errors include those that arise during the coding process:

1. **Assumption coding:** Reporting items or services that are not actually documented, but the coder assumes they were performed
2. Altering documentation after the services are reported
3. Coding without proper documentation
4. Reporting services provided by unlicensed or unqualified clinical personnel
5. Failure to have all necessary documentation available at the time of coding

Errors Relating to the Billing Process

Yet other errors surround the billing process itself:

1. Reporting services that are not covered or have limited coverage
2. Using modifiers incorrectly
3. *Upcoding:* Using a procedure code that provides a higher reimbursement rate than the code that actually reflects the services provided
4. *Unbundling:* Billing the parts of a bundled procedure as separate procedures

National Correct Coding Initiative

The Medicare **National Correct Coding Initiative (NCCI)** (also known as CCI) was implemented to promote national correct coding methodologies and to control improper coding leading to inappropriate payment. NCCI Procedure-to-Procedure (PTP) code pair edits are automated prepayment edits that prevent improper payment when certain codes are submitted together for Part B-covered services. In addition to PTP code pair edits, the NCCI includes a set of edits known as Medically Unlikely Edits (MUEs). An MUE is a maximum number of Units of Service (UOS) allowable under most circumstances for a single Healthcare Common Procedure Coding System/Current Procedural Terminology (HCPCS/CPT) code billed by a provider on a date of service for a single beneficiary.

Accurate coding and reporting of services are critical aspects of proper billing. Service denied based on PTP code pair edits or MUEs may not be billed to Medicare beneficiaries; a provider cannot utilize an Advance Beneficiary Notice of Noncoverage (ABN) to seek payment from a Medicare beneficiary. The NCCI tools found on the CMS website (including the "National Correct Coding Initiative Policy Manual for Medicare Services") help providers avoid coding and billing errors and subsequent payment denials. It is important to understand, however, that the NCCI does not include all possible combinations of correct coding edits or types of unbundling that exist. Providers are obligated to code correctly even if edits do not exist to prevent use of an inappropriate code combination. Should providers determine that claims have been coded incorrectly, they are responsible to contact their Medicare Administrative Contractor (MAC) about potential payment adjustments.

There are four types of edits for NCCI errors:

- *Column I versus Column II edits:* In this group, the first column (formerly known as comprehensive) of codes contains the comprehensive code, and the second column (formerly known as the component column) shows the code. According to the NCCI, Column I code includes all the services that are described by Column II code, so the Column II code cannot be billed together with the Column I code for the same patient on the same day of service.

Example	
Column I	Column II
27370	20610, 76000, 76001

- *Mutually exclusive edits:* Since 1996, the Medicare NCCI procedure-to-procedure (PTP) edits have been assigned to either the Column I/Column II Correct Coding edit file or the Mutually Exclusive edit file based on the criterion for each edit. The Mutually Exclusive edit file included edits where two procedures could not be performed at the same patient encounter because the two procedures were mutually exclusive based on anatomic, temporal, or gender considerations. All other edits were assigned to the Column I/Column II Correct Coding edit file. The edits previously contained in the Mutually Exclusive edit file were *not* deleted but were moved to the Column I/Column II Correct Coding edit file.

Example	
Column I	Column II
50021	49061, 50020

- *Modifier indicators:* This type of NCCI modifier is a number appearing alongside the comprehensive and component code list and the mutually exclusive code list. A provider may include an NCCI modifier to allow payment for both services within the code pair under certain circumstances.
- *Medically Unlikely Edits (MUEs):* An MUE is a maximum number of Units of Service (UOS) allowable under most circumstances for a single Healthcare Common Procedure Coding System/Current Procedural Terminology (HCPCS/CPT) code billed by a provider on a date of service for a single beneficiary. For an example, refer to: The National Correct Coding Initiative Policy Manual may be obtained through the CMS website: www.cms.gov/Medicare/Coding/NationalCorrectCodInitEd/index.html

The student should refer to this manual for more detailed explanation of the tools available for edit. These edits are specific to outpatient or inpatient billing. They will properly show in the coding edit table if the codes are reimbursable. Below is the website on How to Use NCCI Tools.

https://www.cms.gov/Outreach-and-Education/Medicare-Learning-Network-MLN/MLNProducts/Downloads/How-To-Use-NCCI-Tools.pdf

Fraudulent Actions

Healthcare payers base their decision to pay or deny claims only on the diagnosis and procedure codes. The integrity of the request for payment rests on the accuracy and the honesty of the coding. Incorrect coding may be simply an error or may represent deliberate efforts to obtain fraudulent payment. Actions that might be viewed as occasional slips or errors could also be interpreted as establishing a pattern and practice of violations, which constitutes the knowledge meant by "providers knew or should have known."

If a provider has a question as to the legality of an action, the OIG and CMS offer an advisory opinion. An **advisory opinion** is legal advice on any question regarding healthcare business. The requesting party, such as a physician, nursing home, or hospital, formally presents a situation and asks whether the way they intend to handle it is acceptable. The answer is written to the requesting parties and then becomes public so that anyone who needs to know the answer to specific questions can study the opinions. They are published without revealing the requesting parties' name. If the requesting party does not follow the OIG's advice, then they could be prosecuted. If they were in error before the opinion but change their practice to concur with the opinion, then they are immune from investigation. An advisory opinion is the best way to be sure that an intended action will not be subject to investigation.

Federal Compliance

The *Federal Register* publishes the *Compliance Program Guidance for Individual and Small Group Physician Practices* developed by the OIG. The creation of compliance program guidelines is a major initiative of the OIG in its effort to engage the private healthcare community in preventing the submission of erroneous claims and in combating fraudulent conduct. Also available online is the *Medicare Carrier's Manual*, which interprets the guidelines of the Medicare program. The medical office specialist must be familiar with the Medicare website, which provides information on all rules and guidelines for billing.

It is important to emphasize again that the excuse that a billing action was made in error because the provider "didn't know" is not acceptable when billing a government entity. Such actions will be interpreted as violations and may result in penalties and fines for fraud and abuse.

How to Be Compliant

A physician must have a compliance plan in place. The seven components included in the OIG's *Compliance Program Guidance* provide a solid basis on which a physician's practice can create her compliance program:

- Conduct internal monitoring and auditing
- Implement compliance and practice standards

- Designate a compliance officer or contact
- Conduct appropriate training and education
- Respond appropriately to detected offenses and develop corrective actions
- Develop open lines of communication
- Enforce disciplinary standards through well-publicized guidelines

This guidance for physicians' practices does not suggest that physicians' practices implement all seven components of a full-scale compliance program. Instead, the guidance emphasizes a step-by-step approach to follow in developing and implementing a voluntary compliance program.

All healthcare providers have a duty to ensure that the claims submitted to federal healthcare programs are true and accurate. The best way to ensure that an office is honest is to have a compliance plan in place.

Benefits of a Compliance Program

The following are benefits of a compliance program:

- Optimizes the speed of processing and the proper payment of claims
- Minimizes billing mistakes
- Reduces the chances that an audit will be conducted by CMS or the OIG
- Avoids conflicts with the self-referral and anti-kickback statutes

A voluntary compliance plan also shows that the physician's practice is making good-faith efforts to submit claims appropriately. Practices that embrace the active application of compliance principles in their practice culture and make efforts at compliance on a continued basis can help to prevent problems from occurring in the future. A compliance program also sends an important message to the employees of a physician's practice that, although the practice recognizes that mistakes will occur, employees have an affirmative, ethical duty to come forward and report erroneous or fraudulent conduct so that it may be corrected.

Ethics for the Medical Coder

The professional medical office specialist who is responsible for medical coding has a duty to code medical services and procedures to the best of his ability. The guidelines and the codes combined with the regulatory errata change on an almost daily basis. It is important that the coder know his limitations and ask for help from the provider or a more experienced coder when doubts exist as to appropriate coding for a medical situation. The AMA, national specialty medical societies, and local carriers can provide important information regarding coding, governmental regulations, and other payers' policies concerning compliance, coding, and reimbursement.

Accessing patient records is usually a necessary part of the coder's tasks. Patient confidentiality is a patient's right and should never be violated. It is never appropriate to speak of a patient's medical condition with anyone but the medical provider. All such discussions should take place in private areas far from the public ear.

The role of the professional medical office specialist will often be that of emissary and educator to providers and other members of the office staff. The coder's job is to teach and implement strategies for correct coding. When a coder's ability to code services, procedures, and diagnoses is compromised on the job by coding policies deemed fraudulent, then she should try to resolve the problem through the organization's compliance program. Only when all avenues have failed should a coder consider reporting a provider to the authorities. It is the professional coder's job to be a part of a solution, not part of a problem.

A coder should never change billing information marked on an encounter form by a provider without informing the provider of the issue. Good communication skills will serve as an invaluable tool to the professional medical coder. Open dialogue with the provider is the key to success.

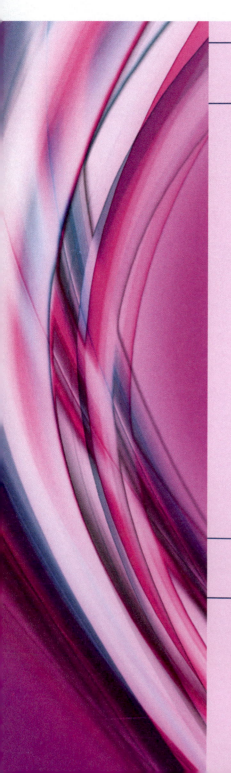

Chapter Summary

- HCPCS is the acronym for the Healthcare Common Procedure Coding System.
- Each of the two HCPCS levels represents a unique coding system.
- Level I is CPT coding.
- Level II is HCPCS national codes, which consist of one alphabetic character (a letter between A and V), followed by four digits.
- The GA modifiers must be used when an ABN is given.
- The HCPCS is organized by code number rather than by service or supply name, so the HCPCS index is invaluable for finding a particular service and its code.
- Payers analyze the connection between the diagnostic and the procedural information, called code linkage, to evaluate the medical necessity of the reported charges.
- When entering CPT or ICD-10-PCS codes on a claim form, the most resource-intensive procedure or service should be listed first.
- The Federal Civil False Claims Act prohibits submitting a fraudulent claim.
- The Health Insurance Portability and Accountability Act of 1996 (HIPAA) created the Healthcare Fraud and Abuse Control Program to uncover fraud and abuse in the Medicare and Medicaid programs.
- Medicare's national policy on correct coding is called the Medicare National Correct Coding Initiative.
- To be compliant, a physician's practice will have a compliance plan in place.
- The coder's job is to teach and implement strategies for correct coding. Problems should be resolved through the facility's compliance program.
- The Stark Law prohibits physicians from self-referral.

Chapter Review

True/False

Identify the statement as true (T) or false (F).

_____ **1.** NCCI is the abbreviation for National Current Coding Initiative.

_____ **2.** Fraud alerts are issued once a year by the Office of Inspector General.

_____ **3.** Work Plans are issued periodically as needed by the Office of Inspector General.

_____ **4.** OIG fraud alerts explain potentially fraudulent or noncompliant billing and reporting practices to providers.

_____ **5.** Overpayments to providers from the Medicare program are always the result of fraud and abuse.

_____ **6.** The OIG Work Plan lists the types of medical billing and reporting practices that the Office of Inspector General intends to investigate in the coming year.

_____ **7.** Coding and billing errors may be considered fraudulent when they are part of a repeated pattern found by an external auditor.

_____ **8.** Having a compliance plan helps a medical practice prevent fraud and abuse relating to reimbursement for services and procedures.

_____ **9.** A medical practice that has a compliance plan demonstrates its desire to be in compliance with rules and regulations.

_____ **10.** Reporting more than one diagnosis code indicates that the procedures are medically necessary.

_____ **11.** A provider who is found guilty of fraud and abuse against the Medicare program can be excluded from further participation as a provider in all government-sponsored healthcare programs.

_____ **12.** Under civil law, large financial penalties and fines can be levied against those guilty of fraud and abuse.

Multiple Choice

Identify the letter of the choice that best completes the statement or answers the question.

_____ **1.** Durable medical equipment (DME), such as wheelchairs, covered by the Medicare program are reported using:
   a. ICD-10-CM codes.   c. HCPCS Level II codes.
   b. CPT codes.   d. local Medicare carrier codes.

_____ **2.** In Medicare's National Correct Coding Initiative, which type of code cannot be billed together with its comprehensive code for the same patient on the same day of service?
   a. Edit   c. Diagnostic
   b. Exclusive   d. Component

_____ **3.** Proposed and final rules from the CMS about the Medicare program are published in:
   a. OIG advisory opinions.
   b. local newspapers.
   c. the _Federal Register_.
   d. the National Correct Coding Initiative.

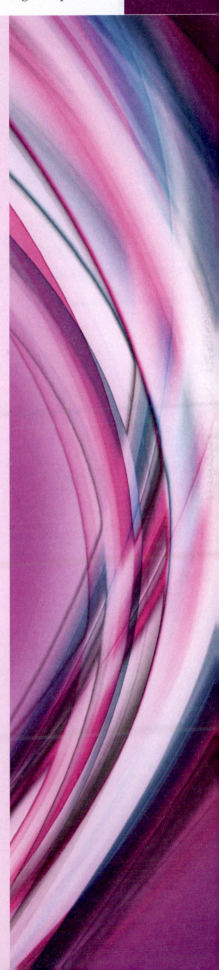

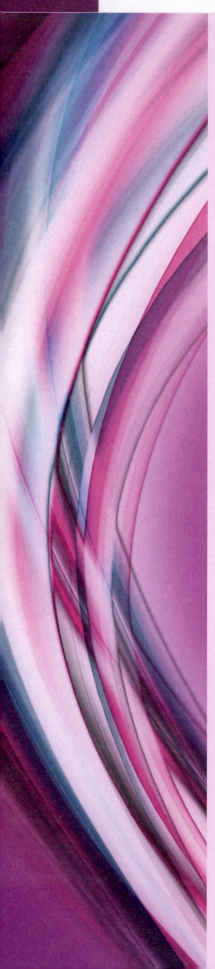

_____ 4. Some possible consequences of inaccurate coding and incorrect billing in a medical practice are:

    a. denied claims and reduced payments.

    b. prison sentences.

    c. fines.

    d. all of the above.

Completion

Complete each sentence or statement.

1. Medicare's National Correct Coding Initiative lists procedures that cannot be billed together for the same _____ on the same _____ of service.

2. To establish compliance plans and follow up on implementation, most medical practices appoint a(n) _____.

3. Healthcare payers base their decision to pay or deny claims only on the _____ and _____ codes.

4. Providers have the ultimate _____ for _____ and _____.

5. Medical practice staff as well as physicians must be aware of, understand, and _____ with all applicable _____ and _____.

6. Each reported service connected to a diagnosis that supports the procedure results in _____.

7. Level I HCPCS codes are found in the _____ book.

8. _____ prohibits submitting a fraudulent claim or making a false statement or representation in connection with a claim.

9. _____ created the Healthcare Fraud and Abuse Control Program to uncover fraud and abuse in the Medicare and Medicaid programs.

10. NCCI means _____.

11. A(n) _____ is legal advice on any question regarding healthcare business.

12. The _____ sets forth the _Compliance Program Guidance for Individual and Small Group Physician Practices_ developed by the Office of Inspector General.

For Additional Practice

Code the following:

1. Ampicillin sodium 500 mg injection: _____

2. Penicillin G benzathine and penicillin procaine 100,000 units: _____

3. Speech screening: _____

4. Ambulatory surgical boot: _____

5. Oxygen tent: _____

6. Roll-about chair with 6-inch casters: _____

7. Hemi-wheelchair with detachable arm desk and swing-away detachable leg rests: _____

Resources

The False Claims Act Legal Center
www.taf.org/top20.htm
www.justice.gov/sites/default/files/civil/legacy/2011/04/22/CFRAUDS_FCA_Primer.pdf

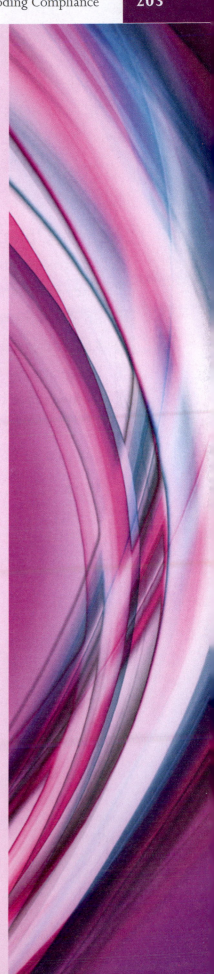

Chapter Objectives

After reading this chapter, the student should be able to:

1. Understand and know how to implement a coding audit.
2. Be able to review and analyze medical records.
3. Know how to use an audit tool.
4. Recognize the content and documentation requirements.
5. Demonstrate the ability to review for coding accuracy.

Key Terms

audit	internal audit	prospective audit
code edits	Patient Protection and	retrospective audit
downcode	Affordable Care Act	upcode
external audit	(PPACA)	

CPT-4 codes in this chapter are from the CPT-4 2017 code set. CPT® is a registered trademark of the American Medical Association.

Dr. Terrance is a family practice physician. He has been practicing for 30 years, and his manner of documentation has been the same for all of that time. With the changes in the documentation regulations, he has had to update the way he dictates. The billing supervisor still has to remind him of the need to document the connection between the level of history and examination and the level of service he wants to bill. This sometimes leads to a difference of opinion.

Questions

1. Why is it important that the medical assistant and/or doctor document precisely and completely for every visit?

2. How can the billing supervisor make the transition easier on Dr. Terrance?

3. Does the use of EMR improve the quality of the medical documentation?

An **audit** is a formal examination or review. It is a process used by health professionals to assess, evaluate, and improve care of patients in a systematic way. With the passage of the **Patient Protection and Affordable Care Act (PPACA)** in 2010, healthcare organizations must develop and implement compliance programs that include a medical documentation and coding audit. An audit, whether it is performed in the office or by an external auditor, examines the documentation to determine whether it adequately substantiates the service billed and shows medical necessity. In addition to facilitating high-quality patient care, an appropriately documented medical record serves as a legal document to verify services provided.

Purpose of an Audit

The following are five of the most important reasons why an office should audit its medical records:

1. To assess the completeness of the medical record
2. To determine the accuracy of the physician's documentation
3. To discover lost revenue
4. To ensure that all HIPAA compliance regulations are being followed
5. To measure current practice against a defined standard.

If audits are not performed on a regular basis, the medical office specialist will not know that the documentation was correct and appropriate for the level of service performed. If an audit is performed, any errors found can be brought to the attention of the provider and corrected for future billing. An audit can help a healthcare provider spot errors and prevent small problems before they become large ones, especially in the area of billing to government healthcare programs. A healthcare provider should regularly monitor records to be in compliance with federal guidelines. Audits help facilitate the maintenance of accurate and complete coding and reimbursement practices. An independent medical record review (i.e., an audit) should be performed a minimum of twice a year to identify coding and documentation errors. Top coding and documentation errors include the following:

- The service is upcoded one level; documentation does not support the level of service, therefore a lower-level code should have been selected. (The term **upcode** means that the procedure code stated is for a procedure that is more involved than the one actually documented in the medical record.)
- The service is downcoded one level; documentation supports a higher level of service, however the coder has chosen a lower-level code to avoid government investigation. (The term **downcode** means that the procedure code stated is for a procedure that is less involved than the one actually documented in the medical record.)
- The chief complaint (the reason for the encounter) is missing.

- Assessment is not clearly documented; the coder cannot use "rule out," "suspected," or "probable."
- No diagnosis is given; the coder must code only signs and symptoms.
- The documentation is not initialed or signed. (e-signatures are accepted in EHRs)
- Tests ordered are not documented but are billed on the encounter form.
- Documentation of medication is not clear.
- The diagnosis is not always referenced correctly.
- Documentation is missing.
- Dictation is lost.
- The encounter form is incomplete or incorrect.
- Documentation is not complete, so the code has no record that an action was taken.
- Documentation is difficult to read; the auditor will disallow the visit when she cannot read the documentation.

Fraud for incorrect billing or coding is prosecuted by the U.S. Attorney's office under Health Care Fraud statutes as well as under theft or embezzlement, false statements, false claims or bribery provisions, mail fraud, wire fraud, and electronic fraud. Penalties for such actions are severe.

For example, a Washington physician and three others were found guilty of healthcare fraud, mail fraud, and conspiracy and received a sentence of 35 months of imprisonment, 3 years of probation, and 5 years of exclusion from practice, plus was ordered to pay $475,710 in restitution. The defendants were owners and operators of clinics located throughout the greater Seattle area. The clinics provided non-covered services, such as acupuncture, nutrition counseling, and massage therapy, but billed Medicare and other insurers for physician office visits.

Types of Audits

The three types of audits are external, internal, and accreditation.

External Audit

An **external audit** is a private payer or government investigator's review of selected patient records of a practice for compliance. Code linkage, completeness of documentation, and adherence to documentation standards, such as signing paper documents and/or e-signature attestation within EHR, and dating of entries by the responsible healthcare professional, may all be studied. The account records are often reviewed as well.

Third-party payers conduct a prepayment audit by reviewing the payments posted on the patient's account. All payments received should be posted and viewable in the provider's accounts receivable software. These edits are reviewed to verify documentation, such as the date of the service provided and the insured's insurance ID number. The documentation regarding the extent of the visit is investigated after payment. A postpayment audit is conducted after payment to ensure that the providers have accurately billed for the visit or procedure. Postpayment audits also investigate the complete documentation regarding the visit, including progress reports, X-rays, laboratory results, scheduling, sign-in sheet, and billing records.

Internal Audit

An **internal audit** is done within the practice to be sure that the practice is coding claims correctly and is compliant. This will reduce the chance of an investigation or of an employee needing to become a whistle-blower. A practice employee or a consultant may be hired to perform this audit. The internal audits should be done routinely and performed without any reason to be suspicious of fraudulent behavior.

Evaluation and management (E/M) codes are important and used widely. Thus, they are always an ongoing focus of audits, which can be used to verify their correct use. For these reasons, an internal audit should be part of the compliance plan in a physician's practice.

An internal audit is used:

- To determine that procedures have been coded correctly based on the documentation
- To analyze the coders' skill and knowledge
- To review any need for further training or review of the practice's compliance plan and policies
- To review the involvement of the billing staff, medical coders, and the office insurance specialist with the physician

A **retrospective audit** is performed retrospectively—that is, after payment. A **prospective audit** is done before the claim is submitted for payment.

A prospective audit would be difficult to do in a physician's office for many reasons. The person conducting the audit would have to wait for the documentation. The majority of claims are sent electronically, and the accounts receivable would be affected if payments or claims submissions were delayed. Many audit tools are available to the medical office staff for performing an internal audit. The documentation for the date of service with the explanation of benefits (EOB) or electronic remittance advice (ERA) is reviewed and checked with the audit tool. The auditor checks the documentation by the physician to determine the correct level of E/M code. An EOB and an ERA both provide detailed payment information and adjustment reason codes from the insurance company (also referred to as the carrier or payer). An EOB is a paper response and an ERA is a digital response. These will be discussed in detail in Chapter 15.

Accreditation Audits

A representative from the managed care organization—for example, a registered nurse—will visit the facility. The provider is informed ahead of time of the upcoming visit. Upon arrival, the nurse will request access to at least 20 medical records of the insured patients in the organization's plan. An audit will be conducted on each record as to any maintenance of the record, patient information, and signed authorizations. Medical auditing will then be assessed as to the proper documentation of the provider for the patient's visits, ordering of tests, prescription drugs, and any follow-up care. Auditors will review claims and corresponding medical records for appropriate coding based on nationally accepted coding guidelines.

If documentation seems inadequate, the provider will be given a warning and asked to be in compliance within a certain amount of time. The auditor will inform the provider of the coding conventions and guidelines used when recommending coding changes. If the provider does not take action to implement changes and be compliant with coding conventions, he may lose his privileges to participate in the plan.

Private Payer Regulations

Private payers require use of the American Medical Association's (AMA's) *Current Procedural Terminology* (CPT) codes and the *International Classification of Diseases, Tenth Revision, Clinical Modification* (ICD-10-CM) codes for reimbursement. They have, however, also developed their own **code edits**, which screen for improperly or incorrectly reported procedure codes. Most states require third-party payers to give a reason for denial of a claim. The software to determine if a clean claim has been submitted may also be different and in error. The medical office specialist must be prepared to appeal a claim if there is no explanation of the reason for denial.

Third-party payers may also have their own rules and policies about submitting a clean claim. One must be familiar with the payers' policies to submit the claim. For example, Blue Cross Blue Shield may want the documentation to include the name of the serum, the dosage, and the route of administration for a hepatitis A immunization. Any third-party payer from which the provider is accepting assignments must follow the third-party payer's policies and procedures as part of their contract agreement. Documentation must also be audited internally to show that the physician's practice is in compliance with all payer regulations.

Medical Necessity for E/M Services

To insure coding is completed correctly, compliance plans focus on training physicians to use the AMA's *Documentation Guidelines for Evaluation and Management Services* and to know the current codes. The key components for selecting E/M codes are the extent of the history documented, the extent of the examination documented, and the complexity of the medical decision making. These guidelines reduce the amount of subjectivity involved in making judgments about E/M codes, such as one person's opinion of an extended examination versus another's definition. This is achieved by describing the specific items that may be documented for each of the three key components: the history documented, the examination documented, and the complexity. The guidelines also explain how many of these items are needed to place the item on the appropriate scale.

The documentation guidelines include precise number counts of these items; these counts can be used to audit as well as to initially code the service. The audit double-checks the selected code based on the documentation in the patient's medical record. The auditor looks at the medical record and, with an auditing tool (Figure 9.1), independently analyzes by number count the services documented. The auditor then compares the code reported to the code selected through the audit. When the results are not the same, the auditor has uncovered a possible problem in interpreting the documentation guidelines.

Federal law requires that all expenses paid by Medicare, including expenses for E/M services, be "medically reasonable and necessary":

- Medical necessity of E/M services is generally expressed in two ways: frequency of services and intensity of service (the CPT level).
- Medicare's determination of medical necessity is separate from its determination that the E/M service was rendered as billed.

E/M Audit Form

Chart #: _____

Patient Name: _____   Date of service: __/__/__   Provider: _____   MR #: _____

Place of Service: _____   Service Type: _____   Insurance Carrier: _____

Code (s) selected: _____   Code(s) audited: _____   ☐ Over ☐ Under ☐ Correct ☐ Miscoded

History

History of Present Illness

☐ Location
☐ Quality
☐ Severity
☐ Duration
☐ Timing
☐ Context
☐ Modifying factors
☐ Associated signs and symptoms
☐ No. of chronic diseases

Review of Systems

☐ Constitutional symptoms
☐ Eyes
☐ Ears, nose, mouth, throat
☐ Cardiovascular
☐ Respiratory
☐ Gastrointestinal
☐ Genitourinary
☐ Integumentary
☐ Musculoskeletal
☐ Neurological
☐ Psychiatric
☐ Endocrine
☐ Hematologic/lymphatic
☐ Allergic/immunologic

Past, Family & Social History

PAST MEDICAL

☐ Current medication
☐ Prior illnesses and injuries
☐ Operations and hospitalizations
☐ Age-appropriate immunizations
☐ Allergies   ☐ Dietary status

FAMILY

☐ Health status or cause of death of parents, siblings, and children
☐ Hereditary or high risk diseases
☐ Diseases related to CC, HPI, ROS

SOCIAL

☐ Living arrangements
☐ Marital status ☐ Sexual history
☐ Occupational history
☐ Use of drugs, alcohol, or tobacco
☐ Extent of education
☐ Current employment ☐ Other

PF=Brief HPI
EPF=Brief HPI, ROS (Pertinent=1)
Detailed= Extended HPI (4+) + ROS=(2-9) PFSH=1
Comprehensive= Extended HPI + ROS (10 + systems) PFSH=2 Established, 3 New Patient
☐ PFSH Form reviewed, no change   ☐ PFSH form reviewed, updated   ☐ PFSH form new

**Extended HPI=Status of 3 chronic illnesses with 1997 DG. Some allow for 1995 as well.

History _____

General Multi-System Examination

Constitutional
☐ 3 of 7 (BP,pulse,respir,tmp,hgt,wgt)
☐ General Appearance
Eyes
☐ Conjunctivae, Lids
☐ Eyes: Pupils, Irises
☐ Ophthal exam -Optic discs, Pos Seg
ENT
☐ Ears, Nose
☐ Oto exam -Aud canals,Tymp membr
☐ Hearing
☐ Nasal mucosa, Septum, Turbinates
☐ ENTM: Lips, Teeth, Gums
☐ Oropharynx -oral mucosa,palates
Neck
☐ Neck
☐ Thyroid
Respiratory
☐ Respiratory effort
☐ Percussion of chest
☐ Palpation of chest
☐ Auscultation of lungs
Cardiovascular
☐ Palpation of heart
☐ Auscultation of heart (& sounds)
☐ Carotid arteries
☐ Abdominal aorta
☐ Femoral arteries
☐ Pedal pulses
☐ Extrem for periph edema/varicoscities
Chest
☐ Inspect Breasts
☐ Palpation of Breasts & Axillae

Gastrointestinal
☐ Abd (+/- masses or tenderness)
☐ Liver, Spleen
☐ Hernia (+/-)
☐ Anus, Perineum, Rectum
☐ Stool for occult blood
GU/Female
☐ Female: Genitalia, Vagina
☐ Female Urethra
☐ Bladder
☐ Cervix
☐ Uterus
☐ Adnexa/parametria
GU/Male
☐ Scrotal Contents
☐ Penis
☐ Digital rectal of Prostate
Lymphatic
☐ Lymph: Neck
☐ Lymph: Axillae
☐ Lymph: Groin
☐ Lymph: Other
Musculoskeletal
☐ Gait (...ability to exercise)
☐ Palpation Digits, Nails
☐ Head/Neck: Inspect, Palp
☐ Head/Neck: Motion (+/-pain,crepit)
☐ Head/Neck: Stability (+/- lux,sublux)
☐ Head/Neck: Muscle strength & tone
☐ Spine/Rib/Pelv: Inspect, Palp
☐ Spine/Rib/Pelv: Motion
☐ Spine/Rib/Pelv: Stability
☐ Spine/Rib/Pelv: Strength and tone
☐ R.Up Extrem: Inspect, Palp

☐ R.Up Extrem: Motion (+/- pain, crepit)
☐ R.Up Extrem: Stability (+/- lux, sublux)
☐ R.Up Extrem: Muscle strength & tone
☐ L.Up Extrem: Inspect, Palp
☐ L.Up Extrem: Motion (+/- pain, crepit)
☐ L.Up Extrem: Muscle strength & tone
☐ R.Low Extrem: Inspect, Palp
☐ R.Low Extrem: Motion (+/-pain, crepit)
☐ R.Low Extrem: Stability (+/- lux, laxity)
☐ R.Low Extrem: Muscle strength & tone
☐ L.Low Extrem: Inspect, Palp
☐ L.Low Extrem: Motion (+/-pain, crepit)
☐ L.Low Extrem: Stability (+/- lux, sublux)
☐ L.Low Extrem: Muscle strength & tone
Skin
☐ Skin: Inspect Skin & Subcut tissues
☐ Skin: Palpation Skin & Subcut tissues
Neuro
☐ Neuro: Cranial nerves (+/- deficits)
☐ Neuro: DTRs (+/- pathological reflexes)
☐ Neuro: Sensations
Psychiatry
☐ Psych: Judgement, Insight
☐ Psych: Orientation time, place, person
☐ Psych: Recent, Remote memory
☐ Psych: Mood, Affect (depression, anxiety)

Exam: _____

1995-1=PF, limited 2-7=EPF, extended
2-7=Detailed, 8+ organ systems=Comprehensive
1997-1-5=PF, 6-11=EPF, 2x6 systems=D
2 from 9 systems=Comp.

Figure 9.1   E/M audit tool.

Number of Diagnoses/Management Options	Points
Self-limited or minor (Stable, improved or worsening) ➔ Maximum 2 points in this category.	1
Established problem (to examining MD); stable or improved	1
Established problem (to examining MD); worsening	2
New problem (to examining MD); no additional work-up planned ➔	3
New problem (to examining MD); additional work-up (e.g. admit/transfer)	4
Total	

Amount and/or Complexity of Data Reviewed	Points
Lab ordered and/or reviewed (regardless of # ordered)	1
X-ray ordered and/or reviewed (regardless of # ordered)	1
Medicine section (90701-99199) ordered and/or reviewed	1
Discussion of test results with performing physician	1
Decision to obtain old record and/or obtain hx from someone other than patient	1
Review and summary of old records and/or obtaining hx from someone other than patient and/or discussion with other health provider	2
Independent visualization of image, tracing, or specimen (not simply review of report)	2
Total	

TABLE OF RISK

Level of Risk	Presenting Problem(s)	Diagnostic Procedure(s) Ordered	Management Options Selected
Minimal	• One self-limited or minor problem, eg, cold, insect bite, tinea corporis	• Laboratory tests requiring venipuncture • Chest x-rays • EKG/EEG • Urinalysis • Ultrasound, eg, echocardiography • KOH prep	• Rest • Gargles • Elastic bandages • Superficial dressings
Low	• Two or more self-limited or minor problems • One stable chronic illness, eg, well controlled hypertension, non-insulin dependent diabetes, cataract, BPH • Acute uncomplicated illness or injury, eg, cystitis, allergic rhinitis, simple sprain	• Physiologic tests not under stress, eg, pulmonary function tests • Non-cardiovascular imaging studies with contrast, eg, barium enema • Superficial needle biopsies • Clinical laboratory tests requiring arterial puncture • Skin biopsies	• Over-the-counter drugs • Minor surgery with no identified risk factors • Physical therapy • Occupational therapy • IV fluids without additives
Moderate	• One or more chronic illnesses with mild exacerbation, progression, or side effects of treatment • Two or more stable chronic illnesses • Undiagnosed new problem with uncertain prognosis, eg, lump in breast • Acute illness with systemic symptoms, eg, pyelonephritis, pneumonitis, colitis • Acute complicated injury, eg, head injury with brief loss of consciousness	• Physiologic tests under stress, eg, cardiac stress test, fetal contraction stress test • Diagnostic endoscopies with no identified risk factors • Deep needle or incisional biopsy • Cardiovascular imaging studies with contrast and no identified risk factors, eg, arteriogram, cardiac catheterization • Obtain fluid from body cavity, eg lumbar puncture, thoracentesis, culdocentesis	• Minor surgery with identified risk factors • Elective major surgery (open, percutaneous or endoscopic) with no identified risk factors • Prescription drug management • Therapeutic nuclear medicine • IV fluids with additives • Closed treatment of fracture or dislocation without manipulation
High	• One or more chronic illnesses with severe exacerbation, progression, or side effects of treatment • Acute or chronic illnesses or injuries that pose a threat to life or bodily function, eg, multiple trauma, acute MI, pulmonary embolus, severe respiratory distress, progressive severe rheumatoid arthritis, psychiatric illness with potential threat to self or others, peritonitis, acute renal failure • An abrupt change in neurologic status, eg, seizure, TIA, weakness, sensory loss	• Cardiovascular imaging studies with contrast with identified risk factors • Cardiac electrophysiological tests • Diagnostic Endoscopies with identified risk factors • Discography	• Elective major surgery (open, percutaneous or endoscopic) with identified risk factors • Emergency major surgery (open, percutaneous or endoscopic) • Parenteral controlled substances • Drug therapy requiring intensive monitoring for toxicity • Decision not to resuscitate or to de-escalate care because of poor prognosis

Medical Decision Making	SF	LOW	MOD	HIGH
Number of Diagnoses or Treatment Options	1	2	3	4
Amount and/or Complexity of Data to be Reviewed	1	2	3	4
Risk of Complications, Morbidity, Mortality	Minimal	Low	Moderate	High
MDM Level=2 out of 3				

MDM _____

Chart Note   **Comments**

☐ Dictated   ☐ Handwritten
☐ Form   ☐ Illegible
☐ Note signed
☐ Signature missing

Other Services or Modalities:

Auditor's Signature

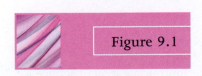

Figure 9.1   (Continued)

Source: E/M Audit Checklist Tool. Copyright by American Academy of Professional Coders (AAPC).

- Medicare determines medical necessity largely through the experience and judgment of clinician coders along with the limited tools provided in the CPT book and by the Centers for Medicare and Medicaid Services (CMS).
- At audit, Medicare will deny or downcode E/M services that, in its judgment, exceed the patient's documented needs.

Information used by Medicare is contained within the medical record documentation of history, examination, and medical decision making. Medical necessity of E/M services is based on the following:

- Number, acuity, and severity/duration of problems addressed through history, physical, and medical decision making
- The context of the encounter among all other services previously rendered for the same problem
- The complexity of documented comorbidities that clearly influenced the physician's work
- Physical scope encompassed by the problems (number of physical systems affected by the problems).

Audit Tool

Because E/M codes are the most widely used codes, they are also the ones that may trigger an audit. The Office of Inspector General (OIG) will announce which codes will be audited, and if a problem in a certain area is found, the audit will then be expanded to all regions.

To prevent errors being found after payment, an internal audit, as discussed, should be performed periodically to determine if the practice is coding properly. This is an objective evaluation, which should be conducted by the office staff or management. Preparing for the audit should include selecting every fifth medical record of patients seen per day over a 1 to 2 week period until reaching 15 to 20 medical records, including new patient visits, established patient visits, consultations, encounter forms, and insurance information. The EOBs or ERAs should be available along with the medical records to determine if the codes billed and paid for were coded to the correct level of an E/M.

Many practices use an audit tool to conduct their internal audits. When an audit is performed either retrospectively or prospectively an audit tool such as that shown in Figure 9.1 should be used to determine the exact E/M code selected by the number count. Trailblazer Health Enterprises, LLC, has published a tool, *Evaluation and Management: Coding and Documentation Pocket Reference*, for auditing physicians' practices billing Medicare Part B. Trailblazer Health Enterprises administers the Medicare program under contracting arrangements with CMS. It develops various publications, such as forms, job aids, manuals, and newsletters.

When conducting an audit with the E/M audit tool in Figure 9.1, the types of information presented in the following sections are analyzed.

Key Elements of Service

To code a claim correctly, the coder must determine the appropriate level of service for a patient's visit. In doing so, it is first necessary to determine whether the patient is new or already established. The physician then uses the presenting illness as a guiding factor and his or her clinical judgment about the patient's condition to determine the extent

Table 9.1	Elements Required for Each Type of History			
Type of History	**Chief Complaint**	**History of Present Illness**	**Review of Systems**	**Past, Family, and/or Social History**
Problem Focused	Required	Brief	N/A	N/A
Expanded Problem Focused	Required	Brief	Problem	N/A
Detailed	Required	Extended	Pertinent Extended	Pertinent
Comprehensive	Required	Extended	Complete	Complete

Source: Department of Health and Human Services, Centers for Medicare and Medicaid, The Medicare Learning Network; Evaluation and Management Services Guide.

of key elements of service to be performed. The key elements of service and documentation of an encounter dominated by counseling and/or coordination of care are history, examination, and medical decision making. Correct code linkage establishes medical necessity for a service or procedure.

History

The elements required for each type of history are depicted in Table 9.1. Note that each history type requires more information as you read down the left-hand column. For example, a problem-focused history requires the documentation of the chief complaint (CC) and a brief history of present illness (HPI), whereas a detailed history requires the documentation of a CC, extended HPI, extended review of systems (ROS), and pertinent past, family, and/or social history (PFSH).

The extent of information gathered for the history is dependent on clinical judgment and the nature of the presenting problem. Documentation of patient history includes some or all of the following elements.

Chief Complaint

A CC is a concise statement that describes the symptom, problem, condition, diagnosis, or reason for the patient encounter. The CC is usually stated in the patient's own words. For example, "Patient complains of upset stomach, aching joints, and fatigue."

History of Present Illness

The HPI is a chronological description of the development of the patient's present illness from the first sign and/or symptom or from the previous encounter to the present. HPI elements include the following:

- *Location:* For example, pain in left leg
- *Quality:* For example, aching, burning, radiating
- *Severity:* For example, 9 on a scale of 1 to 10
- *Duration:* For example, "It started three days ago."
- *Timing:* For example, "It is constant," or "It comes and goes."
- *Context:* For example, "Lifted large object at work."
- *Modifying factors:* For example, "It is better when heat is applied."
- *Associated signs and symptoms:* For example, numbness

There are two types of HPIs:

1. *Brief,* which includes documentation of one to three HPI elements. In the following example, three HPI elements—location, severity, and duration—are documented:
   - CC: A patient seen in the office complains of left ear pain.
   - *Brief HPI:* Patient complains of dull ache in left ear over the past 24 hours.
2. *Extended,* which includes documentation of at least four HPI elements or the status of at least three chronic or inactive conditions. In the following example, five HPI elements—location, severity, duration, context, and modifying factors—are documented:
   - *Extended HPI:* Patient complains of dull ache in left ear over the past 24 hours. Patient states he went swimming two days ago. Symptoms somewhat relieved by warm compress and ibuprofen.

Review of Systems

A review of systems is an inventory of body systems obtained by asking a series of questions in order to identify signs and/or symptoms that the patient may be experiencing or has experienced. The following are the three types of ROS:

1. *Problem pertinent,* which inquires about the system directly related to the problem identified in the HPI. In the following example, one system—the ear—is reviewed:

Example

CC: Earache.
ROS: Positive for left ear pain. Denies dizziness, tinnitus, fullness, or headache.

2. *Extended,* which inquires about the system directly related to the problem(s) identified in the HPI and a limited number (two to nine) of additional systems. In the following example, two systems—cardiovascular and respiratory—are reviewed:

Example

CC: Follow-up visit in office after cardiac catheterization. Patient states, "I feel great."
ROS: Patient states he feels great and denies chest pain, syncope, palpitations, and shortness of breath. Relates occasional unilateral, asymptomatic edema of left leg.

3. *Complete,* which inquires about the system(s) directly related to the problem(s) identified in the HPI plus all additional (minimum of 10) body systems. In the following example, 10 signs and symptoms are reviewed:

Example

CC: Patient complains of "fainting spell."
ROS
   - Constitutional: weight stable; + fatigue.
   - Eyes: + loss of peripheral vision.

- Ear, nose, mouth, throat: no complaints.
- Cardiovascular: + palpitations; denies chest pain; denies calf pain, pressure, or edema.
- Respiratory: + shortness of breath on exertion.
- Gastrointestinal: appetite good, denies heartburn and indigestion; + episodes of nausea. Bowel movement daily; denies constipation or loose stools.
- Urinary: denies incontinence, frequency, urgency, nocturia, pain, or discomfort.
- Skin: + clammy, moist skin.
- Neurological: + fainting; denies numbness, tingling, and tremors.
- Psychiatric: denies memory loss or depression. Mood pleasant.

A sample of medical record notes is shown in Figure 9.2.

Past, Family, and/or Social History

The past, family, and/or social history consist of a review of the patient's:

- Past history including experiences with illnesses, operations, injuries, and treatments.
- Family history including a review of medical events, diseases, and hereditary conditions that may place her at risk.
- Social history including an age-appropriate review of past and current activities.

The following are the two types of PFSH:

1. Pertinent, which is a review of the history areas directly related to the problem(s) identified in the HPI. In the following example, the patient's past surgical history is reviewed as it relates to the current HPI:
   - Patient returns to office for follow-up of coronary artery bypass graft in 2015. Recent cardiac catheterization demonstrates 50% occlusion of vein graft to obtuse marginal artery.

Patient: Summers, Lillian   DOB: 05-23-1945

DOS: 4-15-2015

ROS

+ weight gain—started 2-1-2011, 90 lbs since steroid
+ insomnia due to shortness of breath (SOB)/choking
+ pt complains of (c/o) heat intolerance, alternating with cold spells
+ chronic headache: posterior occipital
+ decreased vision: blurring > 6 months + photophobia, c/o dry eyes
− epistaxis
+ nausea, − vomiting, + constipation with occasional diarrhea
+ polydipsia, + polyuria, + nocturnal uria
+ most recent urinary tract infection (UTI) ~ 1 month ago
+ occasional dysuria
+ lower extremity edema—right ankle swelling
+ skin—dry/itching
+ poor appetite

Figure 9.2

Sample medical record notes.

2. *Complete*, which is a review of two or all three of the areas, depending on the category of E/M service. A complete PFSH requires a review of all three history areas for services that, by their nature, include a comprehensive assessment or reassessment of the patient. A review of two history areas is sufficient for other services. At least one specific item from each of the three history areas must be documented for the following categories of E/M services:

- Office or other outpatient services, established patient
- Emergency department
- Domiciliary care, established patient
- Home care, established patient

At least one specific item from each of the history areas must be documented for the following categories of E/M services:

- Office or other outpatient services, new patient
- Hospital observation services
- Hospital inpatient services, initial care
- Consultations
- Comprehensive nursing facility assessments
- Domiciliary care, new patient
- Home care, new patient

In the following example, the patient's genetic history is reviewed as it relates to the current HPI:

Example

Family history reveals the following:
- Maternal grandparents: both + for coronary artery disease; grandfather deceased at age 69; grandmother still living.
- Paternal grandparents: grandmother, + diabetes, hypertension; grandfather, + heart attack at age 55.
- Parents: mother, + obesity, diabetes; father, + heart attack age 51, deceased age 57 of heart attack.
- Siblings: sister, + diabetes, obesity, hypertension, age 39; brother, + heart attack at age 45, living.

Sample medical record notes for past medical history are shown in Figure 9.3.

Examination

An examination may involve several organ systems or a single organ system. The extent of the examination performed is based on clinical judgment, the patient's history, and nature of the presenting problem.

Table 9.2 depicts the body areas and organ systems that are recognized according to the CPT book.

Two types of examinations can be performed during a patient's visit:

1. A *general multisystem examination*, which involves the examination of one or more organ systems or body areas

Patient: Summers, Lillian   DOB: 05-23-1945

DOS: 4-15-2016

PMH

Status post thyroid resection—1986
Status post splenectomy—1986
    DM/HTN/sickle cell anemia
    Esophagitis status post EGD/OGl

Habits

Smoker 1 pack every 4 days > 29 yrs

No allergies

SHX—disabled

Figure 9.3

Sample medical record notes for past medical history.

2. A *single organ system examination*, which involves a more extensive examination of a specific organ system

Any physician, regardless of specialty, may perform both types of examinations. Table 9.3 compares the elements of the cardiovascular system/body area for both a general multisystem and single organ system examination. The elements required for general multisystem examinations are depicted in Table 9.4.

According to the 1997 *Documentation Guidelines for Evaluation and Management Services*, the following are the 10 single organ system examinations:

- Cardiovascular
- Ear, Nose, and Throat

Table 9.2	Body Areas and Organ Systems Recognized According to the CPT Book	
	Body Areas	**Organ Systems**
	Head, including face	Eyes
	Neck	Ears, Nose, Mouth, and Throat
	Chest, including breast and axilla	Cardiovascular
	Abdomen	Respiratory
	Genitalia, groin, buttocks	Gastrointestinal
	Back	Genitourinary
	Each extremity	Musculoskeletal
		Skin
		Neurologic
		Hematologic/Lymphatic/Immunologic
		Psychiatric

Source: Department of Health and Human Services, Centers for Medicare and Medicaid, The Medicare Learning Network; Evaluation and Management Services Guide.

Table 9.3	Comparison of the Elements of the Cardiovascular System/Body Area for Both a General Multisystem and Single Organ System Examination	
System/Body Area	**General Multisystem Examination**	**Single Organ System Examination**
Cardiovascular	Palpation of heart (e.g., location, size thrills) Auscultation of heart with notation of abnormal sounds and murmurs Examination of: ■ Carotid arteries (e.g., pulse amplitude, bruits) ■ Abdominal aorta (e.g., size, bruits) ■ Femoral arteries (e.g., pulse amplitude, bruits) ■ Pedal pulses (e.g., pulse amplitude) ■ Extremities for edema and/or varicosities	Palpation of heart (e.g., location, size, and forcefulness of the point of maximal impact; thrills; lifts; palpable S3 or S4) Auscultation of heart, including sounds, abnormal sounds, and murmurs Measurement of blood pressure in two or more extremities when indicated (e.g., aortic dissection, coarctation) Examination of: ■ Carotid arteries (e.g., waveform, pulse amplitude, bruits, apical-carotid delay) ■ Abdominal aorta (e.g., size, bruits) ■ Femoral arteries (e.g., pulse amplitude, bruits) ■ Pedal pulses (e.g., pulse amplitude) ■ Extremities for peripheral edema and/or varicosities

Source : Department of Health and Human Services, Centers for Medicare and Medicaid, The Medicare Learning Network; Evaluation and Management Services Guide.

■ Eye
■ Genitourinary
■ Hematologic/Lymphatic/Immunologic
■ Musculoskeletal
■ Neurological
■ Psychiatric
■ Respiratory
■ Skin

Table 9.4 compares the elements that are required for both general multisystem and single organ system examinations.

Some important points that should be kept in mind when documenting general multisystem and single organ system examinations include these:

■ Specific abnormal and relevant negative findings of the examination of the affected or symptomatic body area(s) or organ system(s) should be documented. A notation of "abnormal" without elaboration is insufficient.
■ Abnormal or unexpected findings of the examination of any asymptomatic body area(s) or organ system(s) should be described.
■ A brief statement or notation indicating "negative" or "normal" is sufficient to document normal findings related to unaffected area(s) or asymptomatic organ system(s). (However, an entire organ system should not be documented with a statement such as "negative.")

Figure 9.4 provides a sample of medical record notes for a physical examination.

Type of Examination	Multisystem Examinations	Single Organ System Examinations
Table 9.4	**Comparison of the Elements Required for Both General Multisystem and Single Organ System Examinations**	
Problem Focused	1–5 elements identified by a bullet in 1 or more organ system(s) or body area(s)	1–5 elements identified by a bullet, whether in a box with a shaded or unshaded border
Expanded Problem Focused	At least 6 elements identified by a bullet in one or more organ system(s) or body area(s)	At least 6 elements identified by a bullet, whether in a box with a shaded or unshaded border
Detailed	At least 6 organ systems or body areas; for each system/area selected, performance and documentation of at least 2 elements identified by a bullet expected OR At least 12 elements identified by a bullet in 2 or more organ systems or body areas	At least 12 elements identified by a bullet, whether in a box with a shaded or unshaded border Eye and psychiatric: At least 9 elements identified by a bullet, whether in a box with a shaded or unshaded border
Comprehensive	At least 9 organ systems or body areas. For each system/area selected, all elements of the examination identified by a bullet should be performed, unless specific directions limit the content of the examination. For each area/system, documentation of at least 2 elements identified by bullet is expected.	Perform all elements identified by a bullet, whether in a shaded or unshaded box. Document every element in each box with a shaded border and at least 1 element in a box with an unshaded border.

Source: Department of Health and Human Services, Centers for Medicare and Medicaid, The Medicare Learning Network; Evaluation and Management Services Guide.

Medical Decision Making

Medical decision making refers to the complexity of establishing a diagnosis and/or selecting a management option, which is determined by considering the following factors:

- The number of possible diagnoses and/or the number of management options that must be considered
- The amount and/or complexity of medical records, diagnostic tests, and/or other information that must be obtained, reviewed, and analyzed

Patient: Summers, Lillian DOB: 05-23-1945

DOS: 4-15-2016

PE

Obese BF
Neck—right side mass without bruit
Oropharynx clear
Lung clear
Right extremity edema

Skin—wrinkling in skin of her neck—lateral side

Figure 9.4

Sample medical record notes for a physical examination.

Table 9.5	Elements for Each Level of Medical Decision Making			
Type of Decision Making	**Number of Diagnoses or Management Options**	**Amount and/or Complexity of Data to Be Reviewed**	**Risk of Significant Complications, Morbidity, and/or Mortality**
Straightforward	Minimal	Minimal or None	Minimal
Low Complexity	Limited	Limited	Low
Moderate Complexity	Multiple	Moderate	Moderate
High Complexity	Extensive	Extensive	High

Source: Department of Health and Human Services, Centers for Medicare and Medicaid, The Medicare Learning Network; Evaluation and Management Services Guide.

- The risk of significant complications, morbidity, and/or mortality as well as comorbidities associated with the patient's presenting problem(s), the diagnostic procedure(s), and/or the possible management options

Table 9.5 depicts the elements for each level of medical decision making. To qualify for a given type of medical decision making, two of the three elements must either be met or exceeded.

Number of Diagnoses or Management Options

The number of possible diagnoses and/or the number of management options that must be considered is based on the following:

- The number and types of problems addressed during the encounter
- The complexity of establishing a diagnosis
- The management decisions that are made by the physician

In general, decision making with respect to a diagnosed problem is easier than that for an identified but undiagnosed problem. The number and type of diagnostic tests performed may be an indicator of the number of possible diagnoses. Problems that are improving or resolving are less complex than problems that are worsening or failing to change as expected. Another indicator of the complexity of diagnostic or management problems is the need to seek advice from other healthcare professionals.

Keep these important points in mind when documenting the number of diagnoses or management options:

- For each encounter, an assessment, clinical impression, or diagnosis should be documented, which may be explicitly stated or implied in documented decisions regarding management plans and/or further evaluation.
  - For a presenting problem with an established diagnosis, the record should reflect whether the problem is (1) improved, well controlled, resolving, or resolved or (2) inadequately controlled, worsening, or failing to change as expected.
  - For a presenting problem without an established diagnosis, the assessment or clinical impression may be stated in the form of differential diagnoses or as a "possible," "probable," or "rule out" diagnosis.

- The initiation of, or changes in, treatment should be documented. Treatment includes a wide range of management options, including patient instructions, nursing instructions, therapies, and medications.
- If referrals are made, consultations requested, or advice sought, the record should indicate to whom or where the referral or consultation was made or from whom advice was requested.

Amount and/or Complexity of Data to Be Reviewed

The amount and/or complexity of data to be reviewed are based on the types of diagnostic testing ordered or reviewed. Indications of the amount and/or complexity of data being reviewed include the following:

- A decision to obtain and review old medical records and/or obtain history from sources other than the patient (increases the amount and complexity of data to be reviewed)
- Discussion of contradictory or unexpected test results with the physician who performed or interpreted the test (indicates the complexity of data to be reviewed)
- The physician who ordered a test personally reviews the image, tracing, or specimen to supplement information from the physician who prepared the test report or interpretation (indicates the complexity of data to be reviewed).

Here are some important points that should be kept in mind when documenting amount and/or complexity of data to be reviewed:

- If a diagnostic service is ordered, planned, scheduled, or performed at the time of the E/M encounter, the type of service should be documented.
- The review of laboratory, radiology, and/or other diagnostic tests should be documented. A simple notation such as "White blood count elevated" or "Chest X-ray unremarkable" is acceptable. Alternatively, the review may be documented by initialing and dating the report that contains the test results.
- A decision to obtain old records or obtain additional history from the family, caretaker, or other source to supplement information obtained from the patient should be documented.
- Relevant findings from the review of old records and/or the receipt of additional history from the family, caretaker, or other source to supplement information obtained from the patient should be documented. If there is no relevant information beyond that already obtained, this fact should be documented. A notation of "Old records reviewed" or "Additional history obtained from family" without elaboration is not sufficient.
- Discussion about results of laboratory, radiology, or other diagnostic tests with the physician who performed or interpreted the study should be documented.
- The direct visualization and independent interpretation of an image, tracing, or specimen previously or subsequently interpreted by another physician should be documented.

Risk of Significant Complications, Morbidity, and/or Mortality

The risk of significant complications, morbidity, and/or mortality is based on the risks associated with the following categories:

- Presenting problem(s)
- Diagnostic procedure(s)
- Possible management options

The assessment of risk of the presenting problem(s) is based on the risk related to the disease process anticipated between the present encounter and the next encounter. The assessment of risk of selecting diagnostic procedures and management options is based on the risk during and immediately following any procedures or treatment. The highest level of risk in any one category determines the overall risk.

The level of risk of significant complications, morbidity, and/or mortality can be any of the following:

- Minimal
- Low
- Moderate
- High

Some important points that should be kept in mind when documenting level of risk are as follows:

- Comorbidities/underlying diseases or other factors that increase the complexity of medical decision making by increasing the risk of complications, morbidity, and/or mortality should be documented.
- If a surgical or invasive diagnostic procedure is ordered, planned, or scheduled at the time of the E/M encounter, the type of procedure should be documented.
- If a surgical or invasive diagnostic procedure is performed at the time of the E/M encounter, the specific procedure should be documented.
- The referral for or decision to perform a surgical or invasive diagnostic procedure on an urgent basis should be documented.

Table 9.6 can be used to assist in determining whether the level of risk of significant complications, morbidity, and/or mortality is minimal, low, moderate, or high. Because determination of risk is complex and not readily quantifiable, the table includes common clinical examples rather than absolute measures of risk.

Documentation of an Encounter Dominated by Counseling and/or Coordination of Care

When counseling and/or coordination of care dominates (i.e., is more than 50% of) the physician/patient and/or family encounter (face-to-face time in the office or other outpatient setting, floor/unit time in the hospital or nursing facility), time is considered the key or controlling factor to qualify for a particular level of E/M services. If the level of service is reported based on counseling and/or coordination of care, the total length of time of the encounter should be documented and the record should describe the counseling and/or activities to coordinate care. For example, if 25 minutes were spent face to face with an established patient in the office and more than half of that time was spent counseling the patient or coordinating her care, CPT code 99214 should be selected. Figure 9.5 can be used as a reference to determine the correct code.

Use the following tips to correctly code E/M services based on medical necessity:

1. Identify all of the presenting complaints and or reasons for the visit for which physician work occurred.
   - Demonstrate clearly the history, physician, and extent of medical decision making associated with each problem.

Table 9.6	Table of Risk

Level of Risk	Presenting Problem(s)	Diagnostic Procedure(s) Ordered	Management Options Selected
Minimal	One self-limited or minor problem (e.g., cold, insect bite, tinea corporis)	Laboratory tests requiring venipuncture Chest x-rays Electrocardiogram/ electroencephalogram Urinalysis Ultrasound (e.g., echocardiography) Potassium hydroxide prep	Rest Gargles Elastic bandages Superficial dressings
Low	Two or more self-limited or minor problems One stable chronic illness (e.g., well controlled hypertension, non-insulin-dependent diabetes, cataract, benign prostatic hyperplasia) Acute uncomplicated illness or injury, e.g., cystitis, allergic rhinitis, simple sprain	Physiologic tests not under stress (e.g., pulmonary functions tests) Non-cardiovascular imaging studies with contrast (e.g., barium enema) Superficial needle biopsies Clinical laboratory tests requiring arterial puncture	Over-the-counter drugs Minor surgery with no identified risk factors Physical therapy Occupational therapy Intravenous fluids without additives
Moderate	One or more chronic illnesses with mild exacerbation, progression, or side effects of treatment Two or more stable chronic illnesses Undiagnosed new problem with uncertain prognosis (e.g., lump in breast) Acute illness with systemic symptoms (e.g., pyelonephritis, pneumonitis, colitis) Acute complicated injury (e.g., head injury with brief loss of consciousness)	Physiologic tests under stress (e.g., cardiac stress test, fetal contraction stress test) Diagnostic endoscopies with no identified risk factors Deep needle or incisional biopsy Cardiovascular imaging studies with contrast and no identified risk factors, (e.g., arteriogram, cardiac catheterization) Obtain fluid from body cavity (e.g., lumbar puncture, thoracentesis, culdocentesis)	Minor surgery with identified risk factors Elective major surgery (open, percutaneous, or endoscopic) with no identified risk factors Prescription drug management Therapeutic nuclear medicine Intravenous fluids with additives Closed treatment of fracture or dislocation without manipulation
High	One or more chronic illnesses with severe exacerbation, progression, or side effects of treatment Acute or chronic illnesses or injuries that pose a threat to life or bodily function (e.g., multiple trauma, acute MI, pulmonary embolus, severe respiratory distress, progressive severe rheumatoid arthritis, psychiatric illness with potential threat to self or others, peritonitis, acute renal failure An abrupt change in neurologic status (e.g., seizure, transient ischemic attack, weakness, sensory loss)	Cardiovascular imaging studies with contrast with identified risk factors Cardiac electrophysiological tests Diagnostic endoscopies with identified risk factors Discography	Elective major surgery (open, percutaneous, or endoscopic) with identified risk factors Emergency major surgery (open, percutaneous, or endoscopic) Parenteral controlled substances Drug therapy requiring intensive monitoring for toxicity Decision not to resuscitate or to deescalate care because of poor prognosis

Source: Department of Health and Human Services, Centers for Medicare and Medicaid, The Medicare Learning Network; Evaluation and Management Services Guide.

1 HISTORY

HPI (History of Present Illness): Characterize HPI by considering either the status of chronic conditions or the number of elements recorded.

☐ 1 condition   ☐ 2 conditions   ☐ 3 conditions

OR

☐ Location   ☐ Severity   ☐ Timing   ☐ Modifying factors
☐ Quality   ☐ Duration   ☐ Context   ☐ Associated signs and symptoms

	☐ Status of 1-2 chronic conditions	☐ Status of 1-2 chronic conditions	☐ Status of 3 chronic conditions	☐ Status of 3 chronic conditions
	☐ Brief (1-3)	☐ Brief (1-3)	☐ Extended (4 or more)	☐ Extended (4 or more)

ROS (Review of Systems):

☐ Constitutional (wt loss, etc.)   ☐ Ears, nose, mouth, throat   ☐ GI   ☐ Integumentary (skin, breast)   ☐ Endo
☐ Eyes   ☐ Card/vasc   ☐ GU   ☐ Neuro   ☐ Hem/lymph
☐ Musculo   ☐ Psych   ☐ Resp   ☐ All/immuno

N/A	☐ Pertinent to problem (1 system)	☐ Extended (Pert and others) (2-9 systems)	☐ Complete (Pert and all others) (10 systems)

PFSH (Past Medical, Family, Social History) areas:

☐ Past history (the patient's past experiences with illnesses, operation, injuries and treatments)
☐ Family history (a review of medical events in the patient's family, including diseases that may be hereditary or place the patient at risk)
☐ Social history (an age-appropriate review of past and current activities)

N/A	N/A	☐ Pertinent (1 history area)	☐ *Complete (2 or 3 history areas)

*Complete PFSH: 2 history areas: a) established patients - office (outpatient) care, domiciliary care, home care; b) emergency department; c) subsequent nursing facility care; d) subsequent hospital care; and, e) follow-up consultations.

3 history areas: a) new patients - office (outpatient) care, domiciliary care, home care; b) initial consultations; c) initial hospital care; d) hospital observation; and, e) comprehensive nursing facility assessments.

PROBLEM-FOCUSED	EXP. PROBLEM-FOCUSED	DETAILED	COMPREHENSIVE

Final History requires all 3 components above met or exceeded

2 EXAMINATION

CPT Exam Description	95 Guideline Requirements	97 Guideline Requirements	CPT Type of Exam
Limited to affected body area or organ system	One body area or organ system	1-5 bulleted elements	**PROBLEM-FOCUSED EXAM**
Affected body area or organ system and other symptomatic or related organ systems	2-7 body areas and/or organ systems	6-11 bulleted elements	**EXPANDED PROBLEM-FOCUSED EXAM**
Extended exam of affected body area or organ system and other symptomatic or related organ systems	2-7 body areas and/or organ systems	12-17 bulleted elements for 2 or more systems	**DETAILED EXAM**
General multi-system	8 or more body areas and/or organ systems	18 or more bulleted elements for 9 or more systems	**COMPREHENSIVE EXAM**
Complete single organ system exam	Not defined	See requirements for individual single system exams	

3 MEDICAL DECISION-MAKING

Final Result of Complexity for Medical Decision-Making Level				
A. Number of diagnoses and/or management options	≤ 2 Minimal	3-4 Limited	5-6 Multiple	≥ 7 Extensive
B. Amount and complexity of data reviewed/ordered	≤ 1 None/Minimal	2 Limited	3 Multiple	≥ 4 Extensive
C. Risk	Minimal	Low	Moderate	High
Type of medical decision-making	**Straightforward**	**Low Complexity**	**Moderate Complexity**	**High Complexity**
Final Medical Decision-Making requires 2 of 3 components above met or exceeded				

A. Number of Diagnoses and/or Management Options (see Table A.1)	#DX	#TX	#DX + #TX
New or est problem(s), no evaluation/management mentioned and problem **is not** clearly co-morbid condition.	0	0	0
New or est problem(s), no evaluation/management mentioned and problem **is** a co-morbid condition.		0	
New or established problem(s), evaluation/management mentioned.			
		TOTAL	

Figure 9.5   Tool to determine the correct CPT code.

③ MEDICAL DECISION-MAKING (continued)

A.1 Treatments and Therapeutic Options

DO NOT COUNT AS TREATMENT OPTIONS NOTATIONS SUCH AS Continue "same" therapy or "no change" in therapy (including drug management) without further description (record does not document what the current therapy plan is nor that the physician reviewed it)	0
Continue "same" therapy or "no change" in therapy without further description (record clearly documents what the current therapy plan is and that the physician reviewed it); or scheduled monitoring without specific therapy	1
Drug management, new prescriptions, or changes in dosing for current medications	1
Complex drug management (more than 3 medications/prescriptions and/or over-the-counter) new prescriptions or changes in dosing for current medications	2
Open or percutaneous therapeutic cardiac, surgical, or radiological procedure – minor or major	1
Physical, occupational, or speech therapy or other manipulation	1
Closed treatment for fracture or dislocation	1
IV fluids	1
Complex insulin prescription (SC or combo of SC/IV), hyperalimentation, insulin drip, or other complex IV admix prescription	2
Conservative measures such as rest, ice, bandages, dietary	1
Radiation therapy	1
IM injection/aspiration or other pain management procedure	1
Patient educated on self or home care topics/techniques	1
Hospital admit	1
Hospital admit – other physician(s) contacted	2
Referral to another physician, consultation	1
Other – specify	
TOTAL	

B. Amount and/or Complexity of Data Reviewed or Ordered

Order and/or review results of clinical lab tests	1
Order and/or review results of tests in Radiology section of CPT	1
Order and/or review results of tests in Medical section of CPT	1
Discuss case with consultant or order consultation or discuss case with other physician also managing the patient	1
Discuss test results with performing physician	1
Order (identify specific source of records ordered) and/or summarize old or other health care records (simple statements to the effect that other or old outside records were reviewed is insufficient to count)	1
Physiologic monitoring	1
Independently visualize and report findings from images, tracings, pathological specimens themselves (not the reports) for procedures and tests for which interpretation not separately billed by the provider	1
TOTAL	

C. Risk of Complication and/or Mortality (see Table C.1)

Nature of the presenting illness	Minimal	Low	Moderate	High
Risk conferred by diagnostic options	Minimal	Low	Moderate	High
Risk conferred by therapeutic options	Minimal	Low	Moderate	High

Final Risk determined by highest of 3 components above

C.1 Risk of Complications and/or Morbitity or Mortality

LEVEL OF RISK	PRESENTING PROBLEM(S)	DIAGNOSTIC PROCEDURE(S) ORDERED	MANAGEMENT OPTIONS SELECTED
Minimal	• One self-limited or minor problem, e.g., cold, insect bite, tinea corporis	• Laboratory tests requiring venipuncture • Chest x-rays • EKG/EEG • Urinalysis • Ultrasound, e.g., echo • KOH prep	• Rest • Gargles • Elastic bandages • Superficial dressings
Low	• Two or more self-limited or minor problems • One stable chronic illness, e.g., well-controlled hypertension or non-insulin dependent diabetes, cataract, BPH • Acute uncomplicated illness or injury, e.g., cystitis, allergic rhinitis, simple sprain	• Physiologic tests not under stress, e.g., pulmonary function tests • Non-cardiovascular imaging studies with contrast, e.g., barium enema • Superficial needle biopsies • Clinical laboratory tests requiring arterial puncture • Skin biopsies	• Over-the-counter drugs • Minor surgery with no identified risk factors • Physical therapy • Occupational therapy • IV fluids without additives

C.1 Risk of Complications and/or Morbidity or Mortality

LEVEL OF RISK	PRESENTING PROBLEM(S)	DIAGNOSTIC PROCEDURE(S) ORDERED	MANAGEMENT OPTIONS SELECTED
Moderate	• One or more chronic illnesses with mild exacerbation, progression or side effects of treatment • Two or more stable chronic illnesses • Undiagnosed new problem with uncertain prognosis, e.g., lump in breast • Acute illness with systemic symptoms, e.g., pyelonephritis, pneumonitis, colitis • Acute complicated injury, e.g., head injury with brief loss of consciousness	• Physiologic tests under stress, e.g., cardiac stress test, fetal contraction stress test • Diagnostic endoscopies with no identified risk factors • Deep needle or incisional biopsy • Cardiovascular imaging studies with contrast and no identified risk factors, e.g., arteriogram cardiac cath • Obtain fluid from body cavity, e.g., lumbar procedure, thoracentesis, culdocentesis	• Minor surgery with identified risk factors • Elective major surgery (open, percutaneous or endoscopic) with no identified risk factors • Prescription drug management • Therapeutic nuclear medicine • IV fluids with additives • Closed treatment of fracture or dislocation without manipulation
High	• One or more chronic illnesses with severe exacerbation, progression, or side effects of treatment • Acute or chronic illnesses or injuries that may pose a threat to life or bodily function, e.g., multiple trauma, acute MI, pulmonary embolus, severe respiratory distress, progressive severe rheumatoid arthritis, psychiatric illness with potential threat to self or others, peritonitis, acute renal failure • An abrupt change in neurologic status, e.g., seizure, TIA, weakness or sensory loss	• Cardiovascular imaging studies with contrast with identified risk factors • Cardiac electrophysiological tests • Diagnostic endoscopies with identified risk factors • Discography	• Elective major surgery (open, percutaneous or endoscopic with identified risk factors) • Emergency major surgery (open, percutaneous or endoscopic) • Parenteral controlled substances • Drug therapy requiring intensive monitoring for toxicity • Decision not to resuscitate or to de-escalate care because of poor prognosis

Figure 9.5   (Continued)

4   LEVEL OF SERVICE

OUTPATIENT, CONSULTS (OUTPATIENT AND INPATIENT) AND ER

	New Office/Consults/ER — Requires 3 components within shaded area						Established Office — Requires 2 components within shaded area			
History	PF / ER: PF	EPF / ER: EPF	D / ER: EPF	C / ER: D	C / ER: C	Minimal problem that may not require presence of physician	PF	EPF	D	C
Examination	PF / ER: PF	EPF / ER: EPF	D / ER: EPF	C / ER: D	C / ER: C		PF	EPF	D	C
Complexity of Medical Decision	SF / ER: SF	SF / ER: L	L / ER: M	M / ER: M	H / ER: H		SF	L	M	H
Average Time (minutes) (ER have no average time)	10 New (99201) / 15 Outpt cons (99241) / 20 Inpat cons (99251) / ER (99281)	20 New (99202) / 30 Outpt cons (99242) / 40 Inpat cons (99252) / ER (99282)	30 New (99203) / 40 Outpt cons (99243) / 55 Inpat cons (99253) / ER (99283)	45 New (99204) / 60 Outpt cons (99244) / 80 Inpat cons (99254) / ER (99284)	60 New (99205) / 80 Outpt cons (99245) / 100 Inpat cons (99255) / ER (99285)	5 (99211)	10 (99212)	15 (99213)	25 (99214)	40 (99215)
Level	I	II	III	IV	V	I	II	III	IV	V

INPATIENT

	Initial Hospital/Observation — Requires 3 components within shaded area			Subsequent Inpatient/Follow-up — Requires 2 components within shaded area		
History	D or C	C	C	PF interval	EPF interval	D interval
Examination	D or C	C	C	PF	EPF	D
Complexity of Medical Decision	SF/L	M	H	SF/L	M	H
Average Time (minutes) (Observation care has no average time)	30 Init hosp (99221) / Observ care (99218)	50 Init hosp (99222) / Observ care (99219)	70 Init hosp (99223) / Observ care (99220)	15 Subsequent (99231)	25 Subsequent (99232)	35 Subsequent (99233)
Level	I	II	III	I	II	III

NURSING FACILITY

	Annual Assessment/Admission — Requires 3 components within shaded area			Subsequent Nursing Facility — Requires 2 components within shaded area			
	Old Plan Review	New Plan	Admission				
History	D/C	C	C	PF interval	EPF interval	D interval	C interval
Examination	D/C	C	C	PF	EPF	D	C
Complexity of Medical Decision	SF	M	M	SF	L	M	H
No Average Time Established (Confirmatory consults and ER have no average time)	(99304)	(99305)	(99306)	(99307)	(99308)	(99309)	(99310)
Level	I	II	III	I	II	III	IV

DOMICILIARY (REST HOME, CUSTODIAL CARE) AND HOME CARE

	New — Requires 3 components within shaded area					Established — Requires 2 components within shaded area			
History	PF	EPF	D	C	C	PF interval	EPF interval	D interval	C
Examination	PF	EPF	D	C	C	PF	EPF	D	C
Complexity of Medical Decision	SF	L	M	M	H	SF	L	M	H
Average Time (minutes)	20 Domiciliary (99324) / 20 Home care (99341)	30 Domiciliary (99325) / 30 Home care (99342)	45 Domiciliary (99326) / 45 Home care (99343)	60 Domiciliary (99327) / 60 Home care (99344)	75 Domiciliary (99328) / 75 Home care (99345)	15 Domiciliary (99334) / 15 Home care (99347)	25 Domiciliary (99335) / 25 Home care (99348)	40 Domiciliary (99336) / 40 Home care (99349)	60 Domiciliary (99337) / 60 Home care (99350)
Level	I	II	III	IV	V	I	II	III	IV

PF = Problem focused   EPF = Expanded problem focused   D = Detailed   C = Comprehensive   SF = Straightforward   L = Low   M = Moderate   H = High

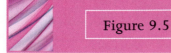

Figure 9.5   (Continued)

- Demonstrate clearly how physician work (expressed in terms of mental effort, physical effort, time spent, and risk to the patient) was affected by comorbidities or chronic problems listed.

2. Ensure that the nature of the patient's presentation corresponds to the CPT book's contributory factors of nature of the presenting problem and/or patient status descriptions for the code reported. For instance:
   - 99231—Usually the patient is stable, recovering, or improving.
   - 99232—Usually the patient is responding inadequately to therapy or has developed a minor complication.
   - 99233—Usually the patient is unstable or has developed a significant complication or a significant new problem.

3. Use clinical examples in Appendix C of the CPT book. Appendix C, located in the back of the CPT book, gives the coder or provider clinical examples for proper E/M coding.
   - The clinical examples established by the CPT coding are intended to represent the physician work that is reasonable and necessary in order to provide appropriate patient care in the specified clinical circumstance of the example.
   - Medicare expects actual documentation of services similar to the ones in the examples to also satisfy CMS documentation requirements to demonstrate that the service billed was provided.

Tips for Preventing Coding Errors with Specific E/M Codes

The medical coder needs to realize that coding mistakes happen. If unsure about which code to use or have not been given enough information in the patient medical record, ask for help. Some common coding errors and how to help prevent them are listed here:

1. *High-level services and the "comprehensive" codes:* Understand the CPT code requirements.
   - All codes in the following code sets require three of the three key components to be documented according to the CMS guidelines to meet published CPT definitions:
     - New patient office services
     - Initial hospital services
     - Initial consultations (inpatient and outpatient)
     - Emergency department services
     - Comprehensive nursing facility assessments
   - All of the following codes require not just three of the three key components to be documented; they also require comprehensive history and comprehensive examination.
     - 99201 and 99205 (New patient office services)
     - 99221 and 99223 (Initial hospital services)
     - 99241 and 99255 (Office consultations)
     - 99251 and 99255 (Initial in-patient consultations)

2. *Emergency department services:* Pay attention to the unique record kept in most emergency departments (EDs). Multiple individuals, including hospital staff, contribute to the ED service and the ED record, but Part B must not pay the physician for services rendered by hospital staff. Physician coding should be based on the physician's E/M work (or work shared by a physician and nonphysician practitioner in the same group). All history obtained and recorded by triage and other hospital nursing

staff must be specifically repeated by the physician and either re-recorded or annotated with specific comments, additions, and/or corrections and notation of the element of work personally performed by the physician.

3. *Subsequent hospital services:* Pay attention to medical necessity. When coding, strongly consider the CPT book's "nature of the presenting problem" contributory factors and/or other patient status descriptions.

> 99231—Usually the patient is stable, recovering, or improving.
>
> 99232—Usually the patient is responding inadequately to therapy or has developed a minor complication.
>
> 99233—Usually the patient is unstable or has developed a significant complication or a significant new problem.

4. *Consultations:* Before coding a consultation, ask and answer questions about the service. If the answer is "no" to any of the following questions, do not report the service as a consultation.

- Did you receive a request for an opinion from another physician?
- Does the documentation of the service clearly demonstrate who made the request and the nature of the opinion requested?
- Has the provider provided a written report of his or her opinion/advice to the referring physician?
- Though the referring physician may have asked for a "consultation," should the E/M service truly be reported as a consultation?
- Will the provider's opinion be used by, and in some manner affect, the requesting physician's own management of the patient?
- Will the referring physician be involved in subsequent decision making about the problem for which the referral has been made?
- For preoperative "consultations," is the service requested specifically for preoperative clearance that is medically necessary considering the patient's condition and the procedure planned?

5. *Critical care:* Before coding critical care, ask and answer the following questions about the service. If the answer is "no" to any of these questions, do not report the service as critical care.

- Does the record demonstrate work performed during the encounter that is more intense than the work of other E/M codes of the same time duration?
- Does the physician's documentation demonstrate all of the following?
  - Direct personal management
  - Frequent personal assessment and manipulation (not generally a once-daily visit)
  - High-complexity decision making to assess, manipulate, and support vital system function(s) to treat multisystem or single organ system failure and/or to prevent further life-threatening deterioration
  - Intervention of a nature such that failure to initiate these interventions on an urgent basis would likely result in sudden clinically significant or life-threatening deterioration in the patient's condition
- What about the time spent providing critical care?
  - Is it specifically recorded?
  - Is it reasonable considering the documented work provided?
  - Does it exclude time spent performing procedures for which separate payment is made?
  - If it includes time spent with family, was the family member operating as a surrogate decision maker because the patient was unable to make decisions?

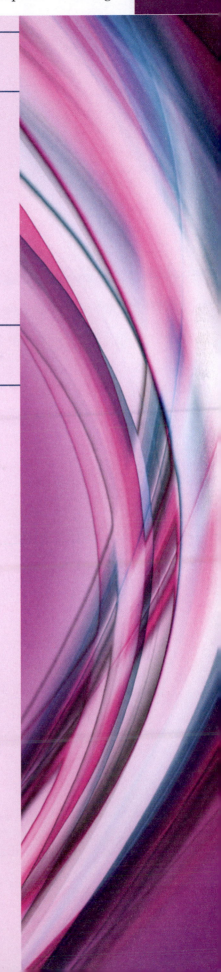

Chapter Summary

■ If audits are not performed on a regular basis, the medical office specialist will not know for a fact that the documentation was correct and appropriate for the level of service performed. If an audit is performed, any errors found can be brought to the attention of the provider and corrected for future billing.

■ The three types of audits are internal, external, and accreditation.

■ The auditor looks at the medical record and with an auditing tool independently analyzes by number count the services documented. The auditor then compares the code reported to the code selected through the audit.

■ The three key elements of service are the history documented, the examination documented, and the medical decision making.

Chapter Review

True/False

Identify the statement as true (T) or false (F).

_____ **1.** There are four types of audits.

_____ **2.** An accreditation audit is performed by the facility before claims submission.

_____ **3.** Code edits are conducted by the medical coder.

_____ **4.** When conducting an internal audit the three key elements reviewed are history, examination, and medical decision making.

_____ **5.** Code edits screen for improperly or incorrectly reported procedure codes.

_____ **6.** Compliance plans focus on training of physicians to use the AMA documentation guidelines for E/M services.

_____ **7.** *Downcoding* refers to a coding method in which lower-level codes are selected to avoid government investigation.

_____ **8.** The term *external audit* may refer to an audit conducted by a consultant that the medical practice has hired.

_____ **9.** Both insurance carriers and agencies of the federal government may conduct external audits of medical practices' claims.

_____ **10.** An internal audit is conducted to verify that a medical practice is in compliance with reporting regulations.

_____ 11. A prospective audit is also called an external audit.

_____ 12. To comply with regulations, all codes that are reported must be current, correct, and complete.

_____ 13. Retrospective internal audits permit the auditor to see which codes have been rejected or downcoded by the payer and to set up ways to avoid making the same errors in the future.

_____ 14. Evaluation and management (E/M) codes are an ongoing focus of internal audits because they are reported by so many medical practices.

_____ 15. Auditors may use an audit tool based on E/M documentation guidelines to determine whether a practice's selection of E/M codes complies with regulations.

Multiple Choice

Identify the letter of the choice that best completes the statement or answers the question.

_____ 1. What type of audit is performed internally after claims are submitted?
   a. Accreditation audit
   b. Routine payer audit
   c. Retrospective audit
   d. Prospective audit

_____ 2. What type of external audit is performed by payers before claims are processed?
   a. Retrospective
   b. Prospective
   c. Prepayment
   d. Postpayment

_____ 3. The term *downcode* means that the procedure code stated is for a procedure that is:
   a. more involved.
   b. in the hospital.
   c. less involved.
   d. less than per diem.

_____ 4. The AMA documentation guidelines set up the rules for the correct selection of:
   a. evaluation and management codes.
   b. anesthesia codes.
   c. surgery codes.
   d. none of the above.

Completion

Complete each sentence or statement.

1. Correct code linkage establishes the medical _____ for a service or procedure.

2. A retrospective is performed _____.

3. Assigning a higher level of CPT code than is warranted by the documented service is called _____.

4. Coding _____ is part of a medical practice's overall effort to follow regulations in many areas.

5. In addition to facilitating high-quality patient care, an appropriately _____ medical record serves as a legal document to verify services provided.

6. A(n) _____ is performed to judge whether a medical practice complies with applicable regulations for correct coding and billing.

Resources

American Academy of Neurology
www.aan.com

When you insert "Audit" in the Search window, you get information on how to perform a physician practice internal billing audit.

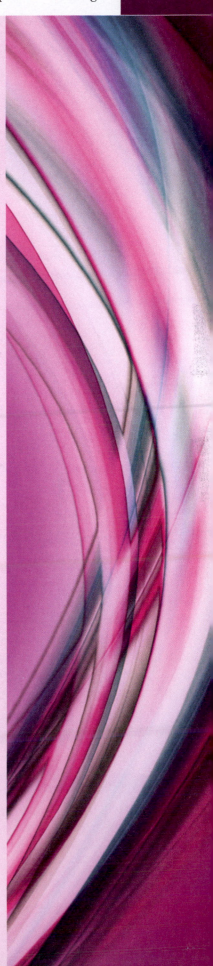

10 Physician Medical Billing

11 Hospital Medical Billing

The medical office specialist must have the knowledge and skills to submit a claim with no errors so that full reimbursement will be received. In the physician's office, as much as 80% of the physician's income can be generated by the submission of insurance claims and the reimbursement received from the insurance carrier. Chapter 10, Physician Medical Billing, will walk the student through the steps necessary to document all services provided accurately and in detail.

In the hospital setting, physicians' bills for inpatient care are much larger than the bills for services rendered in a physician's office. The majority of hospital reimbursement is from insurance companies; however, it is becoming more difficult for patients with insurance coverage to pay their share of the bill. Today's High Deductible Health Plans (HDHP) increase the patient's financial responsibility. As a result, accurate and timely billing with good follow-up and collection techniques are essential. Accurate billing requires correct patient and insurance information; however, the critical aspect of medical billing is diagnostic coding. Chapter 11, Hospital Medical Billing, presents detailed information on the inpatient billing process, coding and reimbursement methods, and the skills required to accurately bill for hospital services.

Chapter 10 / Physician Medical Billing

Chapter Objectives

After reading this chapter, the student should be able to:

1. Differentiate and complete medical claim forms accurately, both manually and electronically.

2. Define claim form parts, sections, and required information.

3. Exhibit the ability to complete claim forms without omitting information.

4. Understand the common reasons why claim forms are delayed or rejected, and submit a claim without payer rejection.

5. File a secondary claim.

Key Terms

assignment of benefits form
audit/edit report
billing services
birthday rule
claim attachment
clean claims
clearinghouse
CMS-1500 claim form
coordination of benefits (COB)
dirty claim
electronic claims, electronic media claims (EMCs)

encryption
employer identification number (EIN)
facility provider number (FPN)
form locators
group provider number (GPN)
guarantor
optical character recognition (OCR)
patient information form
provider identification number (PIN)

release of information form
secondary insurance
state license number
superbills
supplemental insurance
tax identification number (TIN)
UB-04 claim form
verification of benefits (VOB) form

CPT-4 codes in this chapter are from the CPT-4 2017 code set. CPT® is a registered trademark of the American Medical Association.
ICD-10-CM codes in this chapter are from the ICD-10-CM 2017 code set from the Department of Health and Human Services, Centers for Disease Control and Prevention.

**Physician
Medical
Billing**

William arrived at Dr. Spence's office and gave the medical office specialist his insurance cards. Recently, William's wife went back to work and they now have two insurance plans. William asked that his wife's be billed first because it had better coverage. The medical office specialist explained that his insurance would have to be billed primary and his wife's secondary.

Questions

1. Why can't his wife's insurance be primary?

2. What would be the result of billing the wife's insurance as primary?

3. Will there be cases when the spouse's insurance may be primary?

Services that are provided by a physician are generally covered by the patient's health insurance. As much as 80% of a physician's income can be generated by the submission of insurance claims and the reimbursement received from the insurance carrier. A medical office specialist must have the knowledge and skills to submit a claim with no errors so that full reimbursement will be received. The physician and her office staff, both clinical and clerical, must document all services provided accurately and in detail.

Conversion to Electronic Health Records

The material in this chapter will present information for doctors' offices that use basic electronic systems yet still maintain paper charts, and doctors' offices that have implemented Electronic Health Records (EHRs) and are operating using software programs to collect and retain patient demographics, patient care, insurance information, and patient billing electronically. The percentage of doctors' offices that used any EHR for something other than billing grew from 21% in 2004 to 78.4% in 2013 (according to Centers for Disease Control and Prevention). Just half of the offices use EHRs for functions other than billing. Approximately 20% still use paper records.

Whether a doctor's office uses paper charts or is fully integrated into the EHRs, the information such as patient demographics, insurance, guarantor, and patient care documentation is required.

Patient Information

Billing insurance carriers for medical services provided in a medical office setting requires information from many different resources. Because insurance billing provides the majority of a physician's income, it is extremely important to gather accurate information so that claims can be processed without delay.

When a new patient registers at a medical office, he is asked to complete a **patient information** form (Figure 10.1). This form contains patient and guarantor demographics, employment information, and insurance information. The form varies from one practice or facility to another. Some facilities may have a multipage form requesting allergy or personal/family medical history. Although the patient (or parent/guardian) is asked to write his insurance information on the patient information form, it is necessary to obtain a copy (front and back) of the patient's insurance card as well. Some practices also request a copy of the driver's license to confirm the patient/parent identity.

The patient, if an adult, or the guardian (often referred to as the **guarantor**, the person who is ultimately responsible for paying for the services) is also asked to sign an **assignment of benefits form** (Figure 10.2) and a **release of information form** (Figure 10.3)

Assignment of benefits means that the patient/guarantor is asking the insurance carrier to send the money for the services rendered and billed directly to the provider who performed the services instead of to the patient/guarantor. If an assignment of

Figure 10.1

Sample patient information form.

Capital City Medical—123 Unknown Blvd., Capital City,   Patient Information Form

NY 12345–2222 (555)555–1234   Tax ID: 75–0246810

Phil Wells, M.D., Mannie Mends, M.D., Bette R. Soone, M.D.   Group NPI: 1513171216

Patient Information:

Name: (Last, First) _____   ❑ Male   ❑ Female   Birth Date: _____

Address: _____   Phone: (   ) _____

Social Security Number: _____   Full-Time Student: ❑ Yes   ❑ No

Marital Status: ❑ Single   ❑ Married   ❑ Divorced   ❑ Other

- -

Employment:

Employer: _____   Phone: (   ) _____

Address: _____

Condition Related to: ❑ Auto Accident   ❑ Employment   ❑ Other Accident

Date of Accident: _____ State _____

Emergency Contact: _____   **Phone:** (   ) _____

- -

Primary Insurance: _____   **Phone:** (   ) _____

Address: _____

Insurance Policyholder's Name: _____   ❑ M   ❑ F   DOB: _____

Address: _____

Phone: _____ Relationship to Insured: ❑ Self   ❑ Spouse   ❑ Child   ❑ Other

Employer: _____   Phone: (   ) _____

Employer's Address: _____

Policy/I.D. No: _____ Group No: _____ Percent Covered: _____%, Copay Amt: $ ____

- -

Secondary Insurance: _____   **Phone:** (   ) _____

Address: _____

Insurance Policyholder's Name: _____   ❑ M   ❑ F   DOB: _____

Address: _____

Phone: _____Relationship to Insured: ❑ Self   ❑ Spouse   ❑ Child   ❑ Other

Employer: _____   Phone: (   ) _____

Employer's Address: _____

Policy/I.D. No: _____ Group No: _____ Percent Covered: ___%, Copay Amt: $____

- -

Reason for Visit: _____

Known Allergies: _____

Were you referred here? If so, by whom?: _____

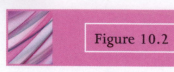

Figure 10.2

Sample assignment of benefits form.

I authorize payment of medical benefits to Allied Medical Center or the specified physician below.

Alison R. Smith, M.D.   Samson Westheimer, M.D.

_____   _____
Patient's Guarantor's Signature   **Date**

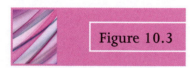

Figure 10.3

Sample release of information form.

**I, _____ ACTING ON
BEHALF OF: (Print Name of Patient or Legally Authorized Representative)**
_____ **HEREBY AUTHORIZE THE RELEASE**
(Print Name of Patient) _____
OF INFORMATION AS INDICATED:

My Healthcare Information

_____ I authorize disclosure of healthcare information (related to my medical history, diagnosis, treatment, or prognosis) to all inquiries or only to the following people or entities (for example, family friends, employer, insurance companies, clergy, etc.):

List Names:
_____
_____

Limited Healthcare Information
_____ I wish to limit disclosure of only certain kinds of healthcare information (related to my medical history, diagnosis, treatment, or prognosis) to the following people or entities:

List Names   **List information that may be released**
_____   _____
_____   _____

No Information
_____ I do not authorize release of any information.

_____   _____
(Signature of Patient or Legally Authorized representative)   (Date)

benefits form is not signed and the office submits the claim to the insurance carrier, the money may be sent directly to the patient. An assignment of benefits form is usually signed once a year.

The release of information form specifies which healthcare information from the patient's medical record may be released and to whom it may be released. If no signed release of information form is on file, the claim may not be submitted to the carrier. A signed release of information form is referred to as the "signature on file" form in most medical offices. This form must be signed once a year; however, some facilities require the patient to sign the release of information every 6 months.

The term *healthcare information* refers to information recorded in any form or medium that identifies the patient and relates to the patient's history, diagnosis, treatment, or prognosis. It is commonly known as the patient's *medical record*.

Generally, a designated person or persons in the office/clinic will verify patients' insurance benefits. One cannot assume that an insurance card is valid just because a patient has one. Verifying the insurance benefits is accomplished by contacting the insurance carrier listed on the patient's insurance card. This can be done by telephone, fax, and sometimes through the carrier's website. There are also software or information technology systems that send information from the facilities registration information system directly to the insurance carrier and verify benefits (eligibility) real-time.

Before the patient's insurance benefits can be verified, the medical office specialist will need to gather basic information about the patient and the policyholder (the person who took out the insurance policy). You will need the patient's name (as it appears on the insurance card) and date of birth, name of the insured/policyholder, insurance identification number (also referred to as certificate number or policy number), insurance group number if applicable, date of service, patient's reason for the visit (routine or problem specific). Different facilities will ask different questions, but every facility needs the following information:

- What is the effective date for this insurance coverage/policy?
- Is this patient and/or type of service subject to a deductible amount and, if so, how much is the deductible amount and has any of it been met?
- Is this type of service subject to a copayment amount and, if so, what is the amount?
- Is this (office visit, test, etc.) a covered benefit?
- Does this plan require a referral or prior authorization?

It is important to document everything. Most facilities have a **verification of benefits (VOB) form** (Figure 10.4) on which to write the answers to these questions when verifying benefits by phone. When a facility is automated, the information may be entered directly into the patient's electronic health record. A VOB form may come in handy if the insurance carrier pays the claim incorrectly or denies the claim after providing information to the contrary when benefits were verified.

Superbills

Superbills, also referred to as encounter forms, charge slips, or routing slips, contain International Classification of Diseases (ICD-10-CM diagnostic) and Current Procedural Terminology (CPT; procedure) codes for the services that the office routinely provides (Figure 10.5). Superbills vary in appearance because they are usually designed by the facility's billing software vendor to meet the specific needs of the practice. As an example, a superbill for a specialty practice will contain ICD-10-CM and CPT codes relating only to that specialty, whereas a family practice will use a superbill with a myriad of ICD and CPT codes dealing with different body systems.

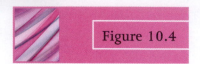

Figure 10.4

Insurance verification of benefits worksheet.

Patient's Name: _____ Medical Record #: _____ Appt. Date: _____
D.O.B. _____ Policy ID # _____ Gr# _____
Policyholder: _____ DOB: _____
Insurance Co. Name: _____ Referral# Required: ❑ No ❑ Yes
Telephone # _____ Referral #: _____
Mailing Address: _____
Employer's Name: _____
Employer's Phone #: _____
Effective Date: _____ Lifetime maximum: _____
Pre-Cert Required: ❑ Yes ❑ No

Deductible Met:
Copay _____ Deductible _____ ❑ No ❑ Yes
Pays @ _____%
Exclusion/Preexisting: _____
Chief Complaint/Diagnosis: _____
Insurance Rep's Name: _____ Ext# _____
Voice Tracking #: _____ Date: _____ Time: _____
Verified by _____ Date: _____

In preparation for a day's activities, the medical office specialist prints a superbill for each patient or when an office is automated prints a scheduling report. The superbill follows the patient throughout the visit. The professional staff (physician, nurse, physician's assistant, etc.) mark on the superbill the procedures and treatments performed during the visit, as well as the diagnosis, and return it to the business office staff to use as the source document for entering data into a computerized accounting system. Because this document contains most of the critical information for the billing process, it serves as a link between the professional staff and the business office staff, which files the insurance claims and bills the patient.

When a patient or physician returns the superbill to the front office or cashier, the medical office specialist opens the patient's account in the computer and keys ("posts") the charge and diagnosis data from the superbill.

To comply with the Health Information Technology for Economic and Clinical Health (HITECH) Act and meaningful use, many physician practices and hospitals have installed electronic medical records. In a medical facility with electronic medical records, the preparation for a day's activities will be electronic oriented and involve less paper preparation. A scheduling report will be generated that lists all appointments for the day and will include the patient's name, type of service, time of appointment, and the doctor the patient will see. Depending on which functions of the electronic medical record system are implemented, the patient's chart may be pulled to document the diagnosis and treatment of the patient, or no paper chart will be pulled and all documentation will be made directly into the electronic medical record software. The advantage of utilizing the full capacity of the EMR is that critical information for patient treatment and billing is available immediately in a physicians' practice or within 24 hours in a hospital setting.

Once the patient demographics, insurance information, diagnosis, and charges are posted to the patient account, it is time to send a claim form to the patient's insurance carrier for the services that were provided. Without the information provided on the patient information form, superbill, insurance card, and verification of benefits

Date of service:	Waiver? ☐	
Patient name:	Insurance:	
	Subscriber name:	
Address:	Group #:	Previous balance:
	Copay:	Today's charges:
Phone:	Account #:	Today's payment: check#
DOB: Age: Sex:	Physician name:	Balance due:

RANK	Office visit	New	Est
	Minimal		99211
	Problem focused	99201	99212
	Expanded problem focused	99202	99213
	Detailed	99203	99214
	Comprehensive	99204	99215
	Comprehensive (new patient)	99205	
	Significant, separate service	-25	-25
	Well visit	**New**	**Est**
	< 1 y	99381	99391
	1-4 y	99382	99392
	5-11 y	99383	99393
	12-17 y	99384	99394
	18-39 y	99385	99395
	40-64 y	99386	99396
	65 y +	99387	99397
	Medicare preventive services		
	Pap		Q0091
	Pelvic & breast		G0101
	Prostate/PSA		G0103
	Tobacco counseling/3-10 min		99406
	Tobacco counseling/>10 min		99407
	Welcome to Medicare exam		G0344
	ECG w/Welcome to Medicare exam		G0366
	Flexible sigmoidoscopy		G0104
	Hemoccult, guaiac		G0107
	Flu shot		G0008
	Pneumonia shot		G0009
	Consultation/preop clearance		
	Expanded problem focused		99242
	Detailed		99243
	Comprehensive/mod complexity		99244
	Comprehensive/high complexity		99245
	Other services		
	After posted hours		99050
	Evening/weekend appointment		99051
	Home health certification		G0180
	Home health recertification		G0179
	Post-op follow-up		99024
	Prolonged/30-74 min		99354
	Special reports/forms		99080
	Disability/Workers comp		99455
	Radiology		

	Diagnoses
1	
2	
3	
4	

Next office visit

Recheck	Prev	PRN	_____	D W M Y

Instructions:

Referral

To:

Instructions:

Physician signature

X _____

RANK	Office procedures	
	Anoscopy	46600
	Audiometry	92551
	Cerumen removal	69210
	Colposcopy	57452
	Colposcopy w/biopsy	57455
	ECG, w/interpretation	93000
	ECG, rhythm strip	93040
	Endometrial biopsy	58100
	Flexible sigmoidoscopy	45330
	Flexible sigmoidoscopy w/biopsy	45331
	Fracture care, cast/splint	29____
	Site: _____	
	Nebulizer	94640
	Nebulizer demo	94664
	Spirometry	94010
	Spirometry, pre and post	94060
	Tympanometry	92567
	Vasectomy	55250

	Skin procedures		**Units**
	Burn care, initial	16000	
	Foreign body, skin, simple	10120	
	Foreign body, skin, complex	10121	
	I&D, abscess	10060	
	I&D, hematoma/seroma	10140	
	Laceration repair, simple	120____	
	Site: _____ Size: _____		
	Laceration repair, layered	120____	
	Site: _____ Size: _____		
	Lesion, biopsy, one	11100	
	Lesion, biopsy, each add'l	11101	
	Lesion, destruct., benign, 1-14	17110	
	Lesion, destruct., premal., single	17000	
	Lesion, destruct., premal., ea. add'l	17003	
	Lesion, excision, benign	114____	
	Site: _____ Size: _____		
	Lesion, excision, malignant	116____	
	Site: _____ Size: _____		
	Lesion, paring/cutting, one	11055	
	Lesion, paring/cutting, 2-4	11056	
	Lesion, shave	113____	
	Site: _____ Size: _____		
	Nail removal, partial	11730	
	Nail removal, w/matrix	11750	
	Skin tag, 1-15	11200	

	Medications		**Units**
	Ampicillin, up to 500mg	J0290	
	B-12, up to 1,000 mcg	J3420	
	Epinephrine, up to 1ml	J0170	
	Kenalog, 10mg	J3301	
	Lidocaine, 10mg	J2001	
	Normal saline, 1000cc	J7030	
	Phenergan, up to 50mg	J2550	
	Progesterone, 150mg	J1055	
	Rocephin, 250mg	J0696	
	Testosterone, 200mg	J1080	
	Tigan, up to 200 mg	J3250	
	Toradol, 15mg	J1885	
	Miscellaneous services		

RANK	Laboratory	
	Venipuncture	36415
	Blood glucose, monitoring device	82962
	Blood glucose, visual dipstick	82948
	CBC, w/ auto differential	85025
	CBC, w/o auto differential	85027
	Cholesterol	82465
	Hemoccult, guaiac	82270
	Hemoccult, immunoassay	82274
	Hemoglobin A1C	85018
	Lipid panel	80061
	Liver panel	80076
	KOH prep (skin, hair, nails)	87220
	Metabolic panel, basic	80048
	Metabolic panel, comprehensive	80053
	Mononucleosis	86308
	Pregnancy, blood	84703
	Pregnancy, urine	81025
	Renal panel	80069
	Sedimentation rate	85651
	Strep, rapid	86403
	Strep culture	87081
	Strep A	87880
	TB	86580
	UA, complete, non-automated	81000
	UA, w/o micro, non-automated	81002
	UA, w/ micro, non-automated	81003
	Urine colony count	87086
	Urine culture, presumptive	87088
	Wet mount/KOH	87210
	Vaccines	
	DT, <7 y	90702
	DTP	90701
	DtaP, <7 y	90700
	Flu, 6-35 months	90657
	Flu, 3 y +	90658
	Hep A, adult	90632
	Hep A, ped/adol, 2 dose	90633
	Hep B, adult	90746
	Hep B, ped/adol 3 dose	90744
	Hep B-Hib	90748
	Hib, 4 dose	90645
	HPV	90649
	IPV	90713
	MMR	90707
	Pneumonia, >2 y	90732
	Pneumonia conjugate, <5 y	90669
	Td, >7 y	90718
	Varicella	90716

	Immunizations & Injections		**Units**
	Allergen, one	95115	
	Allergen, multiple	95117	
	Imm admin, one	90471	
	Imm admin, each add'l	90472	
	Imm admin, intranasal, one	90473	
	Imm admin, intranasal, each add'l	90474	
	Injection, joint, small	20600	
	Injection, joint, intermediate	20605	
	Injection, joint, major	20610	
	Injection, ther/proph/diag	90772	
	Injection, trigger point	20552	
	Supplies		

Figure 10.5   A sample superbill.

form, billing the patient's insurance carrier would be impossible. Physicians bill insurance carriers using the **CMS-1500 claim form**. Hospitals bill carriers using the **UB-04 claim form**. Both the CMS-1500 and UB-04 forms are universal claim forms for filing all medical claims.

Types of Insurance Claims: Paper versus Electronic

Insurance claims are sent by professionals, physicians, and hospitals/facilities to insurance carriers either on paper or electronically. Very few insurance carriers will accept paper claims. The term *encounter record* is a buzz term for a claim. A *paper claim* is one that is submitted on paper, including optically scanned claims that are converted to electronic form by insurance companies. Paper claims may be typed or generated by computer and sent through the U.S. Postal Service. Some claims require additional information for processing. In this instance, the claim is printed to paper and the additional information is sent as a **claim attachment** to the insurance carrier. Claim attachments are forms of documentation that support the medical necessity of a claim, such as an X-ray report or an operative report.

Electronic claims, also called **electronic media claims (EMCs)**, are submitted to the insurance carrier electronically. Electronic claims are never printed on paper. When claims are sent electronically to the insurance carriers for processing, an electronic signature is used to verify that the information received is true and correct. Meaningful use requires that at least 80% of all claims are filed electronically. With few exceptions, Medicare and Medicaid will only accept electronic claims. Electronic claims have a number of advantages:

- Administrative costs are lower because fewer personnel hours are needed to prepare forms, and supply and postage costs are lower.
- Fewer claims are rejected because technical errors are detected and corrected before the claim arrives at the payer.
- Payment is faster. An electronic claim is received by the payer in minutes, and payment can be transferred electronically to the provider's bank, eliminating delays in cash flow. These payments are referred to as *electronic remittances*.

Electronic claims also have disadvantages:

- Claims transmission can be disrupted occasionally due to power failures.
- Computer hardware or software problems might require claims to be resubmitted.
- Many patient billing programs cannot create an electronic attachment, so when a claim attachment is required, the electronic claim must be sent separately from mailed attachments, which sometimes causes problems for the payer in matching up the two. In some cases when the claim must be accompanied by a claim attachment, the claim must instead be submitted on paper.

Electronic claims are submitted through a clearinghouse, a billing service, or directly to the carrier. A physician who plans to use electronic remittance and funds transfer must have a signed agreement with each carrier. A carrier may have special electronic billing requirements with regard to submitting an electronic claim: for example, how to bill for patients who have secondary coverage. Medicare, Medicaid, TRICARE, and many private insurance carriers allow providers to submit insurance claims directly to them with no "middle man." In this type of system, the medical practice must have special software or the physician must lease a terminal from the carrier to key in claims data. Physicians and carriers must meet the HIPAA Version 5010 standards for electronic claims submission.

If the physician is not sending the data directly to the carrier, a clearinghouse may be used. A **clearinghouse** is a company that receives claims from providers, puts them through a series of audits to check for errors, and then forwards them to the appropriate insurance carrier in the carrier's required data format. Clearinghouses may charge a flat fee per claim or charge a percentage of the claim's dollar value. It is very important for physicians' practices to negotiate the best possible fee for using a clearinghouse's services.

The clearinghouse conducts an audit to determine if any data on the claim are incorrect or missing; such a claim is referred to as a **dirty claim**. The results of the audit are sent back to the provider from the clearinghouse in the form of an **audit/edit report**. The audit/edit report shows which claims need corrections and which claims have been forwarded to the appropriate carrier. Figure 10.6 shows a sample

Figure 10.6

Sample acknowledgment report.

Title: Acknowledgment Report

Purpose: To let the submitter know that claims were received and how they were handled (E, D, R)

Comment: None

ACKNOWLEDGMENT REPORT for NAME OF DOCTOR MD - 03-01-2016

E = Submitted Electronically; D = Duplicate; R = Rejected

File: PPSZ–ECS.116

  1 WATSON, BRENDA 922253 SOUTHWEST ADMIN /LA 02-06-16 $42.90 E

  2 RIVERA, ESAU 922318 LAWRENCE HEALTH CAR 02-09-16 $43.80 E

  3 MARTIN, DAN 922582 UNITED HEALTHCARE /02-10-16 $73.20 E

  4 LEGGETT, NEDRA 922621 BLUE CROSS /BLUE CA 02-10-16 $259.80 E

  5 THORERNER, ROBERT 922649 BLUE CROSS /P.B. OX 02-09-16 $43.80 E

  6 DOBALIAN, IVY 922651 BLUE CROSS /OXNARD- 02-09-16 $70.20 E

  7 LEGGETT, NEDRA 922684 BLUE CROSS /BLUE CA 02-06-16 $111.60 E

  8 LEGGETT, NEDRA 922689 BLUE CROSS /BLUE CA 02-06-16 $33.00 E

  9 WATKINS, CHARLES 925031 FIRST HEALTH /KENT 02-16-16 $43.80 E

10 THOMPSON, ANNA 925052 METRAHEALTH /RR–MED 02-18-16 $43.80 E

11 RAMIREZ, VERA 925064 MAXICARE /LA-861059 02-18-16 $43.80 E

TOTAL ELECTRONIC CLAIMS 11 $809.70

TOTAL CLAIMS RECEIVED AND PROCESSED 11 $809.70

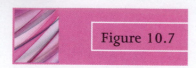

Figure 10.7

Sample accepted claims report.

Title: Accepted Claims Report
Purpose: From Envoy. To let the submitter know that claims for the named people were accepted into the system and sent on to the insurance company.

Comment:
03/02/16 ....

ACCEPTED CLAIMS for NAME OF DOCTOR MD-03/02/16

1. TABB, DONNA   2. ALVAREZ, ELIA   3. REED, ALDOLPHUS
4. JUDD, GEORGE   5. NABER, MIRIAM   6. REED, ALDOLPHUS
7. REED, PATRICIA   8. JUDD, LINDI   9. RAHAL, RIMA
10. RAHAL, RIMA   11. NAMDARKHAN, JAFAR   12. BARRETT, CLEMENTINA
13. BARRETT, CLEMENTINA   14. WATERS, MADALAINE   15. WATERS, MADALAINE
16. BIRD, STACIE   17. SHAO, SEN   18. MANJARREZ, ESTEBAN   19. JR, DARRELL B
20. REYES, MARIO   21. REYES, MARIO   22. AKHAVAN, MOHSEN
23. EHRENPREIS, JACQUELI   24. JOE, BOBBY   25. JOE, BOBBY   26. MONTOYA,
ANTONIO   27. OBERG, CAROL   28. RAUCH, URSULA   29. RAUCH, URSULA
30. CHANDRA, VINOD   31. CHANDRA, VINOD   32. RAHAL, AHMAD
33. RAHAL, AHMAD   34. PHAM, NHUTHUY   35. PHAM, NHUTHUY

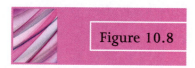

Figure 10.8

Sample rejected claims report.

Title: Rejected Claims Report
Purpose: To let the submitter know which claims were rejected and the reason (sometimes, very cryptic) for the rejection.

Comment: None
03/02/16 ....

REJECTED CLAIMS for NAME OF DOCTOR MD-03/02/16

PATIENT   DATA in ERROR   DESCRIPTION

922387   97118   PROCEDURE INVALID FOR PAYER USE HCPC

acknowledgment report; Figure 10.7 is a sample accepted claims report; Figure 10.8 is a sample rejected claims report; and Figure 10.9 shows a sample claims settlement report. These are the various types of reports generated by a clearinghouse. The medical office specialist will need to correct any claims containing incorrect data (as indicated on the audit/edit report) and resubmit them to the clearinghouse.

Dirty claims will not be transmitted to the carriers. When the claims are corrected and resubmitted to the clearinghouse, they are considered **clean claims**, which are then formatted and forwarded to the carrier. Each time the claim is returned, an additional charge is levied, so the medical office specialist should ensure that clean claims are transmitted initially.

Billing services are companies that provide data processing and claims processing services to physicians' offices for a fee. The provider submits to the billing service the necessary information needed to create the claims that are submitted to the carriers.

Title: Claims Settlement Report

Purpose: To let the submitter know which claims were settled (not necessarily
paid) by the insurance company.

Comment: Some insurance companies will return this report, not all.

03/02/16 ....

CLAIM SETTLEMENT for NAME OF DOCTOR MD - 03/02/16

COMPLETED: EXPENSES INCURRED PRIOR TO COVERAGE

PATIENT	STATEMENT DATES			TOTAL AMOUNT	
	FROM	THRU	PAYER	CHARGES	PAID
911851	06/25/16	07/02/16	METROPOLITAN LIFE	599.00	0.00
911879	08/13/16	08/18/16	METROPOLITAN LIFE	560.00	0.00

COMPLETED: PAYMENT MADE ACCORDING TO PLAN PROVISIONS

PATIENT	STATEMENT DATES			TOTAL AMOUNT	
	FROM	THRU	PAYER	CHARGE	PAID
917914	10/27/16	10/27/16	CIGNA	274.00	0.00
917914	10/27/16	10/27/16	CIGNA	274.00	0.00
917922	10/29/16	10/31/16	CIGNA	560.00	0.00
917922	10/29/16	10/31/16	CIGNA	560.00	0.00
917922	10/29/16	10/31/16	CIGNA	560.00	0.00
917922	10/29/16	10/31/16	CIGNA	560.00	0.00
917922	10/29/16	10/31/16	CIGNA	560.00	0.00
917922	10/29/16	10/31/16	CIGNA	560.00	0.00
917922	10/29/16	10/31/16	CIGNA	560.00	0.00
917922	10/29/16	10/31/16	CIGNA	560.00	0.00
917894	09/29/16	09/29/16	CIGNA	274.00	0.00
917894	09/29/16	09/29/16	CIGNA	274.00	0.00
917922	11/04/16	11/06/16	CIGNA	553.00	0.00
917922	11/04/16	11/06/16	CIGNA	553.00	0.00
917922	11/04/16	11/06/16	CIGNA	553.00	0.00
917922	11/04/16	11/06/16	CIGNA	553.00	0.00

COMPLETED: NO PAYMENT WILL BE MADE FOR THIS CLAIM

PATIENT	STATEMENT DATES			TOTAL AMOUNT	
	FROM	THRU	PAYER	CHARGES	PAID
911851	06/25/16	07/02/16	METROPOLITAN LIFE	599.00	0.00
911851	07/02/16	07/02/16	METROPOLITAN LIFE	371.00	0.00
911879	08/13/16	08/18/16	METROPOLITAN LIFE	560.00	0.00

Figure 10.9

Sample claims settlement
report.

This information includes personal information, the patient's insurance information,
and the patient's procedure(s) and diagnosis at the time of service. The billing company then analyzes the information, requests additional information or clarification if
needed, makes required edits, creates a clean claim, and submits the claim to the
specific carrier(s). Billing companies customarily use a clearinghouse to check the

claims they send out for the physicians. When the carriers adjudicate the claims, reimbursement is sent to the billing service, which then posts the checks to the doctor's accounts.

When the electronic claim is submitted either directly on the website or by computer, the medical office specialist can go to the specified website and view the claim submission report for the first pass. If accepted, the final adjudication will be available within 24 hours of the submission. HIPAA requires that encryption standards for all health care providers, insurance companies and business associates who transmit, store, or access protected health information in electronic format to utilize a standard level of data encryption. **Encryption** is the process of scrambling information during transmission so that it cannot be intercepted and read by anyone except the intended recipient.

Optical Character Recognition

Optical character recognition (OCR) devices (scanners) are being used frequently across the nation for processing paper documents into the doctor's office EHR. A scanner can transfer printed or typed text and bar codes to the EHR with speed and efficiency. Scanners read at such a fast speed that they reduce the cost of data entry and decrease the processing time. More control is gained over data input by using OCR. Optical character recognition can recognize handwriting and text, which helps staff turn paper records into digital records quickly and efficiently.

CMS-1500 Provider Billing Claim Form

The CMS-1500 form was developed by the Centers for Medicare and Medicaid Services (CMS) to facilitate the process of billing by easily arranging diagnoses and services provided that were necessary to treat patients. This information is attached to a claim form that is submitted to insurance carriers—private or government—and used to process claims for billing. The boxes to be completed on the form are referred to as **form locators**.

The CMS-1500 form is divided into two major sections:

Patient and Insured Information (Form locators 1–13)
Physician or Supplier Information (Form locators 14–33)

The CMS-1500 is printed in red ink so that it is recognizable by OCR scanners. Because it was developed by CMS for Medicare claims, Medicare has made it mandatory for all claim submissions. The CMS-1500 is the universal claim form used industry wide and is accepted by most health insurance carriers.

The upper portion of the CMS-1500 form consists of 13 form locators that contain 11 data elements and two signature form locators. The lower portion of the form consists of 20 form locators numbered 14 through 33, which contain 19 data elements, and one signature form locator.

Specific guidelines exist for completing a CMS-1500 claim form. TRICARE, CHAMPVA, Medicare, Medicaid, and workers' compensation carriers have their own rules. Because guidelines vary at the state and local levels for completing the CMS-1500, the medical office specialist should check with his local intermediaries or private carriers. For Blue Cross Blue Shield claims, the medial office specialist should refer to the provider manual for their state's Blue Cross Blue Shield plans for guidelines for completing the CMS-1500 claim form. Blue Cross Blue Shield plans are similar to other insurance carriers, and they do not have their own set of recognized rules for completing the CMS-1500 insurance claim form; therefore, form locators specific to Blue Cross Blue Shield are not listed separately in the text. The difference between Blue Cross Blue Shield and other insurance carriers, such as Aetna, is that BCBS is not a nationwide company in a technical sense of the word. BCBS is comprised of small independent health insurance companies that pay a licensing fee to use the Blue Cross Blue Shield trademark. BCBS of Illinois is totally different from BCBS of Texas, which is totally different from BCBS of Oklahoma. It is the business structure that makes Blue Cross Blue Shield unique. This uniqueness affects where claims are sent for payment but not how the CMS-1500 or UB-04 are completed.

For electronic billing, the Health Insurance Portability and Accountability Act of 1996 (HIPAA) developed standards and regulations that the health industry must follow in order to standardize patient care. The law that regulates electronic billing is known as the Administrative Simplification Subsection of HIPAA, which covers entities such as health plans, clearinghouses, and healthcare providers. When people working with billing in the medical field refer to HIPAA, they are generally referring to this subsection. The Administrative Simplification Subsection contains four distinct components:

1. Transaction and Code Sets
2. Uniform Identifiers
3. Privacy
4. Security

When information is exchanged electronically, both parties must follow the HIPAA 5010 transaction standard, which was in force as of July 1, 2012. Before HIPAA 5010 standards, transactions for every insurance plan used a format that contained variations that made it different from another plan's format. This meant that the plans could not easily exchange or forward claims. Providers were limited when sending electronic claims. HIPAA standardized these formats by requiring specific transaction standards as follows:

- Claims or Equivalent Encounters and Coordination of Benefits
- Remittance and Payment Advice
- Claims Status
- Eligibility and Benefit Inquiry and Response
- Referral Certification and Preauthorization
- Premium Payment
- Enrollment and Un-enrollment in a Health Plan
- Health Claims Attachment
- First Report of Injury
- Retail Drug Claims, Coordination of Drug Benefits, and Eligibility Inquiry

In an electronic transaction, certain portions of the information are sent as codes. For the receiving entity to understand the content of the transaction, both the sender and the receiver must use the same codes. CPT, HCPCS, and ICD-10-CM are examples of the codes required for electronic transmission. Standards have also been set for codes for gender, race, type of provider, relation of the policyholder to the patient, and hundreds of others.

Table 10.1   CMS-1500 Abbreviations

AMA—American Medical Association	HMO—Health maintenance organization
BLK Lung—Black lung	ICD-10-CM– *International Classification of Disease, Tenth Revision, Clinical Modification*
CCYY—Year, indicates entry of four digits for the century (CC) and year (YY)	I.D.—Identification
CHAMPUS—Civilian Health and Medical Program of the Uniformed Services	I.D. #—Identification number
CHAMPVA—Civilian Health and Medical Program of the Department of Veterans Affairs	INFO—Information
	LMP—Last menstrual period
CLIA—Clinical Laboratory Improvement Amendments	M—Male
CMS—Centers for Medicare and Medicaid Services (formerly HCFA)	MM—Month, indicates entry of two digits for the month
COB—Coordination of benefits	NDC—National Drug Code
CPT—*Current Procedural Terminology, 4th Edition*	No.—Number
DD—Day, indicates entry of two digits for the day	NPI—National Provider Identifier
DME—Durable medical equipment	NUCC—National Uniform Claim Committee
EIN—Employer identification number	NUCC-DS—National Uniform Claim Committee Data Set
EMG—Emergency	PH #—Phone number
EPSDT—Early and Periodic Screening, Diagnosis, and Treatment (Medicaid program)	QUAL.—Qualifier
F—Female	REF.—Reference
FECA—Federal Employees' Compensation Act	SOF—Signature on file
GTIN—Global trade item number	SSN—Social Security number
HCFA—Health Care Financing Administration (currently CMS)	UPC—Universal Product Code
HCPCS—Health Care Procedure Coding System	USIN—Unique supplier identification number
HIBCC—Health Industry Business Communications Council	VP—Vendor product number
HIPAA—Health Insurance Portability and Accountability Act of 1996	YY—Year, indicates entry of two digits for the year; may also be noted as CCYY, which allows for entry of four digits to include the century (CC) and year (YY)

General guidelines for filling out each form locator on the CMS-1500 are discussed next. Before learning about the form locators, however, review the abbreviations given in Table 10.1 and the CMS-1500 form itself, shown in Figure 10.10.

A 1500 claim form reference instruction manual published by the National Uniform Claim Committee (NUCC) can be found at www.nucc.org.

Completing the CMS-1500 Claim Form

The areas to be completed on the CMS–1500 claim form are referred to as form locators in this textbook. Additional names for these areas that may be used by other entities are Item Number, Item, Block, and Field.

HEALTH INSURANCE CLAIM FORM

APPROVED BY NATIONAL UNIFORM CLAIM COMMITTEE (NUCC) 02/12

CARRIER

☐☐☐ PICA | PICA ☐☐☐

1. MEDICARE ☒ (Medicare#) MEDICAID ☐ (Medicaid#) TRICARE ☐ (ID#/DoD#) CHAMPVA ☐ (Member ID#) GROUP HEALTH PLAN ☐ (ID#) FECA BLK LUNG ☐ (ID#) OTHER ☐ (ID#) | 1a. INSURED'S I.D. NUMBER (For Program in Item 1)

2. PATIENT'S NAME (Last Name, First Name, Middle Initial) | 3. PATIENT'S BIRTH DATE MM DD YY SEX M☐ F☐ | 4. INSURED'S NAME (Last Name, First Name, Middle Initial)

5. PATIENT'S ADDRESS (No., Street) | 6. PATIENT RELATIONSHIP TO INSURED Self☐ Spouse☐ Child☐ Other☐ | 7. INSURED'S ADDRESS (No., Street)

CITY | STATE | 8. RESERVED FOR NUCC USE | CITY | STATE

ZIP CODE | TELEPHONE (Include Area Code) ( ) | ZIP CODE | TELEPHONE (Include Area Code) ( )

9. OTHER INSURED'S NAME (Last Name, First Name, Middle Initial) | 10. IS PATIENT'S CONDITION RELATED TO: | 11. INSURED'S POLICY GROUP OR FECA NUMBER

a. OTHER INSURED'S POLICY OR GROUP NUMBER | a. EMPLOYMENT? (Current or Previous) YES☐ NO☐ | a. INSURED'S DATE OF BIRTH MM DD YY SEX M☐ F☐

b. RESERVED FOR NUCC USE | b. AUTO ACCIDENT? YES☐ NO☐ PLACE (State) | b. OTHER CLAIM ID (Designated by NUCC)

c. RESERVED FOR NUCC USE | c. OTHER ACCIDENT? YES☐ NO☐ | c. INSURANCE PLAN NAME OR PROGRAM NAME

d. INSURANCE PLAN NAME OR PROGRAM NAME | 10d. CLAIM CODES (Designated by NUCC) | d. IS THERE ANOTHER HEALTH BENEFIT PLAN? YES☐ NO☐ If yes, complete items 9, 9a, and 9d.

READ BACK OF FORM BEFORE COMPLETING & SIGNING THIS FORM.
12. PATIENT'S OR AUTHORIZED PERSON'S SIGNATURE I authorize the release of any medical or other information necessary to process this claim. I also request payment of government benefits either to myself or to the party who accepts assignment below.

SIGNED _____ DATE _____

13. INSURED'S OR AUTHORIZED PERSON'S SIGNATURE I authorize payment of medical benefits to the undersigned physician or supplier for services described below.

SIGNED _____

14. DATE OF CURRENT ILLNESS, INJURY, or PREGNANCY (LMP) MM DD YY QUAL. | 15. OTHER DATE QUAL. MM DD YY | 16. DATES PATIENT UNABLE TO WORK IN CURRENT OCCUPATION FROM MM DD YY TO MM DD YY

17. NAME OF REFERRING PROVIDER OR OTHER SOURCE | 17a. 17b. NPI | 18. HOSPITALIZATION DATES RELATED TO CURRENT SERVICES FROM MM DD YY TO MM DD YY

19. ADDITIONAL CLAIM INFORMATION (Designated by NUCC) | 20. OUTSIDE LAB? YES☐ NO☐ $ CHARGES

21. DIAGNOSIS OR NATURE OF ILLNESS OR INJURY Relate A-L to service line below (24E) ICD Ind. |
A. B. C. D.
E. F. G. H.
I. J. K. L.
| 22. RESUBMISSION CODE ORIGINAL REF. NO.
23. PRIOR AUTHORIZATION NUMBER

24. A. DATE(S) OF SERVICE From To MM DD YY MM DD YY	B. PLACE OF SERVICE	C. EMG	D. PROCEDURES, SERVICES, OR SUPPLIES (Explain Unusual Circumstances) CPT/HCPCS MODIFIER	E. DIAGNOSIS POINTER	F. $ CHARGES	G. DAYS OR UNITS	H. EPSDT Family Plan	I. ID. QUAL	J. RENDERING PROVIDER ID. #
1									NPI
2									NPI
3									NPI
4									NPI
5									NPI
6									NPI

25. FEDERAL TAX I.D. NUMBER SSN☐ EIN☐ | 26. PATIENT'S ACCOUNT NO. | 27. ACCEPT ASSIGNMENT? (For govt. claims, see back) YES☐ NO☐ | 28. TOTAL CHARGE $ | 29. AMOUNT PAID $ | 30. Rsvd. for NUCC Use

31. SIGNATURE OF PHYSICIAN OR SUPPLIER INCLUDING DEGREES OR CREDENTIALS (I certify that the statements on the reverse apply to this bill and are made a part thereof.) SIGNED _____ DATE _____ | 32. SERVICE FACILITY LOCATION INFORMATION a. NPI b. | 33. BILLING PROVIDER INFO & PH # ( ) a. NPI b.

PATIENT AND INSURED INFORMATION / PHYSICIAN OR SUPPLIER INFORMATION

NUCC Instruction Manual available at: www.nucc.org | **PLEASE PRINT OR TYPE** | APPROVED OMB-0938-1197 FORM 1500 (02-12)

Clear Form

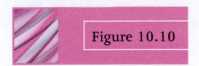

Figure 10.10 CMS-1500 claim form.

Source: Centers for Medicare and Medicaid Services.

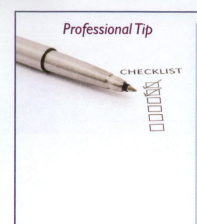

Professional Tip

CHECKLIST

When completing the CMS-1500 form, the medical office specialist should always be consistent in the way he enters the required dates when completing certain form locators. Providers and suppliers have the option of entering either a six- or eight-digit date format. Medicare and many insurance carriers will not accept claims if the date formats are not consistent. In other words, they cannot be used intermittently.

We now take a detailed look at how to complete a CMS-1500 claim form by reviewing how to fill out the information required for each form locator.

Form Locators for the CMS-1500 Form

Form Locator 1: Type of Insurance

Form locator 1 identifies what type of insurance the patient carries. The form lists five government plans: Medicare, Medicaid, TRICARE/CHAMPUS, CHAMPVA, and FECA Black Lung. There are two other options: Group Health Plan and Other. These are used depending on which type of plan the insured is enrolled.

Form Locator 1a: Insured's I.D. Number

Form locator 1a asks for the insured's insurance I.D. number as reflected on the insurance card. The insured could be the patient or someone else, such as a spouse, mother, or father.

Form Locator 2: Patient's Name

In form locator 2, enter the name of the patient who received services. This information is input as full last name, first name, and middle name or initial. The spelling should match the insurance card exactly. Do not use periods within the name.

If the patient's name is the same as the insured's name (i.e., the patient is the insured), then it is not necessary to report the patient's name. If the name on the card is misspelled, then the name in the computer should be misspelled until the patient provides a new card with the correct spelling.

The "Patient's Name" is the name of the person who received the treatment or supplies.

Form Locator 3: Patient's Date of Birth/Gender

In form locator 3, enter the patient's date of birth and gender. The date of birth is entered using the eight-digit format: MMDDYYYY. The patient's gender is identified as either male or female.

Form Locator 4: Insured's Name

Form locator 4 asks for the name of the person who is the insured. This may or may not be the patient. If the patient is the insured, the word "Same" should be entered. The insured's name should be entered full last name, first name, and middle name or initial. Use commas to separate the last name, first name, and middle initial. A hyphen can be used for hyphenated names. Do not use periods within the name. If Medicare is primary, leave the field blank.

Form Locator 5: Patient's Address

Enter the patient's home address and telephone number in form locator 5. This information is taken from the patient information form when the patient registers in the office. The address should include the street name and number, city, state (two-letter abbreviation), and zip code. Do not use commas, periods, or other symbols in the address. When entering a nine-digit zip code, include the hyphen. Do not use a hyphen or space as a separator within the telephone number. If the patient's address is the same as the insured's address, then it is not necessary to report the patient's address.

"Patient's Telephone" does not exist in 5010A1. The NUCC recommends that the phone number not be reported. Phone extensions are not supported.

The "Patient's Address" is the patient's permanent residence. A temporary address or school address should not be used.

Form Locator 6: Patient's Relationship to the Insured

Once form locator 4 has been completed, in form locator 6 enter an X in the correct box to indicate the patient's relationship to the insured. Options include Self, Spouse, Child, or Other. If the patient is the insured person, the "Self" entry is marked here. Only one box can be marked.

Form Locator 7: Insured's Address

Enter the insured's address. If Item Number 4 is completed, then this field should be completed. The first line is for the street address; the second line, the city and state; the third line, the ZIP code.

Do not use punctuation (i.e., commas, periods) or other symbols in the address (e.g., 123 N Main Street 101 instead of 123 N. Main Street, #101). When entering a 9-digit ZIP code, include the hyphen.

Form Locator 8: Reserved for NUCC Use

This field was previously used to report "Patient Status." "Patient Status" does not exist in 5010A1, so this field has been eliminated.

Form Locator 9: Other Insured's Name

If Item Number 11d is marked, complete fields 9, 9a, and 9d; otherwise, leave blank. When additional group health coverage exists, enter other insured's full last name, first name, and middle initial of the enrollee in another health plan if it is different from that shown in Item Number 2. If there is no secondary policy, form locator 9 is left blank.

Form Locator 9a: Other Insured's Policy or Group Number

Enter the policy number or group number of the secondary insurance policy in form locator 9a. The number should be entered exactly as it appears on the insurance card.

Form Locator 9b: Reserved for NUCC Use

This field was previously used to report "Other Insured's Date of Birth, Gender." "Other Insured's Date of Birth, Gender" does not exist in 5010A1, so this field has been eliminated.

Form Locator 9c: Reserved for NUCC Use

This field was previously used to report "Employer's Name or School Name." "Employer's Name or School Name" does not exist in 5010A1, so this field has been eliminated.

Form Locator 9d: Insurance Plan Name or Program Name

Form locator 9d asks for the name of the secondary insurance plan. This information is taken directly from the secondary insurance card. Enter the name exactly as it appears on the card.

Form Locator 10a–c: Is Patient's Condition Related To?

Form locator 10 identifies whether the patient's visit was related to an employment accident, auto accident, or other accident as described in form locator 24. This form locator is used when filing workers' compensation claims, auto accident claims, or claims for other types of injuries. If the patient's visit does not pertain to an accident of any kind, the default answer will be NO. Enter an X in the correct box.

Form Locator 10d: Claim Codes (Designated by NUCC)

When applicable, use to report appropriate claim codes. Applicable claim codes are designated by the NUCC. Please refer to the most current instructions from the public or private payer regarding the need to report claim codes.

When required by payers to provide the subset of Condition Codes approved by the NUCC, enter the Condition Code in this field. The Condition Codes approved for use on the 1500 Claim Form are available at www.nucc.org under Code Sets.

When reporting more than one code, enter three blank spaces and then the next code. "Claim Codes" identify additional information about the patient's condition or the claim.

Form Locator 11: Insured's Policy Group or FECA Number

If form locator 4 is completed, then form locator 11 should be completed. Form locator 11 identifies the insured's policy group number listed on the insurance card. This number should be entered exactly as it appears on the insurance card. A FECA number (nine-digit alphanumeric identifier) is listed here when employees of the federal government are filing workers' compensation claims.

Form Locator 11a: Insured's Date of Birth/Gender

In form locator 11a, list the date of birth of the insured. The date of birth should be listed in the eight-digit format: MMDDYYYY. If the patient and the insured are the same person, this space can be left blank. Choose either male or female accordingly. If gender is unknown, leave the field blank.

Form Locator 11b: Other Claim ID (Designated by NUCC)

When submitting to Property and Casualty payers, e.g. Automobile, Homeowner's, or Workers' Compensation insurers and related entities, the following qualifier and accompanying identifier has been designated for use:

Y4 Agency Claim Number (Property Casualty Claim Number)

Enter the qualifier to the left of the vertical, dotted line. Enter the identifier number to the right of the vertical, dotted line.

Form Locator 11c: Insurance Plan Name or Program Name

Form locator 11c identifies the insurance plan name. Enter the 9-digit PAYERID number or the primary insurer.

Some payers require an identification number of the primary insurer rather than the name in this field.

The "Insurance Plan Name or Program Name" is the name of the plan or program of the insured as indicated in Item Number 1a.

Form Locator 11d: Is There Another Health Benefit Plan?

In form locator 11d, indicate whether there is another health benefit plan. When appropriate, enter an X in the correct box. If marked "YES", complete 9, 9a, and 9d. Only one box can be marked. If there is no additional insurance plan, mark NO.

Form Locator 12: Patient's or Authorized Person's Signature

Form locator 12 is where the patient or guarantor signs, allowing the release of any medical information to the insurance company for billing purposes. Enter "Signature on File," "SOF," or legal signature. When legal signature, enter date signed in 6-digit (MM|DD|YY) or 8-digit format (MM|DD|YYYY) format. If there is no signature on file, leave blank or enter "No Signature on File."

Form Locator 13: Insured's or Authorized Person's Signature

Form locator 13 is where the patient or insured signs, authorizing the insurance company to reimburse the physician or supplier directly. The words "Signature on File" or "SOF" may be added here in place of a written signature when filing claims. If there is no signature on file, leave the field blank or enter "No Signature on File."

Form Locator 14: Date of Current Illness, Injury, Pregnancy

Indicate the first date of the current illness, injury, or pregnancy in form locator 14. The date should be entered in the six-digit (MM/DD/YY) or eight-digit format (MM/DD/CCYY). For a pregnancy, the first day of the woman's last menstrual period (LMP) is used.

Enter the applicable qualifier to identify which date is being reported.
431 Onset of Current Symptoms or Illness
484 Last Menstrual Period
Enter the qualifier to the right of the vertical, dotted line.

Form Locator 15: Other Date

In form locator 15, enter another date related to the patient's condition or treatment for the same or similar illness. The date should be entered in the six-digit (MM/DD/YY) or eight-digit format (MM/DD/YYYY). Enter the applicable qualifier to identify which date is being reported.

454 Initial Treatment
304 Latest Visit or Consultation
453 Acute Manifestation of a Chronic Condition
439 Accident
455 Last X-ray
471 Prescription
090 Report Start (Assumed Care Date)
091 Report End (Relinquished Care Date)
444 First Visit or Consultation
Enter the qualifier between the left-hand set of vertical, dotted lines. If the information is not known, leave the field blank.

Form Locator 16: Dates Patient Unable to Work in Current Occupation

In form locator 16, list the dates the patient is unable to work due to her illness or injury. These dates will be required when filing workers' compensation or disability claims. The dates should be entered in the six-digit (MM/DD/YY) or eight-digit format (MM/DD/YYYY). Date must be shown for the "from–to" dates that the patient is unable to work. An entry in this field may indicate employment-related insurance coverage. If the information is not required, leave the field blank.

Form Locator 17: Name of Referring Provider or Other Source

Form locator 17 requests the name of the provider referring the patient. Some insurance companies, such as health maintenance organizations (HMOs) or exclusive provider organizations (EPOs), require this information to be on a claim. The information entered should include the physician's last name, first name, and credentials. If multiple providers are involved, enter one provider using the following priority order:

1. Referring provider
2. Ordering provider
3. Supervising provider

Enter the applicable qualifier to identify which provider is being reported.

DN Referring Provider
DK Ordering Provider
DQ Supervising Provider

Enter the qualifier to the left of the vertical, dotted line.

If there is no referring physician, leave the field blank.

Form Locator 17a and 17b (Split Field): I.D. Number of Referring Physician 17a: Other ID#

The Other ID number of the referring, ordering, or supervising provider is reported in 17a in the shaded area. The qualifier indicating what the number represents is reported in the qualifier field to the immediate right of 17a.

The NUCC defines the following qualifiers used in 5010A1:

0B State License Number
1G Provider UPIN Number
G2 Provider Commercial Number
LU Location Number (This qualifier is used for Supervising Provider only.)

17b: NPI Number

Enter the NPI number of the referring, ordering, or supervising provider in form locator 17b. The NPI number refers to the HIPAA National Provider Identifier number, which is a 10-digit number.

Form Locator 18: Hospitalization Dates Related to Current Services

Enter the dates the patient has been hospitalized in relation to the current services in form locator 18. If the patient has been discharged from the hospital, the dates should include the day admitted and the day discharged. If the patient is still hospitalized, include only the day admitted. The dates should be entered in the six-digit or eight-digit format. If the patient has not been hospitalized, leave the field blank.

Form Locator 19: Additional Claim Information (Designated by NUCC)

Please refer to the most current instructions from the public or private payer regarding the use of this field. Some payers ask for certain identifiers in this field. If identifiers are reported in this field, enter the appropriate qualifiers describing the identifier. Do not enter a space, hyphen, or other separator between the qualifier code and the number.

The NUCC defines the following qualifiers used in 5010A1:

0B State License Number
1G Provider UPIN Number
G2 Provider Commercial Number
LU Location Number (This qualifier is used for Supervising Provider only.)
N5 Provider Plan Network Identification Number
SY Social Security Number (The social security number may not be used for Medicare.)
X5 State Industrial Accident Provider Number
ZZ Provider Taxonomy (The qualifier in the 5010A1 for Provider Taxonomy is PXC, but ZZ will remain the qualifier for the 1500 Claim Form.)

The above list contains both provider identifiers as well as the provider taxonomy code. The provider identifiers are assigned to the provider either by a specific payer or by a third party in order to uniquely identify the provider. The taxonomy code is designated by the provider in order to identify his/her provider type, classification, and/or area of specialization. Both, provider identifiers and provider taxonomy may be used in this field.

Taxonomy codes reported in this field must not be reportable in other fields, i.e., Item Numbers 17, 24J, 32, or 33.

When reporting a second item of data, enter three blank spaces and then the next qualifier and number/code/information.

Form Locator 20: Outside Lab

Complete this field when billing for purchased services by entering an X in "YES." A "YES" mark indicates that the reported service was provided by an entity other than the billing provider (for example, services subject to Medicare's anti-markup rule). A "NO" mark or blank indicates that no purchased services are included on the claim.

If "Yes" is marked, enter the purchase price under "$Charges" and complete Item Number 32. Each purchased service must be reported on a separate claim form as only one charge can be entered.

When entering the charge amount, enter the amount in the field to the left of the vertical line. Enter number right justified to the left of the vertical line. Enter 00 for cents if the amount is a whole number. Do not use dollar signs, commas, or a decimal point when reporting amounts. Negative dollar amounts are not allowed. Leave the right-hand field blank.

"Outside lab? $Charges" indicates that services have been rendered by an independent provider as indicated in Item Number 32 and the related costs.

Form Locator 21: Diagnosis or Nature of Illness or Injury

In form locator 21, the ICD-10 codes to the highest level of specificity for the date of service are entered. At least one code must be entered, and up to four codes can be used on a claim. Codes are placed in order of precedence, line 1 being the primary diagnosis, and so forth. No written diagnoses are used on a claim form. The ICD-10 codes should be checked for medical necessity to make sure they are used appropriately with the CPT codes used in form locator 24D.

Relate lines A–L to the lines of service in 24E by line number. Do not provide narrative description in this field.

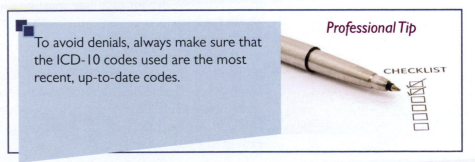

Professional Tip

To avoid denials, always make sure that the ICD-10 codes used are the most recent, up-to-date codes.

CHECKLIST

Form Locator 22: Medicaid Resubmission Code or Original Reference Number

List the original reference number for resubmitted claims. Please refer to the most current instructions from the public or private payer regarding the use of this field (e.g., code).

When resubmitting a claim, enter the appropriate bill frequency code left justified in the left-hand side of the field.

7 Replacement of prior claim

8 Void/cancel of prior claim

This Item Number is not intended for use for original claim submissions.

Form Locator 23: Prior Authorization Number

Some insurance plans, such as those of HMOs, EPOs, and preferred provider organizations (PPOs), require a prior authorization number. If required when preauthorization is obtained from an insurance company for services, the number assigned is input in form locator 23. Also, HMO-required referral numbers are input in this form locator. Any of the following can be entered here: prior authorization number, referral number, mammography precertification number, or Clinical Laboratory Improvement Amendments (CLIA) number, as assigned by the payer for the current service. Do not enter hyphens or spaces within the number. If prior authorization is required and is omitted, the claim will be denied. If no prior authorization is required, leave the field blank.

Form Locator 24

The six date-of-service lines in form locator 24 have been divided horizontally to accommodate submission of both the NPI and another/proprietary identifier and to accommodate the submission of supplemental information to support the billed service. The top area of the six service lines is shaded and is the location for reporting supplemental information. (It is not intended to allow the billing of 12 lines of service.)

The supplemental information is to be placed in the shaded section of form locators 24A through 24G as defined in each item number. Providers must verify this supplemental information with the payer.

Form Locator 24A: Dates of Service

In form locator 24A, enter date(s) of service, both the "From" and "To" dates. If there is only one date of service, enter that date under "From." Leave "To" blank or re-enter "From" date. If grouping services, the place of service, procedure code, charges, and individual provider for each line must be identical for that service line. Grouping is allowed only for services on consecutive days. The number of days must correspond to the number of units in 24G.

When required by payers to provide additional narrative description of an unspecified code, NDC, contract rate, or tooth numbers and areas of the oral cavity, enter the applicable qualifier and number/code/information starting with the first space in the shaded line of this field. Do not enter a space, hyphen, or other separator between the qualifier and the number/code/ information. The information may extend to 24G.

Form Locator 24B: Place of Service

Place of service in form locator 24B is a mandatory field to be completed because it describes the place where the procedure or service was performed. This place could be many places, such as the physician's office, hospital, emergency department, skilled nursing facility, or even the patient's home. A code is used (see the following list) to indicate the place of service. (Note: The CMS has stated that the place of service must also be fully written out in form locator 32.)

Consider this example: The patient was an inpatient (hospital) and the physician saw the patient in the hospital for an E/M service. Therefore, the code 21 (see following list) would be entered in form locator 24B and the following entered in form locator 32:

Allied Hospital
210 Frankford Road
Cheyenne, WY 12345

Common place of service codes include the following:

11 Physician's office
12 Home
13 Assisted living facility
20 Urgent care facility
21 Inpatient hospital
22 On Campus-Outpatient hospital
23 Hospital emergency department
24 Ambulatory surgical center
25 Birthing center
26 Military treatment facility
31 Skilled nursing facility
34 Hospice
81 Independent laboratory

Form Locator 24C: EMG (Emergency)

Form locator 24C is used to indicate whether the service was provided on an emergency basis. This form locator should be marked with a Y for YES or left blank for NO. The definition of an emergency can be defined differently by each payer.

Form Locator 24D: Procedures, Services, or Supplies

In form locator 24D, enter the CPT or HCPCS codes used to identify the procedures, services, or supplies provided. Modifiers are also listed in form locator 24D. This field accommodates the entry of up to four two-digit modifiers. The specific procedure code(s) must be shown without a narrative description.

Form Locator 24E: Diagnosis Pointer

Form locator 24E indicates the number (1, 2, 3, and 4) of the diagnosis code listed in form locator 21 as it relates to each service or procedure. If more than one diagnosis is attached to a single procedure or service, list the primary diagnosis first.

Form Locator 24F: Charges

Form locator 24F lists the charges that are assigned to each CPT or HCPCS code listed. The amount should be entered without a decimal point or dollar sign. If multiple units are entered in form locator 24G, the charges should reflect the amount of the procedure times the number of units. Charges should be updated on a regular basis to follow appropriate billing guidelines.

Form Locator 24G: Days or Units

Enter the number of units per procedure or service provided to a patient in form locator 24G. If billing for anesthesia, the amount entered should be entered in minutes and calculated accordingly. If billing for multiple services, such as liters of oxygen, list the actual number of liters. If multiple units are entered in 24G, the charges should reflect the amount of the procedure multiplied by the number of units.

When required by payers to provide supplemental information such as the National Drug Code (NDC) units in addition to the HCPCS units, enter the applicable NDC units' qualifier and related units in the shaded line. The following qualifiers are to be used when reporting NDC units:

F2	International Unit	ML	Milliliter
GR	Gram	UN	Unit

Form Locator 24H: EPSDT Family Plan

Form locator 24H is used to identify whether the patient is receiving his services through Medicaid's Early and Periodic Screening, Diagnosis, and Treatment (EPSDT) program. If there is no state requirement to report a reason code for EPSDT, enter Y for YES. Only enter Y for yes or N for NO.

If there is a requirement to report a reason code for EPSDT, enter the appropriate reason code as noted below. (Y and N responses are not entered with a code.) The two-character code is entered in the top shaded area of the field.

The following codes are for EPSDT:

AV   Available—Not used (Patient refused referral.)

S2   Under treatment (Patient is currently under treatment for referred diagnostic or corrective health problem.)

ST   New service requested (Referral to another provider for diagnostic or corrective treatment/scheduled for another appointment with screening provider for diagnostic or corrective treatment for at least one health problem identified during an initial or periodic screening service, not including dental referrals.)

NU   Not used (Used when no EPSDT patient referral was given.)

If the service is for family planning, enter Y for YES or N for NO in the bottom, unshaded area of the field.

Form Locator 24I:

Enter in the shaded area of 24I the qualifier identifying if the number is a non-NPI. The Other ID# of the rendering provider should be reported in 24J in the shaded area.

The NUCC defines the following qualifiers used in 5010A1:

0B   State License Number

1G   Provider UPIN Number

G2   Provider Commercial Number

LU   Location Number

ZZ   Provider Taxonomy (The qualifier in the 5010A1 for Provider Taxonomy is PXC, but ZZ will remain the qualifier for the 1500 Claim Form.)

The above list contains both provider identifiers, as well as the provider taxonomy code. The provider identifiers are assigned to the provider either by a specific payer or by a third party in order to uniquely identify the provider. The taxonomy code is designated by the provider in order to identify his provider type, classification, and/or area of specialization. Both provider identifiers and provider taxonomy may be used in this field.

The Rendering Provider is the person or company (laboratory or other facility) who rendered or supervised the care. In the case where a substitute provider (locum tenens) was used, enter that provider's information here. Report the Identification

Number in Items 24I and 24J only when different from data recorded in items 33a and 33b.

Form Locator 24J: Rendering Provider

The individual rendering the service is reported in form locator 24J. Enter the non-NPI I.D. number in the shaded area of the field. Enter the NPI number in the unshaded area of the field.

The NUCC defines the following qualifiers used in 5010A1:

- 0B   State License Number
- 1G   Provider UPIN Number
- G2   Provider Commercial Number
- LU   Location Number
- ZZ   Provider Taxonomy (The qualifier in the 5010A1 for Provider Taxonomy is PXC, but ZZ will remain the qualifier for the 1500 Claim Form.)

Form Locator 25: Federal Tax I.D. Number

List in form locator 25 the physician's federal tax I.D. number or her employer identification number (EIN). Do not enter hyphens with numbers. The appropriate box (SSN or EIN) should be marked with an X.

Form Locator 26: Patient's Account Number

In form locator 26, enter the patient's account number assigned by the medical office. The computer system used in the office will generate the number, and it should be entered on the claim. This in turn will allow for the account number to appear on the Explanation of Benefits (EOB) form, which makes it easier to locate the correct patient to post insurance payments.

Form Locator 27: Accept Assignment?

Form locator 27 is used to indicate whether or not the physician accepts assignment on this claim. If the physician does accept assignment and the patient has signed form locator 13, the insurance carrier will pay the physician directly for services provided. If the physician does not accept assignment, the insurance carrier will send the reimbursement to the patient.

Form Locator 28: Total Charge

Form locator 28 lists the total charges, added together from those listed in form locator 24F. The charges should be checked for accuracy to ensure proper reimbursement. Do not use decimal points or dollar signs in this entry.

Form Locator 29: Amount Paid

Form locator 29 indicates the amount paid on this claim for covered services only. This amount is usually added after the primary EOB/ERA is received and payment is posted. A secondary claim is printed to be sent to the secondary insurance carrier along with a copy of the primary insurance carrier's EOB. Do not use decimal points or dollar signs in this entry.

Form Locator 30: Reserved for NUCC Use

This field was previously used to report "Balance Due." "Balance Due" does not exist in 5010A1, so this field has been eliminated.

Form Locator 31: Signature of Physician or Supplier Including Degrees or Credentials

Form locator 31 identifies the name of the physician or supplier who has provided the services to the patient along with her credentials (M.D., PA-C, or NP).

If a paper claim is submitted, the physician or supplier's name must be typed/printed or the signature of the representative of the physician or supplier included, or enter "Signature on File" or "SOF." Enter a six-digit date (MM/DD/YY), eight-digit date (MM/DD/YYYY), or alphanumeric date. A signature stamp may be used instead of a written signature. The stamp must leave a clear, nonsmeared image on the claim.

Form Locator 32: Name and Address of Facility Where Services Were Rendered

Form locator 32 identifies the name of the facility where services were provided. Enter the name, address, zip code, and NPI number when billing for purchased diagnostic tests. When more than one supplier is used, a separate CMS-1500 form should be used for each supplier.

Form Locator 32a: NPI Number

Enter the NPI number of the service facility location in form locator 32a.

Form Locator 32b: Other I.D. Number

Enter the two-digit qualifier identifying the non-NPI number followed by the I.D. number. Do not enter a space, hyphen, or other separator between the qualifier and number.

The NUCC defines the following qualifiers used in 5010A1:

0B State License Number
G2 Provider Commercial Number
LU Location Number

Form Locator 33: Billing Provider Information and Phone Number

Enter the provider or supplier's billing name, address, zip code, and phone number in form locator 33. The phone number is to be entered in the area to the right of the field title. Enter the name and address information in the following format:

First line: Name
Second line: Address
Third line: City, state, and zip code

Form Locator 33a: NPI Number

Enter the NPI number of the billing provider in form locator 33a. The NPI number refers to the HIPAA National Provider Identifier number, which allows for the entry of 10 characters.

Form Locator 33b: Other I.D. Number

Enter the two-digit qualifier identifying the non-NPI number followed by the I.D. number. Do not enter a space, hyphen, or other separator between the qualifier and number. Refer to form locator 32b for a list of qualifiers.

Remember that the non-NPI I.D. number of the billing provider refers to the payer-assigned unique identifier of the professional.

Physicians' Identification Numbers

Insurance companies and federal and state programs require certain identification numbers on health insurance claim (HIC) forms submitted from individuals and facilities who provide and bill for services to patients. Although the NPI will eventually replace all of these numbers except a few, an understanding of these numbers is imperative for the medical biller. The use of the various numbers can be confusing to the beginner, as well as to someone experienced in insurance billing procedures, so an explanation is provided here.

State license number: To practice within a state, each physician must obtain a physician's **state license number**. Sometimes this number is requested on forms and used as a provider number—for example, Texas Workers' Compensation (form locator 33b).

Employer identification number: In a medical group or solo practice, each physician must have her own federal tax identification number, known as an **employer identification number (EIN)**, or **tax identification number (TIN)**. This number is issued by the Internal Revenue Service for income tax purposes (form locator 25). Each physician may have one or more TIN for financial reasons. Examples of additional TINs would be a group practice that bills from different entities—for example, an orthopedic office that provides physical therapy. An EIN would be used for the physician visits and a TIN for the physical therapy visits. If a group practice has satellite offices, those offices might have different TINs.

Provider numbers: Claims may require three provider identification numbers—one for the referring physician (form locator 17a/b), one for the ordering physician (form locator 17a/b), and one for the performing physician (form locator 24K or form locator 33 for the billing entity). The ordering physician and the performing physician can be the same (form locators 17a/b and 33). On rare occasions, the number may be the same for all three, but more frequently three different numbers are required, depending on the circumstances of the case. For placement on the CMS-1500 claim form, keep in mind what role the physician(s) and their numbers represent in relationship to the provider listed in form locator 33. To assist with claims completion, a reference list of providers' numbers could be compiled for all ordering physicians and physicians who frequently refer patients. Physicians' provider numbers can be obtained by calling their offices or through the Medicare carrier.

Provider identification number: Every physician who renders services to patients may be issued a carrier-assigned **provider identification number (PIN)** by the insurance company.

Group provider number: The **group provider number (GPN)** is used instead of the individual PIN for the performing provider who is a member of a group practice that submits claims to insurance companies under the group name (form locator 33). In this case, the PIN is reported in form locator 24J for the specific performing provider.

National Provider Identifier Number: As of May 2007, all providers have a National Provider Identifier (NPI) number. This number is a lifetime 10-digit number that is recognized by the Medicaid, Medicare, TRICARE, and CHAMPVA programs and will be used by all private insurance carriers. It will replace the existing identification numbers.

Durable medical equipment number: Medicare providers who charge patients a fee for supplies and equipment, such as crutches, urinary catheters, ostomy supplies, surgical dressings, and so forth, must bill Medicare using a durable medical equipment (DME) number.

Facility provider number: Each facility (e.g., hospital, laboratory, radiology office, skilled nursing facility) is issued a **facility provider number (FPN)** to be used by the performing physician to report services done at the location.

Although most facilities send insurance claims electronically, it is necessary to be familiar with the form locators on both the CMS-1500 and the UB-04 claim forms. When submitting an insurance claim, the medical office specialist must make sure that all of the needed information is completed so the claim can be processed by the carrier. As mentioned, a claim without mistakes or missing information is referred to as a clean claim. If needed information is missing from a claim (referred to as a dirty claim), the carrier will not process it, resulting in the added time and expense needed to correct the claim and resend it. Before sending claims electronically, the medical office specialist must look over the claims on the computer screen to make sure they are clean. Being familiar with the locators will assist in this process.

Practice Exercises

The following exercises will familiarize the medical office specialist with the form locators and the information required on the claim forms. By completing claims by hand, the medical office specialist can get a feel for the information that is required on claim forms. Start with the CMS-1500 form in Practice Exercise 10.1.

NOTE: These practice exercises are date sensitive to the date on which the patient presented, which for the student is today's date. Please read the case studies in the exercises and enter the applicable dates. For instance, if the patient was told to return to the office in 3 days, the student would enter a date that is 3 days from today's date, which is the initial date of service.

Practice Exercise 10.1

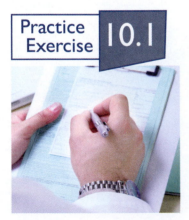

Completion of CMS-1500 (Section I)

Fill out form locators 1 through 13 on the CMS-1500 form based on the information given here. To complete this exercise, copy the CMS-1500 form provided in Appendix D or download the form from MyHealthProfessionsKit or MyHealthProfessionsLab, which accompany this text.

Michael Louis Putnam is a patient in the medical office where you work. This information appears on his patient information form:

Name:	Michael Louis Putnam
Gender:	Male
Birth Date:	May 23, 1945
Phone:	559-555-2233

Address:	765 South Parker
	Fresno, CA 12345
Marital Status:	Single
Employer:	Big Lots
Insurance Carrier:	C 16 NA
Insurance I.D. Number:	459-12-5555
Group Number:	FMR1235
Other Health Insurance:	None

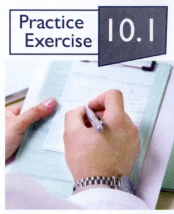

Practice Exercise 10.1

Mr. Putnam has signed an authorization form to release medical records and an assignment of benefits on February 10, 2016. The patient encounter form indicates diagnoses of essential hypertension: ICD-10 (I10). The diagnosis is not related to the patient's previous employment or an accident.

(*Continued*)

Your Practice Exercise 10.1 claim form should look like the one shown in Figure 10.11.

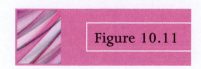

Figure 10.11 Practice Exercise 10.1 CMS-1500 form.

Now complete Practice Exercises 10.2, 10.3, 10.4, 10.5, 10.6, 10.7, 10.8, 10.9, and 10.10.

Practice Exercise 10.2

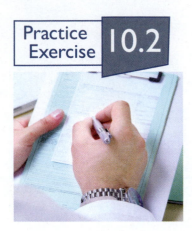

Completion of CMS-1500 (Section I)

Fill out form locators 1 through 13 on the CMS-1500 form based on the information given here. To complete this exercise, copy the CMS-1500 form provided in Appendix D or download the form from MyHealthProfessionsKit or MyHealthProfessionsLab, which accompany this text.

Liz Mary Smith is a patient in the medical office where you work. This information appears on her patient information form:

Name:	Liz Mary Smith
Gender:	Female
Birth Date:	July 1, 1996
Marital Status:	Single
Phone:	480-555-2984
Address:	4591 Explorer Drive
	Phoenix, AZ 12345
Responsible Person:	Harry L. Smith (father)
Insured's DOB:	August 5, 1950
Insured's Gender:	Male
Insured's Home Address:	5419 W. 8th Street, Apt. 306
	Norman, OK 12345
Insured's Employer Address:	Vines Lumber Co.
	6840 Judy Street
	Norman, OK 12345
Insurance Carrier:	BMA
	P.O. Box 7459
	Memphis, TN 12345
Insurance Certificate Number:	78815-080-07-000
Insurance Group Number:	G123456

Treatment and progress notes in the patient medical record indicate diagnosis of left acute otitis media ICD-10 (H66.92), on January 13, 20XX. The medical office collects only the coinsurance and waits for payment directly from the insurance carrier. Guarantor's signature on file for charges to be paid directly to provider, FORM SIGNED January 13, 20XX.

Authorization to release medical information on file.

Completion of CMS-1500 (Section II)

Practice Exercise 10.3

Fill out form locators 14 through 33 on the CMS-1500 form based on the information given here. To complete this exercise, copy the CMS-1500 form provided in Appendix D or download the form from MyHealthProfessionsKit or MyHealthProfessionsLab, which accompany this text.

Physician Information:

Name:	Forrest M. Sherwood, M.D.
	325 Nichols Road, Suite 20B
	Brookfield, Wisconsin 12345
Phone:	414-555-6790
Federal Tax I.D. Number:	52-9753211
NPI:	1226449762

Patient Encounter Form:

Name:	Daniel M. Williams
Date:	Today's date
	T-101 P-90 R-18 BP-132/76 WT-175
CC:	Swollen neck glands, fever, headache, general malaise since yesterday
DX:	Peritonsillar Cellulitis, ICD-10 (J36)
RX:	Rest, fluids, Tylenol for headaches prn. Return in 5 days for recheck.
Date:	Today's date (5 days after initial visit)
	T-98 P-88 R-18 BP-130/60
CC:	Fever, pain, and swelling of tonsils and adenoids
DX:	Hypertrophy of Tonsils and Adenoids, ICD-10 (J35.3)
RX:	#16 Ampicillin 500 mg IM. Return in 2 days
Date:	Today's date (2 days after last visit)
	T-98.8 P-80 R-16 BP-132/74
RX:	Recheck, improvement, continue meds, recheck in 2 weeks.

List of Fees for Services:

Date:	Today's date
DX:	Peritonsillar Cellulitis, ICD-10 (J36)
Services and Charges:	Office visit, expanded problem-focused history & exam, medical decision making of low complexity, $60, CPT (99213)
Date:	Today's date (5 days after initial visit)
DX:	Hypertrophy of Tonsils and Adenoids, ICD-10 (J35.3)

(Continued)

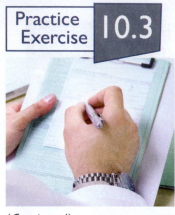

Practice Exercise 10.3

(Continued)

Services and Charges:	Office visit, problem-focused history and exam, straightforward decision making. $35, CPT CODE: 99212 IM Ampicillin 500 mg $20.00, CPT CODE: 96372
Date:	Today's date (2 days after previous visit)
DX:	Hypertrophy of Tonsils and Adenoids, ICD-10 (J35.3)
Services and Charges:	Office visit, problem-focused history and exam, straightforward decision making. $35, CPT CODE: 99212

Patient Ledger:

Insurance Carrier:	United Healthcare
Filing Date:	Today's date
Provider accepts assignment.	

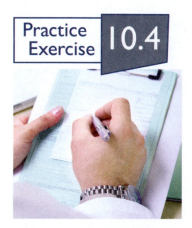

Practice Exercise 10.4

Completion of CMS-1500 (Section II)

Fill out form locators 14 through 33 on the CMS-1500 form based on the information given here. To complete this exercise, copy the CMS-1500 form provided in Appendix D or download the form from MyHealthProfessionsKit or MyHealthProfessionsLab, which accompany this text.

Physician Information:

Name:	Forrest M. Sherwood, M.D.
Address:	325 Nichols Road, Suite 20B Brookfield, WI 12345
Phone:	414-555-6790
Federal Tax I.D. Number:	52-9753211
NPI:	1226449762

Patient Encounter Form:

Name:	Martha M. Butler
Date:	Today's date T-98.8 P-68 R-15 BP-178/98 WT 155
CC:	This a.m. while going to get mail pt fell on sidewalk; a neighbor brought her in c/o pain and disability in left hip area, SOB, chest pain
EXAM:	Pt in distress, X-ray L hip two views—negative, ECG T-wave inversion

LAB:	Cardiac enzymes, electrolytes
DX:	Sprained L Hip, Essential Hypertension, R/O Angina Pectoris
RX:	Injection 2 mL Norflex IM, moist heat, Norflex tablets #12, Inderal capsules 80 mg #30
	Return in 3 days for lab results and recheck
Date:	Today's date (3 days after initial visit) T-98.6 P-68 R-15 BP-150/88
LAB:	Within normal limits
EXAM:	Hip improving, ECG negative
DX:	Essential Hypertension, Angina Pectoris
RX:	Continued prescribed meds. Nitrostat tablets, one tab dissolved under tongue at first sign of angina attack.

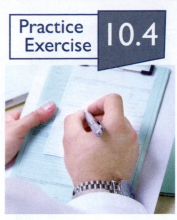

Practice Exercise 10.4

(*Continued*)

List of Fees for Services:

Date:	Today's date
DX:	Sprained L Hip, ICD-10 (S73.102A); Essential Hypertension, ICD-10 (I10)
Services and Charges:	Office visit, detailed history and detailed exam, moderate-complexity decision making $80 (99214); DX: ICD-10 (S73.102A), ICD-10 (I10)
	Venipuncture for collections $18 (36415); DX: ICD-10 (I10)
	Lab (sent to Nottingham Laboratory Services,1435 N. 12th St., Milwaukee, WI 53002).
	X-ray L hip two views $90 (73510); ICD-10 (S73.102A)
	Injection 2 mL Norflex IM $12.00 (96372); DX: ICD-10 (S73.102A)
	ECG routine, 12 leads interpretation & report $55 (93000); DX: ICD-10 (I10)
Date:	Today's date (3 days after initial visit)
DX:	Essential Hypertension, ICD-10 (I10); Angina Pectoris, ICD-10 (I20.9)
Services and Charges:	Office visit, problem-focused history & exam, straightforward decision making $35 (99212)

Patient Ledger:

Patient's Account Number:	BUTMA0 (Date: Today's Date $55)
Insurance Carrier:	US Life
Filing Date:	Today's date

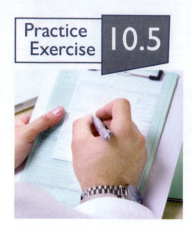

Practice Exercise 10.5

Completion of CMS-1500 (Section II)

Fill out form locators 14 through 33 on the CMS-1500 form based on the information given here. To complete this exercise, copy the CMS-1500 form provided in Appendix D or download the form from MyHealthProfessionsKit or MyHealthProfessionsLab, which accompany this text.

Physician Information:

Name:	Forrest M. Sherwood, M.D.
Address:	325 Nichols Road, Suite 20B
	Brookfield, WI 12345
Phone:	414-555-6790
EIN:	52-9753211
Insurance Carrier:	Cigna
Cigna PIN:	17FMs53
NPI:	1226449762

Patient Encounter Form:

Name:	Audrey Janell Smith
Account Number:	SMIAU
DOB:	2/8/1961
Date:	Today's date
	T-98 P-85 R-15 BP-150/96 WT-164 HT-73
CC:	Patient came in for CPX (complete physical exam) ICD-10 (Z00.00)
HEENT:	Within normal limits
Chest:	Normal
Back:	Normal
Breast:	Normal
Heart:	Normal
Abdomen:	Normal
Pelvic:	Normal
Chest:	X-ray: 2 views—normal
ECG:	Normal
UA Complete-Dip:	Normal
UA-Micro:	Normal
DX:	High Blood Pressure, ICD-10 (R03.0)
RX:	Return tomorrow for recheck on BP
Date:	Today's date (1 day after initial visit)
BP Check:	148/94
Date:	Today's date (1 week after initial visit)
BP:	152/96, reviewed with patient results of exam.
DX:	Essential Hypertension, ICD-10 (I10)
RX:	Maxzide 25 mg one tablet daily, return for recheck in one week

List of Fees for Services:

Date: Today's date

DX: Annual Physical Exam, ICD-10 (Z00.00); High Blood Pressure, ICD-10 (R03.0)

Service and Charges: Initial Preventive Medicine, New Patient: $125, CPT (99386); DX: ICD-10 (Z00.00)

X-ray Chest, 2 Views: $45, CPT (71020); DX: ICD-10 (Z00.00), ICD-10 (R03.0)

ECG routine, 12 lead: $55, CPT (93000); DX: ICD-10 (Z00.00), ICD-10 (R03.0)

Complete UA, $15, CPT (81000); DX: ICD-10 (Z00.00)

Date: Today's date (1 day after initial visit)

DX: High Blood Pressure, ICD-10 (R03.0)

Service and Charges: Follow-up office visit—problem-focused history and exam, straightforward decision making, $35, CPT (99212); DX: ICD-10 (R03.0)

Date: Today's date (1 week after initial visit)

DX: Essential Hypertension, CD-10 (I10)

Services and Charges: Expanded problem-focused history and examination (reviewed results of physical examination), medical decision making of low complexity, $60, CPT (99213); DX: ICD-10 (I10)

Patient Ledger:

Insurance Carrier: Cigna

Date: Today's date, $240

Date: 1 day after initial visit, $35

Date: 1 week after initial visit, $60

Filing Date: 1 week after initial visit

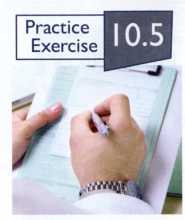

Practice Exercise 10.5

(Continued)

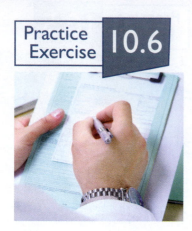

Practice Exercise 10.6

Completion of CMS-1500 (Sections I and II)

Fill out the form locators on the CMS-1500 form based on the information given here. To complete this exercise, copy the CMS-1500 form provided in Appendix D or download the form from MyHealthProfessionsKit or MyHealthProfessionsLab, which accompany this text.

Physician Information:

Name:	Len M. Handelsman, M.D.
Address:	325 Nepperhan Avenue Yonkers, NY 12345
Phone:	914-555-6790
Federal Tax I.D. Number:	52-9683211
Insurance Carrier:	Aetna
Aetna Pin Number:	56991
NPI:	3335224814

Patient Information Form:

Name:	Gloria Poyner-Chin
Gender:	Female
DOB:	July 1, 1945
Marital Status:	Single
Account Number:	POYNEGL0
Address:	1221 Avenue of the Bronx Bronx, NY 12345
Phone Number:	(914) 555-2166
Insured's Employer:	Country Club Bingo Hall
Insurance Carrier:	Aetna
Insurance Carrier Address:	1900 Seventh Avenue New York, NY 12100
Insurance Certificate Number:	445-80-0701
Insurance Group Number:	G020456

Patient Encounter Form:

Date:	Today's date T-99 P-90 R-18 BP-132/76 WT-125
CC:	Pain in elbow and forearms following tennis game, 11-12-15
DX:	Elbow Sprain, ICD-10 (S53.409A)
RX:	Rest

List of Fees for Services:

Date:	Today's date
DX:	Elbow Sprainl; CD-10 (S53.409A)
Services and Charges:	Office visit, problem-focused history and exam, straightforward decision making, $35, CPT (99212)
Signature on File:	Signed today's date

Completion of CMS-1500 (Sections I and II)

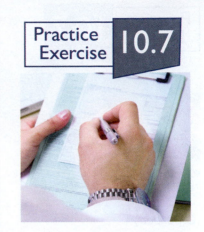

Fill out the form locators on the CMS-1500 form based on the information given here. To complete this exercise, copy the CMS-1500 form provided in Appendix D or download the form from MyHealthProfessionsKit or My-HealthProfessionsLab, which accompany this text.

Physician Information:

Name:	William F. Bonner, M.D.
Corporation Name:	Youngblood and Associates
Address:	2128 East 144th Street, Suite 15
	Chicago, IL 12345
Phone:	312-555-7690
EIN:	56-3342560
NPI:	5524998733
CIGNA Physician I.D. Number:	3266113
Cigna Group Number:	0655872
Group NPI:	6625897130

Patient Information Form:

Name:	Randall Jay Tillman
DOB:	February 19, 1989
Gender:	Male
Marital Status:	Single
Patient Address:	1212 Fry Street
	Des Plaines, IL 12345
	312-555-4993
Account Number:	TILLRA
Responsible Party:	Theresa Mae Tillman (mother)
Insured's DOB:	January 3, 1958
Insured's Gender:	Female
Address:	4225 Benton Avenue, Apt. 6
	Des Plaines, IL 12345
Phone:	312-555-4993
Insured's Employer:	Des Plaines Chevrolet
Insurance Carrier:	Cigna
Insurance Carrier Address:	P.O. Box 3490
	Chicago, IL 60671
Insurance I.D. Number:	753-00865
Insurance Group Number:	DP 139
Signature on File:	Yes, form signed

Patient Encounter Form:

Date:	Today's date
Date of First Symptom:	3 days ago
	WT-45 HT-50 T-100.4 P-94 R-20
	BP- 90/60
CC:	Wheezing, coughing, dyspnea, fever 3 d

(Continued)

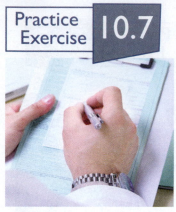

Practice Exercise 10.7

(Continued)

DX:	Bronchitis with Influenza, ICD-10 (J11.1)
RX:	EryPed 200 1 tsp Q.I.D., Tussi-Organidan 1 tsp in AM and 1 tsp at night Return 3 days for recheck

List of Fees for Services:

Date:	Today's date
DX:	Bronchitis with Influenza, ICD-10 (J11.1)
Services and Charges:	Office visit, problem-focused history and exam, straightforward decision making, $50, CPT (99202); DX: ICD-10 (J11.1)
Filing Date:	Today's date

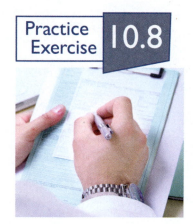

Practice Exercise 10.8

Completion of CMS-1500 (Sections I and II)

Fill out the form locators on the CMS-1500 form based on the information given here. To complete this exercise, copy the CMS-1500 form provided in Appendix D or download the form from MyHealthProfessionsKit or MyHealthProfessionsLab, which accompany this text.

Physician Information:

Name:	Mary Ann Brock, M.D.
Corporation Name:	PCL Medical Associates
Address:	1720 Front Street Philadelphia, PA 12345
Phone:	215-555-3000
Employer I.D. Number:	51-4290642
BS Pin Number:	49-5529-78
Group Number:	BS 0862
NPI:	9998755667
Group NPI:	6666455522

Patient Information Form:

Name:	Amy Louise Lynch
Address:	893 Bay Street Philadelphia, PA 12345
Phone:	215-555-0081
DOB:	January 9, 1999
Student Status:	Full-time Student

Gender:	Female
Marital Status:	Single
Account Number:	LYNAM
Responsible Party:	Fred K. Lynch (father)
Insured's DOB:	June 15, 1947
Insured's Gender:	Male
Insured's Address:	1776 Liberty Road
	Philadelphia, PA 12345
Insured's Phone:	215-555-0704
Insured's Employer:	WDAF Radio
Insurance Carrier:	Blue Cross Blue Shield of Pennsylvania
Insurance Carrier Address:	P.O. Box 7476
	Philadelphia, PA 19174
Insurance I.D. Number:	512-53-9751
Insurance Group Number:	W45980
Signature on File:	Yes, today's date
Insured:	Jessie M. Lynch (mother)
DOB:	August 5, 1950
Gender:	Female
Employer:	Southerland Lumber
Insurance Carrier:	Kindness Healthcare
Insurance Carrier Address:	414 East Franklin Road
	Philadelphia, PA 12345
Insurance I.D. Number:	491-51-0003A
Insurance Group Number:	7989

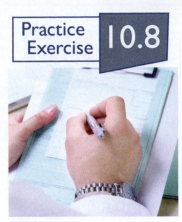

Practice Exercise 10.8

(Continued)

Patient Encounter Form:

Date:	Today's date
Vital Signs:	T-104 P-115 R-25
CC:	Fever, pain in left ear, sensitive to touch, L ear red, tympanic membrane retracted
DX:	Acute Otitis Media, Left Ear, ICD-10 (H66.002)
RX:	Amoxil pediatric suspension 30 mL bottle, 2.5 mL q 8 hrs
	Return 3 days for recheck

List of Fees for Services:

Date:	Today's date
DX:	Acute Otitis Media, ICD-10 (H66.002)
Services and Charges:	Office visit, problem-focused history and exam, straightforward decision making, $40, CPT (99212); DX: ICD-10 (H66.002)
Physician Accepts Assignment—Filing Date:	Tomorrow's Date

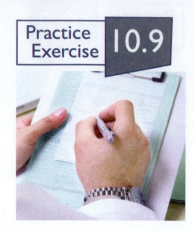

Practice Exercise 10.9

Completion of CMS-1500 (Sections I and II)

Fill out the form locators on the CMS-1500 form based on the information given here. To complete this exercise, copy the CMS-1500 form provided in Appendix D or download the form from MyHealthProfessionsKit or MyHealthProfessionsLab, which accompany this text.

Physician Information:

Name:	Paul Erickson, M.D.
Corporation Name:	Family Medicine, P.C.
Address:	2500 East Avenue, Olathe, KS 12345
	Phone: 913-555-2700
Employer I.D. Number:	53-1919011
Primary Health I.D. Number:	90-ERICKSO-993
Cigna PPO I.D. Number:	04-5657
Cigna Group Number:	567203
NPI:	4531118907
Group NPI:	7221160934

Laboratory Information:

Name:	Johnson County Lab Services
Address:	15107 South Locust
	Olathe, KS 12345
Provider I.D. Number:	528761
NPI:	0325644443
Independent Laboratory:	Johnson County Laboratory Services

Patient Information Form:

Name:	Veronica Lee Bowman
DOB:	June 7, 1961
Gender:	Female
Marital Status:	Single
Account Number:	BOWVE1
Responsible Party:	Self
Address:	25 Elm Street
	Gardner, KS 12345
Phone:	913-555-7779
Employer:	Frito Lay
Insurance Carrier:	Cigna
Insurance Carrier Address:	P.O. Box 16139
	Topeka, KS 12345
Insurance I.D. Number:	26-30254
Insurance Group Number:	FR 2856
Signature on File:	Yes

Patient Encounter Form:

Date:	Today's date
	T-99 P-80 R-16 BP-132/78

CC:	Fever, cough, rhinorrhea X 2 days
DX:	Upper Respiratory Infection, ICD-10 (J06.9)
RX:	Actifed with codeine, Amoxil capsule 500 mg #16 one cap q 8 hrs Return in 2 days for recheck
Date:	Today's date (2 days after initial visit)
Vital Signs:	T-99 P-86 R-18 BP-130/80
CC:	Pt still complains of fever, coughing with sputum, chills, chest pain Auscultation revealed rales Chest X-ray, two views, frontal and lateral, revealed consolidation
Lab:	Sputum culture STAT, WBC 13,000 (Sent to Johnson County Laboratory Services)
DX:	Pneumonia, ICD-10 (J18.9)
RX:	Continue meds, bed rest, fluids, return next day
Date:	Today's date (3 days after initial visit) Sputum culture revealed mycoplasma pneumonia
DX:	Mycoplasma Pneumonia, ICD-10 (J15.7)
RX:	Discontinue previous meds; erythromycin capsules #24 mg one cap, 1 hr before meals q 6 hrs Return 2 days

List of Fees for Services:

Date:	Today's date
DX:	Upper Respiratory Infection, ICD-10 (J06.9)
Services and Charges:	Office visit, problem-focused history and examination, straightforward decision making, $60, CPT (99212); DX: ICD-10 (J06.9)
Date:	Today's date (2 days after initial visit)
DX:	Pneumonia, ICD-10 (B99.9)
Services and Charges:	Office visit, detailed history and examination, moderately complex decision making, $100, CPT (99214); DX: ICD-10 (B18.9) X-ray, chest single view, 2 views, $45 each, CPT (71010); DX: ICD-10 (B18.9) Sputum culture $18, lab fee charge $12, CPT (87015); DX: ICD-10 (B18.9) WBC test $17, lab fee charge $10, CPT (85025); DX: ICD-10 (B18.9)

(Continued)

(Continued)

Practice Exercise 10.9

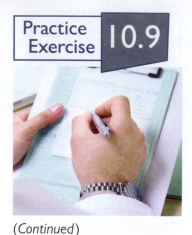

Date:	Today's date (3 days after initial visit)
DX:	Mycoplasma Pneumonia, ICD-10 (J15.7)
Services and Charges:	Office visit, expanded problem-focused history and examination, low-complexity medical decision making, $75, CPT (99213); DX: ICD-10 (J15.7)

Physician Accepts Assignment

(Continued)

Practice Exercise 10.10

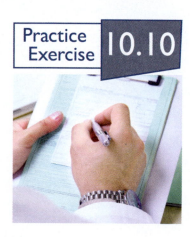

Completion of CMS-1500 (Sections I and II)

Fill out the form locators on the CMS-1500 form based on the information given here. To complete this exercise, copy the CMS-1500 form provided in Appendix D or download the form from MyHealthProfessionsKit or MyHealthProfessionsLab, which accompany this text.

Physician Information:

Name:	Tina Harris, M.D.
Address:	16670 West 95 Terrace
	Overland Park, KS 12345
Phone:	913-555-9706
Employer I.D. Number:	55-1530016
NPI:	8954433148
Referring Physician:	Charles Henderson, M.D.
Referring Doctor NPI:	0815094410

Patient Information Form:

Name:	Kathy Ann Black
Gender:	Female
DOB:	January 20, 1949
Marital Status:	Married
Account Number:	BLAKA
Address:	79 North West Terrace
	Kansas City, KS 12345
Phone:	913-555-1560
Responsible Party:	Jason Darnell Black (husband)
Insured's DOB:	April 1, 1945
Insured's Address:	Same
Insured's Employer:	EDS
Insurance Carrier:	Fortis Insurance Company

Precertification Number: 52521212
I.D. Number: 60923
Group Number: 2222
Signature on File: Yes, form signed 09/15/20XX

Patient Encounter Form:

Date: Today's date
Date of Current Illness: 3 days ago
Vital Signs: T-98.6 P-70 R-16 BP-180/92
CC: Patient has felt lumps in both breasts
Breasts: Masses felt in both R and L breast, breast biopsy bilateral STAT
DX: Breast Mass Bilateral, ICD-10-CM (N63, N63); High Blood Pressure, ICD-10 (I10)
RX: Aldomet tablets 250 mg #100, one tab T.I.D. for first 48 hours
Return tomorrow for BP check and results of biopsy
Date: Today's date (1 day after initial visit)
BP-176/92
Biopsy reveals breast carcinoma
DX: ICD-10 (C50.911, C50.912)
(NOTE: 3 days Pt. admitted to Metropolitan Medical Center, NPI 0066677889, 153 Slater Road, Leawood, KS 66206 for mastectomy bilateral.)
Date: Today's date (3 days after previous visit)
Initial Hospital Admission
Date: Today's date (1 day after admission)
Bilateral Radical Mastectomy performed, no complication.
Date: Today's date (3 days after mastectomy)
Hospital discharge exam. Pt. is to return to office in 1 week for follow-up exam and BP check.

List of Fees for Services:

Date: Today's date
DX: Breast Mass ICD-10 (N63). Elevated Blood Pressure; ICD-10 ((R03.0)
Services and Charges: New patient office visit, expanded history and examination, straightforward decision making, $150, CPT (99204); DX: ICD-10 ((R03.0); ICD-10 (N63).
Breast biopsy (bilateral), $350, CPT (19100-50); DX: ICD-10 ((R03.0); ICD-10 (N63).

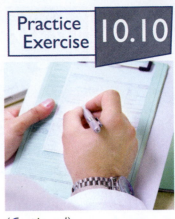

Practice Exercise 10.10

(Continued)

(Continued)

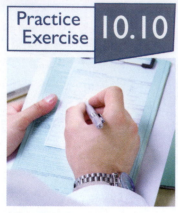

Practice Exercise 10.10

(*Continued*)

Date:	Today's date (1 day after initial visit)
DX:	Breast Carcinoma, Essential Hypertension, ICD-10 (C50.911, C50.912) and ICD-10 (I10).
Services and Charges:	Office visit, problem focused, $40, CPT (99214); DX: ICD-10 (C50.911, C50.912) and ICD-10 (I10).
Date:	Today's date (3 days after previous visit)
DX:	Breast Carcinoma ICD-10 (C50.911, C50.912), Essential Hypertension ICD-10 (I10).
Services and Charges:	Initial Hospital Care, $150, CPT (99221);
DX:	ICD-10 (C50.911, C50.912) and ICD-10 (I10).
Date:	Today's date (1 day after admission)
DX:	Breast Carcinoma, Essential Hypertension, ICD-10 (C50.911, C50.912) and ICD-10 (I10).
Services and Charges:	Bilateral Mastectomy Radical including pectoral muscles, axillary lymph nodes, $3,700, CPT (19305-50);
DX:	ICD-10 (C50.911, C50.912) and ICD-10 (I10).
Date:	Today's date (3 days after mastectomy)
DX:	Breast Carcinoma, Essential Hypertension, ICD-10 (C50.911, C50.912) and ICD-10 (I10).
Services and Charges:	Hospital discharge, day management, $50, CPT (99238); DX: ICD-10 (C50.911, C50.912) and ICD-10 (I10).
Claim Filed:	3 days after discharge with operative report

Common Reasons for Delayed or Rejected CMS-1500 Claim Forms

The medical office specialist should be aware of common billing errors and how to correct them for quicker claims settlements and to reduce the number of appeals. This may help avoid additional administrative burdens, such as making telephone calls, resubmitting claims, and writing appeal letters. Figure 10.12 presents a list of some reasons why claims are rejected or delayed and suggested solutions when completing the CMS-1500 insurance claim form locators.

Problem: Form locator 1. Claim submitted to the secondary insurer instead of the primary insurer.

Solution: Verify with the patient the two carriers and determine which is the primary carrier, either by using the birthday rule, the effective date of coverage, or depending on the illness, injury, or accident during the initial office visit. The birthday rule states that the parent whose day of birth is earlier in the calendar year will be considered the primary insurer. Submit the claim to the primary carrier and then after being paid or denied by the primary carrier submit a claim with the EOB/ERA form to the secondary carrier.

Problem: Form locators 1–13. Information missing on patient portion of the claim form.

Solution: Obtain a complete registration from which information can be extracted. Educate patients on data requirements at the time of the first visit to the physician's office as patients fill out their portion of the form. Review the patient's information before having the patient seen by the physician. If information is missing, ask the patient to provide or verify the missing information.

Problem: Form locator 1a. Patient's insurance number is incorrect or transposed (especially in Medicare and Medicaid cases).

Solution: Proofread numbers carefully from source documents. Always photocopy front and back of insurance identification card.

Problem: Form locator 2. Patient's name and insured's name are entered as the same when the patient is a dependent.

Solution: Verify the insured party and check for Sr., Jr., and correct date of birth.

Problem: Form locator 3. Incorrect gender identification, resulting in a diagnosis or procedure code that is inconsistent with patient's gender.

Solution: Proofread claim before submitting and review patient's medical record to locate gender, especially if the patient's first name could be male or female.

Problem: Form locators 9a and d. Incomplete entry for other insurance coverage.

Solution: Accurately abstract data from the patient's registration form. Telephone the patient if information is incomplete.

Problem: Form locator 10. Failure to indicate whether patient's condition is related to employment or an "other" type of accident.

Solution: Review patient's medical history to find details of injury or illness and proofread claim before mailing. Telephone the employer and verify the injury has been reported as a workers' compensation injury and the employer has workers' compensation insurance.

Problem: Form locator 12 and 13. Patient's signature is missing.

Solution: Always make sure the signature form locators are completed with "Signature on File" or "SOF" except in government (participating physician) or workers' compensation claims. Verify that the signature is on file in the medical record.

Figure 10.12

Suggested solutions to problems that may arise when completing the CMS-1500 form.

(Continued)

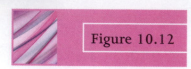

Figure 10.12

(Continued)

Problem: Form locator 14. Date of injury, date of last menstrual period (LMP), or dates of onset of illness are missing. This information is important for determining whether accident benefits apply, patient is eligible for maternity benefits, or there was a preexisting condition.

Solution: Do not list unless dates are clearly documented in the patient's medical record. Read the patient's medical history and call the patient to obtain the date of accident or LMP. Compose an addendum to the record, if necessary. Always proofread the claim before mailing.

Problem: Form locators 17, 17a, and 17b. Incorrect or missing name and/or PIN/NPI numbers of referring physician on claim for consultation or other services requiring this information. The referring physician may also be the ordering physician.

Solution: Check the patient registration form and the chart note for reference to the referring physician. Obtain a list of PIN/NPI numbers for all physicians in the area. Enter the provider's (ordering) name and NPI if there is no referring physician.

Problem: Form locator 19. Refer to the most current instructions from the applicable public or private payer regarding the use of this field.

Solution: Contact the carrier and inquire what information they require. Locator 19 is generally left blank; however, some carriers do require information inserted.

Problem: Form locator 21. The diagnostic code is missing, incomplete, invalid, not coded to the highest level of specificity, certainty (e.g., fourth or fifth digit is missing), or the diagnosis code does not match the CPT code.

Solution: Update encounter forms annually when the addendum comes out in October of each year. Conduct a chart audit every 6 months. Check with physician to verify the diagnosis code that belongs with the CPT code.

Problem: Form locator 22: The Medicaid resubmission number is missing.

Solution: List the original reference number for resubmitted claims and the resubmission code for Medicaid.

Problem: Form locator 23: Prior authorization number missing.

Solution: Enter any of the following: prior authorization number, referral number, mammography precertification number, or CLIA number as assigned by the payer.

Problem: Form locator 24A. Omitted, incorrect, overlapping, or duplicate dates of service.

Solution: Verify against the encounter form or medical record that all dates of services are listed and accurate and appear on individual lines. Date spans for multiple services must be adequate for the number and types of services provided.

Problem: Form locator 24B. Missing or incorrect place of service.

Solution: Verify the place of service from the encounter form or medical record and list the correct code for place of service and submitted procedure.

Problem: Form locator 24C: EMG: Was visit an emergency?—Yes or no.

Solution: NEW: Enter "Y" for YES if emergency; leave blank if not.

Problem: Form locator 24D. Procedure codes are incorrect, invalid, or missing.

Solution: Verify the coding system used by the insurance company and submit correct procedure code(s) by referring to a current CPT book. For Medicare patients and certain private payers, check the HCPCS manual for CMS national and local procedure codes.

Problem: Form locator 24D. Missing or incorrect modifiers.

Solution: Verify the need for modifiers. Submit correct modifiers using a current CPT book or HCPCS.

Problem: Form locator 24E: Diagnosis pointer does not match the CPT.

Solution: Check that the diagnosis pointer refers to the line number in form locator 21 and relates to the reason the service was performed.

Problem: Form locator 24F. Omitted or incorrect amount billed.

Solution: Be certain the fee column is filled in. Check the amounts charged as the UCR, MFS, or workers' compensation fee.

Problem: Form locator 24G. Days do not match dates of service (From and To; e.g., hospital visits); units of time are incorrectly billed (e.g., 1 unit may equal 15 minutes).

Solution: Depending on the error, check the documentation from the encounter form or chart and correct. Check to make sure the third-party payer accepts the units of time, etc.

Problem: Form locator 24I. Provider's NPI is missing.

Solution: Verify the physician's NPI and insert the number in this block if it is different from form locators 33a and 33b.

Problem: Form locator 24J. The number of the individual rendering the service is missing.

Solution: Enter the non–NPI number in the shaded area of the field. Enter the NPI number in the unshaded area of the field.

Problem: Form locator 25. The federal tax ID number is missing.

Solution: Enter the physician's EIN number. Do not use the Social Security number.

Problem: Form locator 27. Accept Assignment not checked.

Solution: Make sure that this box is checked YES. If not, the money will go to the patient.

Problem: Form locator 28. Total amounts do not equal itemized charges.

Solution: Total the charges for each claim and verify amounts with the patients' account. If the number of units in 24G is more than 1, multiply the units by the fee listed in 24F and add to all other charges listed.

Figure 10.12

(*Continued*)

(*Continued*)

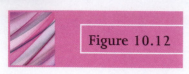

Figure 10.12

(Continued)

Problem: Form locator 31. Physician's signature is missing.

Solution: Have the physician or physician's representative sign the claim form or use an ink stamp with the physician's signature on it.

Problem: Form locator 32. No place of service is recorded.

Solution: Enter the place of service where the procedure was performed, for example, office, hospital, or laboratory.

Problem: Form locator 32a. Missing NPI number.

Solution: Enter the NPI number of the service facility location listed in form locator 32a.

Problem: Form locator 32b. Missing other ID number.

Solution: Enter the two–digit qualifier identifying the non–NPI number followed by the ID number.

Problem: Form locator 33. Provider's billing name, address, or phone number is missing.

Solution: Enter the provider's or supplier's billing name, address, zip code, and phone number. The phone number is to be entered in the area to the right of the field title.

Problem: Form locator 33a. Missing NPI number.

Solution: Enter the NPI number of the billing provider in 33a.

HIPAA Compliance Alert

With the advent of HIPAA, a number of federal laws now apply to insurance claims submissions. HIPAA security standard rules were adopted to safeguard and protect the confidentiality, integrity, and availability of electronic health information. The rules were needed because no standard measures existed in the healthcare industry that addressed all aspects of the security of electronic health information while it is in use, being stored, or exchanged among entities. HIPAA mandated security standards to protect an individual's health information, while permitting the appropriate access and use of that information by healthcare providers, clearinghouses, and health plans without evidence of fraud or abuse issues.

To authorize the release of information, a patient must sign either form locator 12 on the CMS-1500 form or a consent document with similar wording to be retained in the office files. Often the release of information is incorporated into the new patient information form.

Filing Secondary Claims

A patient may have coverage under more than one health insurance plan; additional insurance policies are referred to as **secondary insurance**. For example, a person may have primary insurance through his employer and also be covered under his spouse's insurance, making that his secondary insurance.

Supplemental insurance is an insurance plan that covers part of a patient's expenses, such as coinsurance, for which the policyholder is otherwise responsible. Supplemental insurance is exactly what it sounds like: It supplements the primary insurance. If the primary policy does not cover a service, supplemental insurance does not cover it either. Supplemental insurance is generally limited to Medigap policies. Medigap policies are insurance policies that supplement Medicare payments.

Finding out which policy will be the primary one is important because insurance policies contain a provision called **coordination of benefits (COB)**. The concept of coordination of benefits was originally developed by Blue Cross Blue Shield to prevent overpayment on a claim. If the secondary plan did not know what the primary plan had paid, the amount paid by the two plans could exceed the provider's charge. The COB rule states that when a patient is covered by more than one policy, benefits paid by all policies are limited to 100% of the charge. This clause prevents people from having a number of plans and making a profit by collecting from each one. With coordination of benefits, insurance carriers exchange information with each other regarding payments and payment denials.

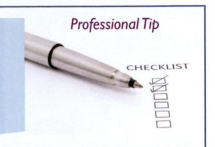

Professional Tip

The difference between supplemental insurance and secondary insurance is that the secondary insurance policy may cover items that the primary insurance does not cover.

Determining Primary Coverage

Various standards are available for determining primary coverage:

- If the patient only has one policy, it is the primary one.
- If the patient has coverage under two plans under which she is the primary policyholder, the plan that has been in effect for the patient for the longest period of time is the primary one. However, if the patient is an active employee of a company and has a plan with her present employer but is still covered by a former employer's plan (as would be the case with, say, a retiree or laid-off employee), the current employer's plan is the primary plan.
- If the patient is covered as a dependent under another insurance policy, such as a spouse's policy, the patient's plan is the primary plan.
- If an employed patient has coverage under the employer's plan and additional coverage under a government-sponsored plan, the employer's plan is the primary one. For example, if the patient is enrolled in a PPO through employment and is also on Medicare, the PPO is primary.
- If a retired patient is covered by a spouse's employer's plan, and the spouse is still employed, the spouse's plan is the primary, even if the retired person has Medicare. Medicare is the primary for individuals and family members who are retired and receiving coverage under a group policy from a previous employer.
- If the patient is a dependent child covered by both parents' plans, and the parents are not separated or divorced (or if they have joint custody of the child), the primary plan is determined by which parent's date of birth is earlier in the calendar year (the **birthday rule**).

■ If two or more plans cover dependent children of separated or divorced parents who do not have joint custody of their children, the children's primary plan is determined in this order:

- The plan of the custodial parent
- The plan of the spouse of the custodial parent (if the parent has remarried)
- The plan of the parent without custody

When two insurance policies are involved, one is considered primary and the other is secondary. The patient's signature should always be acquired for release of information and assignment of benefits for both insurance companies. The initial CMS-1500 is submitted with primary and secondary insurance information in form locators 9a–d. Form locator 11d would be answered "yes." After payment is received from the primary payer, a claim form with a copy of the primary carrier's EOB is submitted to the secondary carrier.

Some physician practices and hospitals will automatically file for secondary insurance benefits, whereas others require the patient to do so. When submitting a secondary claim, you must attach a copy of the primary carrier's EOB to the completed CMS-1500 or UB-04. Most secondary claims are not submitted electronically.

It is important to remember that a referral or prior authorization number may still be required even if that insurance carrier provides secondary coverage for the patient. Without the authorization number and primary carrier's EOB, the claim will be denied.

Practice Exercises

The next group of practice exercises is designed to help the reader learn how to complete claim forms when the patient has secondary insurance. Complete the primary CMS-1500 form manually for each exercise. Then complete the EOB. Complete the secondary CMS-1500 manually, adding the payment from the primary EOB. Hand in the secondary claim and EOB to your instructor.

To complete Practice Exercises 10.11, 10.12, 10.13, 10.14, and 10.15 copy the CMS-1500 form provided in Appendix D or download the form from MyHealthProfessionsKit or MyHealthProfessionsLab, which accompany this text.

Practice Exercise 10.11

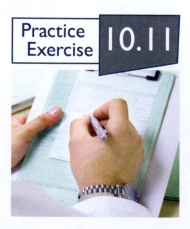

Secondary Claim

Patient Information:

Name:	Barbara Ward
Address:	214 Band Road
	Santa Fe, NM 12345
Phone:	505-555-8943
Gender:	F
DOB:	08/02/56
Marital Status:	M
Employment Status:	Full-time
Employer:	Allied Career Center
Address:	1933 E Frankford Road #110
	Santa Fe, NM 12345
	972-555-3982

Insurance Plan:	Oxford Health
	12030 Plano Parkway
	Plano, VA 43098
	555-800-0302
Insurance I.D./Policy Number:	214689852
Insurance Group Number:	54790012

Other Insured:

Name:	Charles Ward
DOB:	10/09/53
Address:	Same
Relationship:	Spouse
Telephone:	Same
Employer:	Dalmeth Enterprises
Address:	100023 Main Street
	Santa Fe, NM 12345
	214-555-9984
Insurance Plan:	Aetna Health
Address:	PO Box 855
	Irving, TX 75062
	222-889-9751
Insurance I.D./Policy Number:	622648701
Insurance Group Number:	2223389
Provider Information:	James Brown, M.D.
	Phone 555-345-7654
NPI:	5598565422
	1400 Last Street
	Santa Fe, NM 12345
EIN:	16-8749532
Oxford Health Pin:	B0228 Aetna Pin #: AET06
Visit Information:	Barbara Ward

List of Fees for Services:

DOS:	Today's date
DX:	Benign Hypertension, ICD-10 (I10)
	New Patient Expanded Problem
	Focused, 99203, $150

Assignment of benefits on file
Release of information form on file

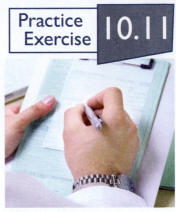

Practice Exercise 10.11

(*Continued*)

For Student Use Only

Payer's Name and Address

Oxford Health
12030 Plano Parkway
Plano, Virginia 43098

Today's Date:
CHECK #287613

Provider's Name and Address

Dr. James Brown
1400 Last Street
Santa Fe, NM 12345

This statement covers payments for the following patient(s):

Claim Detail Section

Patient Name: Ward, Barbara	**Patient Account #:** 0654	
Patient I.D.#: 214689852	**Insured's Name:** Same	**Group #:** 54790012
Provider Name: Dr. Brown	**Inventory #:** 33782	**Claim Control #:** 55502

Service Date(s)	Procedure	Total Billed	Allowed Charges	Contract Adjust	Deduct	Coins	Paid Amt	Total Paid	Remarks
Claim Date	99203	150.00	125.00		00.00		80%		
TOTALS									

BALANCE DUE FROM PATIENT: PT'S DED/NOT COV $_____

PT'S COINSURANCE $_____

PAYMENT SUMMARY SECTION (Totals)

Charges	Adjustment	Allowed	Copay	Deduct/Not Covered	Coins	Total Paid

Secondary Claim

Physician Information:

Name:	Francis J. Boyer, M.D.
	916 E. Frisco Rd.
	Ithaca, NY 12345
	555-888-2233
Employer I.D. Number:	56-3342560
Cigna PIN:	123266
NPI:	5562811442

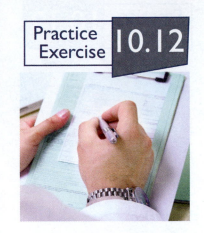

Practice Exercise 10.12

Patient Information Form:

Name:	Jay Wagner (NP)
Date of Birth:	February 19, 1989
Address:	265 First Street
	Ithaca, NY 12345
Phone:	312-555-4993
Gender:	Male
Marital Status:	Single
Responsible Party:	Theresa Wagner (mother)
Address:	Same
Insured's Date of Birth:	January 3, 1958
Insured's Gender:	Female
Phone:	312-555-4993
Insured's Employer:	The Famous Gourmet
	2241 Eatery Avenue
	Ithaca, NY 12345
Insurance Carrier:	Cigna
Insurance Carrier Address:	243 Harrison Avenue
	Hartford, CT 06897
Insurance Phone:	800-678-1212
Insurance I.D./Policy Number:	753-00865
Insurance Group Number:	DP 139
Signature on File:	Yes

Secondary Insurance Information: Father

Name:	Howard Wagner
DOB:	September 21, 1958
Address:	Same as spouse
Phone:	Same as spouse
Employer:	The Print Shop
Address:	6654 Waverly Avenue
	Syracuse, NY 12345
Phone:	555-894-5521

(Continued)

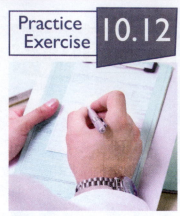

Practice Exercise 10.12

(Continued)

Insurance Carrier:	Allmerica Insurance P.O. Box 123658 Erie, PA 12345
Phone:	215-555-7621
Insurance I.D./Policy Number:	ASD56987
Insurance Group Number:	1256893
Signature on File:	Yes

Patient Encounter Form:

Date:	Today's date
Date of first symptom:	Three days ago
Vital Signs:	WT 45 HT 50 T 100.4 P 94 R 20 BP 90/60
CC:	Wheezing, coughing, dyspnea, fever 3 d.
Auscultation of lungs:	Rales and congestion.
Dx:	Bronchitis, ICD-10 (J40)
Rx:	EryPed 200 1 tsp Q.I.D., Tussi-Organidan 1 tsp in AM and 1 tsp at night, return 3 days for recheck.

List of Fees for Services:

Date:	Today's date
Dx:	Bronchitis, ICD-10 (J40)
Services and Charges:	New Patient Office Visit (99203), $150

Assignment of benefits on file

Release of information form on file

For Student Use Only

Payer's Name and Address

Cigna Health Insurance Company
243 Harrison Avenue
Hartford, CT 06897

Today's Date:
CHECK #8822469

Provider's Name and Address

Francis J. Boyer, M.D.
916 E. Frisco Road
Ithaca, NY 12345

Patient Name: Jay Wagner	**Patient Account #:** WAGJ00	
Patient I.D.#: 753-00865	**Insured's Name:** Theresa Wagner	**Group #:** DP139
Provider: Francis J. Boyer, M.D.	**Inventory #:** 3987540	

Service Date(s)	Procedure	Total Charges	Contract Amount	Copay	Deduct/Not Covered	Coins	Paid Amt	Total Paid	Remarks
Claim Date	99203	150.00	125.00	10.00	0.00	0.00	100%		
TOTALS									

BALANCE DUE FROM PATIENT: PT'S DED/NOT COV $_____

PT'S COINSURANCE $_____

Payment Summary Section (Totals)

Charges	Adjustment	Allowed	Copay	Deduct/Not Covered	Coins	Total Paid

Practice Exercise 10.13

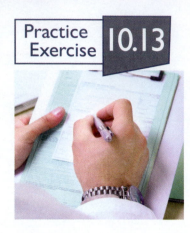

Secondary Claim

Physician Information:

Name:	David Rosenberg, M.D.
Address:	1400 West Center Street
	Toledo, Ohio 12345
Phone:	999-555-2121
Tax I.D. Number:	16-1246791
BCBS Number:	B002
NPI:	5556214735

Patient Information Form:

Name:	Stephanie Gross
	310 Farm Road
	Toledo, Ohio 12345
Phone:	789-555-3641
Insurance Plan:	Blue Cross Blue Shield
	P.O. Box 810
	Columbus, Ohio 44321
Phone:	800-789-1722
I.D. Number:	78235606
Group Number:	ED856
Gender:	F
	Patient's copay is $15.
Birth Date:	08/02/56
Marital Status:	M
Employer:	EDS Company
Employment Address:	2225 Logan Drive
	Toledo, OH 12345
Phone:	800-555-9293
Employment Status:	Full time

Secondary Insurance Information: (Spouse)

Employer:	Stewart's Tuxedos
Address:	1795 Mall Ave
	Toledo, OH. 12345
Phone:	800-555-1234
Husband:	John J. Gross
DOB:	9/4/1953
Phone:	Same
Address:	Same
Insurance Plan:	Cigna
	PO Box 952
	Plano, TX 75022
Phone:	972-380-0880
Policy/I.D. Number:	323542234
Gr Number:	JC7843

Patient Encounter Form:

Date: Today's Date
DX: Upper Respiratory Infection, ICD-10
                          (J06.9)
Service: 99213, $75

Assignment of benefits on file
Release of information form on file

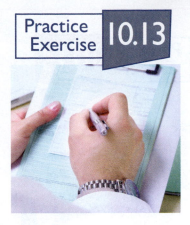

Practice
Exercise **10.13**

(Continued)

For Student Use Only

Payer's Name and Address

| Blue Cross Blue Shield |
| P.O. Box 810 |
| Columbus, Ohio 44321 |

Today's Date:
CHECK #19562

Provider's Name and Address

| David Rosenberg, M.D. |
| 1400 West Center Street |
| Toledo, Ohio 12345 |

This statement covers payments for the following patient(s):

Claim Detail Section

Patient Name: Gross, Stephanie   **Patient Account #:** GROST
Patient I.D. #: 78235606
Provider Name: David Rosenberg, M.D.   **Claim Control #:** 002456

Service Date(s)	Procedure	Charges	Adjustment	Allowed	Copay	Deduct/Not Covered	Coins	Paid Amt.	Total Paid Remarks
Claim Date	99213	75.00	8.75		15.00	0.00	100%		
TOTALS									

BALANCE DUE FROM PATIENT: PT'S DED/NOT COV $_____
                                     PT'S COINSURANCE $_____

Payment Summary Section (Totals)

Charges	Adjustment	Allowed	Copay	Deduct/Not Covered	Coins	Total Paid

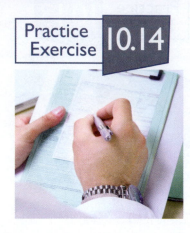

Practice Exercise 10.14

Secondary Claim

Physician Information:	Christopher M. Brown, M.D.
	234 Haverford Road
	Haverford, Ohio 12345
	999-555-3111
Federal Tax I.D.:	34-086541
Physician's Choice	
Services Provider I.D.:	B4321
NPI:	8903789447
Patient Information:	Sandra Henderson
	15 Main Street
	Wadsworth, Ohio 12345
Phone Number:	703-555-6969
Gender:	F
Marital Status:	M
DOB:	06/05/1966
Insurance:	U.S. Life
	2788 Broadway
	New York, NY, 00006
	703-877-0874
Group Number:	931
Policy/I.D. Number:	3317891
Employer:	Compaq Computers
Address:	10 Compaq Way
	Haverford, OH 12345
Phone:	999-555-6543
Employment Status:	Full-time

Secondary Insurance Information (Spouse):

Insured:	Charles Henderson
Gender:	M
Marital Status:	M
Employment:	Full Time
DOB:	08/22/1960
Employer:	Dell Computer
Address:	25 Dell Blvd.
	Haverford, OH 12345
Phone:	999-555-2599
Insurance:	Physicians Choice Services
	900 Blue Rock Turnpike
	Clarkville, Ohio 60817
Group Number:	K 2565
I.D./Policy Number:	5076 241
Phone:	800-793-1257

Patient Encounter Form:

DOS:	Today's Date
DX:	Lateral Epicondylitis ("Tennis Elbow"), ICD-10 (M77.10)
CPT: 99203	$150, New Patient
73070	$50, Radiological view elbow (2 views)
73090	$50 Radiological view forearm (2 views)

Assignment of benefits on file
Release of information form on file

Practice Exercise 10.14

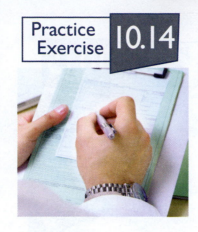

(Continued)

For Student Use Only

Payer's Name and Address

U.S. Life
2788 Broadway
New York, NY 00006

Today's Date:
CHECK #21763

Provider's Name and Address

Christopher M. Brown, M.D.
234 Haverford Road
Haverford, Ohio 12345

This statement covers payments for the following patient(s):

Claim Detail Section (If there are numbers in the REMARKS column, see the Remarks Section for explanation.)

Patient Name: Henderson, Sandra	**Patient Account #:** Hen03
Patient I.D.#: 331779183	**Insured's Name:** Sandra Henderson
Provider Name: Christopher M. Brown, M.D.	**Inventory #:** 25133 **Claim Control** # 55614

Service Date(s)	Procedure	Charges	Adjustment	Allowed	Copay	Deduct/Not Covered	Coins	PaidAmt.	Remarks
Claim Date	99203	150.00	0.00		0.00	100.00		80%	01
Claim Date	73070	50.00	0.00		0.00	0.00		80%	
Claim Date	73070	50.00	0.00		0.00	0.00		80%	
TOTALS									

BALANCE DUE FROM PATIENT: PT'S DED/NOT COV $_____
                              PT'S COINSURANCE $_____

Payment Summary Section (Totals)

Charges	Adjustment	Allowed	Copay	Deduct/Not Covered	Coins	Total Paid

REMARKS SECTION: 01 Deductible

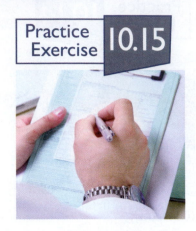

Practice Exercise 10.15

Secondary Claim

Physician Information:

Name:	Mary Ann Brock, M.D.
Address:	1547 Sampson Street
	Philadelphia, PA 12345
Phone:	215-555-3000
Tax Identification Number:	51-4290642
Blue Cross Blue Shield	
Provider I.D. Number:	495529
NPI:	6632588874

Patient Information:

Name:	Amy Louise Lynch
Address:	1776 Liberty Road
	Philadelphia, PA 12345
Phone:	215-555-9632
Date of Birth:	January 9, 1998
Gender:	Female
Marital Status:	Single
Employer:	Full-time student

Responsible Party (Both parents are insured):

Name:	Fred K. Lynch (father)
Insured's Address:	1776 Liberty Road
	Philadelphia, PA 12345
Phone:	215-555-9632
Insured's DOB:	July 15, 1967
Insured's Gender:	Male
Insured's Employer:	WDAF Radio
	200 Ester Lane
	Philadelphia, PA 12345
Phone:	215-555-9321
Insurance Carrier:	Blue Cross Blue Shield of Pennsylvania
	P.O. Box 354
	Philadelphia, PA 19174
Phone:	215-668-2334
Insured's I.D./Policy Number:	512-53-9751
Insured's Group Number:	W45980

Additional Insurance:

Name:	Jessie M. Lynch (mother)
	Insured's Address 1776 Liberty Road
	Philadelphia, PA 12345
	215-555-9632
Date of Birth:	May 6, 1969
Gender:	Female
Employer:	Southerland Lumber
	5145 Frontier Lane
	Philadelphia, PA 12345
Phone:	215-555-1722
Insurance Carrier:	Metropolitan Family Insurance Company
	414 East Franklin Road
	Philadelphia, PA 19111
Phone:	800-555-4141
Insured's I.D./Policy Number:	491-51-0003
Insured's Group Number:	7989

Patient Encounter Form/List of Fees for Services:

Date of Service:	Today's date
DX:	Annual Physical Examination, ICD-10 (Z00.00)
Services:	99385 Physical Examination Preventive Medicine Visit: $85

Assignment of benefits on file
Release of information form on file

Practice Exercise 10.15

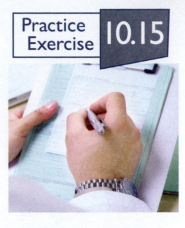

(*Continued*)

For Student Use Only

The charges are being paid at 80%.

Payer's Name and Address

| |
| |
| |

Today's Date:
CHECK #24466

Provider's Name and Address

| Mary Ann Brock, M.D. |
| 1547 Sampson Street |
| Philadelphia, PA 12345 |

This statement covers payments for the following patient(s): Lynch, Amy

Claim Detail Section (If there are numbers in the SEE REMARKS column, see the Remarks Section for explanation.)

Patient Name: Lynch, Amy	**Patient Account #:** Lyncham1
Patient I.D.#:	**Insured's Name:**
Group #:	
Provider Name: Mary Ann Brock, M.D. **Inventory #:** 44562 **Claim Control #:** 28081	

Service Date(s)	Procedure	Charges	Adjustment	Allowed	Copay	Deduct/Not Covered	Coins	Paid Amt.	Remarks
Claim Date	99385	85.00	0.00		0.00	0.00		80%	
TOTALS									

BALANCE DUE FROM PATIENT: PT'S DED/NOT COV $_____

                                                    PT'S COINSURANCE $_____

Payment Summary Section (Totals)

Charges	Adjustment	Allowed	Copay	Deduct/Not Covered	Coins	Total Paid

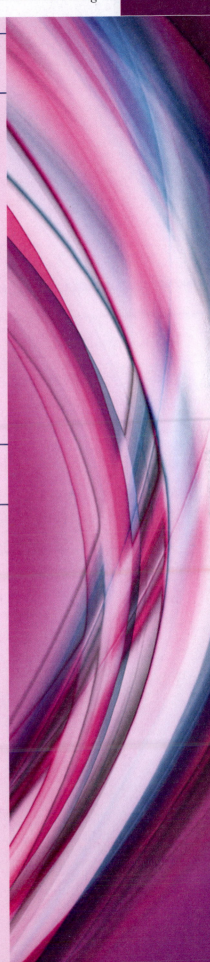

Chapter Summary

- Electronic claims have a number of advantages, such as low administrative costs, reduced claim rejection, and faster payment.
- Specific guidelines are available for completing a CMS-1500 form. Because guidelines vary by carriers for completing the CMS-1500, the medical insurance specialist should check with her local intermediaries or private carriers.
- Insurance companies and federal and state programs require certain identification numbers on health insurance claim forms submitted from individuals and facilities who provide and bill for services to patients.
- The medical office specialist should be aware of common billing errors and how to correct them for quicker claims settlements and to reduce the number of appeals.
- A patient may have coverage under more than one group insurance plan; additional insurance policies are referred to as secondary insurance. For example, a person may have primary insurance through his employer and also be covered under his spouse's insurance, making that his secondary insurance.

Chapter Review

True/False

Identify the statement as true (T) or false (F).

_____ **1.** If the patient is the insured person, the "Self" entry is marked under Patient Relationship to Insured on the CMS-1500 claim form.

_____ **2.** If the patient has additional insurance through a spouse, this information must be provided on the CMS-1500 claim form.

_____ **3.** Form locator 15 on the CMS-1500 is where the physician's unique identification number is entered.

_____ **4.** An audit of an electronic CMS-1500 claim by a clearinghouse tells the submitter if required data is missing.

_____ **5.** The birthday rule states that the parent whose day of birth is earlier in the calendar year will be considered the primary insurer.

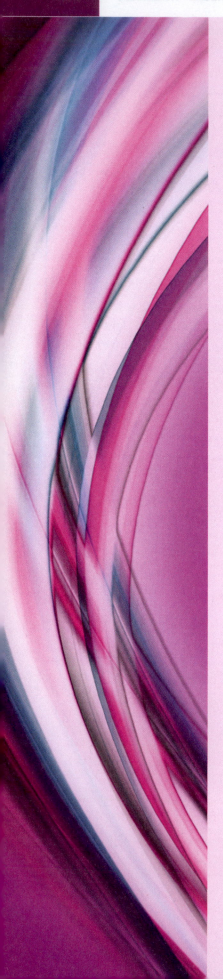

_____ **6.** Assignment of benefits refers to the minor giving the guarantor authority to see her medical records.

_____ **7.** The CMS-1500 is a universal claim form for filing all professional medical claims.

Multiple Choice

Identify the letter of the choice that best completes the statement or answers the question.

_____ **1.** The first 13 form locators on the CMS-1500 form refer to the:
   a. patient.
   b. provider.
   c. authorization to release information.
   d. medical practice.

_____ **2.** Form locators 14 through 33 on the CMS-1500 form refer to the:
   a. patient.
   b. physician or supplier.
   c. third-party payer.
   d. secondary insurance plan.

_____ **3.** The patient's birth date on the CMS-1500 form is entered in which of the following formats?
   a. MM/DD/YY
   b. DD/MM/YY
   c. MM/DD/YYYY
   d. DD/MM/YYYY

_____ **4.** HIPAA developed standards and regulations to be used by all providers, carriers, billing services, and clearinghouses in order to:
   a. standardize patient care.
   b. protect patient confidentiality.
   c. expedite claims processing.
   d. eliminate errors.

_____ **5.** Where is the facility information located on the CMS-1500 form?
   a. form locator 32
   b. form locator 14
   c. form locators 20–25
   d. form locators 1 and 5

_____ **6.** Locator 24B requires a place of service to be identified. Which of the following is a common place-of-service code?
   a. Urgent care facility
   b. Hospice
   c. Birthing center
   d. All of the above

Matching

Match the acronym with the correct definition.

a. FPN   f. TIN
b. EIN   g. NPI
c. GPN   h. HIC
d. EMG   i. PIN
e. SOF   j. LMP

_____ **1.** Also known as federal tax identification number

_____ **2.** Provider identification number, issued by the carrier

_____ **3.** National Provider Identifier issued by the CMS

_____ **4.** Member of a group practice who submits claims under the group's name

_____ **5.** Denotes signature on file

_____ **6.** Emergency

_____ **7.** Health insurance claim

_____ **8.** Last menstrual period

_____ **9.** Number issued by the Internal Revenue Service for income tax purposes

_____ **10.** A facility provider number used by the performing physician to report services done at that location

For Additional Practice

Complete the CMS-1500 form based on the information given here. To complete this exercise, copy the CMS-1500 form provided in Appendix D or download the form from MyHealthProfessionsKit or MyHealthProfessionsLab, which accompany this text.

Physician Information:

Physician Name: Ralph Wiggum, M.D.
Address: 333 Forrest Lane
                       Dallas, TX 75225
Phone: 214-388-5050
EIN: 72-5786322
NPI: 2222233333
Aetna PIN: CNC041

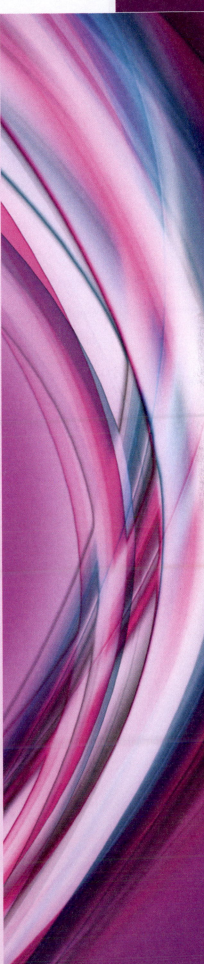

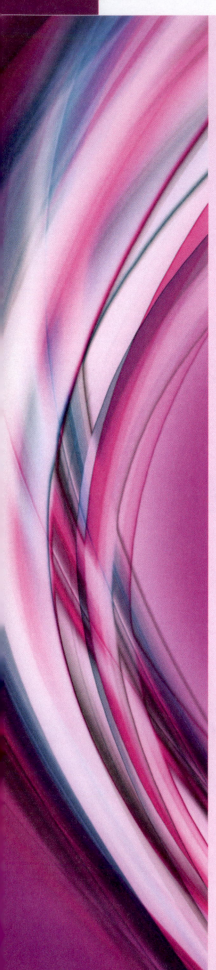

Patient Information Form:

Name:	Charlotte Watson
	124 Dallas Dr.
	Dallas, TX 75201
Phone:	214-388-5072
DOB:	07/08/44
Gender:	Female, Single
Patient Account Number:	WATCH101
Employer:	GPX Incorporated
Insurance Carrier:	Aetna (HMO)
Insurance Address:	5555 Walkway Ave.
	New York, NY 10000
Insurance I.D. Number:	555-88-8888
Insurance Group Number:	56885

Patient Encounter Form:

Date:	Today's date
	T-98 P-85 R-15 BP-150/96 WT-164 HT -73
CC:	No complaints, physical examination

List of Fees for Services:

Date:	Today's date
DX:	Physical Exam, ICD-10 (Z00.00)

Initial preventive medicine, new patient, $80 (99386); DX: ICD-10 (Z00.00)

X-ray, chest, 2 views, $45 each (71020); DX: ICD-10 (Z00.00)

ECG routine, 12 leads, $55 (93000); DX: ICD-10 (Z00.00)

Complete UA, $15 (81000); DX: ICD-10 (Z00.00)

Assignment of benefits and release of information on file, form signed today's date, claim submitted to carrier on today's date.

Resources

AAFP
aafp.org
800.274.2237
American Academy of Family Practices
11400 Tomahawk Creek Parkway
Leawood, KS 66211-2680

AAFP was founded in 1947 to promote and maintain high quality standards for family doctors. It is a resource for current topics, information, and education.

Healthcare Financial Management Association
www.hfma.org
800.252.4362
3 Westbrook Corporate Center
Suite 600
Westchester, IL 60154

A membership organization for healthcare finance leaders.
www.ICD10Data.com

An excellent tool for students, this is a resource where you can search for an ICD-10-CM diagnosis code and convert it to an ICD-10-CM diagnosis code. The conversion information should not be used as a tool to choose the final diagnostic code.

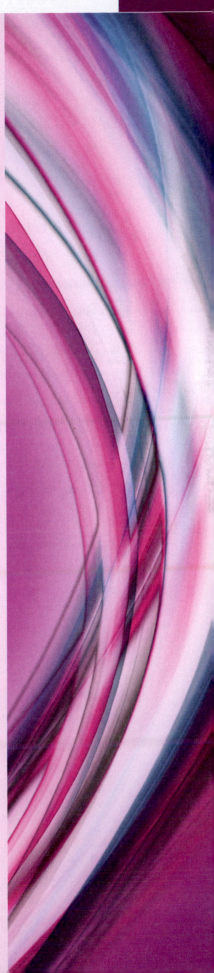

Chapter 11 / Hospital Medical Billing

Chapter Objectives

After reading this chapter, the student should be able to:

1 Understand the inpatient billing process used by hospitals.

2 Submit accurate and timely hospital claims and practice good follow-up and collection techniques.

3 Identify the different types of facilities and differentiate between inpatient and outpatient services.

4 Understand that hospital billing and coding are based on revenue.

5 Recognize that hospital reimbursement is not a fee for service but a fixed fee payment based on the diagnosis, rather than on time or services rendered.

6 Complete the UB-04 hospital billing claim form.

Key Terms

admitting physician	emergency care	Outpatient Prospective
Ambulatory Payment	grouper	Payment System
Classification (APC)	hospice	(OPPS)
ambulatory surgical	occurrence span	patient control number
center (ASC)	codes	(PCN)
ambulatory surgical unit	health information system	present on admission
(ASU)	(HIS)	(POA)
attending physician	inpatient care	principal diagnosis
charge description master	master patient index	prospective payment
(CDM)	Medicare DRG	system
comorbidity	(CMS-DRG &	registration
cost outlier	MS-DRG)	rendering physician
Diagnosis Related Group	operating physician	skilled nursing facility (SNF)
(DRG)	outpatient care	urgent care

CPT-4 codes in this chapter are from the CPT-4 2017 code set. CPT® is a registered trademark of the American Medical Association.

ICD-10 codes in this chapter are from the ICD-10-CM 2017 code set from the Department of Health and Human Services, Center for Disease Control and Prevention.

Stacy has recently suffered from appendicitis. The morning it began, she contacted her physician's office and was sent directly to the emergency room. After several procedures, including CAT scans and examinations, she was scheduled for an appendectomy. She stayed in the hospital for several days because of the severity of her case. After everything was complete, she received several bills. She was confused as to why she received so many bills from so many different places, some that she had never even heard of. She contacted the hospital and spoke with a billing manager who explained everything.

Questions

1. What types of bills might Stacy have received?
2. Why would she not recognize all of the offices from which the bills originated?
3. In general, what types of codes may have been used to bill the hospital visit?

Hospital inpatient and outpatients can accrue a much larger bill than for services rendered in a physician's office. Patients are admitted to hospitals for severe health problems and many require major surgery, resulting in considerable expense to the patient. The majority of most hospitals' reimbursement comes from insurance companies. However, it is becoming more difficult for patients with insurance coverage to pay their share of the bill. Consequently, accurate and timely claim submission, good follow-up, and effective collection techniques are in demand.

Inpatient Billing Process

The insurance billing functions are often centralized and referred to as the hospital's business office or patient financial services (PFS).

The hospital's billing process involves many employees and departments inside and outside the hospital. Each hospital has a **master patient index**, which is the main database of all of the hospital's patients. As a patient arrives and goes through the registration or admission process, the patient is assigned a **patient control number (PCN)** or medical record number, which is a unique number provided for each hospital admission. All charges and payments are posted to this number. **Registration** or admission is the process of collecting a patient's personal information, including insurance information, and entering it into the hospital's **health information system (HIS)**. Health information system refers to any technical system used to enter, store, manage, or transmit information related to the patient demographics, health insurance, billing, and care of patient. This information integrates with electronic health records. Registration information, all authorization and signature documents, a copy of the insurance card(s), and the emergency department's report, if the patient was admitted through the emergency department, are entered in the HIS system and retained in the electronic medical records. All physicians associated with the patient can access the patient's records to coordinate care through the EMR.

Hospital records should be completed and signed within 3 to 4 days and no more than 14 days after the patient is discharged, otherwise a cash flow problem could result. A discharge analyst checks the completeness of each patient's medical record for dictated reports and signatures. She submits a deficiency notation that alerts the appropriate physician indicating any documentation deficiencies or missing signature. Physicians may have access to a patient's medical record remotely, which allows physicians to address any deficiencies from their office, home, or most mobile devices. Physicians are expected to complete a patient's medical record and sign off before or at the time of the patient's discharge. When an analyst or coder requests additional information or a signature, the request is generated electronically. The physician will complete the record online or will sign electronically. A medical office specialist will not have direct access to the hospital's electronic medical record as the physician does but will have access to reports that reflect what deficiencies the physician has. The medical office specialist can help by reviewing the report with the physician to prompt him to complete the deficiencies. This is normally the responsibility of the office manager, but in some physician offices it is delegated to a designated medical office specialist.

Charge Description Master

All services and items provided to the patient are keyed into HIS system to assist with a high volume of billing for services received by hospital patients. Hospital charges are entered as services are provided. All services are listed in **charge description master (CDM)**, also commonly referred to as a charge master (Figure 11.1). The CDM is loaded into HIS and includes the following information:

1. *Procedure code:* CPT and HCPCS codes appear on a detail bill, outpatient bill, or outpatient uniform bill claim form UB-04, but not usually on the inpatient form.
2. *Procedure description:* This is a detailed narrative of each procedure (surgery, laboratory test, radiological test, etc.).
3. *Service description:* This is a detailed narrative of each service (E/M, observation, emergency department visits, clinical visits, etc.).
4. *Charge:* The dollar amount for each service or procedure is recorded. This is the standard fee for the item and not the actual amount paid by the third-party payer.
5. *Revenue code:* This is a three-digit code representing a specific accommodation, ancillary service, or billing calculation related to the service.

Each patient's data, consisting of revenue codes, procedure codes, descriptions, charges, and medical record data, are organized by the CDM and printed onto a hospital Uniform Bill claim form, commonly known as a UB-04 form or sometimes a CMS 1450 form. The CDM must be kept current and accurate to obtain proper reimbursement. It must be regularly audited; otherwise, negative impacts such as overpayment,

Department Number	Service Code	HCPCS Code	Description	Revenue Code	Charge
100	001	99281	ER Visit Level I	450	$100.00
100	002	99282	ER Visit Level II	450	$125.00
100	003	99283	ER Visit Level III	450	$150.00
100	004	99284	ER Visit Level IV	450	$200.00
100	005	99285	ER Visit Level V	450	$250.00
100	006		Room/Board/Pvt	110	$500.00
100	007		Intensive Care	190	$750.00
200	001	71010	Chest X-ray, AP	324	$100.00
200	002	71020	Chest X-ray, AP & Lat	324	$125.00
200	006	76705	Limited Ultrasound	320	$275.00
300	001	93005	IV Therapy	260	$350.00
400	001	Q0081	EKG	730	$250.00

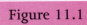

Figure 11.1

Examples of charge master entries.

underpayment, undercharging for services, claim rejections, fines, and/or penalties may result. There is usually a lag time—for example, 4 days after patient discharge—to be sure that all charges have been entered before claim submission. A sample charge master is shown in Figure 11.1.

Types of Payers

Hospitals negotiate their fees through different types of payers, including health maintenance organizations (HMOs), preferred provider organizations (PPOs), exclusive provider organizations (EPOs), point-of-service (POS) plans, commercial and indemnity plans, Medicare, Medicaid, TRICARE Prime (HMO), TRICARE Extra (PPO), TRICARE Standard, CHAMPUS, CHAMPVA, and workers' compensation.

Coding and Reimbursement Methods

Three basic reimbursement methods are used for inpatient and outpatient hospital services:

1. Prospective payment system
2. Fee for service
3. Per diem

The **prospective payment system** is the most recognized method, but a number of carriers use other methods. The prospective payment system was initiated by Medicare, which established payment rates to hospitals prospectively, which means before services are rendered.

Fee for services is the oldest method for which actual charges rendered to the patient are paid if found to be medically necessary. This is based on the diagnosis as related to the treatment rendered the patient.

The third type of reimbursement is the per diem type, which pays a fixed rate per day for all services performed or provided by the hospital facility. This is based on a daily rate for the type of admission and level of service provided to the patient. This method is used by rehabilitation centers and other facilities for negotiating reimbursement by third-party carriers.

An outpatient classification system developed by Health Systems International and used by the Centers for Medicare and Medicaid Services (CMS) is the **Ambulatory Payment Classification (APC)** system. This system is based on procedures rather than diagnoses. Services associated with a specific procedure or visits are bundled into the APC reimbursement. More than one APC may be billed if more than one procedure is performed, but discounts may be applied to any additional APCs. APCs are applied to the following:

■ Ambulatory surgical procedures
■ Chemotherapy
■ Clinic visits
■ Diagnostic services and diagnostic tests
■ Emergency department visits
■ Implants

- Outpatient services furnished to nursing facility patients not packaged into a nursing facility consolidated billing (These are services commonly furnished by hospital outpatient departments that nursing facilities are not able to provide, e.g., computed tomography, magnetic resonance imaging, or ambulatory surgery.)
- Partial hospitalization services for community mental health centers
- Preventive services (colorectal cancer screening)
- Radiology, including radiation therapy
- Services for patients who have exhausted Medicare Part A benefits
- Services to hospice patients for treatment of a nonterminal illness
- Surgical pathology

CMS provides a list of reimbursement rates for the APC system. CMS refers to it as the **Outpatient Prospective Payment System (OPPS)**. When a patient undergoes multiple processes and services, multiple APCs are generated and the payments are added together. APC software automatically discounts multiple APCs when appropriate.

Diagnosis Related Group System

Another form of the prospective payment system is the **Diagnosis Related Group (DRG)** system, which categorizes diagnoses and treatments into groups.

The DRG reimbursement system is a patient classification method that categorizes patients who are medically related with respect to diagnosis and treatment and who are statistically similar in terms of their length of hospital stay. The DRG system is used both to classify past cases to measure the relative resources hospitals have expended to treat patients with similar illnesses and to classify current cases to determine payment. The classifications were formed from more than 10,000 *International Classification of Diseases, Tenth Revision, Clinical Modification* (ICD-10-CM) codes that are divided into 25 major diagnostic categories (MDCs).

The diagnoses were assigned a specific DRG number from 001 to 511 and specific values commensurate with geographic area, type of hospital, depreciation value, teaching status, and other specific criteria. TRICARE and other private insurance companies that use DRGs use DRG numbers 600 to 900. Most MDCs are based on a particular organ system of the body. Payments for each DRG are based on a "relative weight" assigned to each case and on the hospital's individual rate. The relative weight represents the average resources necessary to provide services for a specific diagnosis. Within MDCs, DRGs are either medical or surgical. Seven variables are responsible for DRG classifications:

- Principal diagnosis
- Secondary diagnosis (up to eight)
- Surgical procedures (up to six)
- Comorbidity and complications
- Age and sex
- Discharge status
- Trim points (number of hospital days for a specific diagnosis)

When a patient is admitted to the hospital, the admission process can be done by either the attending physician or the admitting physician. The **admitting physician** only admits the patient to the hospital. An example of this would be an emergency department physician who admits a patient. An **attending physician** is primarily responsible for the patient's care. A **rendering physician** is a provider who renders a service—for example, a radiologist. If the patient requires an operation, the physician who conducts the operation is referred to as the **operating physician**. Throughout the patient's stay, diagnoses are established and coded from the **principal diagnosis** to the secondary diagnosis. The UB-04 form allows up to ten diagnoses, including the principal and admitting diagnoses. The assignment of the DRG is not performed by the facility. It is assigned by the carrier at the time the claim is processed, much like the billing of the APC. The facility has the ability to determine the DRG that should be assigned and the expected reimbursement based on the seven variables of the DRG classification given in the preceding list.

The facility may determine its charges for DRGs by using a case mix index (CMI). Each facility has a standardized dollar amount assigned to it by Medicare, determined by factors such as the CMI, local wage index, type of facility, number of low-income patients, type of institution, and so forth. A case mix is simply an average of all the DRG weights. Other factors that contribute to the facility's case mix are:

- Severity of illness
- Prognosis
- Treatment difficulty
- Need for intervention
- Resource intensity

Although the DRG is assigned by the carrier at the time the claim is processed, the facility can determine its reimbursement by working with the DRGs. To determine the reimbursement, a coder will view the pertinent patient case history information and code the principal and secondary diagnoses and operative procedures. Using a computer software program called a **grouper**, this information is keyed in and the program calculates and assigns the DRG payment group. The grouper is not able to consider any differences between chronic and acute conditions. Looping is the grouper process of searching all listed diagnoses for the presence of any comorbid conditions or complications or searching all procedures for operating room procedures or more specific procedures. If any factors that affect the DRG assignment change or are added, the new information is entered and the case is assigned the new DRG.

Let's look at an example of a patient with chronic bronchitis who is admitted to the hospital with pneumonia. His medical record shows that he has had emphysema for many years, and it lists chronic obstructive pulmonary disease (COPD) as the principal diagnosis with pneumonia as a secondary diagnosis; this DRG assignment, however, is inaccurate. As stated, the assignment entitles the hospital to receive $2,723.66. However, if the pneumonia diagnostic code were listed as the principal diagnosis with two secondary diagnoses, emphysema and chronic bronchitis, then the hospital would be entitled to $3,294.17—an additional $570.00 when the DRGs are assigned correctly.

Cost Outliers

A case that cannot be assigned an appropriate DRG because of an atypical situation is called a **cost outlier**. These atypical situations are as follows:

- Unique combinations of diagnoses and surgeries causing high costs
- Very rare conditions

Alcoholism	Diabetes mellitus, insulin-dependent
Anemia, due to blood loss, acute/chronic	Furuncles
Angina pectoris	Hematemesis
Atelectasis	Hematuria
Atrial fibrillation	Hypertensive heart disease
Cachexia	Malnutrition
Cardiomyopathy	Pneumothorax
Cellulitis	Renal failure; acute/chronic
Chronic obstructive pulmonary disease	Respiratory failure
Decubitus ulcer	Urinary retention
Dehydration	Urinary tract infection

Figure 11.2

Examples of comorbidities that could change the amount of a reimbursement.

- Long length of stay (referred to as a day outlier)
- Low-volume DRGs
- Inliers (in which the hospital case falls below the mean average or expected length of stay)
- Death
- Leaving against medical advice
- Admitted and discharged on the same day

The current federal reimbursement plan for outliers is to pay the full DRG rate plus an additional payment for services provided. An unethical practice, DRG creep or upcoding, is to code a patient's DRG category for a more severe diagnosis than indicated by the patient's condition. The amount of payment may be increased by documenting in the patient's medical record any comorbid conditions or complications. When referring to DRGs, the abbreviation CC is used to indicate such complications or comorbidities. **Comorbidity** is defined as a preexisting condition that, because of its effect on the specific principal diagnosis, will require intensive therapy or cause an increase in length of stay by at least 1 day in approximately 75% of cases (Figure 11.2).

If a patient is admitted because of two or more conditions and the physician fails to indicate the "most resource-intensive" or "most specific" diagnosis as the principal diagnosis—which is the diagnosis established after study or testing—the DRG assessment will be incorrect, resulting in decreased reimbursement to the healthcare facility. It is the responsibility of the attending physician to decide on a principal diagnosis based on her best judgment.

Several different DRG systems have been developed in the United States. One of the DRG systems is **Medicare DRG (CMS-DRG & MS-DRG)**. MS-DRG Grouper version 32 took effect as of October 1, 2015. Certain conditions are no longer considered complications if they were not **present on admission (POA)**, which will cause reduced reimbursement from Medicare for conditions apparently caused by the hospital. The rationale for the use of POA indicators, according to the Healthcare Cost and Utilization Project in 2013 (HCUP), is that it will distinguish preexisting conditions from complications and help to improve the design and fairness of pay-for-performance programs.

UB-04 Hospital Billing Claim Form

The UB-04 form is divided into four sections and includes 81 different form locators. The four sections are:

1. Patient information (form locators 1–41)
2. Billing information (form locators 42–49 and claim line 23)
3. Payer information (form locators 50–65)
4. Diagnosis information (form locators 66–81)

The numbering system begins with 1 at the top of the form and moves from left to right and top to bottom to form locator 81. Each form locator name describes the type of information that is to be input into the field. The form is printed in red ink on white paper for processing with optical scanning equipment. Figure 11.3 is an example of a blank UB-04. Figure 11.4 is a sample of a completed outpatient UB-04.

The UB-04 is considered a summary document supported by an itemized or detailed bill. The UB-04 is required by CMS and is accepted by private payers. It is used by institutional facilities to submit claims for inpatient and outpatient services. Let's take a look at the types of facilities that use the UB-04 form.

Inpatient care refers to a hospital confinement of more than 24 hours. Hospice facilities, which care for patients with terminal illnesses such as cancer and liver disease, also use the UB-04 for billing. **Hospice** is a type of coordinated care that can be delivered to either outpatients or inpatients to provide palliative services for terminally ill patients and their families.

The **skilled nursing facility (SNF)** is another type of inpatient care. SNF units care for patients who have been in the hospital and do not require a hospital stay any longer but are still unable to take care of themselves at home. The services provided to patients in an SNF unit are given by licensed nurses under the direction of a physician. An SNF may be in the hospital or in an independent facility. A rehabilitation center is an independent facility that also provides care for patients who have been in the hospital. An example would be a patient who was treated for a cerebrovascular accident (CVA) or stroke in the hospital and is recovering well. The patient may not have complete use of his limbs yet so, instead of being discharged home, the physician refers the patient to a rehabilitation center.

Outpatient care or ambulatory care does not require the patient to stay overnight. Different types of outpatient centers exist. An **ambulatory surgical center (ASC)** is a designated center where outpatient services are offered to patients. It may be affiliated with a particular hospital but is a freestanding building away from the hospital. An **ambulatory surgical unit (ASU)** is a department in a hospital that performs outpatient services for patients. **Emergency care** is also considered outpatient care because patients receive their treatment and are sent home. If, at the time, the emergency department physician feels the patient needs further care, the patient will be admitted to the hospital for inpatient services. Emergency situations are ones that require immediate attention to avoid the loss of life or limb. **Urgent care** is slightly different from emergency care. Although urgent care may require immediate attention, there is no risk of losing life or limb.

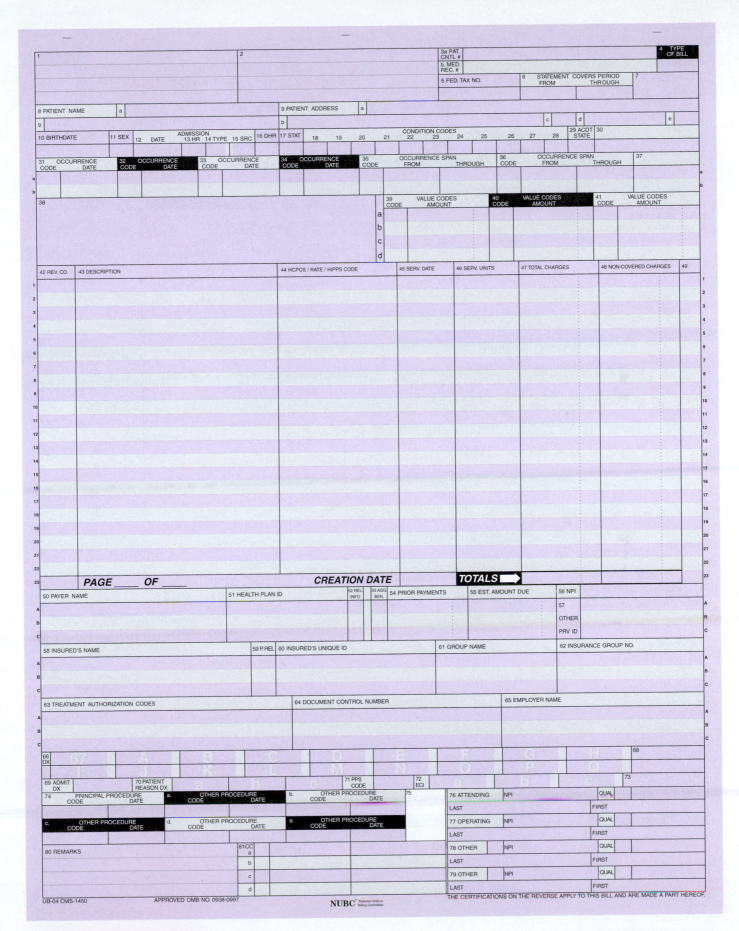

Figure 11.3   Sample UB-04 form.

1 ALLIED RADIOLOGY CENTER	2 ALLIED RADIOLOGY CENTER	3a PAT. CNTL. # 348501		4 TYPE OF BILL
1 BELMONT AVE SUITE 400	1 BELMONT AVE SUITE 400	b. MED. REC. # 5194		321
DENVER, CO 80415		5 FED. TAX NO.	6 STATEMENT COVERS PERIOD	7
806–511–4555	DENVER, CO 80415	342011578	FROM 05/15/16 THROUGH 05/15/16	

8 PATIENT NAME a		9 PATIENT ADDRESS a 9555 N SAINT BERNARD ST		
b WELCH, RUTH ANN		b	c CO d 80411	e US

10 BIRTHDATE	11 SEX	12 DATE	ADMISSION 13 HR 14 TYPE 15 SRC	16 DHR	17 STAT	18 19 20 21	CONDITION CODES 22 23 24 25 26 27 28	29 ACDT STATE	30
12/26/1955	F	08/18/14	9		30				

31 OCCURRENCE CODE DATE	32 OCCURRENCE CODE DATE	33 OCCURRENCE CODE DATE	34 OCCURRENCE CODE DATE	35 OCCURRENCE SPAN CODE FROM THROUGH	36 OCCURRENCE SPAN CODE FROM THROUGH	37
a						a
b						b

38		39 VALUE CODES CODE AMOUNT	40 VALUE CODES CODE AMOUNT	41 VALUE CODES CODE AMOUNT
UHC COMMUNITY PLAN -PA		a		
P.O. BOX 5200		b		
KINGSTON, NY 12402–5250		c		
800–600–9997		d		

	42 REV. CD.	43 DESCRIPTION	44 HCPCS / RATE / HIPPS CODE	45 SERV. DATE	46 SERV. UNITS	47 TOTAL CHARGES	48 NON-COVERED CHARGES	49	
1	0330	X-RAY	74000	05/15/16	500.00	500 : 00			1
23	PAGE 1 OF 1		CREATION DATE		TOTALS	500 : 00	0 : 00		23

50 PAYER NAME	51 HEALTH PLAN ID	52 REL INFO	53 ASG BEN	54 PRIOR PAYMENTS	55 EST. AMOUNT DUE	56 NPI	
A UHC COMMUNITY PLAN -PA	54704	Y	Y			57 OTHER PRV ID	A
B							B
C							C

58 INSURED'S NAME	59 P.REL	60 INSURED'S UNIQUE ID	61 GROUP NAME	62 INSURANCE GROUP NO.	
A WELCH, RUTH ANN	18	104159700		10041455	A
B					B
C					C

63 TREATMENT AUTHORIZATION CODES	64 DOCUMENT CONTROL NUMBER	65 EMPLOYER NAME	
A 0620580317			A
B			B
C			C

66 DX R1030	A B C D E F G H		68
0	I J K L M N O P Q		
69 ADMIT DX 4441	70 PATIENT REASON DX a b c	71 PPS CODE	72 ECI a b c	73

74 PRINCIPAL PROCEDURE CODE DATE	a. OTHER PROCEDURE CODE DATE	b. OTHER PROCEDURE CODE DATE	75	76 ATTENDING NPI 1972544788	QUAL 1G
c. OTHER PROCEDURE CODE DATE	d. OTHER PROCEDURE CODE DATE	e. OTHER PROCEDURE CODE DATE		LAST MAPLE	FIRST NATHAN
				77 OPERATING NPI	QUAL
				LAST	FIRST

80 REMARKS	81CC a B3 251E00000X	78 OTHER NPI	QUAL
	b	LAST	FIRST
	c	79 OTHER NPI	QUAL
	d	LAST	FIRST

UB-04 CMS-1450   APPROVED OMB NO. 0938-0997   NUBC National Uniform Billing Committee   THE CERTIFICATIONS ON THE REVERSE APPLY TO THIS BILL AND ARE MADE A PART HEREOF.

Figure 11.4   Sample completed outpatient UB-04 form.

Instructions for Completing the UB-04 Claim Form

Because hospital billing happens after the patient is discharged, it is important for the medical office specialist to know what information is required in each form locator so that it can be gathered before the claim is submitted. The medical office specialist must choose the correct selection from the different types of codes in order for the claim form to be completed with the correct data. Table 11.1 explains each form locator and the information required to complete each of them. (Note: "N/A" means not applicable.)

Table 11.1	UB-04 Claim Form Instructions
Form Locator Name	**Instructions**
1. Billing Provider Name & Address	Enter the name and address of the hospital/facility submitting the claim.
2. Pay to Address	Pay to address if different than field 1.
3a. Patient Control Number	Enter your facility's unique account number assigned to the patient, up to 20 alpha/numeric characters. This number will be printed on the RA and will help you identify the patient.
3b. Medical Record Number	Number assigned to patient's medical record by provider. Up to 30 alpha/numeric characters.
4. Type of Bill	Enter the four digit code that identifies the specific type of bill and frequency of submission. The first digit is a leading zero. 2nd Digit – <u>Submitting Facility</u> 1 = Hospital 2 = Skilled Nursing 3 = Home Health 4 = Christian Science (Hospital) 5 = Christian Science (Extended Care) 6 = Intermediate Care 7 = Clinic (Use "2nd Digit – Clinics Only" below) 8 = Special Facility (Use "2nd Digit – Special Facilities Only" below) 2nd Digit – <u>Bill Classification</u> (*Except Clinics and Special Facilities*) 1 = Inpatient (Including Medicare Part A) 2 = Inpatient (Medicare Part B Only) 3 = Outpatient 4 = Other 5 = Intermediate Care – Level I 6 = Intermediate Care – Level II 7 = Intermediate Care – Level III 8 = Swing Beds 2nd Digit – <u>Clinics Only</u> 1 = Rural Health 2 = Hospital Based or Independent Renal Dialysis Center 3 = Free Standing 4 = Outpatient Rehabilitation Facility (ORF) 5 = Comprehensive Outpatient Rehabilitation Facility (CORF) 9 = Other

(Continued)

Table 11.1	UB-04 Claim Form Instructions (Continued)

Form Locator Name	Instructions
	<u>2nd Digit</u> – <u>Special Facilities Only</u>
	1 = Hospice (Non-Hospital Based)
	2 = Hospice (Hospital Based)
	3 = Ambulatory Surgery Center
	4 = Free Standing Birthing Center
	9 = Other
	<u>3rd Digit</u> – <u>Frequency</u>
	0 = Non-Payment/Zero Claim
	1 = Admit Through Discharge Date (one claim covers entire stay)
	2 = First Interim Claim
	3 = Continuing Interim Claim
	4 = Last Interim Claim
	5 = Late Charge(s) Only Claim
	6 =
	7 = Replacement of Prior Claim
	8 = Void/Cancel of Prior Claim
5. Federal Tax Number	Enter the facility's tax identification number.
6. Statement Covers Period	Enter the beginning and ending service dates of for the period covered on the claim in MMDDCCYY format.
7. Administrative Necessary Days	Enter the number of Administratively Necessary Days (AND).
8. Patient Name	Enter the recipient's name exactly as it is spelled on the Medical Assistance ID card.
9. Patient Address	Enter the recipient's mailing address including street address, city, state and zip code.
10. Birth Date	Enter the recipient's date of birth in MMDDCCYY format.
11. Sex	Enter "M" for Male, "F" for Female or "U" for unknown.
12. Admission Date	Enter the start date of this episode of care. Use the MMDDCCYY format.
13. Admission Hour	Enter the hour (using a two-digit code below) that the patient entered the facility.
	1:00 a.m. - 01 2:00 a.m. - 02
	3:00 a.m. - 03 4:00 a.m. - 04
	5:00 a.m. - 05 6:00 a.m. - 06
	7:00 a.m. - 07 8:00 a.m. - 08
	9:00 a.m. - 09 10:00 a.m. - 10
	11:00 a.m. - 11 12:00 noon - 12
	1:00 p.m. - 13 2:00 p.m. - 14
	3:00 p.m. - 15 4:00 p.m. - 16
	5:00 p.m. - 17 6:00 p.m. - 18
	7:00 p.m. - 19 8:00 p.m. - 20
	9:00 p.m. - 21 10:00 p.m. - 22
	11:00 p.m. - 23 12:00 a.m. - 24/00
14. Admit Type	Enter one of the following primary reason for admission codes:
	1 = Emergency
	2 = Urgent
	3 = Elective
	4 = Newborn
	5 = Trauma
	9 = Information Not Available

Table 11.1	UB-04 Claim Form Instructions (Continued)

Form Locator Name	Instructions
15. Source of Admission	Enter one of the following source of admission codes: 1 = Physician Referral 2 = Clinic Referral 3 = HMO Referral 4 = Transfer from Hospital 5 = Transfer from SNF 6 = Transfer From Another Health Care Facility 7 = Emergency Room 8 = Court/Law Enforcement 9 = Information Not Available In the Case of Newborn 1 = Normal Delivery 2 = Premature Delivery 3 = Sick Baby 4 = Extramural Birth
16. Discharge Hour	Enter the hour (using a two-digit code below) that the patient entered the facility. 1:00 a.m. - 01 2:00 a.m. - 02 3:00 a.m. - 03 4:00 a.m. - 04 5:00 a.m. - 05 6:00 a.m. - 06 7:00 a.m. - 07 8:00 a.m. - 08 9:00 a.m. - 09 10:00 a.m. - 10 11:00 a.m. - 11 12:00 noon - 12 1:00 p.m. - 13 2:00 p.m. - 14 3:00 p.m. - 15 4:00 p.m. - 16 5:00 p.m. - 17 6:00 p.m. - 18 7:00 p.m. - 19 8:00 p.m. - 20 9:00 p.m. - 21 10:00 p.m. - 22 11:00 p.m. - 23 12:00 a.m. - 24/00
17. Patient Discharge Status	Enter one of the following two-digit codes for the patient's status (as of the "through" date): 01 = Discharged to home or self care (routine discharge) 02 = Discharged/transferred to another short-term general hospital 03 = Discharged/transferred to skilled nursing facility (SNF) 04 = Discharged/transferred to an intermediate care facility (ICF) 05 = Discharged/transferred to another type of institution 06 = Discharged/transferred to home under care of organized home health service organization 07 = Left against medical advice 08 = Reserved 09 = Admitted as an inpatient to this hospital (Medicare Outpatient Only) 20 = Expired (or did not recover – Christian Science patient) 21–29 Reserved 30 = Still a patient 40 = Expired at home

(Continued)

Table 11.1	UB-04 Claim Form Instructions (Continued)

Form Locator Name	Instructions
	41 = Expired in a medical facility; e.g., hospital, SNF, ICF, or free-standing hospice (Medicare Hospice Care Only)
	42 = Expired – place unknown (Medicare Hospice Care Only)
	43 = Discharged to Federal Health Care Facility
	50 = Hospice – Home
	51 = Hospice – Medical Facility
	52–60 Reserved
	61 = Discharge to Hospital Based Swing Bed
	62 = Discharged to Inpatient Rehab
	63 = Discharged to Long Term Care Hospital
	64 = Discharged to Nursing Facility
	65 = Discharged to Psychiatric Hospital
	66 = Discharged to Critical Access Hospital
18–28. Condition Codes	Enter two digit alpha numeric codes up to eleven occurrences to identify conditions that may affect processing of this claim. See National Uniform Billing Committee for guidelines.
29. Accident State	Enter two-digit state abbreviation.
30. Accident	Date Date accident occurred.
31–34. Occurrence Codes and Dates	Enter up to four code(s) and associated date(s) for any significant event(s) that may affect processing of this claim.
	01 = Auto Accident
	02 = Auto Accident – No Fault Insurance
	03 = Accident – Tort Liability
	04 = Accident – Employment Related
	05 = Other Accident
	06 = Crime Victim
	09 = Start of Infertility Treatment
	11 = Illness – Onset of Symptoms
	12 = Date of Onset For Chronically Dependant
	16 = Date of Last Therapy
	17 = Date Outpatient Occupational Therapy
	18 = Date of Retirement
	20 = Date Guarantee of Payment Began
	21 = Date UR Notice Received
	22 = Date Active Care Ended
	24 = Date Insurance Denied
	25 = Date Benefits Terminated By Primary Payer
	26 = Date Skilled SNF Became Available
	27 = Date Hospice Certification
	28 = Date Comprehensive Outpatient Rehab
	29 = Date Outpatient Physical Therapy
	30 = Date Outpatient Speech Pathology
	31 = Date Beneficiary Notified of Intent to Bill (procedures)
	32 = Date Beneficiary Notified of Intent to Bill
	33 = First Day of COB for ESRD
	34 = Date of Election of Extended Care
	35 = Date Treatment for Physical Therapy

Table 11.1	UB-04 Claim Form Instructions (Continued)

Form Locator Name	Instructions
	36 = Date of Inpatient Discharge for Covered Transplant
	37 = Date of Inpatient for Non-Covered Transplant
	38 = Date Treatment for Home IV
	39 = Date Discharged on Continuous IV
	40 = Scheduled Date of Admission
	41 = Date of First Test Pre-Admit
	42 = Date of Discharge
	43 = Cancelled Surgery
	44 = Inpatient Admit Changed to Outpatient
	44 = Date Treatment Started Occupational
	45 = Date Treatment Started Speech
	46 = Date Treatment Started Cardiac Rehab
	47 = Date Cost Outlier Begins
	A1 = Birth Date – Insured A
	A2 = Effective Date – Insured A Policy
	A3 = Benefits – Exhausted
	A4 = Split Bill Date
	B1 = Birth Date – Insured B
	B2 = Effective Date – Policy B
	B3 = Benefits Exhausted – Payer B
	C1 = Birth Date – Insured C
	C2 = Effective Date – Insured C
	C3 = Benefits Exhausted – Payer C
35–36. Occurrence Span	Enter the span of occurrence dates as indicated in 31–35.
38. Responsible Party Name and Address	Enter the responsible party name and address.
39–41. Value Code and Amount	Enter up to three value codes to identify special circumstances that may affect processing of this claim. See NUBC manual for specific codes.
	In the Amount box, enter the number, amount, or UCR value associated with that code.
42. Revenue Code	Enter a four digit Revenue Code beside each service described in column 43.
	(See Section 800, "Revenue Codes.")
	After the last Revenue Code, enter "0001" corresponding with the Total Charges amount in column 47. (PAPER CLAIMS ONLY)
43. Description	Enter a brief description that corresponds to the Revenue Code in column 42. List applicable NDC if location 44 is a J code.
	Report the N4 qualifier in the first two (2) positions, left justified, followed immediately by the 11 character NDC number. Immediately following the last character of the NDC (no space) the Unit of Measurement Qualifier immediately followed by the quantity with a floating decimal with a limit of 3 characters to the right of the decimal point.
	Unit of Measurement:
	F2 - International Unit
	GR - Gram
	ML - Milliliter
	UN - Unit

(Continued)

Table 11.1	UB-04 Claim Form Instructions (Continued)

Form Locator Name	Instructions
	To report more than one NDC per HCPC use the NDC attachment form.
	Enter "Total Charges" after the last description in this column to correspond with the total of all charges amount in column 47.
44. HCPC	Utilized for outpatient bills. If billing for an injectable code must display an NDC in location 43.
45. Service Date	Enter the date this service was provided (MMDDCCYY format).
46. Service Units	Enter the number of hospital accommodation days or units of service (such as pints of blood) which were rendered. AND days must correspond to the number of days in form locator 7.
47. Total Charges	Enter the total amount charged for each line of service. Also, enter the total of all charges after the last amount in this column.
48. Non-Covered Charges	Enter the amount, if any that is not covered by the primary payer for this service.
50. Payer	Enter the name and three-digit carrier code of the primary payer on line A and other payers on lines B and C. (Medical Assistance is always the payer of last resort.) **If the patient has Medical Assistance only, enter "RI Medicaid" on line A.** If Medicare is the primary payer, indicate Part A or Part B coverage.
51. Health Plan ID	The number used by the health plan to identify itself.
52. Release of Information	Enter "Y" for yes or "N" for no.
53. Assignment of Benefits	Enter "Y" for yes.
54. Prior Payments	Enter the amounts paid by the other insurance payers listed in form locator 50. If payment is made by other insurance, proof of payment (e.g., EOB) must be attached to the claim form.
55. Estimated Amount Due	The amount estimated to be due.
56. National Provider Identifier Billing Provider (NPI)	Unique identifier assigned to the provider. Seven digit RI Medical Assistance Provider ID if not submitting NPI.
57. Other Provider Identifier	**Taxonomy must be entered if NPI is entered in location 56**. This id **must** be entered in line A,B,C that corresponds to the line in which the "RI Medicaid" payer information is entered in locator 50.
58. Insured's Name	If other health insurance is involved, enter the insured's name.
59. Patient's Relation to Insured	Enter the code for the patient's relationship to the insured. 01 = Spouse 18 = Self 19= Child 20 = Employee 21 = Unknown 39 = Organ Donor 40 = Cadaver Donor 53 = Life Partner G8 = Other Relationship

Table 11.1	UB-04 Claim Form Instructions (Continued)

Form Locator Name	Instructions
60. Insured's Unique Identifier	Enter recipient's nine-digit Medical Assistance ID. This id **must** be entered in line A,B,C that corresponds to the line in which the RI Medicaid payer information is entered in locator 50.
61. Group Name	Enter the name of insured's other group health coverage, if applicable.
62. Insurance Group Number	Enter insured's group number, if applicable.
63. Treatment Authorization Number	Number that designates that treatment has been authorized.
64. Document Control Number	Control number assigned to the original bill.
65. Employer Name	Name of employer providing health coverage.
66. Diagnosis and Procedure Code Qualifier	Enter 10 for ICD 10 coding.
67. Principal Diagnosis Code on Admission	Enter the ICD-10 CM diagnosis code that describes the nature of the illness or injury.
67A - Q Other Diagnosis Codes	Enter up to 16 ICD-10 CM codes for other diagnoses.
68. Admitting Diagnosis Code	Enter the ICD-10 CM diagnosis code that describes the patient's condition at the time of admission.
70. Patient's Reason for Visit	Enter the ICD-10 CM diagnosis code that describes the patient's reason for visit.
71. PPS Code	The PPS code assigned to the claim.
72. External Cause of Injury Code	Enter the ICD-10 CM diagnosis code pertaining to external cause of injuries.
74. Principal Procedure Code and Date	Enter the ICD code that identifies the principal procedure performed. Enter the date of that procedure.
74A–E. Other Procedure Codes	Enter other ICD codes identifying all significant procedures performed. Enter the date of those procedures.
76. Attending Provider Name and Identifiers	Enter NPI of individual in charge of patient care. If UPIN number is entered, qualifier must be 1G. Enter the last and first name below.
77. Operating Physician Name and Identifiers	Required when surgical procedure is performed. Enter the NPI. If UPIN number is entered, qualifier must be 1G. Enter the last and first name.
78–79. Other Provider Name and Identifiers	Enter the NPI. If UPIN number is entered, qualifier must be 1G. Enter the last and first name.
80. Remarks Field/**Signature**	**Enter provider signature or authorized agent.**
81cc. Code-Code Field	Enter B3 in the qualifier if locations 76–79 contain an NPI. **Enter the corresponding provider taxonomy of provider NPI's entered in locations** 76a – 81CCa 77b – 81CCb 78c – 81CCc 79d – 81CCd

Source: Centers for Medicare and Medicaid Services.

Codes for Use on the UB-04 Claim Form

The UB-04 requires different codes for specifying the fiscal intermediary, type of bill, patient condition and cause, responsible party, rooms, occurrences, dates, times of admission and discharge, and other pertinent details. Revenue codes identify the department in which the services were rendered or from which supplies came. Value codes identify services and benefit days for Medicare patients. The following information and tables refer to specific form locators and provide examples of the information the code represents.

Revenue codes were originally three-digit codes. The need for additional codes mandated that the revenue codes become four-digit codes. The first digit should be a 0 followed by the three-digit code. The first two digits indicate which department rendered the service or supply.

Revenue codes are grouped into the following major categories:

- Room and Board—Private (0100)
- Pharmacy (0250)
- Physical Therapy (0420)

Revenue codes correspond with procedure codes. When placing a revenue code in a charge master, the correct revenue code must be placed with the correct CPT code that is used for a particular department. The revenue codes allow a hospital to use the same CPT code in multiple departments because the revenue code shows in which department the services are provided.

An example of a single code is CPT code 99282, the code for an emergency room visit of low to moderate severity. Revenue code 0450 is the code for emergency room. Revenue code 0450 is the only code that could be used for this CPT code because the CPT code and Revenue code both represent emergency room services.

An example of a procedure code that can be used in multiple locations is CPT code 12001, a simple laceration repair of a wound on the scalp, trunk of the body, or extremities such as hands and feet. This procedure could be done in multiple locations, including a treatment room (0761), clinic (0510), or emergency room (revenue code 0450).

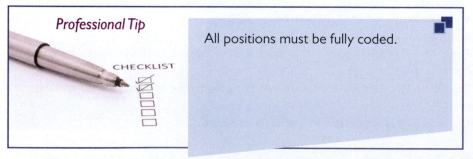

Professional Tip

CHECKLIST

All positions must be fully coded.

Type of Bill Codes (Form Locator 4)

The type of bill code is a three-digit code that provides information about the type of bill, type of care, and episode of care. The type of bill code is a four-digit alphanumeric code that gives three specific pieces of information after a leading zero. CMS will ignore the leading zero. The second digit identifies the type of facility. The third classifies the type of care. The fourth indicates the sequence of this bill in this particular episode of care. It is referred to as a "frequency" code. Table 11.2 lists the acceptable types of bill codes.

NOTE: This three-digit code requires one digit of each, in the following sequence:

Table 11.2	UB-04/CMS-1450 Reference Material

Type of Bill Codes (Field 4)
This is a three-digit code; each digit is defined below.

1st Digit – Type of Facility	Code
Hospital	1
Skilled Nursing Facility	2
Home Health	3
Christian Science (Hospital)	4
Christian Science (Extended Care)	5
Intermediate Care	6
Clinic	7

2nd Digit – Bill Classifications (Excluding Clinics & Special Facilities)	Code
Inpatient	1
Outpatient	3
Other (For Hospital Referenced Diagnostic Services, or Home Health Not Under a Plan of Treatment)	4
Intermediate Care, Level I	5
Intermediate Care, Level II	6
Intermediate Care, Level III	7
Swing Beds	8

2nd Digit – Bill Classifications (Clinics Only)	Code
Rural Health	1
Hospital Based or Independent Renal Dialysis Center	2
Free Standing	3
Other Rehabilitation Facility (ORF)	4
Other	9

2nd Digit – Bill Classifications (Special Facility Only)	Code
Hospice (Non-Hospital Based)	1
Hospice (Hospital Based)	2
Ambulatory Surgery Center (ASC)	3
Freestanding Birthing Center	4

3rd Digit – Frequency	Code
Admit through Discharge Claim	1
Interim – First Claim	2
Interim – Continuing Claims	3
Interim – Last Claim	4
Late Charge only	5
Adjustment of Prior Claim	6
Replacement of Prior Claim	7
Void/Cancel of Prior Claim	8

For Medicare use a 0 before the three digits.

1. Type of facility
2. Bill classification
3. Frequency

Sex Codes (Form Locator 11)

The type of sex code is a one-digit code that is used to complete form locator 11, which must be filled out. See Table 11.3 for a list of sex codes.

Admission/Discharge Hour Codes (Form Locators 13 and 16)

The admission/discharge hour codes are listed in military time. Table 11.4 lists the admission/discharge hour codes.

Admission Type Codes (Form Locator 14)

The types of admission codes establish the level of urgency for admission. Admission type codes are required on inpatient bills only. See Table 11.5.

Table 11.3	Sex Codes for Use with Form Locator 11	
	Code	**Definition**
	M	Male
	F	Female
	U	Unknown

Source: https://www.thehealthplan.com/documents/providers/ub04_instructions.pdf.

Table 11.4	Admission/Discharge Hour Codes for Use with Form Locators 13 and 16			
	Code	**Time (A.M.)**	**Code**	**Time (P.M.)**
	00	12:00–12:59 Midnight	12	12:00–12:59 Noon
	01	01:00–01:59	13	01:00–01:59
	02	02:00–02:59	14	02:00–02:59
	03	03:00–03:59	15	03:00–03:59
	04	04:00–04:59	16	04:00–04:59
	05	05:00–05:59	17	05:00–05:59
	06	06:00–06:59	18	06:00–06:59

Table 11.4	Admission/Discharge Hour Codes for Use with Form Locators 13 and 16 (continued)			
	Code	**Time (A.M.)**	**Code**	**Time (P.M.)**
	07	07:00–07:59	19	07:00–07:59
	08	08:00–08:59	20	08:00–08:59
	09	09:00–09:59	21	09:00–09:59
	10	10:00–10:59	22	10:00–10:59
	11	11:00–11:59	23	11:00–11:59
			99	Hour Unknown

Source: Geisinger Health Plan site, https://www.geisinger.org, https://www.thehealthplan.com/documents/providers/ub04_instructions.pdf.

Table 11.5	Admission Type Code Examples for Use with Form Locator 14	
Code	**Definition**	
1	Emergency	The patient requires immediate medical intervention as a result of severe, life-threatening, or potentially disabling condition(s).
2	Urgent	The patient requires immediate attention for the care and treatment of a physical or mental disorder.
3	Elective	The patient's condition permits adequate time to schedule the service.
4	Newborn	Use of this code necessitates the use of special source of admission codes (Form Locator 15).
5	Trauma	Center Visit to a trauma center/hospital as licensed or designated by the state or local government authority authorized to do so, or as verified by the American College of Surgeons and involving trauma activation. (Use revenue code 068 to capture trauma activation charges.) Reserved for National Assignment.
9	Information	Not Available Information not available.

Source: Geisinger Health Plan site, https://www.geisinger.org, https://www.thehealthplan.com/documents/providers/ub04_instructions.pdf.

Source of Admission (Form Locator 15)

The source of admission tells the payer how the patient was admitted and from where. For newborn admissions only, the source would be the type of delivery.

Table 11.6 provides admission source code examples.

Discharge Status Codes (Form Locator 17)

The type of discharge status defines to where the patient was discharged. This is especially important for Medicare patients for determining a covered benefit period. Table 11.7 includes discharge status code examples.

Table 11.6	Admission Source Code Examples for Use with Form Locator 15	
	Code	**Definition**
	1	Physician Referral
	2	Clinic Referral
	3	HMO Referral
	4	Transfer from a Hospital
	5	Transfer from an SNF
	6	Transfer from Another Facility
	7	Emergency Room
	8	Court/Law Enforcement
	9	Information Not Available
	A	Transfer from a Critical Access Hospital (CAH)
	B	Transfer from Another Home Health Agency
	C	Readmission to Same Home Health Agency
	D	Transfer from Hospital Inpatient to Same Facility Resulting in a Separate Claim to the Payer
	E–Z	Reserved for national assignment

Source: Geisinger Health Plan site, https://www.geisinger.org, https://www.thehealthplan.com/documents/providers/ub04_instructions.pdf.

Condition Codes (Form Locators 18–28)

If applicable, enter specific condition codes pertaining to the patient's admission. Up to 11 conditions may be entered. These codes identify conditions that may affect the payer's processing of the bill because they identify special circumstances, events, room accommodations, or conditions that surround the services provided. Condition codes should be entered in alphanumeric sequence. See Table 11.8 for a list of condition codes.

Occurrence Code Examples (Form Locators 31–34)

Form locators 31 through 34 are used to describe the accident or mishap responsible for the patient's admission to the hospital and the date. The occurrence codes are used to determine liability, coordinate benefits, and administer subrogation clauses. Please note that the **occurrence span codes** listed in Table 11.10 refer to dates only and do not relate to the occurrence codes in Table 11.9. The from/through dates are used for repetitive Part B services to show a period of inpatient hospital care or outpatient surgery during this billing period. These codes also determine the patient's liability period.

Table 11.7	Discharge Status Code Examples for Use with Form Locator 17

Code	Definition
01	Discharged to home or self-care (routine discharge)
02	Discharged/transferred to a short-term general hospital for inpatient care
03	Discharged/transferred to an SNF with Medicare certification in anticipation of covered skilled care
05	Discharged/transferred to another type of healthcare institution not defined elsewhere in this code list
06	Discharged/transferred to home under care of an organized home health service organization in anticipation of covered skilled care
07	Left against medical advice or discontinued care
08	Discharged/transferred to home under care of home IV therapy provider
09	Admitted as an inpatient to this hospital
20	Expired (or did not recover)
30	Still a patient or expected to return for outpatient services
31–39	Still a patient to be defined at state level, if necessary
40	Expired at home (for hospice care only)
41	Expired in a medical facility such as a hospital, SNF, ICF, or freestanding hospice (for hospice care only)
42	Expired, place unknown (for hospice care only)
50	Discharged to hospice-home
51	Discharged to hospice-medical facility

Source: Geisinger Health Plan site, https://www.geisinger.org, https://www.thehealthplan.com/documents/providers/ub04_instructions.pdf.

Table 11.8	Condition Codes for Use with Form Locators 18 through 28

Code	Description	Definition
01	Military Service Related	Medical condition was incurred during military service.
02	Employment Related	Condition is employment related.
03	Ins Coverage Not Listed	Indicates that patient/patient representative has stated that coverage may exist beyond that reflected on this bill.
04	Information Only Bill	Indicates bill is submitted for information only and the Medicare beneficiary is enrolled in a risk-based managed care plan and the provider expected to receive payment from the plan.
05	Lien Has Been Filed	Provider has filed legal claim for recovery of funds potentially due a patient as a result of legal action initiated by, or on behalf of, the patient.
06	ESRD Patient in First 18 months by Employer Group Health Insurance	Code indicates Medicare may be a secondary insurer if the patient is also covered by employer group health insurance during patient's first 18 months of end-stage renal disease (ESRD) entitlement.
07	Treatment of Nonterminal Condition for Hospice Patient	Code indicates the patient is a hospice enrollee, but the provider is not treating patient's terminal condition and is, therefore, requesting regular Medicare.

(Continued)

Table 11.8	Condition Codes for Use with Form Locators 18 through 28 (Continued)	

Code	Description	Definition
08	Pt Refuses Other Payer Info	Beneficiary would not provide information concerning coverage.
09	Neither Patient nor Spouse Employed	Indicates that the patient and spouse, in response to registration questions, have denied any employment.
10	Patient and/or Spouse Employed but No EGHP Exists	Code indicates that in response to development questions, the patient and/or spouse have indicated that one or both are employed but have no group health insurance from an employer group health plan (EGHP) or other employer-sponsored or -provided health insurance that covers the patient.
17	Patient Is Homeless	The patient is homeless.
20	Beneficiary Requested Billing	
21	Billing for Denial Notice	
31	Full-Time Student (Full-Time Day)	
ACCOMMODATIONS		
37	Ward Accommodation at Patient Request	Patient assigned to ward accommodations at patient's request.
38	Semi-Private Room Not Available	Indicates that either private or ward accommodations were assigned because semiprivate accommodations were not available.
39	Private Room Medically Necessary	Patient needs a private room for medical requirements.
40	Same-Day Transfer	Patient transferred to another facility before midnight on the day of admission.

Source: Geisinger Health Plan site, https://www.geisinger.org, https://www.thehealthplan.com/documents/providers/ub04_instructions.pdf.

Value Codes (Form Locators 39–41)

Value codes are two-digit codes that give the number of services provided and the amount. These form locators are also used for Medicare patients with regard to covered days, non-covered days, coinsurance days, and the lifetime reserve days. Table 11.11 includes value code examples for use in completing form locators 39 through 41.

Revenue Codes (Form Locator 42)

Revenue codes describe the specific accommodation and/or ancillary charges. The revenue code in form locator 42 must explain each charge in form locator 47. The provider must list revenue codes in ascending numeric sequence and not repeat the same to the extent possible. A maximum of 22 services may be billed on one claim form. Table 11.12 lists revenue code examples.

Table 11.9	Occurrence Codes for Use with Form Locators 31 through 34

Code	Description	Definition
01	Accident/Medical Coverage	Code indicating the date of an accident/injury for which there is medical payment coverage.
02	No-Fault Insurance Involved (Including Auto Accident/Other)	Code indicating the date of an accident including auto or other where state has applicable no-fault liability laws (i.e., legal basis for settlement without admission or proof of guilt).
03	Accident/Tort Liability	Code indicating the date of an accident resulting from a third party's action that may involve a civil court process in an attempt to require payment by the third party, other than no-fault liability.
04	Accident/Employment Related	Code indicating the date of an accident allegedly relating to the patient's employment.
11	Onset of Symptoms/Illness	Code indicating the date patient first became aware of symptoms/illness.
18	Date of retirement for patient/beneficiary	
24	Insurance denied	Date insurance was denied.

Source: Geisinger Health Plan site, https://www.geisinger.org, https://www.thehealthplan.com/documents/providers/ub04_instructions.pdf.

Table 11.10	Occurrence Span Codes

Code	Description	Definition
74	Non-covered Level of Care	The from/through dates of a period at a non-covered level of care in an otherwise covered stay, excluding any period reported by occurrence span code 76, 77, or 79. These codes are also used for repetitive Part B services to show a period of inpatient hospital care or outpatient surgery during the billing period. This code is also used for home health agency or hospice services billed under Part A.
76	Patient Liability Period	The from/through dates of a period of non-covered care for which the provider is permitted to charge the Medicare beneficiary. Code should be used only where the Peer Review Organization (PRO) or intermediary has approved such charges in advance and patient has been notified in writing at least 3 days before the from date of this period.
77	Provider Liability	The from/through dates of a period of non-covered care for which the provider is liable. The beneficiary's record is charged with Part A days, Part A or Part B deductible, and/or Part B coinsurance. The provider may collect the Part A or Part B deductible and coinsurance from the beneficiary.

Source: Geisinger Health Plan site, https://www.geisinger.org, https://www.thehealthplan.com/documents/providers/ub04_instructions.pdf.

Table 11.11	Value Code Examples for Use with Form Locators 39 through 41

Code	Description
12	Working aged beneficiary spouse with an EGHP
37	Pints of blood furnished
50	Physical therapy visits
53	Cardiac rehabilitation visits
80	Covered days
81	Non-covered days
82	Coinsurance days
83	Lifetime reserve days

Source: Geisinger Health Plan site, https://www.geisinger.org, https://www.thehealthplan.com/documents/providers/ub04_instructions.pdf.

Patient Relationship (Form Locator 59)

The patient relationship form locator determines the relationship to the insured listed in form locator 58. Table 11.13 includes patient relationship code examples.

Practice Exercises

Complete Practice Exercises 11.1, 11.2, 11.3, 11.4, and 11.5 by filling out the form locators on a UB-04 form based on the information given in each exercise and this chapter. This form can be located in Appendix D of the text or it can be downloaded from MyHealth-ProfessionsKit or MyHealthProfessionsLab, which accompany this text.

Table 11.12	Revenue Code Examples for Use with Form Locator 42

Code	Definition
0100	All-Inclusive Rate
0110	R&B (Private/Med/Gen)
0450	Emergency Room
0200	Intensive Care
0210	Coronary Care
0320	Radiology-Diagnostic

Source: Geisinger Health Plan site, https://www.geisinger.org, https://www.thehealthplan.com/documents/providers/ub04_instructions.pdf.

Table 11.13	Patient Relationship Code Examples for Use with Form Locator 59	
Code	**Definition**	
01	Spouse	
18	Patient Is Insured	
19	Natural Child-Insured Has Financial Responsibility	
43	Natural Child-Insured Does Not Have Financial Responsibility	
22	Handicapped Dependent	
29/53	Life Partner	
32	Mother	
33	Father	

Source: Geisinger Health Plan site, https://www.geisinger.org, https://www.thehealthplan.com/documents/providers/ub04_instructions.pdf.

Fill out the form locators on a UB-04 form based on the information given here. To complete this exercise, copy the UB-04 form provided in Appendix D or download the form from MyHealthProfessionsKit online or MyHealthProfessionsLab, which accompany this text.

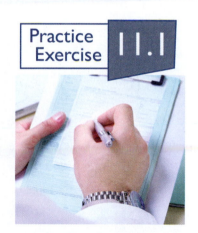

Practice Exercise 11.1

Patient Information:

	Marion K. Perry
	1601 Amber Way
	Lancaster, TX 12345
	214-555-3456
DOB:	12-14-1970
Patient I.D.:	450-10-4320
	Single, Female
Employer:	Benefits Assistance
	1710 Firman St., #400
	Lancaster, TX 12345
	214-555-1928
	Full-time

Insurance Information:

	Great West Life Insurance Co.
	2300 Main Street
	Dallas, TX 75234
I.D. Number:	450104320
Group Number:	G12345

(Continued)

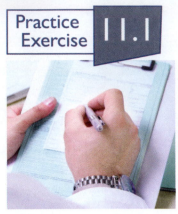

Practice Exercise 11.1

(*Continued*)

History of Present Illness (HPI): Marion Perry was seen in the emergency room on January 3, 2016, at 1:15 P.M. She presented with severe chills for 3 hours. Patient has a past history of being hospitalized for pneumonia. She has had past difficulties with shortness of breath and respiratory difficulties that required steroids and antibiotics. Patient denies nausea, vomiting, diarrhea, or cough. She was admitted to the hospital for fever of unknown origin. Discharged at 3:30 P.M. on January 7, 2016.

Attending Provider:	William F. Bonner, M.D.
NPI:	2556622146
Facility:	Presbyterian Hospital Dallas
	2600 Walnut Hill Lane Dallas,
	TX 12345 214-555-0001
NPI:	3671824096
Federal Tax Number:	75-1234567 3 days approved by carrier
Patient Control Number:	0100045
Medical Record Number:	INI001PE
Treatment Authorization Code:	2323444
Health Plan I.D. Number:	5985561421

List of Fees:

Revenue Codes			Date of Service
110	Room/Board/Semi.	$ 650.00	01/03/2016 to 01/07/2016
320	X-ray	$ 100.00	01/03/2016
324	X-ray/Chest	$ 275.00	01/03/2016
301	Lab Chemistry	$ 200.00	01/03/2016
981	ER Doctor	$ 300.00	01/03/2016
730	EKG	$ 175.00	01/03/2016
260	IV Therapy (4) (left arm)	$ 250.00	01/03/2016 to 01/05/2016
262	IV Solutions (4)	$ 800.00	01/03/2016 to 01/05/2016
264	IV Supplies (4)	$ 400.00	01/03/2016 to 01/05/2016
001	TOTAL	$3150.00	

Principal DX:	(ICD-10-CM) J44.1,
	(ICD-10-CM) I25.10,
	(ICD-10-CM) E78.5,
	(ICD-10-CM) F34.1
Admitting DX:	(ICD-10-CM) R50.9
Principal Procedure Code:	(CPT) 99.21, (ICD-10-PCS) 3E00X29
	(01/03/2016)

Assignment of benefits/release of information on file.

Fill out the form locators on a UB-04 form based on the information given here. To complete this exercise, copy the UB-04 form provided in Appendix D or download the form from MyHealthProfessionsKit online or MyHealthProfessionsLab, which accompany this text.

Patient Information:

	Janet K. Stephens
	6589 Ridge Crest Lane
	Las Vegas, NV, 87041
	836-555-9894
DOB:	3-21-55
Social Security number:	555-89-9877
	Married, female
Employer:	Homemaker

Insurance Information:

Insured's Name:	John D. Stephens (spouse)
Address:	Same
DOB:	11-14-54
Carrier:	Blue Cross Blue Shield
Carrier Address:	4899 S. Insurance Processing Blvd.
	Bluespring, MO 45898
I.D. Number:	658-88-3328
Group Number:	65432
Employer:	Jane's Video
	1616 Lovers Lane
	Las Vegas, NV, 87044
	836--555-6544

History of Present Illness (HPI): Janet Stephens showed up at Trinity Medical Center emergency room on May 1, 2016, at 7:05 P.M. She was complaining of severe head pain and shortness of breath. She was admitted to the hospital for further evaluation and discharged on May 3, 2016, at 1:30 P.M.

Attending Physician:

	Francis J. Brown, M.D.	
NPI:	2348810011	
BCBS I.D.:	551012	
Facility:	Trinity Medical Center	
	1234 Avenue	
	Las Vegas, NV , 87036	
	836-555-4300	
NPI:	5519822376	
Federal Tax Number:	75-1215977	
Medical Record Number:	695247	
Treatment Authorization Code:	1012559	Approved: 3 days
Health Plan I.D. Number:	9876223551	

(Continued)

Practice Exercise 11.2

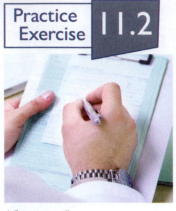

(*Continued*)

List of Fees:

Revenue Codes

110	Room/Board/Semi (2)	$ 615.00	05/01/2016 to 05/03/2016
740	EEG	$ 400.00	05/01/2016
351	CT Scan	$ 940.00	05/02/2016
610	MRI	$1050.00	05/01/2016
250	Pharmacy	$ 630.00	05/01/2016
900	Respiratory Services (10)	$ 456.00	5/1/2016, 5/2/2016
450	Emergency Room	$ 770.50	05/01/2016
990	Personal Items	$ 25.50	05/01/2016

Principal DX:	(ICD-10-CM) I67.1
Admitting DX:	(ICD-10-CM) R06.02
Principal Procedure Code:	Frontal lobe, (HCPCS) G8819 (05/01/2016)
Patient Control Number:	0010015

Assignment of benefits/release of information on file.

Practice Exercise 11.3

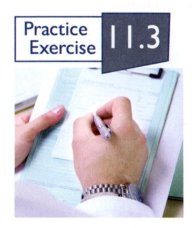

Fill out the form locators on a UB-04 form based on the information given here. To complete this exercise, copy the UB-04 form provided in Appendix D or download the form from MyHealthProfessionsKit online or MyHealthProfessionsLab, which accompany this text.

Patient Information:

	Michael R. James
	5489 Slow Bend Drive
	Denver, CO 80215
	806-555-9458
DOB:	7-1-1968
Social Security number:	555-55-5544
	Married, male
Employer:	Jim's Wholesale Club
	1698 Forest Lane
	Denver, CO 80215
	806-555-4900
	Full-time

Insurance Information:

Insured's Name:	Jennifer M. James (spouse)
Address:	same
DOB:	4-11-1968
Carrier:	Cigna PPO
Carrier Address:	4899 S. Insurance Processing Blvd. East Insurance City, MO 45898

I.D. Number: 555-66-6548
Group Number: 8488
Employer: NASTEC, Inc.
                          222 Career Center
                          Denver, CO 80215
                          806-555-2525

History of Present Illness (HPI): Michael James arrived at University Medical Center Emergency Room at 11:15 P.M. on January 21, 2016, complaining of severe lower abdominal pain. He was admitted to the hospital and released on January 23, 2016, at 10:00 A.M.

Attending Physician: Dennis J. O'Connor, M.D.
NPI: 4589854428
Cigna Pin: 27069
Facility: University Medical Center
                          1700 Jose Lane
                          Denver, CO 80216
                          806-555-4400
NPI: 9126485410
Federal Tax Number: 75-251487
Medical Record Number: 232774
Treatment Authorization
    Code: 551478   Approved: 2 days
Health Plan I.D. Number: 5874446251

List of Fees:

Revenue Codes (1 unit each)			Dates of Service
110	Room/Board Private	$615.00	01/21/2016 through 01/23/2016
320	X-ray	$275.00	01/21/2016
305	Lab/Chemistry	$180.00	01/22/2016
260	IV Therapy	$125.00	01/22/2016
250	Pharmacy	$208.00	01/23/2016
730	EKG/ECG	$210.00	01/23/2016

Principal DX: (ICD-10-CM)
                          K25.0 Acute Gastric Ulcer with hemorrhage without obstruction
Admitting DX: (ICD-10-CM)
                          R10.30 Abdominal Pain
Principal Procedure Code: (ICD-10-PCS) 0DQ60ZZ
                          Repair Stomach, Open Approach (01/21/2016)
Patient Control Number: 0030087

Assignment of benefits/release of information forms on file.

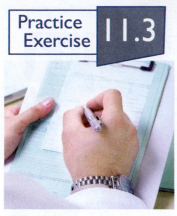

Practice Exercise 11.3

(*Continued*)

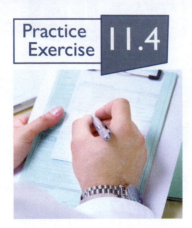

Practice Exercise 11.4

Fill out the form locators on a UB-04 form based on the information given here. To complete this exercise, copy the UB-04 form provided in Appendix D or download the form from MyHealthProfessionsKit or MyHealthProfessionsLab, which accompany this text.

Patient Information:

	Olive Westcot
	5 Apple Lane
	West Hartford, CT 12345
	860-555-2269
DOB:	3-2-49
Social Security number:	144-40-1442
	Single, Female
Employer:	Jamison Casket
	68 West Avenue
	Hartford, CT 12345
	860-555-8956
	Full-time

Insurance Information:

	Aetna
	215 Sisson Avenue
	Hartford, CT 06106
I.D. Number:	005598JA
Group Number:	JAM908
Admitting Physician:	Charles W. Henderson, M.D.
PIN:	56891T
NPI:	0006667999

History of Present Illness (HPI): Ms. Westcott presented herself to the emergency room complaining of abdominal pain. She was evaluated and admitted to the hospital at 1:35 P.M. on 02/26/2016. She was discharged at 9:45 A.M. on 02/28/2016.

Facility:	Presbyterian Hospital Hartford
	2600 Walnut Hill Lane
	West Hartford, CT 12345
	860-555-0001
NPI:	3671824096
Federal Tax Number:	75-1234567 3 days are approved by carrier
Patient Control Number:	987625941
Medical Record Number:	OLIWES0226
Treatment Authorization Code:	900ASC
Health Plan I.D. Number:	5985561421

List of Fees:

Revenue Codes			Date of Service
110	Semiprivate room	$ 340.00	02/26/2016
730	ECG	$ 95.00	02/27/2016
997	Admission Kit	$ 25.00	02/26/2016
351	CT Scan	$1,536.00	02/27/2016
300	Lab	$ 356.00	02/26/2016
981	ER Doctor	$ 300.00	02/26/2016
001	TOTAL	$2,992.00	

Principal DX: (ICD-10-CM) K80.50   Hepatolithiasis
Admitting DX: (ICD-10-CM) R10.10   Abdominal Pain
Principal Procedure
   Code: (ICD-10-PCS) 0FC90ZZ   (02/26/2016)

Assignment of benefits/release of information forms on file.

Practice Exercise 11.4

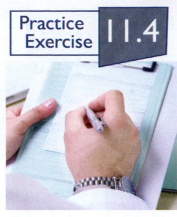

(*Continued*)

Fill out the form locators on a UB-04 form based on the information given here. To complete this exercise, copy the UB-04 form provided in Appendix D or download the form from MyHealthProfessionsKit online or MyHealthProfessionsLab, which accompany this text.

Practice Exercise 11.5

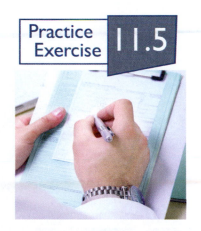

Patient Information:

	Alyssa M. Smith
	10552 Candlewood
	Las Cruces, NM 12345
	505-555-0669
DOB:	4-2-1971
Social Security number:	563-88-5691
	Single, Female
Employer:	Olive's Garden
	10305 Gateway West
	Las Cruces, NM 12345
	505-555-3611
	Full-time

Insurance Information:

	BCBS HMO
	6933 Coit
	Las Cruces, NM 12345
I.D. Number:	ZGY563885691
Group Number:	00063952
Admitting Physician:	Francis J. Bonner, M.D.
PIN:	110992F
NPI:	5555555555

(*Continued*)

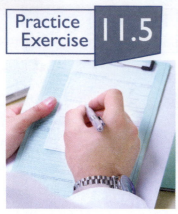

Practice Exercise 11.5

(Continued)

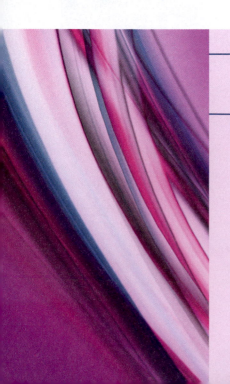

History of Present Illness (HPI): Alyssa Smith was given orders from her physician to have an outpatient radiology procedure done. She came to the outpatient registration department at 8:00 A.M. on 1/10/2016 for her procedure. She was registered and sent to the radiology department for her test.

Facility:	University Medical Center
	1700 Josey Lane
	Las Cruces, NM 12345
	505-555-4400
NPI:	9126485410
Federal Tax Number:	75-251487 I visit approved by carrier
Patient Control Number:	36249967
Medical Record Number:	SMI4291ALY
Treatment Authorization Code:	693358924
Health Plan I.D. Number:	5116523337

List of Fees:

Revenue Codes (1 unit each)		**Date of Service**
341 Radioisotope scan of the liver (78205)		01/10/2016
001 TOTAL	$ 756.50	
Principal DX:	(ICD-10-CM) K76.7	Hepatorenal Syndrome
Principal Procedure Code:	Planar Nuclear Medicine Imaging of Liver using Technetium 99m (Tc-99m) ICD-10-PCS (CF151ZZ)	(01/10/2016)

Assignment of benefits/release of information forms on file.

Chapter Summary

- Each hospital maintains a master patient index, which is the main database of all the hospital's patients. As a patient arrives and goes through the registration or admission process, the patient is assigned a patient control number (PCN), which is a unique number given for each hospital admission.
- Each patient's data, consisting of revenue codes, procedure codes, descriptions, charges, and medical record data, are organized by the charge description master and transferred onto a hospital Uniform Bill claim form, the UB-04, also known as the CMS-1450.
- Hospitals contract with managed care organizations and government health plans and negotiate fees for reimbursement.
- Three basic reimbursement methods are used for inpatient hospital services: prospective payment system, fee for service, and per diem.

- The DRG prospective payment system is a patient classification method that categorizes patients who are medically related with respect to diagnosis and treatment and who are statistically similar in terms of their length of hospital stay.
- ICD-10-CM codes are used for all inpatient and outpatient diagnosis. ICD-10-PCS is only used by hospital for inpatient procedures. CPT is used by all healthcare providers for outpatient procedures.
- The UB-04 is considered a summary document supported by an itemized or detailed bill. It is used by institutional facilities (e.g., inpatient and outpatient departments, rural health clinics, chronic dialysis services, and adult day healthcare) to submit claims for inpatient and outpatient services.
- The four sections of the UB-04 are patient information, billing information, payer information, and diagnosis information.

Chapter Review

True/False

Identify the statement as true (T) or false (F).

_____ **1.** The DRG indicates the medications the patient is taking while in the hospital.

_____ **2.** Hospitals bill for services only after the patient is discharged.

_____ **3.** An occurrence code describes the accident or mishap responsible for the patient's admission.

_____ **4.** The revenue code is a five-digit code number representing a specific accommodation, ancillary service, or billing calculation related to the service.

_____ **5.** The Ambulatory Payment Classification (APC) system is based on procedures rather than diagnoses.

_____ **6.** An inpatient is one who has been seen in the emergency department.

_____ **7.** A case that cannot be assigned an appropriate DRG because of an atypical situation is called a budget outlier.

_____ **8.** The type of discharge status defines to where the patient was discharged.

_____ **9.** The rendering provider is the provider who attended the patient.

_____ **10.** The PCN is the unique number given to the patient at admission.

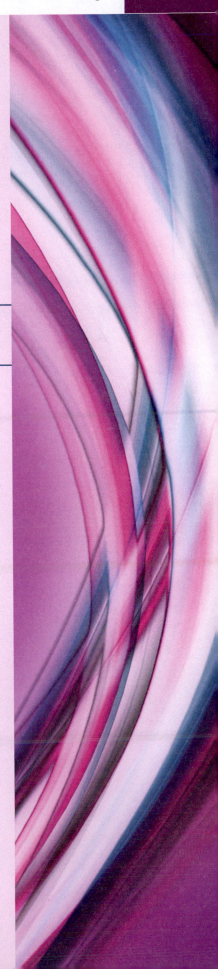

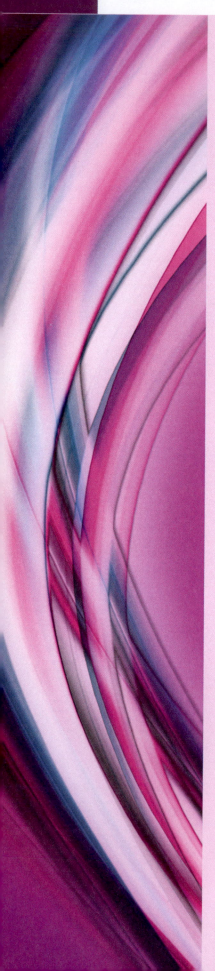

_____ **11.** The patient's reason for a visit is required on scheduled outpatient visits for outpatient bills.

_____ **12.** Birth dates on the UB-04 form should be shown in the MMDDCCYY format.

_____ **13.** The UB-04 form requires information about the source of a patient's admission.

_____ **14.** A charge master contains a hospital's list of services, codes, and charges.

Multiple Choice

Identify the letter of the choice that best completes the statement or answers the question.

_____ **1.** A hospice is a facility that cares for:
   a. auto accident victims.
   b. patients with a terminal illness.
   c. Medicare patients.
   d. individuals without insurance.

_____ **2.** A charge description master or charge master includes which of the following information?
   a. Patient's demographics   c. Procedure codes
   b. Number of clinic visits   d. Superbill

_____ **3.** Which term describes the patient's condition that is the diagnosis established after study or testing?
   a. Inpatient   c. Principal procedure
   b. Principal diagnosis   d. Admitting diagnosis

_____ **4.** Which term describes the patient's condition upon hospital admission?
   a. Inpatient   c. Admitting diagnosis
   b. Principal diagnosis   d. Principal procedure

Matching

Choose the best word or phrase that matches the description.

a. Admitting physician   h. Ambulatory payment classification
b. ASC   i. ASU
c. Attending physician   j. Comorbidity
d. DRG   k. Grouper
e. Rendering Physician   l. Principal diagnosis
f. Prospective Payment System   m. Outpatient Prospective Payment System
g. Patient Control Number   n. Charge master

_____ **1.** Unique number given to the patient for each hospital admission

_____ **2.** Sheet that contains the following information: procedure code, procedure, description, service description, charge, and the revenue code

_____ **3.** Outpatient payment classification system based on procedures

_____ **4.** Established payment rates for hospitals before services being rendered

_____ **5.** A form of PPS that categorizes diagnoses and treatments into groups

_____ **6.** OPPS

_____ **7.** A program that calculates and assigns the DRG payment group

_____ **8.** The physician who only admits the patient to the hospital

_____ **9.** Pre-existing condition that affects the principal diagnosis

_____ **10.** Department in the hospital that performs outpatient services for patients

_____ **11.** Designated center where outpatient services are offered to patients

_____ **12.** A provider who is primarily responsible for the patient's care

_____ **13.** The reason for the hospital stay

_____ **14.** Provider who renders a service

For Additional Practice

Complete a UB-04 form (located in Appendix D or available from MyHealth ProfessionsKit or MyHealthProfessionsLab, which accompany this text) with the following information:

Physician Information:

Name:	Charlotte Webb
	6589 Slow Curve Lane
	Dallas, TX 12345
	214-555-9874
Social Security number:	555-89-9877
DOB:	3-14-36
	Married, Female
Employer:	Bob's Crab Shack
	1629 Lovers Lane
	Dallas, TX 12345
	214-555-6786
	Employed Full-Time

Primary Insurance:

Insured's Name:	Michael Webb (Husband)
Employer:	ABC Incorporated
Employer address:	2222 Stillwater Blvd Dallas, TX 12345
Blue Cross Blue	
Shield I.D. Number:	XYC555
Group Number:	551489

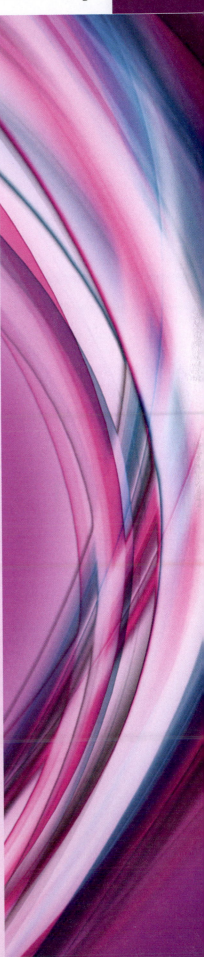

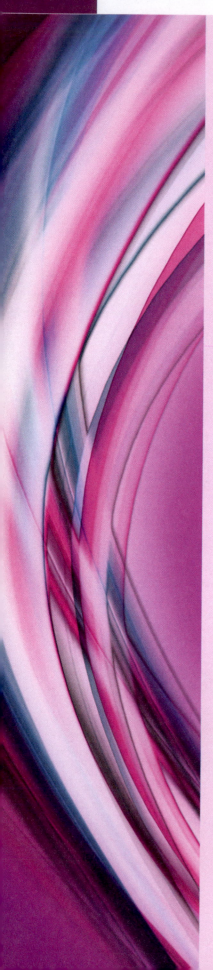

Case Information

Patient arrived at the Presbyterian Hospital emergency room on January 9, 2016, at 10:45 P.M. She presented with symptoms of low abdominal pain. She has been complaining of pain to her right side. She was admitted to the hospital on January 9, 2016, at 10:45 P.M. and discharged on January 12, 2016, at 1:00 P.M.

Attending Physician:

	Dr. William Fredrickson
NPI:	5555005555
BCBS I.D. Number:	665599
Facility:	

Presbyterian Hospital Dallas   3 days are approved
2600 Walnut Hill Lane
Dallas, TX 12345
214-555-8989

NPI:	2354498762
Federal Tax I.D. Number:	74-1258923
Patient Control Number:	9877773 Claim filed to carrier on 01/12/2016
Medical Record Number:	CW1515633
Treatment Auth Code:	1973888
Health Plan I.D. Number:	2354498762

Assignment of Benefits and Release of Information are on file.

List of Fees:

Revenue Codes:

010	Room & Board	$300.00 per day (3)	01/09/2016
320	X-ray: 2 views	$250.00	01/09/2016
981	ER Doctor	$200.00	01/09/2016
300	Lab	$375.00	01/10/2016

Principal Dx:	(ICD-10-CM) K35.2
Admitting Dx:	(ICD-10-CM) R10.30
Principal Procedure:	(ICD-10-PCS) 0DTJ0ZZ
Principal Procedure Date:	1/10/2016

Resources

National Uniform Billing Committee (NUBC)
www.nubc.org

The website for the National Uniform Billing Committee (NUBC) should be visited frequently to be aware of any changes in the billing form. The reader should go to the following website and click on "What's New" in the menu to find any new information.

UB-04 Data Specifications Manual
www.cms.gov/transmittals/downloads/R1104CP.pdf

This document is located on the CMS website and provides detailed information on how to complete the UB-04 claim form.

Section V / Government Medical Billing

12 Medicare Medical Billing

13 Medicaid Medical Billing

14 TRICARE Medical Billing

This section will provide the student with the knowledge to accurately file Medicare, Medicaid, and TRICARE claims. Medicare is a federal health insurance program established by Congress for the elderly, people with disabilities, and individuals who have end-stage renal disease. A large percentage of elderly Americans and those with disabilities are covered by the Medicare program, so it is important that the medical office specialist have a thorough understanding of Medicare claims processing. Chapter 12 discusses Medicare billing in detail.

Medicaid is a federal/state entitlement program that pays for medical assistance for certain individuals and families with low incomes and resources. Medicaid is the largest source of funding for medical and health-related services for low-income individuals, some of whom may have no medical insurance or inadequate medical insurance. Medicaid is also available for individuals who have disabilities or are blind and for pregnant women and children, though certain requirements must be met. Chapter 13 provides detailed information on Medicaid guidelines and claims filing.

TRICARE is the Department of Defense's medical entitlement program. It covers eligible uniformed services beneficiaries for medically necessary care. Chapter 14 provides an in-depth look at TRICARE and CHAMPVA, submitting claims to TRICARE on the Internet, and completing the CMS-1500 claim form for TRICARE.

Professional Vignette

My name is Sharon Goucher-Norris. I started working at Medicare 3 months after the Medicare program came into existence in 1966. After 6 years there, I went to work for a plastic surgeon, then a community hospital. I eventually ended up at Blue Cross, first in customer service, then in training, where I spent the majority of my career. Today I am teaching the next generation of medical billers and claims processors.

I have seen the industry go from entirely paper based, to terminals, to PCs, to complete electronic claims processing. The job insurance specialists today are more specialized and require more knowledge than in the past. The easy claims are processed entirely by the computer. The ones that edit out for human intervention are the more complex cases, requiring more investigation and a greater understanding of medical procedures and insurance rules. Education and training are essential in today's environment.

The keys to success in this field are openness to change and being a good communicator, with both internal and external customers. There is much opportunity for growth and advancement in the insurance side of the business, as larger companies conduct internal training and support external education as well. It really makes my day when I see one of my students get a new job.

Chapter 12 / Medicare Medical Billing

Chapter Objectives

After reading this chapter, the student should be able to:

1. Discuss government billing guidelines.

2. Determine the amount due from the patient for a participating provider.

3. Understand the different Medicare fee schedules.

4. Examine and complete accurate Medicare claims forms.

5. Identify the types of Medicare fraud and abuse that can occur.

Key Terms

benefit period
Consolidated Omnibus
   Budget Reconciliation
   Act of 1985 (COBRA)
crossover
end-stage renal disease
   (ESRD)
Electronic Remittance
   Advice (ERA)
Healthcare Common
   Procedure Coding
   System (HCPCS)
intermediaries
limiting charge
Local Coverage
   Determinations (LCDs)

Medicare abuse
Medicare Advantage
   (MA)
Medicare Administrative
   Contractor (MAC)
Medicare Development
   Letter
Medicare fraud
Medicare Part A
Medicare Part B
Medicare Part C
Medicare Part D
Medicare Remittance
   Notice (MRN)
Medicare Secondary
   Payer (MSP)

Medicare Summary
   Notice (MSN)
Medigap
non-par MFS
Office of Inspector
   General (OIG)
Program of All-Inclusive
   Care for the Elderly
   (PACE)
Recovery Audit
   Contractor (RAC)
scrubbing
Tax Relief and Health
   Care Act (TRHCA)
Telemedicine
   (telehealth)

CPT-4 codes in this chapter are from the CPT-4 2017 code set. CPT is a registered trademark of the American Medical Association.
ICD-10-CM codes in this chapter are from the ICD-10-CM 2017 code set from the Department of Health and Human Services, Centers for Disease Control and Prevention.

Ramon has received a bill for his recent visit to the doctor's office. He is confused because he has Medicare and American Association of Retired Persons (AARP) insurance and does not believe he should owe anything. He called AARP and was told that a bill for the visit had never been received. He had been told that all claims would come directly from Medicare. He then called Medicare and asked why the claim had not been sent to AARP. Medicare stated that the physician's office had not listed AARP as a secondary insurance carrier on the claim. Ramon realized that he had not given the office his AARP card at his visit.

Questions

1. How could his physician's office have prevented this problem?
2. What is it called when Medicare forwards a claim to the secondary insurance?
3. If this claim had fallen under the Medicare deductible, would the secondary insurance pick up the change?

Medicare is a federal health insurance program established by Congress for the elderly, people with disabilities, and individuals afflicted with **end-stage renal disease (ESRD)**. A large percentage of elderly Americans and those with disabilities are covered by the Medicare program. The network of Medicare administrators, contractors, and providers throughout the United States is kept quite busy serving the needs of Medicare beneficiaries.

Medicare History

Since the beginning of the 20th century, healthcare issues have continued to escalate in importance in the United States. There has long been broad agreement in the United States on the real need for some form of universal health insurance to alleviate the unpredictable and uneven costs associated with medical care.

In 1965, Congress acted to create a comprehensive program called Medicare that would provide medical insurance for elderly people who needed assistance with medical expenses. In 1972, Medicare benefits were also given to individuals with disabilities and those with ESRD. Today, more than 55 million Americans are enrolled in the Medicare program.

Medicare is divided into two main programs: **Medicare Part A**, which is hospital insurance, and **Medicare Part B**, which is medical insurance. In 1997 a new option was added called Medicare+Choice. This is now known as **Medicare Advantage (MA)**.

Medicare Advantage offers expanded benefits for a fee through private health insurance programs such as health maintenance organizations and preferred provider organizations that have contracts with Medicare. This program is commonly referred to as Part C, although the Medicare administration does not label it as such. In 2006 **Medicare Part D** became available to participants for prescription drug coverage.

Medicare Administration

The Medicare program is administered by the Centers for Medicare and Medicaid Services (CMS), a division of the U.S. Department of Health and Human Services (HHS or DHHS). CMS (formerly called the Health Care Financing Administration) was created in 1977 by Congress to serve as a consolidated agency that would administer both Medicare and Medicaid: the two largest healthcare programs in the United States. CMS serves the Medicare program and Medicare beneficiaries in many ways. Its roles include the following:

- Establishing policy for the reimbursement of providers
- Conducting research into healthcare management and treatment
- Assessing the quality of healthcare facilities and services

The agency's primary function is to ensure that its contractors and state agencies properly administer Medicare. CMS has ten Regional Offices (ROs) reorganized in a Consortia structure based on the agency's key lines of business: Medicare Health Plans Operations, Financial Management and Fee-For-Service Operations, Medicaid and

Children's Health Operations, and Quality Improvement and Survey & Certification Operations.

The Social Security Administration (SSA) also assists CMS to administer Medicare by enrolling new Medicare beneficiaries into the program. The SSA also collects Medicare premiums and maintains the Medicare master beneficiary record.

A Medicare Administrative Contractor (MAC) is a private healthcare insurer that has been awarded a geographic jurisdiction to process (adjudicate) Medicare Part A and Part B (A/B) medical claims or Durable Medical Equipment (DME) claims for Medicare Fee-For-Service (FFS) beneficiaries. Adjudicate is to make a formal judgment or decision. CMS relies on a network of MACs to serve as the primary operational contact between the Medicare FFS program and the healthcare providers enrolled in the program. MACs are multi-state, regional contractors responsible for administering both Medicare Part A and Medicare Part B claims. A list of the **Medicare Administrative Contractor (MAC)** entities can be found online by visiting the CMS website (www.cms.gov) and searching for "Medicare Administrative Contractors" by state.

CMS currently has 12 MAC Part A and Part B contractors but has planned to have 10 A/B MAC) jurisdictions throughout the United States. These MACs may administer Medicare Part A or Medicare Part B for their jurisdiction.

Some of the roles and responsibilities of Medicare Administrative Contractors include the following:

- Determining costs and reimbursement amounts
- Establishing controls
- Safeguarding against fraud and abuse or excess use
- Conducting reviews and audits
- Making the payments to providers for services
- Assisting both providers and beneficiaries as needed
- Maintaining quality of performance records
- Assisting in fraud and abuse investigations
- Assisting both suppliers and beneficiaries as needed

The primary responsibility of **intermediaries** and carriers is to process and reimburse Medicare claims submitted by providers.

The **Recovery Audit Contractor Program (RAC)** was implemented in all states in 2010 for Medicare Administrative Contractors who process the claims. This program was included in the Tax Relief and Healthcare Act of 2006. The RAC contractors are tasked with identifying improper payments made on claims of healthcare services provided to Medicare beneficiaries. These errors include the following:

- Duplicate claims
- Fiscal intermediaries' mistakes
- Medical necessity errors
- Coding errors

RACs are paid for these audits by receiving a percentage of the recouped Medicare payments and underpayments they collect from providers. A RAC may request medical records for its audit. In fact, the requests for these records have increased from 300 to 400 in a 45-day period. This has added an additional expense and burden to the providers. MAC will send out a demand on the automated and complex Recovery Audit review. When completed, the RAC will send review results letters, which include the results of the audit and information on how to correct these errors.

Medicare Part A Coverage and Eligibility Requirements

Medicare Part A coverage (also known as *hospital insurance*) includes the following:

- Inpatient hospital care (Staying overnight in the hospital does not automatically mean inpatient; the physician must write an order for the patient to be admitted.)
- Inpatient care in a skilled nursing facility (SNF) (after a minimum of three medically necessary inpatient hospital stays)
- Home healthcare
- Hospice care
- Blood
- Organ transplants

The intermediary determines payment and processes claims for Part A facilities for covered items and services provided by the facility. Part A provides benefits for inpatient services provided at hospitals and SNFs. There is no premium if the beneficiary is eligible for Medicare. Individuals who are prior to three months of age 65 or younger who do not receive Social Security benefits may enroll in Medicare Part A by paying a premium.

To qualify for Medicare Part A, individuals must meet Medicare's eligibility requirements under one of the following beneficiary categories:

1. *Individuals 65 or older:* Individuals age 65 or older who have paid or the beneficiary's spouse has paid FICA taxes or Railroad Retirement Board taxes for at least 40 calendar quarters.
2. *Adults with disabilities:* Individuals who have been receiving Social Security disability benefits or Railroad Retirement Board disability benefits for more than 2 years. Coverage begins 5 months after the 2 years of entitlement. If the patient has Lou Gehrig's disease, benefits begin the first month that disability benefits are received.
3. *Individuals who became disabled before age 18:* Individuals under the age of 18 who meet the disability criteria of the Social Security Act.
4. *Spouses of entitled individuals:* Spouses of deceased or retired individuals or individuals with disabilities who were or still are entitled to Medicare benefits.
5. *Retired federal employees enrolled in the Civil Service Retirement System (CSRS):* Retired CSRS employees and their spouses.
6. *Individuals with ESRD:* Individuals of any age who receive dialysis or a renal transplant for ESRD. Coverage typically begins on the first day of the month following the start of dialysis treatments. In the case of a transplant, entitlement begins the month the individual is hospitalized for the transplant (the transplant must be completed within 2 months). The donor is covered for services related to the donation of the organ only.
7. *Permanent Residents:* Foreign nationals who have permanent resident status may qualify to "buy" Medicare coverage if they have lived in the United States continuously for at least 5 years and if they are at least 6 years old. Most people who have worked and paid taxes in the United States will receive basic Medicare (Part A) at no additional cost when they reach age 65. Older people who have not worked or paid FICA taxes in the United States will usually be required to pay the Medicare Part A premium.

Inpatient Hospital Care

Medicare Part A provides coverage for inpatient hospital care. A patient is eligible for 90 days of hospital care in a **benefit period**, as long as medical necessity for the admission and the number of days has been proven. Coverage includes semiprivate rooms, meals, general nursing, and other hospital services and supplies. This does not include private-duty nursing or a television or telephone in the room. It also does not include a private room, unless medically necessary. The patient also has a lifetime reserve of 60 days that may be used once the 90 days have been exhausted. Once the reserve days have been used, they are not replenished.

Skilled Nursing Facility

Part A provides coverage for a skilled nursing facility. A patient is eligible for 100 days of care in an SNF during a benefit period, as long as medical necessity for the admission and the number of days has been proven. Semiprivate room, meals, skilled nursing and rehabilitative services, and other services and supplies (after a related 3-day inpatient hospital stay) are also covered.

Home Healthcare

Part A provides coverage for home healthcare. Home healthcare is defined as part-time or intermittent skilled nursing care and home health aide services, physical therapy, occupational therapy, speech–language therapy, medical social services, durable medical equipment (such as wheelchairs, hospital beds, oxygen, and walkers), medical supplies, and other services. There is no time limit on home healthcare as long as medical necessity has been proven.

Hospice Care

Part A provides coverage for hospice care. Hospice care is for individuals

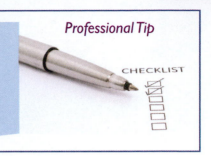

Professional Tip

The deductible for 2017 is $1,316 per benefit period (see example of benefit period).

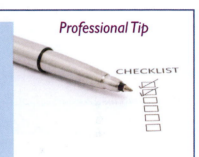

Professional Tip

As of 2017, the SNF coinsurance fees are as follows:

- $0 for the first 20 days of each benefit period
- $164.50 per day for days 21–100 of each benefit period
- All costs for each day after day 100 in a benefit period

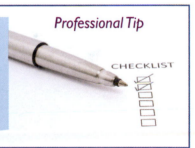

Professional Tip

As of 2017, the coinsurance due from the patient is as follows:

- $0 for home healthcare services.
- 20% of the Medicare-approved amount for durable medical equipment.

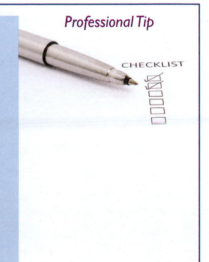

Professional Tip

As of 2017, the patient is responsible for the following coinsurance:

- $0 for hospice care.
- A copayment of up to $5 per prescription for outpatient prescription drugs for pain and symptom management.
- 5% of the Medicare-approved amount for inpatient respite care.
- Medicare does not cover room and board when you get hospice care in your home or in another facility where you live (such as a nursing home).

with a terminal illness and includes drugs for symptom control and pain relief, medical and support services from a Medicare-approved hospice, and other services not otherwise covered by Medicare. Hospice care can be given in the home. However, Medicare covers short-term hospital and inpatient respite care (care given to a hospice patient so that the usual caregiver can rest).

Blood

In most cases, the hospital gets blood from a blood bank at no charge, and the patient does not have to pay for it or replace it. If the hospital has to buy blood for the patient, the patient must either pay the hospital for the first 3 units of blood received in a calendar year or have the blood donated.

Organ Transplants

A transplant program is defined as a component within a transplant hospital that provides transplantation of a particular type of organ.

Types of organ transplant programs include the following:

- Heart
- Lung
- Heart/lung (The program must be located in a hospital with an existing Medicare-approved heart and Medicare-approved lung program.)
- Liver
- Intestine (The program must be located in a hospital with a Medicare-approved liver program. This program includes multivisceral and combined liver–intestine transplants.)
- Kidney
- Pancreas (The program must be located in a hospital with a Medicare-approved kidney program. This program includes combined kidney–pancreas transplants.)

All organ transplant programs must be located in a hospital that has a Medicare provider agreement. In addition to meeting the transplant Conditions of Participation, the transplant program must also comply with the hospital Conditions of Participation (specified in 42 CFR 482.1 through 482.57).

Inpatient Benefit Days

A benefit period is a period of time during which medical benefits are available to an insurance beneficiary. For Medicare Part A, a benefit period:

- Starts the day a patient enters the hospital if the patient has not been an inpatient or an SNF patient in the last 60 days.
- Ends when the patient has not been an inpatient or SNF patient for 60 consecutive days.

With Medicare Part A, a patient may be allowed up to 150 days of coverage when the regular 90-day benefit period (60 basic days and 30 coinsurance days) and the 60 lifetime reserve days are included. The different types of days are discussed next.

Table 12.1	Changes in Deductibles for Medicare Patients for Days 1 through 60 of Each Benefit Period	
	Year	**Deductible**
	2009	$1,068
	2010	$1,100
	2011	$1,132
	2012	$1,156
	2013	$1,184
	2014	$1,216
	2015	$1,260
	2016	$1,288
	2017	$1,316

Basic Days

Basic days are the first 60 days of acute inpatient care provided to a beneficiary during a benefit period. Medicare Part A criteria for the basic days are as follows:

- The beneficiary's financial responsibility is limited to the benefit period deductible.
- There is no coinsurance.
- If exhausted, these days are recycled once a new benefit period begins.

Table 12.1 illustrates how the deductibles for Medicare patients have been changed in recent years.

Coinsurance Days

Medicare patients hospitalized for more than 60 days in a benefit period must pay coinsurance if they remain in the hospital.

Example

Days 1–60   Full benefits
Days 61–90   Coinsurance ($329 per day, 2017)
Days 91–150   Lifetime reserve ($658 after day 90 of each benefit period, 2017)

Coinsurance is a daily charge of one-quarter of the current Part A deductible:

$1,316 (2017)
× 0.25
―――――――
$329 per day

Lifetime Reserve Days (LTR)

Once a patient with Medicare Part A has used 90 days in one benefit period (60 basic days and 30 coinsurance days), he or she becomes eligible to start using 60 lifetime reserve days for the 91st through 150th day of acute inpatient care during that same benefit period.

- Once the reserve days have been used, they cannot be renewed. That is, if the beneficiary elects to use these days, they can never be reused.
- The charge to the beneficiary for using reserve days is one-half of the current Part A deductible.

An example of the cost of using lifetime reserve days is calculated in the following example.

Example

Lifetime reserve days include a daily charge (coinsurance) of one-half of the current Medicare Part A deductible:

$1,316 (2017)
× 0.5
—————
$658 per day

Medicare Part B Coverage and Eligibility Requirements

Medicare Part B insurance helps pay for physician services in both hospital and nonhospital settings, outpatient hospital services, emergency departments, diagnostic tests, clinical laboratory services, wellness visits, outpatient physical therapy, speech therapy services, durable medical equipment, ambulance transportation, rural health clinic services, and telemedicine. **Telemedicine**, also called **telehealth**, has become an option for urban areas with populations up to 100,000 with limited access to healthcare providers.

Telemedicine

Medicare historically only provided limited coverage for telemedicine services, which has included coverage for interactive audio and video telecommunications that provide real-time communications between a practitioner and a Medicare beneficiary while the beneficiary is present at the encounter. Medicare only covered the provision of telehealth services if the beneficiary was seen at an approved "originating site" (e.g., physician offices, hospitals, skilled nursing facilities) for a small, defined set of services (e.g., consultations, office visits, pharmacological management, and individual and group diabetes self-management training services). The services could only be provided by these approved providers:

- physicians
- nurse practitioners
- clinical psychologists

The Medicare Telehealth Parity Act of 2015 extended Medicare coverage of remote patient monitoring services (RPM) for covered chronic health conditions, and home dialysis services for those with end-stage renal disease. The 2015 act represented federal lawmakers' continued and increasing support for expanding Medicare telehealth reimbursement. CMS added certified registered nurse anesthetists to the list of qualified telehealth providers for healthcare services. Medicare reimbursement for telehealth services remains strictly limited by statutory requirements; however, CMS continues to review the benefits of Telemedicine and how the technology can improve the cost and quality of healthcare delivery. For 2016, CMS added the following CPT codes:

- 99356 and 99357 for prolonged inpatient or observation care.
- 90963 through 90966 for services related to home dialysis for patients with end-stage renal disease.

To qualify for Medicare Part B, individuals must meet Medicare's eligibility requirements under one of its beneficiary categories:

- Must meet requirements for Medicare Part A, or
- Must have purchased Medicare Part A

To obtain Medicare Part B, a qualified individual must choose to enroll and pay a monthly premium which is required even if the beneficiary is Medicare Part A eligible. Medicare Part B covers a portion of the cost of physicians' services, outpatient hospital services, certain home health services, durable medical equipment, and other items after the beneficiary pays the yearly deductible, which is $183 in 2017. By law, the standard premium is set to cover one-fourth of the average cost of Part B services incurred by beneficiaries aged 65 and over, plus a contingency margin. The contingency margin is an amount to ensure that Part B has sufficient assets and income to:

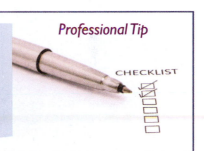

Professional Tip

Medicare Part B also covers diagnostic and emergency department services for inpatients if the beneficiary does not have or has exhausted Part A coverage.

CHECKLIST

- cover Part B expenditures during the year.
- cover incurred-but-unpaid claims costs at the end of the year.
- provide for possible variation between actual and projected costs.
- amortize any surplus assets.

The 2017 standard Part B premium amount is $134 (or higher depending on income). However, most people who get Social Security benefits will pay less than this amount ($109 on average). As required in the Medicare Prescription Drug, Improvement, and Modernization Act of 2003, beginning in 2007 the Part B premium a beneficiary pays each month is based on his or her annual income. Specifically, if a beneficiary's "modified adjusted gross income" is greater than the legislated threshold amounts, the beneficiary is responsible for a larger portion of the estimated total cost of Part B benefit coverage. In addition to the standard Part B premium, affected beneficiaries must pay an income-related monthly adjustment amount.

Medicare Part C

In 1997, Congress created a set of healthcare options known as **Medicare Part C**, or Medicare+Choice, now known as Medicare Advantage plans. These plans offer the same benefits as Medicare Parts A and B. In addition, many of the plans offer benefits for services not covered by the "traditional" Medicare programs, such as hearing aids, dentures, and prescription drugs (Medicare Part D). The scope of additional coverage is based on the individual policy and plan; the individual has the option to choose additional coverage with Medicare Part C, which can include vision, dental, hearing, and health and wellness programs. Most Medicare Advantage plans also include Medicare Part D (prescription coverage).

The following are the types of Medicare Part C plans:

- Health maintenance organization (HMO)
- Competitive medical plan (CMP)
- Point-of-service (POS) option
- Provider sponsored organization (PSO)
- Preferred provider organization (PPO)
- Medical savings account (MSA)
- Fee-for-service (FFS) plan
- Religious fraternal benefit society plan

Medicare Part D

Medicare Part D provides prescription drug coverage to everyone who has Medicare. If Medicare Part D is not purchased at the time of initial enrollment and the enrollee does not have creditable prescription drug coverage or does not have Extra Help, a late penalty will be assigned. The enrollee must pay a premium depending on the coverage chosen. Each Medicare Plan D has a list of drugs, which are called formularies. The plans put these drugs into different tiers of their formularies, which determine the patient's responsibility for their coinsurance. The coinsurance will be higher or lower, depending on the tier drug.

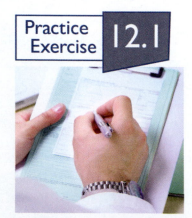

Practice Exercise 12.1

Indicate whether the following statements about Medicare are true or false:

_____ **1.** Medicare is a state health insurance program for the poor and medically indigent.

_____ **2.** Medicare is a federal health insurance program for the elderly, people with disabilities, and ESRD patients.

_____ **3.** Medicare is a health insurance program enacted by Congress in 1965 that today serves more than 55 million elderly Americans and people with disabilities.

_____ **4.** Medicare is a federal health insurance program created to alleviate the unpredictable and uneven costs associated with medical care for the elderly, people with disabilities, and ESRD patients.

(Program of All-Inclusive Care for the Elderly) PACE is a joint Medicare–Medicaid program that gives the patient the Medicare drug plan. There is no need to apply for Medicare Part D if the patient has PACE. The patient will be disenrolled from PACE upon applying for Medicare Part D. To qualify for the Extra Help benefit, a person must be receiving Medicare, have limited resources and income, and reside in one of the 50 states or the District of Columbia.

Services Not Covered by Medicare Parts A and B

Medicare doesn't cover everything. Items and services that are not covered include, but are not limited to, the following:

- Acupuncture
- Deductibles, coinsurance, or copayments when a beneficiary receives health-care services
- Dental care and dentures (with only a few exceptions)
- Cosmetic surgery
- Custodial care (help with bathing, dressing, using the bathroom, and eating) at home or in a nursing home
- Eye refractions
- First 3 pints of blood if they cannot be replaced in some manner
- Healthcare received while traveling outside of the United States
- Hearing aids and hearing exams for the purpose of fitting a hearing aid
- Hearing tests (other than for fitting a hearing aid) that have not been ordered by a physician
- Long-term care, such as custodial care in a nursing home
- Orthopedic shoes (with only a few exceptions)
- Prescription drugs
- Private-duty nursing care
- Routine foot care such as cutting of corns or calluses (with only a few exceptions)
- Routine eye care and most eyeglasses

There are exceptions to the rules on Medicare Part A and Part B covered services. Items and services that are covered include the following:

- Services provided in Canada when the beneficiary travels between Alaska and another state while on board a ship in U.S. territorial waters
- One pair of eyeglasses with standard frames after cataract surgery that includes implanting an intraocular lens
- A one-time physical exam within the first 6 months of receiving Part B benefits and once every 12 months
- Tests such as bone mass measurements once every 24 months, or more if medically necessary; cardiovascular screenings every 5 years to test cholesterol, lipid, and triglyceride levels; colorectal cancer screenings (screening colonoscopy) once every 120 months unless patient is at high risk, in which case every 24 months; diabetes screening up to two screenings every year based on history and test results; Pap test and pelvic exam every 24 months except for women at high risk, in which case every 12 months; prostate

screening once every 12 months for the prostate-specific antigen (PSA) test; and mammograms once every 12 months

■ Pneumococcal vaccinations, hepatitis B shots, and flu shots. Hepatitis shots are covered for patients with high or medium risk for hepatitis B, such as a patient with hemophilia, ESRD, or a condition that lowers resistance to infection

■ Syringes or insulin, unless the insulin is used with an insulin pump or the patient has Medicare Part D

Medigap, Medicaid, and Supplemental Insurance

A Medicare beneficiary may obtain additional coverage to pay for any parts of a claim not covered by Medicare. In these cases, Medicare is always primary for Medigap and Medicaid.

Medigap is a privately offered, supplemental health insurance policy designed to provide additional coverage for services that Medicare does not pay for. It also helps to satisfy deductibles or any coinsurance payments. Medigap is not available to patients enrolled in HMOs.

Be aware that not all Medicare supplemental insurance is Medigap. Only certain insurance companies are authorized to offer Medigap insurance to Medicare beneficiaries. The Medigap policies offered by these companies are regulated by Medicare law. When a Medicare beneficiary has elected to purchase a Medigap policy, Medicare must be informed that the beneficiary wishes to have his claims information sent to a Medigap insurer. The notification is made by the information provided on the claim. The reassignment of the gaps in coverage is called **crossover** and eliminates the need for the beneficiary to file a separate claim with his Medigap insurer. To enable the crossover process, beneficiaries must sign a release-of-information/assignment of benefits form with each of their providers. This authorization is kept in the patient's medical file. An authorization for payment to the participating provider must be signed by the patient for the physician to receive direct payment from the secondary payer. If the provider is not accepting assignment, the Medicare payment will be sent directly to the patient. An Advance Beneficiary Notice should be given to the patient if the provider believes that Medicare may deny the service. If this is on file, the patient is responsible for the payment for the service; if not on file, the patient is not responsible.

Medicaid is a federally and state-funded program through which certain categories of the United States's population that falls under the eligibility level of 133% of the federal poverty level under age 65 and individuals with disabilities are entitled to medical and health-related benefits. The federal government provides broad guidelines for eligibility, but it allows each state to do the following:

■ Dictate more defined eligibility standards
■ Determine the coverage of services
■ Set rates of payment
■ Administer the program

MediMedi is Medicare Medicaid coverage. Medicare is always primary with Medicaid being the payer of last resort. If the patient has any additional coverage, Medicaid will always be secondary. Medicaid is discussed in detail in Chapter 13.

Requirements for Medical Necessity

For a service to be considered medically necessary, the following criteria must be met:

- Matches the diagnosis
- Is not an elective procedure
- Is not an experimental or investigational procedure
- Is an essential treatment—that is, not performed for the patient's convenience
- Is delivered at the most appropriate level that can be safely and effectively administered to the patient

Medicare Coverage Plans

Medicare beneficiaries may receive benefits in two ways:

1. *Fee-for-service benefits:* Benefits that require patients to pay a deductible (if not previously met) and any applicable coinsurance each time a service is rendered. Patients are also responsible for paying non-covered services (program exclusion), or any items for which they signed an advance beneficiary notice (ABN).
2. *Managed care plan:* A plan in which the beneficiaries prepay a set amount (usually a copayment) for items or services provided by physicians or other healthcare providers. Most managed care programs today are run by HMOs, although some are also competitive medical plans.

Fee-for-Service: The Original Medicare Plan

The type of insurance coverage offered under the original Medicare plan was a fee-for-service plan. A fee-for-service plan is a method of reimbursement that paid the provider her standard charge for each procedure. Medicare uses the *resource-based relative value scale* (RBRVS) reimbursement method to determine its fees for service. This plan pays 80% of the Medicare fee.

Medicare Advantage Plans or Medicare Part C

Medicare Advantage plans (Medicare Part C) are health plan options that are part of the Medicare program. Except in emergencies, beneficiaries who choose a managed care plan typically receive all of their care from the doctors, hospitals, and other healthcare providers who are a part of that plan. This coverage includes prescription drug coverage. Medicare pays a set amount of money every month to these private health plans for the care of plan enrollees whether the services are rendered or not. Most of these plans generally provide extra benefits and have lower copayments than the original fee-for-service Medicare plan.

The types of Medicare Advantage plans include HMOs and PPOS. In an HMO, patients must choose a primary care physician (PCP) and usually pay a copayment at each visit. A primary care physician is the medical provider chosen by an insured or subscriber to provide initial medical care before seeing a specialist. Patients also have the choice of receiving services from providers outside the network for an additional fee.

In a PPO, patients are given a financial incentive to use doctors within a network but may choose to go outside the network. Visits outside the network incur additional costs that may include a higher copayment or coinsurance. The following are the two types of PPOs:

1. Local PPOs that serve individual counties
2. Regional PPOs that serve an entire region, which may be a single state or multistate area. In a regional PPO, members have added protection for Medicare Part A and Medicare Part B benefits. They have an annual limit on their out-of-pocket costs; the limit varies depending on the plan

Value-Based Payment Modifier Program

The **value-based payment (VBP)** modifier program competitively rates Medicare Part B professionals on quality measures to determine upward or downward payment adjustments to their reimbursements. Part A hospital and Part C Medicare Advantage payments are not impacted by VBP. CMS developed the value-based payment program in an effort to move physician reimbursement toward a system that rewards value rather than volume. It rewards high-performing providers with increased payments and reduces payments to low-performing providers. The value modifier uses **Physician Quality Reporting System (PQRS)** quality data and Medicare cost data to determine a provider's overall value score. The Physician Value-Based Payment Modifier adjusts a group practice's or solo practitioner's MPFS payments during a given year based on performance on specific quality and efficiency measures 2 years earlier. According to the Patient Protection and Affordable Care Act, the modifier must be applied to all physicians and physician groups by January 1, 2017.

Medicare Providers

A healthcare person or organization that supplies beneficiaries with healthcare services and products is called a *provider*. A participating provider is a physician or an organization that agrees to provide medical service to a payer's policyholders according to the terms of a contract. All providers (regardless of participation) must file claims on behalf of Medicare patients; however, not all physicians have to be participating providers in the Medicare program.

Part A Providers

Part A providers are healthcare facilities such as hospitals, skilled nursing facilities, nursing homes, and others.

All Part A providers must become certified with Medicare to be able to provide services to Medicare patients. Part A provider certification occurs through formal inspections by state agencies that verify whether or not a healthcare facility has the appropriate staff, equipment, facility, and medical licensing to perform quality medical services for Medicare patients.

Part B Providers

Part B providers are physicians, nonphysician practitioners, or suppliers who have agreed with Medicare to supply services for their Medicare patients and accept the Medicare fee as payment in full. The Medicare fee includes the amount paid by the patient and the amount paid to the provider by Medicare. Physicians who are not using EHR (electronic health records) will be penalized in their reimbursement: 1% in 2015, 2% in 2016, 3% in 2017, and 4% in 2018.

Physician

For Medicare purposes, a physician is a doctor of medicine or osteopathy, dental medicine, dental surgery, podiatric medicine, optometry, or chiropractic medicine legally authorized to practice by the state in which he performs. The **Tax Relief and Health Care Act (TRHCA)** of 2006 authorized the establishment of a physician quality reporting system by CMS. The Physician Quality Reporting Initiative (PQRI) establishes a financial incentive for eli-

gible professionals to participate in a voluntary quality reporting program. No registration or enrollment is required to participate. Those who successfully report a designated set of quality measures on claims may earn a 1.5% bonus, subject to a cap.

Nonphysician Practitioner

A nonphysician practitioner includes, but is not limited to, an anesthesia assistant, an independent billing psychologist, an independent billing audiologist, a certified clinical nurse specialist, a family nurse practitioner, a clinical psychologist, a certified registered nurse practitioner, and a licensed clinical social worker.

Supplier

Suppliers include, but are not limited to, organizations such as a screening mammography center, an ambulance service supplier, a portable X-ray supplier, an independent diagnostic testing facility, and an independent laboratory.

Participating versus Nonparticipating Medicare Part B Providers

A nonparticipating provider is a physician who chooses not to participate in a Medicare plan. A nonparticipating provider can treat Medicare patients and choose to accept assignment or not accept assignment.

Accepting assignment refers to a provider who has agreed to accept the allowed charge of a rendered service as payment in full. *Not accepting assignment* refers to a provider who will not accept the allowed charge as payment in full.

When the provider does not accept assignment, the payment will be sent directly to the patient. The medical office specialist should collect payment at the time of service.

A participating provider is a physician who contracts with Medicare to provide treatment for beneficiaries of Medicare Part B. Medicare participating providers receive benefits that nonparticipating providers do not. These benefits include the following:

- Timely reimbursement comes directly from Medicare rather than from the patient.
- Reimbursement is 5% higher than for the nonparticipating provider.

- Medigap insurance automatically crosses over (if the requirements for cross-over are met).
- Access is provided to beneficiary eligibility information.

If a nonparticipating provider accepts assignment, then she:

- Must still file all Medicare claims on behalf of Medicare patients.
- Accepts a 5% lower fee allowances for services.
- Understands that Medigap/supplemental insurance does not automatically cross over.
- Does not have access to beneficiary eligibility information.

Part B providers who choose not to participate and not to accept assignment may charge a limiting charge, as discussed next.

Limiting Charge

Physicians who are not participating and not accepting assignment may charge a limiting charge. The **limiting charge** is 115% more than the nonparticipating provider's Medicare Fee Schedule (MFS). To calculate this number, take the **non-par MFS** and multiply it by 115%. The limiting charge does not apply to immunizations, supplies, or ambulance service.

The Medicare Comprehensive Limiting Charge Compliance Program was created to prevent nonparticipating physicians from collecting the balance from Medicare patients. Physicians who collect amounts in excess of the limiting charge are subject to financial penalties.

Patient's Financial Responsibility

Patients who choose the fee for service benefits can choose their providers. The amount due by patients will depend on what type of provider they choose.

1. *Par Provider Accepting Assignment:* Patient pays 20% of the Medicare Fee Schedule after the deductible has been met.
2. *Non-Par Provider Accepting Assignment:* Patient pays 20% of the Non-Par Medicare Fee Schedule after the deductible has been met.
3. *Non-Par Provider, Not Accepting Assignment:* Patient is responsible for the limiting charge. The patient will only be reimbursed by Medicare at 80% of the Non-Par Medicare Fee Schedule. Patient out-of-pocket expense will be the difference between the limiting charge and the reimbursement of 80% of the Nonparticipating Fee. The payment will be made directly to the patient.

Determining the Medicare Fee and Limiting Charge

Complete Practice Exercises 12.2, 12.3, 12.4, and 12.5 to determine the amount owed by the patient to a participating provider, a nonparticipating provider who accepts assignment, and a nonparticipating provider who does not accept assignment.

Determine the amount owed by the patient after deductible has been met in the following situations:

Participating Provider:

Physician's standard fee: $175.00
Medicare fee: $140.00

1. Medicare pays 80%:   _____
2. Patient or supplemental plan pays 20%:   _____
3. Provider adjustment (write-off):   _____

Nonparticipating Provider Accepting Assignment:

Physician's standard fee: $175
Medicare fee: $140

1. Medicare non-par fee: _____
2. Medicare pays 80%:   _____
3. Patient or supplemental plan pays 20%:   _____
4. Provider adjustment (write-off):   _____

Nonparticipating Provider Not Accepting Assignment:

Physician's standard fee: $175
Medicare fee: $140

1. Medicare non-par fee: _____
2. Limiting charge: _____
3. Patient billed: _____
4. Medicare pays patient: _____
5. Total provider can collect: _____
6. Patient out-of-pocket expense: _____

Determine the amount owed by the patient after the deductible has been met in the following situations:

Procedure Code	Physician's Fee	Medicare Fee
99212	$75.00	$38.32

Participating Provider:

1. Physician's standard fee: _____
2. Medicare fee: _____
3. Medicare pays 80%:   _____

(Continued)

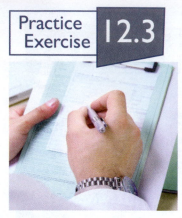

Practice Exercise 12.3

(*Continued*)

4. Patient or supplemental plan pays 20%: _____
5. Provider adjustment (write-off): _____

Nonparticipating Provider Accepting Assignment:

1. Physician's standard fee: _____
2. Medicare non-par fee: _____
3. Medicare pays 80%: _____
4. Patient or supplemental plan pays 20%: _____
5. Provider adjustment (write-off): _____

Nonparticipating Provider Not Accepting Assignment:

1. Physician's standard fee: _____
2. Medicare non-par fee: _____
3. Limiting charge: _____
4. Patient billed: _____
5. Medicare pays patient: _____
6. Total provider can collect: _____
7. Patient out-of-pocket expense: _____
8. Patient out-of-pocket with Medigap: _____
9. Provider adjustment: _____

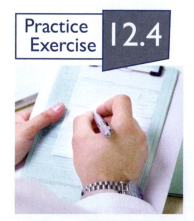

Practice Exercise 12.4

Determine the amount owed by the patient after the deductible has been met in the following situations:

Procedure Code	Physician's Fee	Medicare Fee
99213	$100.00	$52.12

Participating Provider:

1. Physician's standard fee: _____
2. Medicare fee: _____
3. Medicare pays 80%: _____
4. Patient or supplemental plan pays 20%: _____
5. Provider adjustment (write-off): _____

Nonparticipating Provider Accepting Assignment:

1. Physician's standard fee: _____
2. Medicare non-par fee: _____
3. Medicare pays 80%: _____
4. Patient or supplemental plan pays 20%: _____
5. Provider adjustment (write-off): _____

Nonparticipating Provider Not Accepting Assignment:

1. Physician's standard fee: _____
2. Medicare non-par fee: _____
3. Limiting charge: _____
4. Patient billed: _____
5. Medicare pays patient: _____
6. Total provider can collect: _____
7. Provider adjustment (write-off):   _____

Practice Exercise 12.4

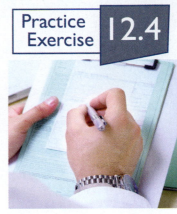

(Continued)

Determine the amount owed by the patient after the deductible has been met in the following situations:

Procedure Code	Physician's Fee	Medicare Fee
99203	$150.00	$95.75

Practice Exercise 12.5

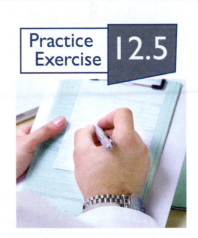

Participating Provider:

1. Physician's standard fee: _____
2. Medicare fee: _____
3. Medicare pays 80%:   _____
4. Patient or supplemental plan pays 20%: _____
5. Provider adjustment (write-off):   _____

Nonparticipating Provider Accepting Assignment:

1. Physician's standard fee: _____
2. Medicare non-par fee: _____
3. Medicare pays 80%:   _____
4. Patient or supplemental plan pays 20%: _____
5. Provider adjustment (write-off):   _____

Nonparticipating Provider Not Accepting Assignment:

1. Physician's standard fee: _____
2. Medicare non-par fee: _____
3. Limiting charge: _____
4. Patient billed: _____
5. Medicare pays patient: _____
6. Total provider can collect: _____
7. Provider adjustment (write-off):   _____

Patient Registration

The medical office specialist should check patients' Medicare eligibility at each visit. For a medical office specialist who receives initial patient information, four major tasks are vital to the efficiency and financial welfare of the healthcare organization:

1. Copying the Medicare card
2. Copying the driver's license
3. Obtaining essential patient information through the use and completion of medical information/history and insurance forms
4. Determining if Medicare is the primary or secondary insurance

Copying the Medicare Card

The Medicare enrollee receives a health insurance card (Figure 12.1). It is very important for the medical office specialist to obtain a copy of the beneficiary's card during a patient's first visit with the facility. Medicare also recommends that the beneficiary's insurance information be verified periodically to determine if any changes have occurred. If changes have occurred, patient records should be updated accordingly.

The pieces of information to record from the patient's card are as follows:

■ Exact name
■ Claim number, including all numbers and letters
■ Type of coverage
■ Effective dates of coverage for Part A and Part B

Recording the information from the Medicare card accurately is extremely important because that information will be used on many claims forms and medical documentation materials throughout the patient's history with the facility. The need for recording

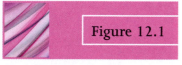

Figure 12.1

Medicare card.

Medicare.gov

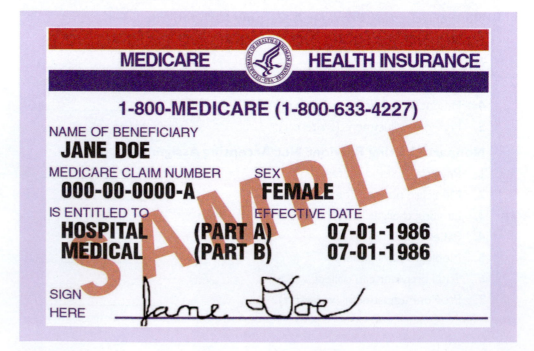

MEDICARE   HEALTH INSURANCE

1-800-MEDICARE (1-800-633-4227)

NAME OF BENEFICIARY
JANE DOE
MEDICARE CLAIM NUMBER   SEX
000-00-0000-A   **FEMALE**
IS ENTITLED TO   EFFECTIVE DATE
HOSPITAL   (PART A)   07-01-1986
MEDICAL   (PART B)   07-01-1986

SIGN
HERE   _Jane Doe_

the information exactly as it appears on the card even extends to misspelling the patient's name in the computer if it is misspelled on the Medicare card! It is the patient's responsibility to call Medicare and have any misspelling corrected.

If the medical office specialist makes a mistake when recording information from the Medicare card, these mistakes can carry over to Medicare claims forms, causing claim rejections, delays in processing, and even denials. These mistakes cause more work and can be quite costly for the practice.

Eligibility and verification of benefits can be done online. This can be done individually and also if there are multiple patients to verify in a batch. The medical office specialist also calls and verifies through the Interactive Voice Response (IVR) system, which is a self-service tool that allows providers to quickly and easily access most Medicare information. This makes it easy for the medical office specialist to keep a record of verification at the time of each visit.

Copying the Driver's License

Another important practice to incorporate during patient screening is to validate the person's identity. Identity theft is a crime that includes identity theft and identity fraud. Both are considered crimes when someone wrongfully obtained and used another person's personal data in some way that involved fraud or deception, typically for economic gain.

Validating the patient's identity by copying the driver's license photo I.D. and maintaining a copy on file will allow the office to ensure that the patient is not a victim of identity theft or participating in an identity scam in some way. Validation of the patient's identity will also provide the office with valuable information in the event that multiple patients have the same or a similar name. The photo I.D. on file can assist the insurance specialist in making sure that an incorrect patient's records are not pulled in error.

Obtaining Patient Signatures

Having the appropriate patient signatures on Medicare claim forms or on file is essential. Rather than have patients sign each time a claim is processed, Medicare provides a document that patients can sign and which lasts a lifetime: the Lifetime Beneficiary and Claim Authorization Form. A facility may use its own form to obtain authorization for release of information and payments. When the Medicare claim is submitted, the signature of the patient or the signature on file (SOF) must be noted on form locator 12. If the patient has Medigap coverage, the signature or SOF must be noted on form locator 13 in order for the provider to receive payment instead of the patient. If the provider is nonparticipating, the Medigap payment will always be paid directly to the patient.

The UB-04/CMS-1450 and CMS-1500 claims forms are good references to use for developing a release-of-information form for the office. The information on the release-of-information form should at least encompass the information necessary to fill out the Medicare claims forms correctly.

Determining Primary and Secondary Payers

When registering a hospital patient, the medical office specialist will be required to have the patient complete a Medicare questionnaire similar to that shown in Appendix D.

A patient can be covered by a wide range of insurance plans in addition to Medicare. In cases where a patient has additional coverage, Medicare may be considered the secondary payer and the additional insurance carrier the primary payer.

You should ask patients some specific questions to ensure that you have obtained complete and correct information about their insurance coverage:

1. Is your injury/illness due to:
   - A work-related accident or condition?
   - A condition covered under the federal Black Lung Program?
   - An automobile accident?
   - An accident other than an automobile accident?
   - The fault of another party?
2. Are you eligible for coverage under the Veterans Administration?
3. Are you employed?
   - Do you have coverage under an employer group health insurance plan?
4. Is your spouse employed?
   - Do you have coverage under the group health insurance plan of your spouse's employer?
5. Are you a dependent covered under a parent or guardian's employer group health plan?

The preceding questions will help the medical office specialist determine if the beneficiary is:
   - Covered under another policy or government program.
   - Potentially eligible for coverage by a different insurer because of an accident or injury that makes a third party liable for medical expenses.
   - Eligible for coverage of all expenses over the amount that Medicare covers.

6. Have you had outpatient or emergency department services in the last 3 days? This question is asked to determine if any outpatient charges occurred within the last 3 days before an inpatient admission (72 hours). This is called the *72-hour rule* (also the *3-day payment window rule*). The Medicare rule states that if a patient receives diagnostic tests and hospital outpatient services within 72 hours of admission to a hospital, then all such tests and services are combined with inpatient services. The preadmission services become part of the MS-DRG payment to the hospital and may not be billed or paid separately.
7. Do you currently reside in a nursing home? If the patient answers yes, list the name of the nursing home.
8. Has the patient given up his Medicare and replaced it with an HMO? If yes, the HMO is primary. If no, the HMO is secondary.

Plans Primary to Medicare

When an individual is employed and receives coverage through the employer's group health plan, Medicare is the secondary payer. Medicare is also the secondary payer when an individual age 65 or older receives coverage through a spouse's employer (the spouse does not have to be 65 or older).

Medicare is the primary payer for individuals 65 or older:

- Who are working for an employer with 20 employees or fewer.
- Who are covered by another policy that is not a group policy.
- Who are enrolled in Part B, but not Part A, of the Medicare program.
- Who must pay premiums to receive Part A coverage.
- Who are retired and receiving coverage under a group policy from a previous employer.
- Who are retired and receiving coverage under a group policy from a previous employer.
- Who are receiving coverage under COBRA.

Consolidated Omnibus Budget Reconciliation Act of 1985

The **Consolidated Omnibus Budget Reconciliation Act of 1985 (COBRA)** requires employers to allow employees, their spouses, and their dependents to continue group health insurance coverage for a minimum of 18 months after their employment ends. The employee pays premiums without any contribution from the employer. COBRA is primary to Medicare.

People with Disabilities

If an individual has a disability, is under age 65, and receives coverage through an employer's group health plan (which may be held by the individual, a spouse, or another family member), Medicare is the secondary payer. If the individual or family member is not actively employed, Medicare is the primary payer.

People with End-Stage Renal Disease

During a coordination of benefits period (currently 30 months), Medicare is the secondary payer for individuals with ESRD who receive coverage through an employer-sponsored group health plan and who fail to apply for ESRD-based Medicare coverage. The coordination of benefits period begins the first month the individual is eligible for or entitled to Part A benefits based on an ESRD diagnosis. This rule is in effect regardless of whether the individual is employed or retired.

Workers' Compensation

If an individual is receiving treatment for a work-related job injury, Medicare is not filed. The workers' compensation claim is paid in full for the allowed amount for that injury only by the employer's workers' compensation carrier.

Automobile, No-Fault, and Liability Insurance

Medicare is always the secondary payer when treatment is for an accident-related claim. Medicare is not responsible for any payment until the patient has reached her maximum allowed benefits from the primary payer. In that case, a copy of the letter of denial is sent to Medicare with the claim.

Veteran Benefits

If a veteran is entitled to Medicare benefits, he may choose whether to receive coverage through Medicare or through the Veterans Benefits Administration.

Medicare Coordination

Information on eligibility and benefits entitlement can be obtained from the Coordination of Benefits (COB) Central File Contractor. This is a service that is used to facilitate accurate payment. The COB contractor is not affiliated with the local Medicare carrier or

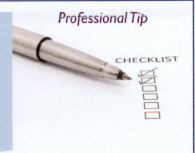

Professional Tip

All Medicare secondary payer (MSP) inquiries, including the reporting of potential MSP situations, changes in a beneficiary's insurance coverage, changes in employment, and general MSP questions or concerns, should be directed to the COB contractor. The toll free number is 800-999-1118.

CHECKLIST

intermediary. The COB contractor will provide customer service to all callers from any source, including but not limited to beneficiaries, attorneys, or other beneficiary representatives, employers, insurers, providers, and suppliers.

When contacting the COB contractor, have the following information available:

- Patient's name
- Patient's Medicare or Social Security number
- Date of incident
- Date of illness
- Name and address of the other insurance
- Name of injured
- Policy/claim number
- Medicare provider number

Medicare as the Secondary Payer

When Medicare is clearly the secondary payer, the provider's organization needs to follow certain steps when submitting the claim. The medical office specialist must complete the required form locator fields in the computer, and the claim will be processed without any attachment. Medicare does not require the primary insurance remittance notice when submitting **Medicare Secondary Payer (MSP)** claims electronically. The medical office specialist will need to keep the remittance notice on file and make it available to Medicare on request. The fields that need to be completed are these:

1. The primary insurance allowed amount (form locator 28)
2. The primary insurance paid amount (form locator 29)
3. The Obligated to Accept as Payment in Full (OTAF) amount, if any (form locator 30)

Medicare will no longer accept paper attachments.

Conditional Payment

In liability cases where the beneficiary's medical expenses may be covered by a third party's insurance, the provider has a choice of actions. These choices include the following:

1. *Bill the insurer:* The provider can bill the liability insurer directly. If it is determined that the primary payer will not pay promptly (within 120 days after billing the liability insurer), the provider may file a claim with Medicare for conditional primary payment. If a Medicare conditional payment is made, providers or suppliers may no longer bill the primary insurer or the beneficiary for services that were covered by the Medicare conditional payment. They may only bill the beneficiary for applicable Medicare deductibles and coinsurance.
2. *File a lien:* When the patient sues the liability insurer for damages, the provider may file a lien against the settlement proceeds of the liability case. If it is determined that the primary payer will not pay promptly (within 120 days after billing the liability insurer), the provider may file a claim with Medicare for conditional primary payment. If a Medicare conditional payment is made, the provider or supplier may no longer bill the primary insurer or the beneficiary for services that were covered

by the Medicare conditional payment. They may only bill the beneficiary for applicable Medicare deductibles and coinsurance.

Medicare Documents

As discussed, some Medicare documents need to be signed by the insured. The documents that require the insured's signature—the Advance Beneficiary Notice and the Lifetime Beneficiary Claim Authorization and Information Release (lifetime release form)—can be copied from the Medicare website, which ensures that the documents are worded correctly.

The Advance Beneficiary Notice (ABN) is proof that the office has given patients notice that the services about to be provided may not be covered by Medicare because they are not medically reasonable or necessary, and that the patient is responsible for the charges. If a procedure, service, or supply that the patient is receiving is questionable as to its coverage under Medicare, an ABN form should be given to the patient to sign before services are rendered. An ABN should also be given to the patient before receiving a non-covered or excluded service. Use this link to obtain the updated form, CMS-R-131: www.cms.gov/BNI/02_ABN.asp#TopOfPage.

For Medicare to determine if the patient has been notified in advance that she will be responsible for payment, a GA modifier is used with the procedure. This is defined to mean "Waiver of Liability Statement Issued as Required by Payer Policy" and should be used when a required ABN was issued for a service. The GZ modifier is defined as "Waiver of Liability Issued Voluntarily under the Payer's Policy" and is used to report when a voluntary ABN was given to report a service. If the provider chooses to make an ABN, rather than use the one from the Medicare website, the notice must include the following information:

- The patient's name
- Date(s)
- Description of item or service
- Reason(s) why the item or service may not be considered medically necessary

Refer to the ABN in Appendix D. An ABN notice must be signed and dated by the patient each time an item is given or service is rendered that may not be deemed "medically necessary." In contrast, a lifetime release form is signed once by the patient and filed in her record.

Medicare Development Letter

A **Medicare Development Letter** is sent from Medicare to a provider when a claim is filed that needs additional information or documentation. These letters usually detail what information is necessary in order for Medicare to resume processing a specific claim or claims. The medical office specialist may be responsible for gathering and sending the information that Medicare requests. A time limit is usually placed on return of the requested information. If the additional information is not sent to Medicare within the time frame communicated in the development letter, the services at issue will be denied payment by Medicare.

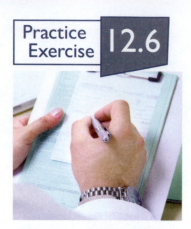

Practice Exercise 12.6

Indicate whether the following statements about Medicare are true or false:

_____ 1. The Advance Beneficiary Notice is a notice from Medicare that a claim submitted by a provider organization cannot be processed without additional information and/or documentation.

_____ 2. A Medicare Development Letter is sent to a provider when a claim is filed that needs additional information or documentation. There is no time limit on responding, but a claim may be denied if the wrong information is sent.

_____ 3. The Advance Beneficiary Notice must include the patient's name, date(s), a description of the item or service provided, and the reason(s) why the item or service may not be considered medically necessary.

Medicare Insurance Billing Requirements

The **Healthcare Common Procedure Coding System (HCPCS)** is used to report procedures and services for Medicare patients. This system is also used to report services for Medicaid patients. HCPCS is divided into two principal subsystems, referred to as Level I and Level II of HCPCS. Level I of HCPCS is comprised of the Current Procedural Terminology (CPT), a numeric coding system maintained by the American Medical Association (AMA).

Level II of HCPCS is a standardized coding system that is used primarily to identify products, supplies, and services not included in the CPT codes, such as ambulance services and durable medical equipment, prosthetics, orthotics, and supplies (DMEPOS) when used outside a physician's office. Because Medicare and other insurers cover a variety of services, supplies, and equipment that are not identified by CPT codes, the Level II HCPCS codes were established for submitting claims for these items. Level II codes are referred to as alphanumeric codes because they consist of a single alphabetical letter followed by four numeric digits, whereas CPT codes are identified using five numeric digits.

The Health Insurance Portability and Accountability Act (HIPAA) Transaction and Code Set Rule requires providers to use the medical code set that is valid at the time that the service is provided.

Completing Medicare Part B Claims

Providers are required by law to submit electronically all Medicare claims for services performed on Medicare beneficiaries. The CMS-1500 claim form is used to file Medicare Part B claims. A paper CMS-1500 claim form can be used to bill Medicare carriers when a provider qualifies for a waiver from the Administration Simplification

Compliance Act (ASCA) requirement for electronic submission of claims. The medical office specialist should check the electronic billing address, or the payer I.D., for the region under which to bill. These addresses are numbers that must be entered under Medicare in the medical practice software system for billing. Every carrier has a specific electronic "billing address." Electronic claims clearinghouses were devised by Medicare and the insurance companies to prescreen for claim errors and act as controllers of electronic claim transmittal.

The following is an example of a payer I.D.:

> 04102   MEDICARE B COLORADO x x 4* x Please call 866.749.4302 for Electronic Data Interchange (EDI) enrollment.
>
> 09102   MEDICARE B FLORIDA x x x 4* x
>
> 05130   MEDICARE B IDAHO x x x 4* x
>
> 00952   MEDICARE B ILLINOIS x x x 4* x Contact 877.567.7261 to enroll in EDI. The Availity Assigned Submitter ID is 70000
>
> 00953   MEDICARE B MICHIGAN x x 4* x Contact 877.567.7261 to enroll in EDI. The Availity Assigned Submitter ID is 70000

The billing software on the medical office specialist's desktop creates the electronic file (electronic claim), which is then sent by uploading to the clearinghouse account. The clearinghouse then scrubs the claim, checking it for errors.

There are two components in **scrubbing** claims. As the most common error for denied claims is data entry errors, the patient demographic data are reviewed for the most common mistakes. For instance, keying in an incorrect procedure code that is age specific would make the claim invalid, and the scrubber flags those types of errors for correction before submission. This is the easy part of the automation.

The complicated portion of scrubbing involves a thorough review of the codes and modifiers to ensure complicity with specific guidelines. This is commonly referred to as the *rules engine*. In some fashion, every data element of the claim is analyzed. If a physician submits a claim for a hysterectomy and the scrubber sees a male gender, obviously the claim will be flagged. The scrubber verifies that a procedure performed is associated with a diagnosis code that justifies the medical necessity of that procedure along with variables such as gender, age, date and place of service, and any required modifiers.

The complexity of scrubbing should not be underestimated. By the time one multiplies the total number of local and national Medicare coverage determinations, along with data from the Correct Coding Initiative (CCI), ICD-10-CM codes, and modifiers, the potential number of editable combinations surpasses 10 million. Once the claim is accepted, the clearinghouse securely transmits the electronic file to Medicare, with which it has established a secure connection that meets the strict HIPAA 5010 standards. HIPAA x12 standards version 5010 is a new standard that regulates the electronic transmission of specific healthcare entities. The American National Standards Institute (ANSI) implementation guides

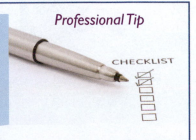

Professional Tip

Always make sure that the ICD-10-CM codes used are the most recent, up-to-date codes used to avoid denials. Codes used should be coded to the highest level of specificity.

CHECKLIST

have been established as the standards for all services, supplies, equipment, and health-care claims other than pharmacy retail prescription drugs. Submission 5010 has replaced the ANSI X 12N version 4010 for electronic data interchange (EDI). As of January 1, 2012, all software programs for electronic submissions were to be formatted to adapt to the 5010 version that accommodates ICD-10.

Filing Guidelines

The rules and regulations for Medicare claims are complex. The medical office specialist must be familiar with the rules and regulations for the provider's Medicare carrier. For instance, a medical necessity claim can be denied if it is billed too often during the allowed time period.

Local Coverage Determination

Local Coverage Determinations (LCDs) are notices sent to physicians on a regular basis that contain detailed and updated information about the coding and medical necessity of a specific service.

Medicare Remittance Notice

If the Medicare claims processing computer determines that payment is due on a claim, the beneficiary or provider will receive payment in approximately 14 days for electronic claims. Every 30 days, the Medicare contractor (carrier) sends Medicare patients a **Medicare Summary Notice (MSN)** itemizing what services were billed to Medicare by the provider, the amount Medicare paid, and the amount the beneficiary is responsible for paying the provider, if any.

Providers will receive a **Medicare Remittance Notice (MRN)** or an **Electronic Remittance Advice (ERA)** from a Medicare contractor on assigned claims. A Medicare Remittance Notice is received electronically. It informs the provider what payment he will receive, what adjustments were made, and what the patient owes. It will also notify the provider if the claim has been forwarded to a Medigap payer.

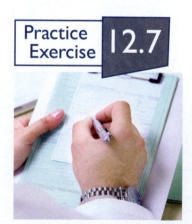

Practice Exercise 12.7

Complete a Medicare claim based on the information provided below. To complete this exercise, copy the CMS-1500 form provided in Appendix D or download the CMS-1500 form from MyHealthProfessionsKit or MyHealthProfessionsLab, which accompany this text.

Physician Information:

Physician Name:	Mallard and Associates, P.A.
	J. D. Mallard, M.D.
License Number:	TX54308
Address:	19333 Forrest Haven
	Owingsville, KY 12345–2222
Phone Number:	613-555-5040

Group Identification Numbers:

Group NPI:	7777788888
Referring Physician:	William F. Bonner, M.D.

Dr. William F. Bonner Identification Numbers

NPI: 11111199999

Dr. J. D. Mallard Identification Numbers

EIN: 72-5727222
NPI: 8888877777

Patient Information Form:

Name: Your Name
                                              1884 Dallas Way
                                              Preston, KY 12345
Phone Number: 972-555-4572
DOB: 06-25-44
Sex: Female, Single
Patient Account Number: Your Name (first three letters of your last
                                              name and first two letters of your first name)
Employer: Allied Health Corporation
Insurance Carrier: Medicare
Payer I.D.:   04001
Insurance I.D. number: 145-87-5988A

Patient Encounter Form:

Date: Today's date
Date of first symptoms: Two days ago
CC: Patient complaining of Left Lower Quadrant
                                              Abdominal Pain, ICD-10-CM (R10.32)
Lungs: Normal
Heart: Normal
Abdomen: Normal
Pelvic: Normal
Chest X-ray: 2 Views—Normal
ECG: Normal
DX: LLQ Abdominal Pain;
ICD-   ICD-10-CM (R10.32)

List of Fees for Services:

Date: Today's date
DX: Left Lower Quadrant Pain: ICD-10-CM
                                              (R10.32); Essential Primary Hypertension:
                                              ICD-10-CM (I10)
99203:   Expanded problem-focused history, exami-
                                              nation, and MDM of low complexity—$80
Diagnosis: ICD-10-CM (R10.32)
71020:   Radiological Exam, chest, frontal and
                                              lateral—$75
Diagnosis: ICD-10-CM (R10.32)
93000:   Electrocardiogram, routine ECG with at least
                                              12 leads with interpretation and report $65
Diagnosis: ICD-10-CM (I10)
TOTAL CHARGES: $220

Practice Exercise 12.7

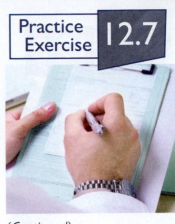

(*Continued*)

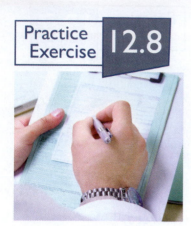

Practice Exercise 12.8

Utilizing the information in Practice Exercise 12.7 along with the following Medigap information, complete a CMS-1500 form for supplemental insurance. Copy the CMS-1500 form provided in Appendix D or download the form from MyHealthProfessionsKit or MyHealthProfessionsLab, which accompany this text.

Medigap:

United Healthcare
123 My Street
Baltimore, MD 21204
MG number 223546721

Medicare Fraud and Abuse

Medicare fraud and abuse affect everybody. Fraud is a ploy to receive unearned reimbursement for services not rendered. The funds come from the taxes that each of us contribute. This in turn leads to increased Medicare premiums and less payment to the provider. As a result, providers choose not to participate in the Medicare programs.

Medicare Fraud

Medicare fraud is defined by CMS as "Knowingly and willfully executing, or attempting to execute a scheme or artifice to defraud any health care benefit program or to obtain, by means of false or fraudulent pretenses, representations, or promises, any of the money or property owned by, or under the custody or control of, any health care benefit program." Figure 12.2 illustrates the four most common types of Medicare fraud.

Inappropriate actions or behaviors against the Medicare program that are identified by the provider but not remedied may be considered fraudulent by Medicare. All healthcare providers who participate in the Medicare program are expected to furnish and report services in accordance with the established regulations and policies.

Fraud Scenarios

The following are examples of fraud scenarios:

- A clinical laboratory receives orders from a physician for specific clinical laboratory tests. The lab performs and bills for the tests indicated on the order, but then also bills for additional tests that were not ordered or rendered.

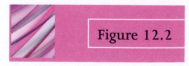

Figure 12.2

The four most common types of Medicare fraud.

1. Billing for services that were not rendered.
2. Misrepresenting as medically necessary any non-covered or screening services by reporting covered procedure/revenue codes.
3. Signing blank records or certification forms or falsifying information on records or certification forms for the sole purpose of obtaining payment.
4. Consistently using procedure/revenue codes that describe more extensive services than those actually performed.

- A patient recruiter convinces unsuspecting beneficiaries to reveal their Medicare numbers to him. The recruiter then sells the Medicare numbers to a fictitious provider who, in turn, bills for services/items that were never furnished. (Providers should ensure that only the services/items they order are furnished.)
- Nursing home patients are offered free exercise and/or social activities. However, the free services are billed to Medicare as covered partial hospitalization services at a community mental health center or as covered physical therapy at a rehabilitation facility.
- A durable medical equipment supplier has a financial arrangement with a physician who completes Certificates of Medical Necessity (CMNs) for patients he has never treated. The completed CMNs are used to falsely document the medical necessity of equipment given to patients who do not need the equipment. A physician unwittingly signs blank certification forms for a home health agency that falsely represents that skilled nursing services are needed for patients who would not have qualified for home health services. (In these two scenarios, both providers are committing Medicare fraud. The durable medical equipment company committed fraud by filing false prescriptions and the physician committed fraud by signing incomplete or blank prescription forms for the purpose of obtaining Medicare payments.)
- A physician routinely bills for high-level E/M services procedure codes although many of the visits she furnishes do not meet the requirements for the codes reported.
- A hospital falsely reports pneumonia as the diagnosis for a majority of the inpatient hospital stays billed to Medicare. As a result, its diagnostic-related group payment was significantly higher than it should have been.

Be aware of other types of Medicare fraud:

- Using an incorrect or invalid provider number in order to be paid or to be paid at a higher rate of reimbursement
- Selling or sharing Medicare health insurance claim numbers so that false Medicare claims can be filed
- Routinely waiving coinsurance and/or deductibles for Medicare patients when no effort has been made to collect the amounts due or when the patient *does* have the ability to pay
- Falsifying information on applications, medical records, billings statements, and/or cost reports, or on any document filed with the government
- Offering, accepting, or soliciting bribes, rebates, or kickbacks

Medicare Abuse

Medicare abuse is legally defined by CMS as "Abuse may, directly or indirectly, result in unnecessary costs to the Medicare or Medicaid program, improper payment for services which fail to meet professionally recognized standards of care, or that are medically unnecessary. . . . Abuse involves payment for items or services when there is no legal entitlement to that payment and the provider has not knowingly and/or intentionally misrepresented facts to obtain payment."

The following are the two common types of Medicare abuse:

- Billing for services/items in excess of those needed by the patient
- Routinely filing duplicate claims, even if doing so does not result in duplicate payment

Abuse Scenarios

The following are examples of Medicare abuse scenarios:

- Laboratory equipment is calibrated to run additional indices with every CBC test. Physician orders may only be for a CBC, but claims filed to Medicare include charges for the CBC and the additional indices. A hospital has a standard protocol that requires all patients admitted through the emergency room to have the following tests performed, regardless of the patient's condition: EKG, chest X-ray, urinalysis, and lab panel. This is abuse; not all patients require these tests.
- A provider's electronic billing program automatically refiles its claims if payment is not received within a 3-week period from the submission date.
- A hospital reports salaries paid to its administrators that have been determined to be excessive in prior cost report settlements.
- An outpatient rehabilitation facility includes non-covered charges in its "allowable costs" section of the cost report.

Protecting Against Medicare Fraud and Abuse

An important aspect of protecting the medical office from Medicare fraud and abuse is knowing when and how the practice may be liable as a provider. Keep the following three points in mind when considering liability:

1. Providers are liable for Medicare fraud when their intent to purposely obtain money or property owned by Medicare through false or fraudulent pretenses has been clearly determined.
2. Providers are liable for Medicare abuse for all claims submitted that violate the Medicare program guidelines.
3. Providers may also be held responsible for fraudulent or abusive claims submitted where they are listed as referring physicians for services performed, such as claims submitted by clinical laboratories.

Provider Liability Cases

Consider the following situations and discussions about provider liability:

- **Q:** An external billing service set up as the payee of the provider (on Medicare's file) commits fraud by billing for additional services not rendered by the provider. Is the provider liable?

  A: The provider would be liable for the Medicare fraud committed by the billing service in this case if his intent to commit fraud had definitely been established by the results of an investigation. If that were the case, the provider would be responsible for returning all overpayments to Medicare and may also be criminally liable.

- **Q:** An employee of a provider commits fraud without the provider knowing it. Is the provider liable?

  A: All providers are responsible for the actions of their employees. Prosecution of the provider in this case for her employee's Medicare fraud is unlikely if the provider's lack of intent has been definitely established by the results of an investigation. The provider will, however, be responsible for returning all overpayments to Medicare.

■ **Q:** A physician refers a patient to another provider for diagnostic tests. The other provider bills medically unnecessary services as covered services for the referred patient. Is the referring physician liable?

A: The referring physician, in this case, is not liable for the other provider's Medicare fraud as long as his referral information concerning the medical necessity of the test is appropriately documented.

■ **Q:** A provider uses incorrect billing procedures when billing Medicare for services that result in overpayment by Medicare. Is the provider liable?

A: Providers are responsible for incorrect billing practices. Providers are expected to correct mistakes and return overpaid monies to Medicare. If providers fail to correct mistakes and return overpaid monies, they may be suspected of fraud.

A provider's actions may be considered fraudulent and the provider would be considered liable in the following situations:

- Claims are submitted that contain mistakes resulting in an overpayment.
- Claims are submitted in which the provider intentionally upcoded charges.
- Claims are submitted that contain mistakes resulting in an overpayment that the provider identifies but does not correct.

The Department of Health and Human Services (HHS or DHHS), which includes CMS and the **Office of Inspector General (OIG)**, has the authority to impose remedial action or administrative sanctions against individuals who consistently fail to comply with Medicare law or are deemed abusive to the Medicare program. Sanctions include the following:

- Provider education and warning
- Revocation of assignment privileges
- Withholding of provider's Medicare payments and recovery of Medicare's overpayments
- Exclusion of provider from the Medicare program
- Posting of provider's name on national Sanctioned Provider list that is sponsored by the U.S. government

The penalties that may be imposed on convicted individuals and/or entities include loss of medical license; criminal penalties, fines, restitution, and/or imprisonment; and civil penalties, plus triple damages.

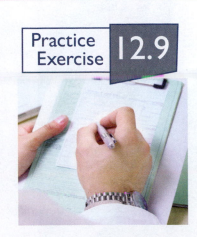

Practice Exercise 12.9

Identify whether each of the providers in the following situations is guilty of upcoding, fraud, or abuse:

1. A radiologist routinely bills for chest X-rays with two views, although most of the chest X-rays performed are for single views.

2. A fictitious provider bills for services that were never furnished.

3. A physician uses a nonphysician practitioner to perform follow-up visits, but bills the practitioner's services as comprehensive initial evaluations.

(Continued)

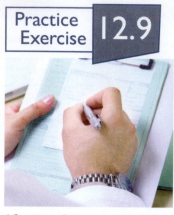

Practice Exercise 12.9

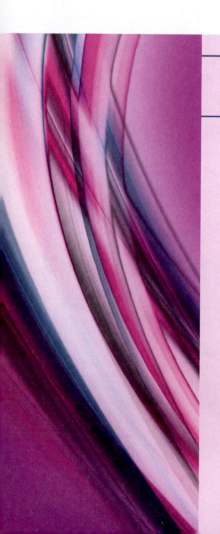

(Continued)

Identify whether each of the providers in the following situations is guilty of misrepresentation in terms of medically necessary, non-covered, or screening services:

4. A home health agency bills for covered home health services for an unqualified patient.
5. An ambulance company bills for emergency transportation for scheduled trips from a nursing home to a clinic.
6. A physician falsifies the diagnosis for a service that would otherwise be denied coverage if it were correctly reported.

Answer the following question:

7. Which of the following definitions is the correct definition of nonrendered services?

    A. Services/items furnished to a patient but not billed to Medicare
    B. Non-covered services under Medicare
    C. Services/items not furnished to a patient but billed to Medicare

Chapter Summary

■ Medicare is divided into two main programs: Medicare Part A, which is hospital insurance, and Medicare Part B, which is medical insurance.

■ The fee-for-service method is a method of charging for healthcare services under which each procedure is based on a specific amount of reimbursement. Medicare determines its fees for service using the resource-based relative value scale reimbursement method.

■ Recording the information from the Medicare card accurately is extremely important because that information will be used on many claims forms and medical documentation materials throughout the patient's history with the facility.

■ A provider may choose to participate or not participate in the Medicare program. Medicare reimbursement depends on participation and nonparticipation.

■ Medigap is a supplemental insurance sponsored by Medicare. It is an optional policy available to individuals who qualify for Medicare.

■ Medicare fraud is knowingly and willfully executing, or attempting to execute, a scheme to defraud any healthcare benefit program. Medicare abuse involves payment for items or services when there is no legal entitlement. The four most common types of Medicare fraud include the following:

1. Billing for services that were not rendered
2. Misrepresenting as medically necessary any non-covered or screening services by reporting covered procedure/revenue codes

3. Signing blank records or certification forms or falsifying information on records or certification forms for the sole purpose of obtaining payment

4. Consistently using procedure/revenue codes that describe more extensive services than those actually performed

Chapter Review

True/False

Identify the statement as true (T) or false (F).

_____ 1. The Medicare 2017 deductible for Part B is $200.00.

_____ 2. A MAC is a company that is paid to process claims for Medicare.

_____ 3. The medical office specialist should check patients' Medicare eligibility each time an appointment is made.

_____ 4. Care in a skilled nursing facility is covered under Medicare Part B.

_____ 5. Medicare Part A is administered by the CMS.

_____ 6. The benefit period Medicare Part A is the period during which a patient is insured.

_____ 7. Medicare Part A provides coverage for physician services and procedures.

_____ 8. Medicare Part B provides coverage for durable medical equipment.

_____ 9. Medicare covers an annual physical examination.

_____ 10. Medicare Part B covers eyeglasses.

_____ 11. Scrubbing means to return denied claims.

Multiple Choice

Identify the letter of the choice that best completes the statement or answers the question.

_____ 1. Individuals who are prior to 3 months of age 65 who do not receive Social Security benefits may enroll in Medicare Part A by:
a. paying a deductible.
b. paying into a Medical Savings Account.
c. paying a premium.
d. enrolling in a Medicare HMO.

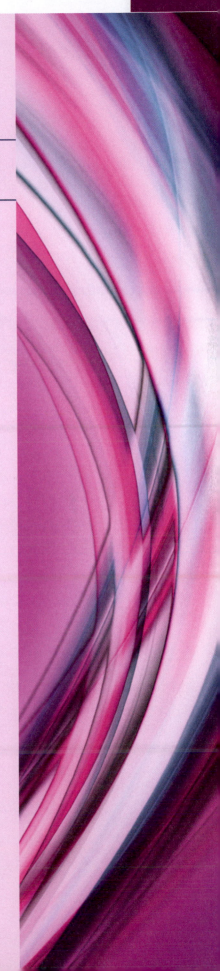

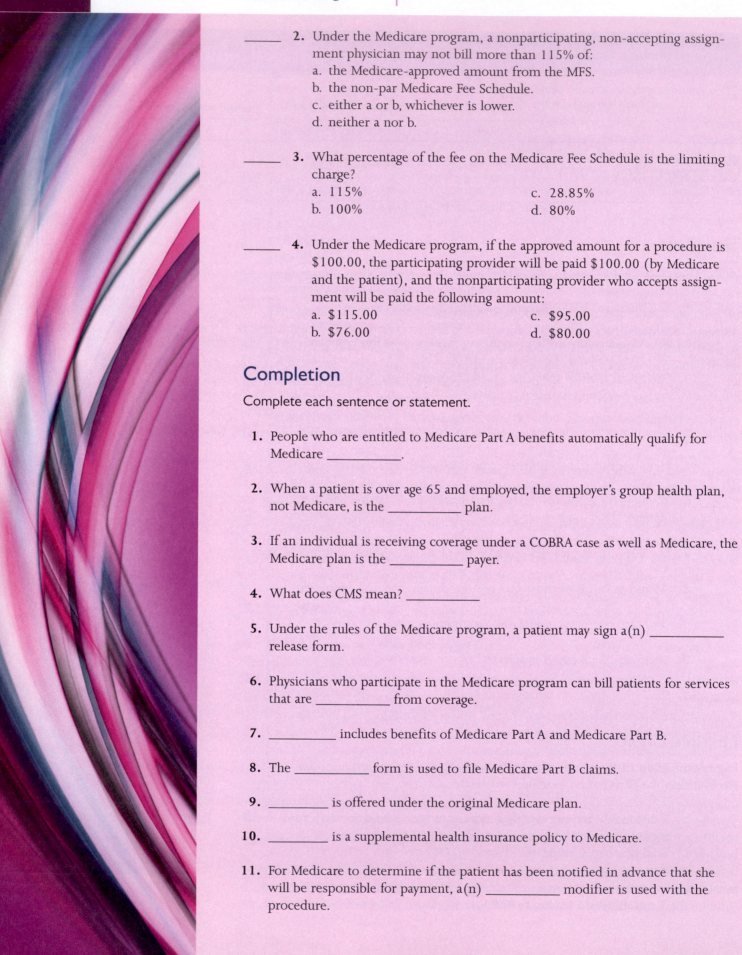

_____ **2.** Under the Medicare program, a nonparticipating, non-accepting assignment physician may not bill more than 115% of:
    a. the Medicare-approved amount from the MFS.
    b. the non-par Medicare Fee Schedule.
    c. either a or b, whichever is lower.
    d. neither a nor b.

_____ **3.** What percentage of the fee on the Medicare Fee Schedule is the limiting charge?
    a. 115%   c. 28.85%
    b. 100%   d. 80%

_____ **4.** Under the Medicare program, if the approved amount for a procedure is $100.00, the participating provider will be paid $100.00 (by Medicare and the patient), and the nonparticipating provider who accepts assignment will be paid the following amount:
    a. $115.00   c. $95.00
    b. $76.00   d. $80.00

Completion

Complete each sentence or statement.

1. People who are entitled to Medicare Part A benefits automatically qualify for Medicare _____.

2. When a patient is over age 65 and employed, the employer's group health plan, not Medicare, is the _____ plan.

3. If an individual is receiving coverage under a COBRA case as well as Medicare, the Medicare plan is the _____ payer.

4. What does CMS mean? _____

5. Under the rules of the Medicare program, a patient may sign a(n) _____ release form.

6. Physicians who participate in the Medicare program can bill patients for services that are _____ from coverage.

7. _____ includes benefits of Medicare Part A and Medicare Part B.

8. The _____ form is used to file Medicare Part B claims.

9. _____ is offered under the original Medicare plan.

10. _____ is a supplemental health insurance policy to Medicare.

11. For Medicare to determine if the patient has been notified in advance that she will be responsible for payment, a(n) _____ modifier is used with the procedure.

12. If the patient refuses to sign the ABN for a nonassigned claim, use a(an) _____ modifier.

13. MA is the abbreviation for _____.

14. Medicare Part D covers _____.

15. CMS has stated that the place of service must also be fully written out in form locator _____.

Resources

www.Novitas-solutions.com
This website may be used to obtain the latest information on CMS and Novitas for Medicare.

Advance Beneficiary Notice of Non-coverage (ABN) Booklet
www.cms.gov/MLNProducts/downloads/ABN_Booklet_ICN006266.pdf
This website allows providers to download the forms the patient must sign if a service is non-covered by Medicare.

Beneficiary Notice Initiative (BNI)
https://www.cms.gov/Medicare/Medicare-General-Information/BNI/index.html?redirect=/BNI/
These notices for patient financial rights and protection under the Fee For Service Medicare and Medicare Advantage Programs are to be given to the patients or beneficiaries before services are given.

A/B MAC Workload Implementation Handbook (for contractors)
www.cms.gov/Medicare/Medicare-Contracting/Medicare-Administrative-Contractors/MedicareAdministrativeContractors.html

A/B MAC Jurisdiction Information
www.cms.gov/medicare-coverage-database/indexes/national-and-local-indexes.aspx

A/B MAC Procurement and Implementation Documents
www.cms.gov/Medicare/Medicare-Contracting/Medicare-Administrative-Contractors/Downloads/CycleOne-CycleTwo/CycleTwoABMACBackgroundSheet.pdf

Part A/Part B MAC
www.cms.gov/Medicare/Medicare-Contracting/Medicare-Administrative-Contractors/What-is-a-MAC.html

GAO Report on Medicare Contracting Reform
www.gao.gov/new.items/d05873.pdf

MMA Assignment of Physicians, Providers, and Suppliers to the Medicare Administrative Contractors (MACs)
https://www.cms.gov/Medicare/Medicare-Contracting/Medicare-Administrative-Contractors/Who-are-the-MACs.html

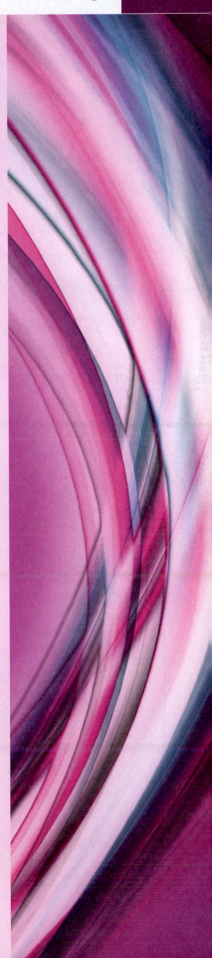

Chapter Objectives

After reading this chapter, the student should be able to:

1 Understand the requirements for qualifying to receive Medicaid benefits.

2 Determine the schedule of benefits the Medicaid recipient will receive.

3 Discuss the method of verifying Medicaid benefits.

4 Submit a Medicaid claim and decipher claim status.

Key Terms

categorically needy
Children's Health
  Insurance Program
  (CHIP)
Children's Health
  Insurance Program
  Reauthorization Act
  (CHIPRA)
Early and Periodic
  Screening, Diagnostic,

and Treatment
  (EPSDT)
Federal Medical
  Assistance Percentages
  (FMAP)
medically needy
Medi-Medi
payer of last resort
restricted status
spend-down program

State Children's Health
  Insurance Program
  (SCHIP)
Supplemental Security
  Income (SSI)
Temporary Assistance for
  Needy Families
  (TANF)
Welfare Reform Bill

CPT-4 codes in this chapter are from the CPT-4 2017 code set. CPT® is a registered trademark of the American Medical Association.

ICD-10 codes in this chapter are from the ICD-10-CM 2017 code set from the Department of Health and Human Services, Centers for Disease Control and Prevention.

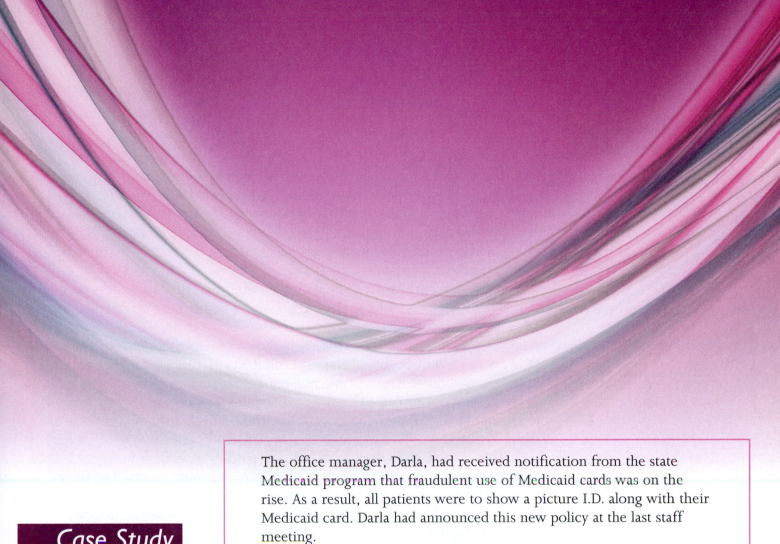

Case Study

Medicaid

The office manager, Darla, had received notification from the state Medicaid program that fraudulent use of Medicaid cards was on the rise. As a result, all patients were to show a picture I.D. along with their Medicaid card. Darla had announced this new policy at the last staff meeting.

While Ginger was working as the receptionist, a patient arrived and showed her Medicaid card. Ginger explained that she needed to see a picture I.D. because of increased fraud. The patient became indignant and refused to comply because she felt she was being accused of doing something illegal. Ginger asked Darla to explain the situation to the patient.

Questions

1. Should the patient be required to comply with the new policy in order to be seen by the physician? Why?

2. Could Ginger have handled the situation differently?

3. What should Darla tell the patient in order to calm her down?

Introduction

Authorized by Title XIX of the Social Security Act, Medicaid was signed into federal law in 1965 and is an optional program for the states. Currently all states, the District of Columbia, and all U.S. territories have Medicaid programs.

The federal government establishes certain requirements for each state's Medicaid program. The states then administer their own programs, determining the eligibility of applicants, deciding which health services to cover, setting provider reimbursement rates, paying for a portion of the total program, and processing claims.

Eligibility for enrollment in Medicaid is determined by both federal and state law. Title XIX specifies which groups of people must be eligible, and states have considerable flexibility to extend coverage to additional groups. In addition to income, eligibility is typically based on several other factors, including financial resources (or assets), age, disability status, other government assistance, and other health or medical conditions such as pregnancy. Beginning in 2014, the Affordable Care Act expanded Medicaid eligibility to all individuals under age 65 in families with income below 138% of the Federal Poverty Level (FPL), $16,243 individual and $33,465 for a family of four in 2015. This amount is adjusted for inflation in January of each year.

Title XIX specifies that certain medical services must be covered under Medicaid, while also granting the states flexibility to cover many other benefits. Services typically covered include hospital care, physician services, laboratory and other diagnostic tests, prescription drugs, dental care, and many long-term-care services. The states also have options to use managed care plans to provide and manage benefits and to apply for waivers that allow the states more flexibility in developing specialized benefit packages for specific populations. With limited exceptions—such as the use of waivers, demonstration projects, and benchmark benefit plans—states must provide the same benefit package to all Medicaid enrollees. In addition, states must extend eligibility to all mandatory populations and cover all mandatory services defined by Title XIX in order to receive federal matching funds for their Medicaid programs. The federal government and the states share the responsibility for funding Medicaid. States pay providers or managed care organizations for Medicaid costs and then report these payments to the Centers for Medicare and Medicaid Services (CMS). The federal government pays for a percentage of the costs of medical services by reimbursing each state; this percentage, known as the **Federal Medical Assistance Percentage (FMAP)**, is calculated annually for each state based on a statutory formula that takes into account state per capita income with some adjustments prescribed by legislation. Notably, the Affordable Care Act specifies FMAPs for beneficiaries who are newly eligible as a result of the Medicaid expansion beginning in 2014. In addition, the federal government pays for a portion of each state's administration costs. Beneficiary cost sharing, such as deductibles or copayments, and beneficiary premiums are very limited in Medicaid and do not represent a significant share of the total cost of healthcare services for Medicaid enrollees.

Medicaid Guidelines

Within broad national guidelines established by federal statutes, regulations, and policies, each state:

1. Establishes its own eligibility standards.
2. Determines the type, amount, duration, and scope of services.
3. Sets the rate of payment for services.
4. Administers its own program.

Medicaid policies for eligibility, services, and payment are complex and vary considerably, even among states of similar size or geographic proximity. Thus, a person who is eligible for Medicaid in one state may not be eligible in another state, and the services provided by one state may differ considerably in amount, duration, or scope from services provided in a similar or neighboring state. In addition, state legislatures may change Medicaid eligibility, services, and/or reimbursement during any given year. Most Medicaid plans do not require a premium.

Eligibility Groups

States are required to include certain types of individuals or eligibility groups under their Medicaid plans, and they may include others. States' eligibility groups include the following:

1. Categorically needy
2. Medically needy
3. Special groups

Categorically Needy

Persons who qualify as categorically needy under the Medicaid program include the following:

- Families who meet states' TANF eligibility requirements (See definition below.)
- Pregnant women and children under age 6 whose family income is at or below 133% of the federal poverty level (Services to these pregnant women are limited to those related to pregnancy, complications of pregnancy, birth, and postpartum care.)
- Infants born to Medicaid-eligible women. Medicaid eligibility must continue throughout the first year of life as long as the infant remains in the mother's household and she remains eligible or would be eligible if she were still pregnant. Pregnant women remain eligible for Medicaid throughout the end of the calendar month in which the 60th day after the end of the pregnancy falls.
- Recipients of adoption assistance and foster care under Title IV-E of the Social Security Act
- Children ages 6 to 19 with family income up to 100% of the federal poverty level

- Caretakers (relatives or legal guardians who take care of children under age 18 or 19 if still in high school)
- People who lose SSI payments because of earnings from work or increase of Social Security benefits. (**Supplemental Security Income [SSI]** is a federal income supplement program funded by general tax revenues designed to help the elderly and people who are blind or have a disability and who have little or no income.)
- Individuals and couples who are living in medical institutions and who have monthly income up to 300% of the SSI income standard (federal benefit rate)

Medically Needy

People who are termed **medically needy** have too much money (and in some cases resources such as savings accounts) to be categorized as **categorically needy**. If a state has a medically needy program, it must include pregnant women through a 60-day postpartum period, children under age 18, certain newborns for 1 year, and certain protected people who are blind.

The medically needy (MN) option allows states to extend Medicaid eligibility to additional people. These people would be eligible for Medicaid under one of the mandatory or optional groups, except that their income and/or resources are above the eligibility level set by their state. Persons may qualify immediately or may spend down by incurring medical expenses that reduce their income to or below their state's MN income level. A **spend-down program** is one in which the individual is required to spend a portion of her income or resources until she is at or below the state's income level. The concept is similar to an annual deductible, except that it resets at the beginning of every month. Each month, the enrollee pays a portion of incurred medical bills, up to a certain amount, before the Medicaid fee schedule takes effect and Medicaid takes over the payments.

Medicaid eligibility and benefit provisions for the medically needy do not have to be as extensive as for the categorically needy and, in fact, they may be quite restrictive. Federal matching funds are available for MN programs. However, if a state elects to have an MN program, the federal government requires that certain *groups* and certain *services* must be included; that is, children under age 19 and pregnant women who are medically needy must be covered, and prenatal and birth care for pregnant women, as well as ambulatory care for children, must be provided. A state may elect to provide MN eligibility to certain additional groups and may elect to provide certain additional services within its MN program.

Example

A patient who has a spend down of $100 per month visits the physician on June 5 and the fee is $75. The patient is responsible for the $75. Ten days later, on June 15, the patient returns to the physician and the fee is $75. The patient is responsible for $25, and Medicaid will pay the remaining $50. At the beginning of July, the patient is again responsible for $100 of medical services incurred during July.

Special Groups

States' eligibility groups may also include immigrants, families that need temporary assistance, and children with disabilities.

Immigrants

The Personal Responsibility and Work Opportunity Reconciliation Act of 1996 (Public Law 104-193), known as the **Welfare Reform Bill**, made restrictive changes regarding eligibility for SSI coverage that impacted the Medicaid program. For example, legal resident aliens and other qualified aliens who entered the United States on or after August 22, 1996, are ineligible for Medicaid for 5 years. Medicaid coverage for most aliens entering before that date and coverage for those eligible after the 5-year ban are state options; emergency services, however, are mandatory for both of these alien coverage groups. For aliens who lose SSI benefits because of the new restrictions regarding SSI coverage, Medicaid can continue only if these persons can be covered for Medicaid under some other eligibility status (again with the exception of emergency services, which are mandatory). The welfare reform bill also affected a number of children with disabilities who lost SSI as a result of the restrictive changes; however, their eligibility for Medicaid was reinstituted by the Balanced Budget Act.

TANF

Welfare reform also repealed the open-ended federal entitlement program known as Aid to Families with Dependent Children (AFDC) and replaced it with **Temporary Assistance for Needy Families (TANF)**, which provides states with grants to be spent on time-limited cash assistance. TANF generally limits a family's lifetime cash welfare benefits to a maximum of 5 years and permits states to impose a wide range of other requirements as well—in particular, those related to employment. Although most persons covered by TANF will receive Medicaid, it is not required by law. Eligibility for TANF is determined at the county level. The following questions are taken into account:

- Is the family's income below set limits?
- Are the family's resources (including property) equal to or less than set limits?
- Is there at least one child under 18 in the household?
- Is at least one parent unemployed, incapacitated, or absent from the home?
- Does the individual have a Social Security number and birth certificate?
- Does the individual receive adoptive or foster care assistance?

Children's Health Insurance Program Reauthorization Act (CHIPRA)

The **Children's Health Insurance Program Reauthorization Act (CHIPRA)** went into effect on April 1, 2009, providing healthcare to millions of children across the country. CHIPRA renewed and expanded coverage of the **Children's Health Insurance Program (CHIP)** from 7 million children to 11 million children. CHIP was previously known as the **State Children's Health Insurance Program (SCHIP)**.

Originally created in 1997, CHIP is Title XXI of the Social Security Act and is a state and federal partnership that targets uninsured children and pregnant women in families with incomes too high to qualify for most state Medicaid programs, but often too low to afford private coverage. CHIPRA finances CHIP through FY 2013. It will preserve coverage for the millions of children who rely on CHIP today and provide the resources for states to reach millions of additional uninsured children from families with higher incomes and uninsured low-income pregnant women.

CMS administers CHIP. The program is jointly financed by the federal and state governments and is administered by the states. Within broad federal guidelines, each state determines the design of its program, eligibility groups, benefit packages, payment levels for coverage, and administrative and operating procedures. CHIP provides a capped amount of funds to states on a matching basis. The Affordable Care Act extended CHIP through most of 2015. Beginning October 1, 2015, the already enhanced CHIP federal matching rate increased by 23 percentage points, bringing the average federal matching rate for CHIP to 93%. The enhanced federal matching rate continues until September 30, 2019. (For more information on federal funding in the Affordable Care Act see https://www.medicaid.gov/chip/financing/financing.html)

Scope of Medicaid Services

Title XIX of the Social Security Act allows considerable flexibility within the states' Medicaid plans. However, some federal requirements are mandatory if federal matching funds are to be received. A state's Medicaid program *must* offer medical assistance for certain *basic* services to most categorically needy populations. These services generally include the following:

- Inpatient hospital services
- Outpatient hospital services
- Prenatal care
- Vaccines for children
- Physician services
- Nursing facility services for persons age 21 or older
- Family planning services and supplies
- Rural health clinic services
- Home healthcare for persons eligible for skilled nursing services
- Laboratory and X-ray services
- Pediatric and family nurse practitioner services
- Nurse-midwife services
- Federally qualified health center (FQHC) services and the ambulatory services of an FQHC that would be available in other settings
- **Early and Periodic Screening, Diagnostic, and Treatment (EPSDT)** services for children under age 21

States may also receive federal matching funds to provide certain *optional* services. The following are the most common of the 34 currently approved optional Medicaid services:

- Diagnostic services
- Clinic services
- Intermediate care facilities for people with mental retardation
- Prescribed drugs and prosthetic devices
- Optometrist services and eyeglasses
- Nursing facility services for children under age 21

- Transportation services
- Rehabilitation and physical therapy services
- Home and community-based care to certain persons with chronic impairments

PACE

The Balanced Budget Act (BBA) of 1997 made sweeping changes to Medicare and generated savings that are critical to extending the life of the Medicare Trust Fund. It established the new state Children's Health Insurance Program, which provides another landmark opportunity to improve the health of children. In Medicaid, the BBA created new eligibility options, expanded assistance for low-income Medicare beneficiaries, and set new quality standards for Medicaid managed care plans.

BBA implementation is an enormous effort that requires CMS to balance many competing priorities within existing resources. CMS has already fully implemented more than half of the more than 300 individual BBA provisions affecting CMS programs.

The Balanced Budget Act included a state option known as Programs of All-Inclusive Care for the Elderly (PACE). PACE provides an alternative to institutional care for persons age 55 or older who require a nursing-facility level of care. The PACE team offers and manages *all* health, medical, and social services and mobilizes other services as needed to provide preventive, rehabilitative, curative, and supportive care. This care, provided in day health centers, homes, hospitals, and nursing homes, helps the person maintain independence, dignity, and quality of life. PACE functions within the Medicare program as well. Regardless of the source of payment, PACE providers receive payment only through the PACE agreement and must make available all items and services covered under both Titles XVIII and XIX, without amount, duration, or scope limitations and without application of any deductibles, copayments, or other cost sharing. The individuals enrolled in PACE receive benefits solely through the PACE program.

Amount and Duration of Medicaid Services

Within broad federal guidelines and certain limitations, states determine the amount and duration of services offered under their Medicaid programs. States may limit, for example, the number of days of hospital care or the number of physician visits covered. Two restrictions apply: (1) Limits must result in a sufficient level of services to reasonably achieve the purpose of the benefits, and (2) limits on benefits may not discriminate among beneficiaries based on medical diagnosis or condition.

In general, states are required to provide comparable amounts, duration, and scope of services to all categorically needy and categorically related eligible persons, with two important exceptions:

1. Medically necessary healthcare services that are identified under the EPSDT program for eligible children under age 21, and that are within the scope of mandatory or optional services under federal law, must be covered even if those services are not included as part of the covered services in that state's plan. States are required by federal law to inform all Medicaid-eligible persons in the state who are under age 21 of the availability of EPSDT and immunizations. Patients are not charged a fee for EPSDT services; however, some families do

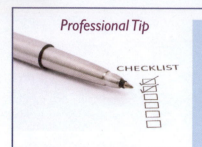

Professional Tip

CHECKLIST

Medicaid mandates procedures and regulations to follow for receiving reimbursement. Each state has its own guidelines, which need to be reviewed for reimbursement.

pay a premium. This program emphasizes preventive care. Health screenings (known as well-child checkups) for medical, vision, hearing, and dental are performed at regular intervals.

2. States may request "waivers" to pay for otherwise uncovered home- and community-based services (HCBS) for Medicaid-eligible persons who might otherwise be institutionalized. As long as the services are cost effective, states have few limitations on the services that may be covered under these waivers (except that, other than as a part of respite care, states may not provide room and board for the beneficiaries). With certain exceptions, a state's Medicaid program must allow beneficiaries to have some informed choices among participating providers of healthcare and to receive quality care that is appropriate and timely.

Payment for Medicaid Services

Medicaid operates as a vendor payment program. States may pay healthcare providers directly on a fee-for-service basis, or states may pay for Medicaid services through various prepayment arrangements, such as health maintenance organizations (HMOs). If Medicaid does not cover a service, the patient may be billed if the following conditions have been met:

- The physician informed the patient before the service was performed that the procedure was not covered by Medicaid.
- The medical office specialist had the patient sign an Advance Beneficiary Notice (ABN) form before the service was rendered, which states the amount of the procedure and why it will not be covered.

If a claim is denied by Medicaid for the following reasons, the physician may not bill the patient for the amount:

- Necessary preauthorization was not obtained before the procedure.
- The service was not medically necessary.
- The claim was not filed within the allotted time period.

Within federally imposed upper limits and specific restrictions, each state, for the most part, has broad discretion in determining the payment methodology and payment rate for services. Generally, payment rates must be sufficient to enlist enough providers so that covered services are available at least to the extent that comparable care and services are available to the general population within that geographic area. Providers participating in Medicaid must accept Medicaid payment rates as payment in full; that is, providers are not allowed to bill patients for the unpaid balance. States must make additional payments to qualified hospitals that provide inpatient services to a disproportionate number of Medicaid beneficiaries and/or to other low-income or uninsured persons under what is known as the *disproportionate share hospital* (DSH) adjustment.

States may impose nominal deductibles, coinsurance, or copayments on some Medicaid beneficiaries for certain services. The following Medicaid beneficiaries, however, must be excluded from cost sharing: pregnant women, children under age 18 years, and hospital or nursing home patients who are expected to contribute most of their income to institutional care. In addition, all Medicaid beneficiaries must be exempt from copayments for emergency services and family planning services.

The federal government also reimburses states for 100% of the cost of services provided through facilities of the Indian Health Service, provides financial help to the 12 states that furnish the highest number of emergency services to undocumented aliens, and shares in each state's expenditures for the administration of the Medicaid program. Most administrative costs are matched at 50%, although higher percentages are paid for certain activities and functions, such as development of mechanized claims processing systems.

Except for the CHIP program, the Qualifying Individuals (QI) program, and DSH payments, federal payments to states for medical assistance have no set limit (cap). Rather, the federal government matches (at FMAP rates) state expenditures for the mandatory services, as well as for the optional services that the individual state decides to cover for eligible beneficiaries, and matches (at the appropriate administrative rate) all necessary and proper administrative costs. The Balanced Budget Refinement Act of 1999 increased the amount that certain states and the territories can spend on DSH and CHIP payments, respectively.

Medicaid Growth Trends

From program inception, the cost of Medicaid has generally increased at a significantly faster pace than the U.S. economy. This growth pattern is not unique to Medicaid. Costs for virtually every form of health insurance, public and private, have increased rapidly, reflecting growth in the number of insured persons, wage increases, and price inflation in the medical sector; provision of a greater number of medical services; and the development of new, better, more complex, and generally more expensive services. Together, these cost factors have increased at a faster rate than the number of workers, general inflation, and productivity underlying economic growth. Determining how to optimally balance our collective demand for the best possible healthcare with our not-unlimited ability to fund such care through private and public efforts represents one of the most challenging policy dilemmas facing the United States.

The Patient Protection and Affordable Care Act, as amended by the Health Care and Education Reconciliation Act of 2010, substantially reduced the number of people in the United States without health insurance. Much of this reduction occurred as a result of expanded eligibility criteria for Medicaid, which the Congressional Budget Office (CBO) estimates will increase the number of Medicaid enrollees by about 20 million in 2019. Medicaid provides a relatively low-cost way to increase the number of people with health coverage because its payment rates for healthcare services and health plans are low compared with other forms of health insurance. Even so, aggregate Medicaid costs will increase significantly as a result of the Patient Protection and Affordable Care Act because of the very large number of additional enrollees starting in 2014. According to CMS, the total number of individuals enrolled in Medicaid and CHIP in January 2015 in all states reporting January data was nearly 70 million. Among states that had implemented the Medicaid expansion and were covering newly eligible adults in January 2015, Medicaid and CHIP enrollment rose by over 26.1%, compared to the July–September 2013 baseline period, while states that have not, to date, expanded Medicaid reported an increase of over 7.8% over the same period.

With the passage of this health act in 2010, the Recovery Audit Contractor (RAC) was expanded to include Medicaid. Section 6411 of this act required states and territories to establish Medicaid RAC programs. Medicaid RACs are tasked with identifying and recovering Medicaid overpayments and identifying underpayments.

Affordable Care Act Projections

The Affordable Care Act is projected to increase Medicaid expenditures by a total of $455 billion for FY 2010 through FY 2019, an increase of about 8% over projections of Medicaid spending without the impact of the legislation. Almost all of this increase is projected to be paid by the federal government ($434 billion, or about 95%). The most significant change to Medicaid was the expansion of Medicaid eligibility beginning in 2014.

Another significant development in Medicaid is the growth in managed care as an alternative service delivery concept different from the traditional fee-for-service system. Under managed care systems, HMOs, prepaid health plans (PHPs), or comparable entities agree to provide a specific set of services to Medicaid enrollees, usually in return for a predetermined periodic payment per enrollee. Managed care programs seek to enhance access to quality care in a cost-effective manner. Waivers may provide the states with greater flexibility in the design and implementation of their Medicaid managed care programs. Waiver authority under Sections 1915(b) and 1115 of the Social Security Act is an important part of the Medicaid program. Section 1915(b) waivers allow states to develop innovative healthcare delivery or reimbursement systems. Section 1115 waivers allow statewide healthcare reform experimental demonstrations to cover uninsured populations and to test new delivery systems without increasing costs. Finally, the BBA provided states with a new option to use managed care.

The Medicaid–Medicare Relationship (Medi-Medi)

Medicare beneficiaries who have low incomes and limited resources may also receive help from the Medicaid program. For such persons who are eligible for full Medicaid coverage, the Medicare healthcare coverage is supplemented by services that are available under their state's Medicaid program, according to eligibility category. These additional services are known as **Medi-Medi** and may include nursing facility care beyond the 100-day limit covered by Medicare, prescription drugs, eyeglasses, and hearing aids. People with Medicare and Medicaid automatically qualify (and do not need to apply) for Extra Help paying for Medicare prescription drug coverage. Each fall, Medicare uses data from the states to decide whether a person will continue to automatically qualify for Extra Help for the coming year.

For persons enrolled in both programs, any services that are covered by Medicare are paid for by the Medicare program before any payments are made by the Medicaid program because Medicaid is always the **payer of last resort**. CMS estimates that Medicaid currently provides some level of supplemental health coverage for about 6.5 million Medicare beneficiaries. Medicaid pays last on a claim when a patient has other effective insurance coverage.

Medicaid Managed Care

Managed care refers to a health system in which all healthcare providers in a network agree to coordinate and provide healthcare to a designated or specific population. The following are two different managed care models:

- HMOs, which receive a monthly "capitation" or fixed payment for each person enrolled based on an average projection of medical expenses for the typical patient. Some Medicaid managed care programs use the fee-for-service reimbursement methodology for participating providers.
- Primary care case management (PCCM), which is a noncapitated model. Each PCCM participant is assigned to a single primary care provider (PCP) who must authorize most other services, such as specialty physician care, before Medicaid can reimburse the specialty physician care. The state sets up physician networks and contracts directly with providers. Providers receive fee-for-service reimbursement, plus PCPs receive a small monthly case management fee for each patient.

Managed care programs are intended to reduce service fragmentation, increase access to care, reduce costs, and stimulate the development of more appropriate use of services. Medicaid clients are required to select a PCP. The PCP serves as the *medical home* and is responsible for 24-hour coverage when the patient requires access or care coordination. The medical home potentially gives enrollees a provider who knows their needs and can coordinate their healthcare. PCPs provide preventive checkups, treat the majority of conditions that enrollees experience, and refer the patient out of office for specialty care when necessary. The medical home was intended as a method for delivering coordinated care and a means to control costs. Some managed care Medicaid programs are designed to integrate delivery of acute and long-term care services through a managed care system. Participants receive all Medicaid services from their choice of HMOs. The HMOs provide all Medicaid primary, acute, and long-term care services through one service delivery system. This includes ensuring that each Medicaid-only member has a primary care doctor. Other acute care services include specialists, home health, medical equipment, laboratory, X-ray, and hospital services. If enrollees meet the medical necessity criteria to be in a nursing facility, they may choose to receive community-based alternatives and waiver services.

Enrollees with complex medical conditions are assigned a care coordinator, an HMO employee who is responsible for coordinating acute and long-term care services. The care coordinator develops an individual plan of care with the enrollee, family members, and providers, and can authorize services. The emphasis is on providing home- and community-based services to avoid the need for institutionalization.

Medicaid Verification

Medicaid cards may be issued to qualified individuals. Most states are changing to electronic verification of eligibility. Patients' eligibility should be checked *before each time they see the physician*. To verify eligibility monthly for Medicaid patients, a list of current patients can be kept on the Medicaid website under a facility's Medicaid Provider Identifier/NPI (National Provider Identifier) number. When patients present with their Medicaid card, verification can be done by scanning the card or going directly to the website. To verify on the website, enter the Medicaid number and check eligibility from 3 months past to today's date. If you do not know the recipient's Medicaid I.D. number, enter the recipient's Social Security number or card control number from the front of the recipient's Medicaid identification card. Verification shows if the patient has regular Medicaid, a managed care plan, or private insurance.

To keep this information on the website for future verification, add it to the list. Each month, this list of patients can be checked through the website for current eligibility.

The medical office specialist should always verify patient eligibility because it may change on a monthly basis. During the verification process, check to see if the patient is on **restricted status**, which requires him to see a specific physician (e.g., PCP) and/or pharmacy.

Medicaid Claims Filing

For claims payment to be considered, providers must adhere to the time limits described in this section. Claims received after the time limits have expired are not payable because the Medicaid program does not provide coverage for late claims.

Unless otherwise stated below, claims must be received within 95 days from each date of service (DOS). A 95- or 180-day filing deadline that falls on a weekend or holiday is extended to the next business day following the weekend or holiday. For submission of prior authorization requests, refer to the specific Medicaid manual section for that program.

Time Limits for Submitting Claims

Review the following time limits for submitting claims:

- Inpatient claims filed by the hospital must be received by Medicaid within 95 days from the discharge date.
- Although not recommended, hospitals reimbursed according to diagnostic-related group (DRG) payment methodology may submit an interim claim if the client has been in the facility 30 consecutive days or longer. A total stay claim is needed to ensure accurate calculation for potential outlier payments for people younger than age 21.
- Children's hospitals reimbursed according to Tax Equity and Fiscal Responsibility Act (TEFRA) methodology may submit interim claims before discharge and must submit an interim claim if the client remains in the hospital past the hospital's fiscal year end.
- When medical services are rendered to a Medicaid client, claims must be received within 95 days of the date of service (DOS). The DOS is the date the service is provided or performed. If the provider's enrollment is not complete, the claim will be denied. However, by ensuring that the claims are received within the 95-day filing limit, the provider has established the right to appeal for reimbursement once the enrollment process has been completed. To be considered for payment, an appeal must be received within 180 days of the date of denial notification.

Appeal Time Limits

All appeals of denied claims and requests for adjustments on paid claims must be received within 180 days from the date of disposition, the date of the Remittance and

Status (R&S) report on which that claim appears. As mentioned, if the 180-day appeal deadline falls on a weekend or holiday, the deadline will be extended to the next business day.

Claims with Incomplete Information and Zero Paid Claims

Claims lacking the information necessary for processing are listed on the R&S report with an explanation of benefits (EOB) code requesting the missing information. Providers must resubmit a signed, completed/corrected claim with a copy of the R&S on which the denied claim appears within 180 days from the date of the R&S to be considered for payment.

Newborn Claim Hints

When filing a claim for a newborn, if the mother's name is "Jane Jones," use "Boy Jane Jones" for a male child and "Girl Jane Jones" for a female child.

Enter "Boy Jane" or "Girl Jane" in the first name field and "Jones" in the last name field. Always use "Boy" or "Girl" first and then the mother's full name. An exact match must be submitted or the claim will not be processed. Do not use "NBM" for newborn male or "NBF" for newborn female.

Medicaid participating physicians file claims electronically using the CMS-1500 claim format. Medicaid participating hospitals and other inpatient facilities file claims electronically using the UB-04 format. Healthcare Common Procedure Coding System (HCPCS) codes are required for both claims. Be sure to submit the claim to the appropriate Medicaid claims payer. Medicaid managed care plans are not sent to the state Medicaid payer but are instead sent to the managed care carrier for payment.

Completing the CMS-1500 Form for Medicaid (Primary)

This section reviews each form locator on the CMS-1500 and what information should be entered when filing a Medicaid claim. There are only a few differences for claim completion for Medicaid claims. The Patient is always the Insured unless it is a newborn so the Insured Name in Locator 4 should be left blank. As with other insurance plans, input last name, first name, and middle name or initial. *The spelling should match the insurance card exactly.* If the name on the card is misspelled, then the name in the computer should be misspelled until the patient provides a new card with the correct spelling. Because the patient is the insured, the Self box is marked in **Form Locator 6: Patient's Relationship to the Insured**, unless the claim is for a newborn, then choose Child.

If required, form locator 22, **Medicaid Resubmission Code**, is where the Medicaid resubmission code used for Medicaid claims is entered. List the original reference number and the code for resubmitted claims.

Professional Tip

CHECKLIST

If a problem occurs with provider enrollment and the process is expected to take more than 180 days to complete, the original claims must be resubmitted and received before the 180-day appeals deadline has lapsed. Although this results in another denial of the claim, it will reestablish the provider's right to appeal.

Form locator 24H **EPSDT Family Plan** is used to identify whether the patient is receiving services through Medicaid's EPSDT program. If there is no requirement (e.g., state requirement) to report a reason code for EPSDT, enter "Y" for "YES" or "N" for "No" only.

If there is a requirement to report a reason code for EPSDT, enter the appropriate reason code as noted below. (A "Y" or "N" response is not entered with a code.) The two-character code is right justified in the top shaded area of the field.

The following codes for EPSDT are used:

AV   Available—Not used (Patient refused referral.)

S2   Under treatment (Patient is currently under treatment for referred diagnostic or corrective health problem.)

ST   New service requested (Referral to another provider for diagnostic or corrective treatment/scheduled for another appointment with screening provider for diagnostic or corrective treatment for at least one health problem identified during an initial or periodic screening service, not including dental referrals.)

NU   Not used (Used when no EPSDT patient referral was given.)

If the service is for family planning, enter "Y" for "YES" or "N" for "NO" in the bottom, unshaded area of the field.

Professional Tip

CHECKLIST

To avoid denials, always make sure that the ICD-10-CM codes used are the most recent, up-to-date codes. Codes used should be coded to the highest level of specificity.

Example

22. Medicaid Resubmission	ORIGINAL REF NO.
Code 123	ABC1234567890

Form Locator 27: Accept Assignment? No assignment required for Medicaid.

Practice Exercises

Complete Practice Exercises 13.1, 13.2, 13.3, and 13.4 by completing a CMS-1500 claim form using patient information forms and encounter forms. The practice exercises in this chapter are to be answered with ICD-10-CM codes.

Fill out a CMS-1500 form based on the information given here. To complete this exercise, copy the CMS-1500 form provided in Appendix D or download the form from MyHealthProfessionsKit or MyHealthProfessionsLab, which accompany this text.

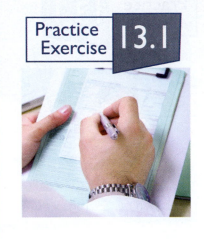

Practice Exercise 13.1

Allied Medical Center, 2145 Frankford Rd.	Patient Information Form
Baltimore, MD 12345 (555) 214-6500	Tax I.D.: 75-0246810
Phil Wells, M.D. (NPI: 1513171216; Medicaid ID: 51750)	Group NPI: 1234567890

Patient Information:

Name: (Last, First) **Shelton, Margaret** ❏ Male ☒ Female Birth Date: **03/25/2010**

Address: **12 Bonnie Lane, Baltimore, MD 12345** Phone: **(214) 555-1212**

Full-Time Student: ❏ Yes ☒ No

Marital Status: ☒ Single ❏ Married ❏ Divorced ❏ Other

Employment:

Employer: _____ Phone: ( )_____

Address: _____

Condition Related to: ❏ Auto Accident ❏ Employment ❏ Other Accident

Date of Accident: _____ State _____

Emergency Contact: Sheila Shetton, Mother **Phone: (214) 555-6958**

Primary Insurance: Medicaid Phone: **(800) 333-4563**

Address: **P.O. Box 200555, Baltimore, MD 12345**

Insurance Policyholder's Name: **Shelton, Margaret** ❏ M ❏ F DOB: _____

Address: **Same**

Phone: **Same** Relationship to Insured: ☒ Self ❏ Spouse ❏ Child ❏ Other

Employer: _____ Phone: ( )_____

Employer's Address: _____

Policy/I.D. No: **558479630** Group No: ___ Percent Covered: **100** %, Copay Amt: $ ___

Secondary Insurance: _____ Phone: ( ) _____

Address: _____

Insurance Policyholder's Name: _____ ❏ M ❏ F DOB: _____

Address: _____

Phone: _____ Relationship to Insured: ❏ Self ❏ Spouse ❏ Child ❏ Other

Employer: _____ Phone: ( ) _____

Employer's Address: _____

Policy/I.D. No: _____ Group No: ___ Percent Covered: ___ %, Copay Amt: $ ___

Reason for Visit: Routine well-child examination

Known Allergies: _____

Were you referred here? If so, by whom?: _____

(Continued)

Practice Exercise 13.1

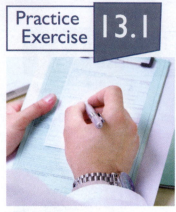

(*Continued*)

ALLIED MEDICAL CENTER

Patient: Shelton, Margaret **Chart#:** **Date:** Today's date
Address: 12 Bonnie Lane, Baltimore, MD 12345 **Phone:** 214-555-1212

Code	Description	Fee
	New Patient Codes	
99201	New Patient Focused	
99202	New Patient Expanded	
99203	New Patient Complete Physical	
99204	New Patient Comprehensive	
	Established Patient Codes	
99213	Established Patient Expanded	
99214	Established Patient Routine	× 95.00
99215	Established Patient Complex	
99211	Established Patient Minimal	
99212	Established Patient Focused	
	Procedures	
85007	Manual WBC	
85651	ESR-Erythrocyte Sed Rate	
86403	Strep Test, Rapid	
86580	Tine Test	
87880	Strep Screen	
87086	Urine, bacterial culture	
93000	Electrocardiogram-ECG-Intrp/Rprt	
93015	Treadmill Stress Test	
90471	Injection	
90707	MMR Vaccination	
	Other Codes:	

DIAGNOSIS: Encounter for routine child health examination without abnormal findings, ICD-10-CM (Z00.129)

NOTES/REMARKS:

Today's Charges: 95.00

Next Appt: **Amt Paid:** 0.00

Fill out a CMS-1500 form based on the information given here. To complete this exercise, copy the CMS-1500 form provided in Appendix D or download the form from MyHealthProfessionsKit or MyHealthProfessionsLab, which accompany this text.

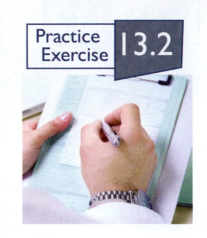

Allied Medical Center, 1933 Frankford Rd.	Patient Information Form
Baltimore, MD 12345 (555) 214-6500	Tax I.D.: 75-0246810
Phil Wells, M.D. (NPI: 1513171216; Medicaid ID: 51750)	Group NPI: 1234567890

Patient Information:

Name: (Last, First) **Churchill, Shawn L.** ☒ Male ☐ Female Birth Date: **07/29/2005**

Address: **6580 Belt Line Road, #12B, Rosedale, MD 12345** Phone: **(469) 555-7406**

Full-Time Student: ☐ Yes ☒ No

Marital Status: ☒ Single ☐ Married ☐ Divorced ☐ Other

Employment:

Employer: _____ Phone: ( )_____

Address: _____

Condition Related to: ☐ Auto Accident ☐ Employment ☐ Other Accident

Date of Accident: _____ State _____

Emergency Contact: **Edward Churchill, father** Phone: **(214) 555-8652**

Primary Insurance: **Medicaid** Phone: **(800) 333-4563**

Address: **P.O. Box 65921, Baltimore, MD 12345**

Insurance Policyholder's Name: **Same as patient** ☐ M ☐ F DOB: _____

Address: _____

Phone: _____ Relationship to Insured: ☒ Self ☐ Spouse ☐ Child ☐ Other

Employer: _____ Phone: ( )_____

Employer's Address: _____

Policy/I.D. No: **599630014** Group No: ___ Percent Covered: **100** %, Copay Amt: $ ___

Secondary Insurance: _____ Phone: ( ) _____

Address: _____

Insurance Policyholder's Name: _____ ☐ M ☐ F DOB:_____

Address: _____

Phone: _____ Relationship to Insured: ☐ Self ☐ Spouse ☐ Child ☐ Other

Employer: _____ Phone: ( )_____

Employer's Address: _____

Policy/I.D. No: _____ Group No: ___ Percent Covered: ___ %, Copay Amt: $ ___

Reason for Visit: Flu shot

Known Allergies: Feather

Were you referred here? If so, by whom? _____

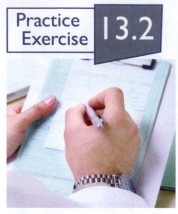

Practice Exercise 13.2

(Continued)

ALLIED MEDICAL CENTER

Patient: Churchill, Shawn L.   **Chart#:**   **Date:** Today's date
Address: 6580 Belt Line Road, #12B, Rosedale,   **Phone:** 469-555-7406
MD 12345

Code	Description	Fee
	New Patient Codes	
99201	New Patient Focused	
99202	New Patient Expanded	
99203	New Patient Complete Physical	
99204	New Patient Comprehensive	
	Established Patient Codes	
99213	Established Patient Expanded	
99214	Established Patient Routine	
99215	Established Patient Complex	
99211	Established Patient Minimal	
99212	Established Patient Focused	
	Procedures	
85007	Manual WBC	
85651	ESR-Erythrocyte Sed Rate	
86403	Strep Test, Rapid	
86580	Tine Test	
87880	Strep Screen	
87086	Urine, bacterial culture	
93000	Electrocardiogram-ECG-Intrp/Rprt	
93015	Treadmill Stress Test	
90471	Injection	× 5.00
90707	90707	
	Other Codes: 90658 FLU Vaccine	× 15.00

DIAGNOSIS: Encounter for immunizationl: CD-10-CM (Z23)

NOTES/REMARKS:

Next Appt:

Today's Charges: 20.00
Amt Paid: 0.00

Fill out a CMS-1500 form based on the information given here. To complete this exercise, copy the CMS-1500 form provided in Appendix D or download the form from MyHealthProfessionsKit or MyHealthProfessionsLab, which accompany this text.

Practice Exercise 13.3

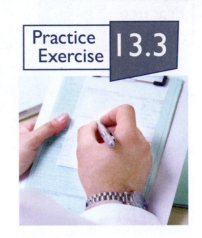

Allied Medical Center, 1933 W. Pearl City Rd.

Freeport, IL 12345 (555) 214-6500

Phil Wells, M.D. (NPI: 1513171216; Medicaid ID: 51750)

Patient Information Form

Tax I.D.: 75-0246810

Group NPI: 1234567890

Patient Information:

Name: (Last, First) **Bradford, Luella M.**   ❏ Male   ☒ Female Birth   Date: **03/17/1988**

Address: **2594-B N. Cedarville Rd, Cedarville, IL 12345**   Phone: **(214) 555-0147**

Full-Time Student: ❏ Yes   ☒ No

Marital Status: ☒ Single   ❏ Married   ❏ Divorced   ❏ Other

Employment:

Employer: **None**   Phone: ( )

Address:

Condition Related to: ❏ Auto Accident   ❏ Employment   ❏ Other Accident

Date of Accident: _____ State _____

Emergency Contact: **Mary Beth Bradford, mother**   **Phone: (972) 555-8733**

Primary Insurance: **Amerigroup**   Phone: **(800) 600-4441**

Address: **P.O. Box 61117, Freeport, IL 12345**

Insurance Policyholder's Name: **Same as patient**   ❏ M   ❏ F   DOB: _____

Address:

Phone: _____ Relationship to Insured: ☒ Self   ❏ Spouse   ❏ Child   ❏ Other

Employer: _____ Phone: ( ) _____

Employer's Address: _____

Policy/I.D. No: **515301607**   Percent Covered: _____%,   Copay Amt: $**5**

Secondary Insurance: _____ Phone: ( ) _____

Address: _____

Insurance Policyholder's Name: _____   ❏ M   ❏ F DOB:_____

Address: _____

Phone: _____ Relationship to Insured: ❏ Self   ❏ Spouse   ❏ Child   ❏ Other

Employer: _____ Phone: ( ) _____

Employer's Address: _____

Policy/I.D. No: _____ Group No: ___ Percent Covered: ___ %, Copay Amt: $ ___

Reason for Visit: Pregnancy Test

Known Allergies: _____

Were you referred here? If so, by whom? _____

(Continued)

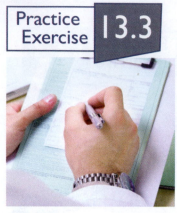

Practice Exercise 13.3

(Continued)

ALLIED MEDICAL CENTER

Patient: Bradford, Luella   **Chart#:**   **Date:** Today's date

Address: 2594-B N. Cedarville Rd,   **Phone:** 214-555-0147
Cedarville, IL 12345

Code	Description	Fee
	New Patient Codes	
99201	New Patient Focused	
99202	New Patient Expanded	
99203	New Patient Complete Physical	
99204	New Patient Comprehensive	
	Established Patient Codes	
99213	Established Patient Expanded	
99214	Established Patient Routine	
99215	Established Patient Complex	
99211	Established Patient Minimal	
99212	Established Patient Focused	
	Procedures	
85007	Manual WBC	
85651	ESR-Erythrocyte Sed Rate	
86403	Strep Test, Rapid	
86580	Tine Test	
87880	Strep Screen	
87086	Urine, bacterial culture	
93000	Electrocardiogram-ECG-Intrp/Rprt	
93015	Treadmill Stress Test	
90471	Injection	
90707	MMR Vaccination	
	Other Codes: 81025 Urine pregnancy test	× 20.00

DIAGNOSIS: Pregnancy Test: ICD-10-CM (Z32.00)

NOTES/REMARKS:

	Today's Charges:	20.00
Next Appt:	**Amt Paid:**	5.00

Fill out a CMS-1500 form based on the information given here. To complete this exercise, copy the CMS-1500 form provided in Appendix D or download the form from MyHealthProfessionsKit or MyHealthProfessionsLab, which accompany this text.

Practice Exercise 13.4

Allied Medical Center, 1933 Merrick Rd.

Massapequa, NY 12345 (555) 214-6500

Phil Wells, M.D. (NPI: 1513171216; Medicaid ID: 51750)

Patient Information Form

Tax I.D.: 75-0246810

Group NPI: 1234567890

Patient Information:

Name: (Last, First) **Nguyen, Thuy** ☐ Male ☒ Female Birth Date: **05/01/2017**

Address: **7619 Seaview Ave, Massapequa, NY 12345** Phone: **(214) 555-6488**

Full-Time Student: ☐ Yes ☒ No

Marital Status: ☒ Single ☐ Married ☐ Divorced ☐ Other

Employment:

Employer: _____ Phone: ( )_____

Address: _____

Condition Related to: ☐ Auto Accident ☐ Employment ☐ Other Accident

Date of Accident: _____ State _____

Emergency Contact: **Josie Thuy, mother** Phone: **(800) 333-4563**

Primary Insurance: **Medicaid** Phone: _____

Address: **P.O. Box 4601, Rensselaer, NY 12345**

Insurance Policyholder's Name: **Same as patient** ☐ M ☐ F DOB: _____

Address: _____

Phone: _____ Relationship to Insured: ☒ Self ☐ Spouse ☐ Child ☐ Other

Employer: _____ Phone: ( )_____

Employer's Address: _____

Policy/I.D. No: **999528741** Group No: ____ Percent Covered: **100** %, Copay Amt: $ ____

Secondary Insurance: _____ Phone: ( )_____

Address: _____

Insurance Policyholder's Name: _____ ☐ M ☐ F DOB: _____

Address: _____

Phone: _____ Relationship to Insured: ☐ Self ☐ Spouse ☐ Child ☐ Other

Employer: _____ Phone: ( )_____

Employer's Address: _____

Policy/I.D. No: _____ Group No: ____ Percent Covered: ____ %, Copay Amt: $ ____

Reason for Visit: **Low birth weight**

Known Allergies: _____

Were you referred here? If so, by whom? _____

(Continued)

Practice Exercise 13.4

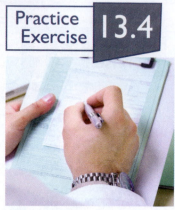

(Continued)

ALLIED MEDICAL CENTER

Patient: Nguyen, Thuy   **Chart#:**   **Date:** Today's date

Address: 7619 Seaview Ave., Massapequa   **Phone:** 214-555-6488
NY 12345

Code	Description	Fee
	New Patient Codes	
99201	New Patient Focused	
99202	New Patient Expanded	
99203	New Patient Complete Physical	
99204	New Patient Comprehensive	
	Established Patient Codes	
99213	Established Patient Expanded	
99214	Established Patient Routine	
99215	Established Patient Complex	
99211	Established Patient Minimal	
99212	Established Patient Focused	
	Procedures	
85007	Manual WBC	
85651	ESR-Erythrocyte Sed Rate	
86403	Strep Test, Rapid	
86580	Tine Test	
87880	Strep Screen	
87086	Urine, bacterial culture	
93000	Electrocardiogram-ECG-Intrp/Rprt	
93015	Treadmill Stress Test	
90471	Injection	
90707	MMR Vaccination	
	Other Codes: 99381 NP infant under 1 year of age.	× 175.00

DIAGNOSIS: Low Birth Weight newborn, 2,000–2,499 grams: ICD-10-CM (PO7.18)

NOTES/REMARKS:

Today's Charges: 175.00

Next Appt: **Amt Paid:**   0.00

Chapter Summary

- Medicaid is the largest source of funding for medical and health-related services for certain low-income people, some of whom may have no medical insurance or inadequate medical insurance.
- States may pay healthcare providers directly on a fee-for-service basis, or states may pay for Medicaid services through various prepayment arrangements, such as HMOs.
- If Medicaid does not cover a service, the patient may be billed if certain conditions have been met.
- A significant development in Medicaid is the growth in managed care as an alternative service delivery concept different from the traditional fee-for-service system.
- For claims payment to be considered, providers must adhere to claim filing time limits.
- All appeals of denied claims and requests for adjustments on paid claims must be received within 180 days from the date of disposition, the date of the Remittance and Status (R&S) report on which that claim appears.
- Claims lacking the information necessary for processing are listed on the R&S report with an Explanation of Benefits (EOB) code requesting the missing information. Providers must resubmit a signed, completed/corrected claim with a copy of the R&S on which the denied claim appears within 180 days from the date of the R&S to be considered for payment.
- When filing a claim for a newborn, if the mother's name is "Jane Jones," use "Boy Jane Jones" for a male child and "Girl Jane Jones" for a female child.
- Medicaid-participating physicians file claims electronically using the CMS-1500 format. Medicaid-participating hospitals and other inpatient facilities file claims electronically using the UB-04 format. Healthcare Common Procedure Coding System (HCPCS) codes are required for both claims.

Chapter Review

True/False

Identify the statement as true (T) or false (F).

_____ 1. Under the payer-of-last-resort regulation, Medicaid pays last on a claim when a patient has other effective insurance coverage.

_____ 2. The medical office specialist should check patients' Medicaid eligibility before they see the physician.

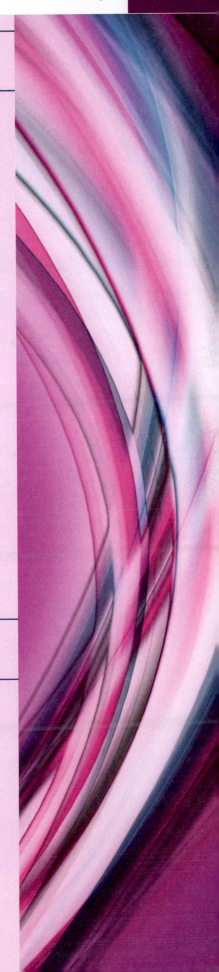

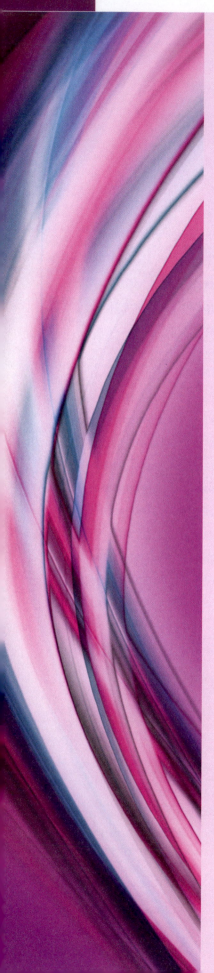

_____ **3.** Under a Medicaid spend-down program, individuals are required to spend all of their discretionary income on health costs before Medicaid begins to contribute.

_____ **4.** Children under 6 years old who meet TANF requirements or whose family income is below 133% of the poverty level must be offered state Medicaid benefits.

_____ **5.** A person eligible for Medicaid in a given state is also eligible in all states that border on that state.

_____ **6.** Individuals receiving financial assistance under TANF because of low incomes and few resources must be covered by state Medicaid programs.

_____ **7.** TANF is the abbreviation for Temporary Assistance for Needy Families.

_____ **8.** Inpatient claims filed by the hospital must be received by Medicaid within 95 days from the discharge date.

_____ **9.** All appeals of denied claims and request for adjustments on paid claims must be received within 180 days from the date of the R&S report.

_____ **10.** The federal government makes payments to states under the Federal Medical Assistance Percentages (FMAP) program.

_____ **11.** Immigrants are automatically excluded from state medical programs.

_____ **12.** The managed care PCP serves as the medical home and the liaison between the Medicaid recipient and the state.

Multiple Choice

Identify the letter of the choice that best completes the statement or answers the question.

_____ **1.** Within broad national guidelines established by federal statutes, regulations, and policies, each state:
a. follows the Medicare eligibility standards.
b. receives the type, amount, duration, and scope of services.
c. sets the rate of payment to receive from the federal government.
d. administers its own program.

_____ **2.** States' eligibility groups will be considered one of the following:
a. Income needy
b. Medically needy
c. Geographic groups
d. Education level

_____   **3.** If a state has a medically needy program, it must include:
     a. college students who qualify for financial aid.
     b. pregnant women.
     c. children under age 18.
     d. certain protected elderly persons.

_____   **4.** Which of the following provides states with grants to be spent on time-limited cash assistance?
     a. TANF
     b. SIS
     c. CMS
     d. Welfare reform

_____   **5.** Medi-Medi benefits may include:
     a. hospital care beyond the 100-day limit covered by Medicare.
     b. over-the-counter drugs.
     c. eyeglasses and hearing aids.
     d. orthopedic care.

_____   **6.** When filing a claim for a male newborn, if the mother's name is "Jane Jones," then the claim would be filed as:
     a. Boy Jane Jones.
     b. Jane Jones Boy.
     c. Jones, Jane Boy.
     d. Jones, Baby Boy.

Completion

Complete each sentence or statement.

1. Medicaid, by law, is the _____ of last resort.

2. The _____ program under Medicaid offers health insurance coverage for uninsured children.

3. Persons may qualify immediately or may _____ by incurring medical expenses that reduce their income to or below their state's MN income level.

4. _____ determine the amount and duration of services offered under their Medicaid programs.

5. Two different managed care models are _____ and _____.

6. An R&S report is the _____ and _____ report.

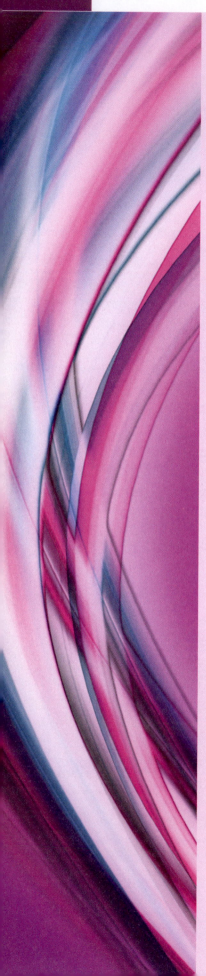

For Additional Practice

Fill out a CMS-1500 form based on the information given here. To complete this exercise, copy the CMS-1500 form provided in Appendix D or download the form from MyHealthProfessionsKit or MyHealthProfessionsLab, which accompany this text.

Physician Information:	Charles H. Borden, M.D.
	980 Newton Memorial
	Dr. Forsyth, GA 12345
Phone:	899-555-2276
EIN:	22-9872767
Professional License:	TX2056
Medicaid PIN :	K00J879
NPI:	1234568901
Patient Information:	Katherine Becker
	254 W. Adams St.
	Forsyth, GA 12345
	999-555-3457
DOB:	06/23/1954
Patient Account:	12358
Status:	Married
Sex:	Female
Patient's Insurance Information:	Medicaid I.D.#5555211106
	1123 High Point
	Tucker, GA 12345
	800-973-1123

Date of Service: Today's date

CC: Patient CC of back pain. Leaned over to pick up 2-yr-old toddler and felt sharp pain in low back.

- DX: Lumbar Sprain. Sprain of ligaments of lumbar spine, initial encounter: ICD-10-CM (S33.5XXA)
- 99203—NP Office Visit, Problem focused-history and examination, straight-forward decision making, $85, DX code: Sprain of ligaments of lumbar spine, ICD-10-CM (S33.5XXA)

Plan: Rx for Relafen one tab daily. Return in one week.

Resources

Centers for Medicare & Medicaid Services
www.cms.gov/cmsforms
Many CMS program-related forms are available in pdf format at this site.
New York State Education Department/Medicaid in Education/Billing/Claiming
Guidance
www.oms.nysed.gov/medicaid/billing_claiming_guidance
Billing/Claiming guidance materials to be used as both instructions and reference
tools for the preschool/school supportive health services program (SSHSP) are
available at this site.

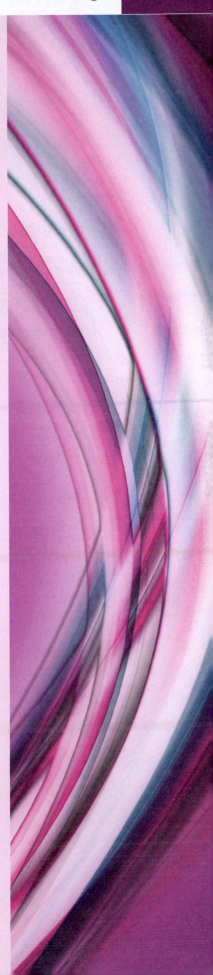

Chapter Objectives

After reading this chapter, the student should be able to:

1. Determine eligibility for TRICARE participants.

2. Identify different types of benefits available to veterans and their family members.

3. Submit claims to TRICARE using the CMS-1500 and the UB-04 (CMS-1450) form.

Key Terms

beneficiary

catastrophic cap

Civilian Health and Medical Program of the Uniformed Services (CHAMPUS)

Civilian Health and Medical Program of the Department of Veterans Affairs (CHAMPVA)

cost share

Defense Enrollment Eligibility Reporting System (DEERS)

military treatment facility (MTF)

nonavailability statement (NAS)

Palmetto Government Benefits Administrators (PGBA)

primary care manager (PCM)

sponsor

TRICARE

TRICARE Extra

TRICARE for Life (TFL)

TRICARE Prime

TRICARE Prime Remote (TPR)

TRICARE Reserve Retired (TRR)

TRICARE Reserve Select (TRS)

TRICARE Senior Prime

TRICARE Standard

TRICARE Young Adult (TYA)

Wisconsin Physicians Service (WPS)

CPT-4 codes in this chapter are from the CPT-4 2017 code set. CPT® is a registered trademark of the American Medical Association.

ICD-10-CM codes in this chapter are from the ICD-10-CM 2017 code set from the Department of Health and Human Services, Centers for Disease Control and Prevention.

Kerry Kosh had a new patient appointment with Dr. Lader. She is covered by TRICARE under the sponsorship of her husband, Carl. She presented her insurance card.

At the visit, the doctor gave Kerry three prescriptions for long-term medications. Each prescription was written for a year's worth of refills. As the medical assistant handed the prescriptions to Kerry, she noticed the number of refills. She told the patient that she could mail the prescriptions to the military base that was approximately 40 miles away, but that she probably wouldn't receive the refills for more than a week. She then offered to call in a week's worth of medications to a local pharmacy.

Questions

1. What is the term used for the policyholder of a TRICARE plan?

2. What would be the advantage of sending the prescriptions to the military base?

3. How does this show the medical office assistant's concern for the patient's healthcare?

TRICARE is the U.S. Department of Defense (DoD) medical entitlement program that covers medically necessary care for eligible uniformed services beneficiaries (active duty, retirees, family members, and survivors). In this chapter, you will learn how to determine eligibility for TRICARE participants and how to file claims under the TRICARE program.

TRICARE

The U.S. Congress created the **Civilian Health and Medical Program of the Uniformed Services (CHAMPUS)** in 1966 under Public Law 89-614 because individuals in the military were finding it increasingly difficult to pay for the medical care required by their families. CHAMPUS was a congressionally funded comprehensive health benefits program. Beginning in 1988, CHAMPUS beneficiaries had a choice of retaining their benefits under CHAMPUS or enrolling in a managed care plan called CHAMPUS Prima, a plan to control escalating medical costs and standardize benefits for active duty families, military retirees, and their dependents. In January 1994, TRICARE became the new title for CHAMPUS. Individuals can choose from the following different TRICARE health plans:

1. **TRICARE Standard** is a fee-for-service, cost-sharing option.
2. **TRICARE Prime** is a health maintenance organization (HMO) option. TRICARE Prime options include the following:
   - TRICARE Prime Remote (TPR)
   - TRICARE Prime Overseas
   - TRICARE Global Remote Overseas
3. **TRICARE Extra** is a preferred provider organization (PPO) option.
4. **TRICARE Senior Prime** (also referred to as **TRICARE for Life [TFL]**) is a program for Medicare-eligible beneficiaries age 65 and older that pays patient liability after Medicare payment.
5. **TRICARE Reserve Select (TRS)** is a premium-based healthcare plan.
6. **TRICARE Reserve Retired (TRR)** is a premium-based healthcare plan.
7. **TRICARE Young Adult (TYA)** is a premium-based healthcare plan.

Eligible TRICARE beneficiaries may receive care at either a **military treatment facility (MTF)** or from TRICARE-authorized civilian providers. (Authorization of civilian providers is discussed in a later section.)

TRICARE Eligibility

An individual who qualifies for TRICARE is known as a **beneficiary**; the active duty service member is called the **sponsor**. A person who is retired from a career in the armed forces is known as a *service retiree* or *military retiree*. At age 65, the individual becomes eligible for the Medicare program. At that point, Medicare becomes the primary insurance policy and TRICARE becomes the secondary policy. Beneficiaries who have Medicare

Part A must have Medicare Part B to remain TRICARE eligible. The only exceptions are the following:

1. The sponsor is on active duty.
2. The beneficiary is enrolled in the US Family Health Plan.
3. The beneficiary is enrolled in TRICARE Reserve Select.

No further family benefits are provided in the event that an active duty military person served from 4 to 6 years and then chose to leave the armed services, thereby giving up a military career. **Civilian Health and Medical Program of the Department of Veterans Affairs (CHAMPVA)** beneficiaries are not eligible for TRICARE. CHAMPVA is for veterans with 100% service-related disabilities and their families. As the result of a recent policy change, if the eligible CHAMPVA sponsor is the spouse of another eligible CHAMPVA sponsor, both may now be eligible for CHAMPVA benefits.

To be eligible for TRICARE, all uniformed services sponsors and family members must be enrolled in the **Defense Enrollment Eligibility Reporting System (DEERS)**. Sponsors needing to enroll themselves or family members may contact or visit their personnel office, their nearest identification card–issuing facility, or the Defense Manpower Data Center Support Office (DSO). A TRICARE beneficiary may check status by contacting the nearest personnel office of any branch of the service or by calling the toll-free number of the DEERS center.

Patient's Financial Responsibilities

The TRICARE fiscal year begins October 1 and ends September 30. TRICARE's treatment of deductibles is different from that of most other healthcare programs. The medical office specialist should be aware of these differences when collecting deductibles. Generally, insurance deductibles renew (or start over) on January 1; however, because of the TRICARE fiscal year, TRICARE deductibles renew on October 1 each year. Another way TRICARE differs from other health plans is that instead of *coinsurance*, TRICARE uses the term **cost share** to refer to the charges that are the responsibility of the patient. (Other differences are discussed later in the discussion of how to complete the CMS-1500 form.)

Timely Filing

Professional and institutional TRICARE claims must be submitted within 30 days from the date of service, or inpatient discharge date, but no later than 1 year from the date of service or discharge. Claims older than 1 year must be submitted with a detailed explanation why the claim is being filed late. Each case is reviewed by a claims processor and given individual consideration.

Penalties and Interest Charges

Penalties and interest charges may not be billed to a beneficiary by a physician or supplier because of TRICARE's failure to make payment on a timely basis.

Authorized Providers

An authorized provider may treat a TRICARE Standard patient. Only providers who meet TRICARE's licensing and credentialing process can be reimbursed by TRICARE for its share of costs for patient care. Beneficiaries who use nonauthorized providers may be responsible for their entire bill, and there are no legal limits on the amounts these providers can bill beneficiaries. Examples of nonauthorized providers are most chiropractors and acupuncturists and those physicians who do not meet state licensing or training requirements or were rejected for authorization by TRICARE. Authorized providers include the following:

- Doctor of medicine (MD)
- Doctor of osteopathy (DO)
- Doctor of dental surgery (DDS)
- Doctor of dental medicine (DDM)
- Doctor of podiatry (DPM)
- Doctor of optometry (DO)
- Psychologist (PhD)

Other authorized nonphysician providers include audiologists, certified nurse midwives, clinical social workers, licensed practical nurses, licensed vocational nurses, registered nurses, registered physical therapists, and speech therapists.

A participating provider is assigned a personal identification number (PIN) and agrees to accept the TRICARE allowable charge in full for services, which is the Medicare fee. A nonparticipating provider cannot charge more than 115% of the TRICARE allowed charge (Medicare fee).

Preauthorization

TRICARE enforces certain referral and preauthorization requirements for TRICARE Standard patients when specialty care or hospitalization is necessary. A military treatment facility must be used if services are available; otherwise, a **nonavailability statement (NAS)** must be obtained so that the patient may see a civilian provider. NAS request forms are submitted electronically to the DEERS database before any treatment by a civilian provider. An NAS request is an electronic document stating that the service the patient requires is not available at the nearby MTF. Once approved by DEERS, NASs are valid for 30 days after they are issued and for 15 days after hospital discharge for treatment related to the original condition. If an NAS is not filed and approved, TRICARE will not pay any claims associated with the non-MTF treatment.

A healthcare finder (HCF) will assist the patient with a referral or preauthorization process. HCFs are available at TRICARE service centers along with beneficiary representatives.

All admissions, ambulatory surgical procedures, and other selected procedures require preauthorization. Certain types of healthcare services require prior approval from the TRICARE health contractor, including the following:

- Arthroscopy
- Breast mass or tumor removal
- Cardiac catheterization
- Cataract removal
- Cystoscopy
- Dental care
- Dilation and curettage (D&C)
- Durable medical equipment (DME) purchases
- Gastrointestinal endoscopy
- Gynecologic laparoscopy
- Hernia repair

- Laparoscopic cholecystectomy
- Ligation or transection of fallopian tubes
- Magnetic resonance imaging (MRI) services
- Mental healthcare
- Myringotomy or tympanostomy
- Neuroplasty
- Rhinoplasty or septoplasty
- Strabismus repair
- Tonsillectomy and adenoidectomy
- Physical therapy

TRICARE Standard and TRICARE Extra

TRICARE Standard and TRICARE Extra are two of the Prime plans offered to active duty service members and retired service members and their families. Note: When retired service members and their families become eligible for TRICARE for Life they are no longer able to enroll in TRICARE Prime. The key difference between TRICARE Standard and TRICARE Extra is choice of providers. With TRICARE standard a TRICARE-authorized provider outside of TRICARE network can be selected and the sponsor will pay higher cost shares. With TRICARE Extra only a TRICARE network provider can be selected and the sponsor will pay lower cost shares. TRICARE Standard and TRICARE Extra are fee-for-service programs.

Under TRICARE Standard and TRICARE Extra, medical expenses are shared between TRICARE and the beneficiary. When using TRICARE Standard and TRICARE Extra, the patient is responsible, under law, to pay an annual deductible and cost share with their care. The law prohibits healthcare providers from waiving the deductible or cost shares and requires providers to make reasonable efforts to collect these amounts. Providers who offer to waive the deductible and cost shares, or who advertise that they will do so, can be suspended or excluded as TRICARE-authorized providers. In addition to the deductible, families of active duty members pay 15% in-network and 20% non-network for outpatient visits. Retirees and their families, former spouses, and families of deceased personnel pay 20% in-network and 25% non-network for outpatient visits. If a beneficiary is treated by a provider who does not accept assignment (non-network provider), he or she is also responsible for the provider's additional charges up to 15% above of the TRICARE-allowable charge (i.e., the limiting charge; see Chapter 12). Patient cost share payments are subject to an annual **catastrophic cap** (i.e., a limit on the total medical expenses) that beneficiaries are required to pay within 1 fiscal year. The fiscal year begins October 1 each calendar year. For retired members' families, the annual cap is $1,000. For a family using TRICARE Reserve Select the annual cap is $1,000 per family, per fiscal year. For all others, the annual cap is $3,000 per family, per fiscal year. Once this cap has been met, TRICARE pays 100% of additional charges for that year. The catastrophic cap does not apply to active duty service members. The following is a list of services that are not covered under the TRICARE Standard plan:

- Chiropractic care
- Cosmetic surgery
- Custodial care
- Unproven procedures or treatments
- Routine physical examinations
- Routine foot care

If a TRICARE Standard beneficiary needs treatment that is not available at an MTF, the person must file an NAS with DEERS.

TRICARE Prime

TRICARE Prime is a managed care plan, similar to an HMO. In addition to most of the benefits offered by TRICARE Standard, the program offers additional preventive care, including routine physical examinations.

The TRICARE Prime option requires enrollment. After enrolling in the plan, each individual is assigned a **primary care manager (PCM)** who coordinates and manages that patient's medical care. The PCM may be a single military or civilian provider or a group of providers. All referrals for specialty care must be arranged by the PCM to avoid point-of-service charges.

TRICARE Prime enrollees receive the majority of their healthcare services from MTFs, and they receive priority at these facilities. TRICARE Prime results in fewer out-of-pocket costs than any other TRICARE option. Active duty members and their families do not pay enrollment fees, annual deductibles, or copayments for care provided within the TRICARE network.

Retired service members may also take advantage of the TRICARE Prime plan, but they must pay an annual enrollment fee of $282.60 for an individual or $565.20 for individual and a family, and minimal copays apply for care within the TRICARE network. (These enrollment fees were effective October 1, 2016; fees may change each fiscal year.) TRICARE Prime also offers a *point-of-service* option for care received outside of the TRICARE Prime network, but point-of-service care requires payment of significant out-of-pocket costs. Visits to civilian network providers require a $6 or $12 copayment, depending on the grade (military rank; e.g., E4) of the sponsor. Charges for visits to providers outside the TRICARE Prime network are paid 50% by TRICARE and 50% by the beneficiary.

TRICARE Prime enrollees are guaranteed certain access standards for care, as listed in Table 14.1.

TRICARE Prime Remote

TRICARE Prime Remote (TPR) is a healthcare program for active duty service members who are assigned to permanent-duty stations that are not near sources of military

Table 14.1	Access Standards for TRICARE Prime Enrollees			
	Urgent Care	**Routine Care**	**Referred Specialty Care**	**Wellness/ Preventive Care**
Appointment wait time	Not to exceed 24 hours	Not to exceed 7 days	Not to exceed 4 weeks	Not to exceed 4 weeks
Drive time	Within 30 minutes of home	Within 60 minutes of home	Within 60 minutes of home	Within 60 minutes of home
Wait time in office	Not to exceed 30 minutes for nonemergency situations			

care, typically 50 miles or more from a military treatment facility. TPR is offered in the 50 U.S. states only and requires enrollment. The benefits under TRICARE Prime Remote are the same as TRICARE Prime, with no out-of-pocket costs for TPR enrollees.

Enrollees must select or be assigned a local PCM. If no network PCMs are available in the area, beneficiaries may use any TRICARE-authorized provider for primary care. PCMs provide preventive services, care for routine illnesses or injuries, and manage referrals to specialists or hospitals if needed.

All specialty care must be coordinated through the TRICARE regional healthcare finder. Network PCMs will coordinate specialty care directly with the regional HCF. The regional HCF will coordinate active duty TRICARE Prime Remote specialty-care referrals through the service point of contact (SPOC) to determine if the specialty care must be received from a military provider for a "fitness for duty" determination. Specialty-care referrals for TPR active duty family members are managed by the HCF and are not coordinated through the SPOC.

A brief comparison of the four TRICARE plans discussed thus far is shown in Table 14.2. Sample military I.D. cards and TRICARE cards are shown in Figure 14.1. ID

Table 14.2	A Brief Comparison of TRICARE Plans	
	TRICARE Standard/Extra	**TRICARE Prime/Prime Remote**
Type of program	A fee-for-service program with the option of using a preferred provider network under the TRICARE Extra benefit	A managed care program, similar to an HMO
Availability	Throughout the United States and overseas	Only available in TRICARE Prime service areas (PSAs); active duty families eligible for TRICARE Prime Remote can enroll outside a PSA
Enrollment	Not required	Required
Enrollment fees	No fee	*Active duty families:* None *Retirees/others:* $260/individual $520/individual and family
Costs	$150/individual or $300/family for (Active Duty) E-5 & above; $50/$100 for E-4 & below	*Active duty families:* None *Retirees/others:* Small copays per service
Provider choices	Any TRICARE authorized provider	Limited to MTFs and TRICARE network providers
MTF priority	Only limited space-availability access	Priority access to MTFs
Primary care managers	No designated PCM required	All care coordinated through a designated PCM
Referral and authorization requirements	No referrals required; only a few types of services require prior authorization	Most care requires referral by the PCM; more authorization requirements than TRICARE Standard/Extra
Clinical preventive care	Limited benefits compared with TRICARE Prime	Various preventive benefits such as routine eye exams and routine preventive care exams

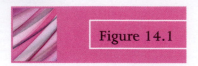

Figure 14.1

Sample military and TRICARE patient cards.

Source: From showing your ID to Providers published by TRICARE.

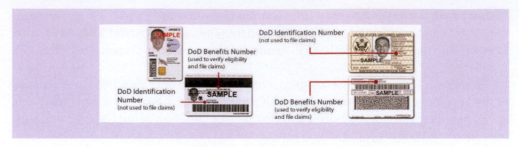

cards will have a DoD ID Number. If the beneficiary is eligible for DoD Tricare benefits, there will also be an 11-digit DoD Benefits Number printed on the ID card.

TRICARE Senior Prime/TRICARE for Life

Individuals over the age of 65 who are eligible for Medicare and TRICARE may receive healthcare at a military treatment facility. Benefits offered through TRICARE Senior Prime, also known as TRICARE for Life (TFL), are similar to those of a Medicare HMO, with an emphasis on preventive and wellness services. Prescription drug benefits are also included in TRICARE Senior Prime/TRICARE for Life.

All enrollees in TRICARE Senior Prime/TRICARE for Life must be enrolled in Medicare Parts A and B and must have Part B premiums deducted from their Social Security checks. Other than Medicare costs, TRICARE Senior Prime/TRICARE for Life beneficiaries pay no enrollment fees and no cost share fees for inpatient or outpatient care at a military facility. TRICARE acts as a second payer to Medicare for benefits payable by both Medicare and TRICARE. Claims will automatically be forwarded to TRICARE after Medicare pays. TRICARE is the primary payer if benefits are not covered under Medicare, such as pharmacy benefits.

TRICARE Reform

In Feburary 2016, a TRICARE reform packet was submitted by the Department of Defense (DoD) to overhaul TRICARE. It is projected to save TRICARE about $1 billion annually, starting in 2018 by raising beneficiary fees and copays, particularly for retirees, their family members, and their survivors. For the first time, Medicare-eligible retirees using TRICARE for Life as supplemental insurance would pay an annual enrollment fee. For 2018, it would be set at 1% of gross retired pay, but not to exceed $300. It would climb to 2% of gross retired pay, not to exceed $600, by 2020. General and flag officer retirees using TRICARE for Life would face slightly higher fee ceilings.

Catastrophic caps on total out-of-pocket health costs, which haven't been raised in a decade, would be reset to $1,500 a year, from $1,000, for active duty families and to $4,000 a year, from $3,000, for retiree families. The new participation fee paid by retirees would not count toward the caps.

CHAMPVA

CHAMPVA is a comprehensive healthcare program in which the U.S. Department of Veterans Affairs (VA) shares the cost of covered healthcare services and supplies with veterans with 100% service-related disabilities and their families. The program is administered by the Health Administration Center, which has offices in Denver, Colorado.

Because of the similarity between CHAMPVA and the DoD TRICARE program, the two are often mistaken for each other. While the benefits are similar, the programs are administered separately, with significant differences in claim filing procedures and preauthorization requirements. CHAMPVA is a Department of Veterans Affairs program, whereas TRICARE is a regionally managed healthcare program for active duty and retired members of the uniformed services, their families, and survivors. An eligible CHAMPVA sponsor may be entitled to receive medical care through the VA healthcare system based on his or her own veteran status. In addition, as the result of a recent policy change, if the eligible CHAMPVA sponsor is the spouse of another eligible CHAMPVA sponsor, both may now be eligible for CHAMPVA benefits. In each instance where the eligible spouse requires medical attention, she or he may choose the VA healthcare system or coverage under CHAMPVA for healthcare needs.

Veterans requesting medical care through the VA healthcare system should first seek to obtain care in VA facilities. Sometimes, however, VA facilities cannot provide the necessary medical care and services. In such cases, the VA may authorize medical care provided in the community for those veterans who meet the eligibility requirements. The VA authorization will specify the following:

- Medical services approved by the VA
- Length of period for treatment
- Amount the VA will pay

Each individual veteran's eligibility status and medical care needs are reviewed to decide whether community treatment can be approved. All VA-authorized services *must be approved* before the veteran receives treatment. However, it may not be possible to contact the VA before treatment in life-threatening emergency situations.

CHAMPVA is always the last payer after Medicare and any other health insurance.

Submitting Claims to TRICARE

Physicians submit claims to TRICARE using the CMS-1500 form. Hospitals and other inpatient facilities submit claims on the UB-04 (CMS-1450) claim form. Figure 14.2 lists the information that must be on the submitted claim form. Most claims are submitted electronically, but when it is necessary to submit a paper claim, submission addresses vary depending on the provider's location. Members can use www.tricareonline.com to determine the appropriate claims mailing address. TRICARE claims are managed in four separate regions. The three U.S. regions are north, south and west. Information on which carrier and contact information for the medical office specialist to reference can be located at www.tricare.mil/about/regions.aspx. **Wisconsin Physicians Service (WPS)** is the claims processor for all TRICARE Senior Prime/TRICARE for Life claims. The Medicare provider submits a claim to Medicare first. After

> **Professional Tip**
>
> The term *sponsor* refers to the member who is/was active in the military. The terms *beneficiary* and *patient* are synonymous.
>
> CHECKLIST

Figure 14.2

Information that must appear on the submitted TRICARE claim forms.

All claims must include the following information:

- Patient's name as it appears on his or her military ID card
- Sponsor's Social Security Number (SSN) or Department of Defense Benefits Number (DBN) (eligible former spouses should use their SSN)
- Patient's date of birth
- Other health insurance (OHI) information
- Appropriate HCPCS, CPT, and ICD-10 codes on CMS-1500 claim forms
- Appropriate HCPCS, CPT ICD-10, and revenue codes on UB-04 claim forms

- Admitting diagnosis on UB-04 claim forms
- Care approval number if applicable
- Provider's tax ID number or SSN
- Referring physician
- Rendering physician
- Beneficiary's signature (or indicate "signature on file" if the beneficiary's signature is on a "release of information" document)
- The provider's or representative's signature

adjudicating the claim, Medicare will forward the claim to WPS TRICARE Senior Prime (aka TRICARE for Life, TFL).

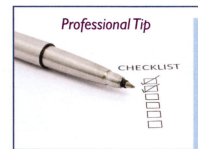

Professional Tip

CHECKLIST

To register for online CMS-1500 claim submission through XPressClaim, providers can go online to www.mytricare.com. The site has a demo available to show how easy it is to submit a claim.

Claims for CHAMPVA patients are sent electronically through the VA's clearinghouse, Change Healthcare, formerly Emdeon Inc., or submitted on paper. Paper claims for CHAMPVA are submitted to the Fee Department of the VA facility that authorized payment of services in advance or to Chief Business Office Purchased Care, CHAMPVA, P.O. Box 4690634, Denver, Colorado 80246-9063.

Completing the CMS-1500 Form for TRICARE (PRIMARY)

When completing the claim, mark an X in the TRICARE/CHAMPUS box. Enter the sponsor's Social Security number or Department of Defense Benefits Number (DBN) in the Insured's ID Number locator box. The sponsor is the person who qualifies the patient for TRICARE benefits. (Former spouses should use their own SSN.) Enter the patient's name as it is written on the ID card. Complete all other claim locator boxes per instructions in Chapter 10 for physician claims and Chapter 11 for hospital claims.

Figure 14.3 represents a completed CMS-1500 claim form for TRICARE.

HEALTH INSURANCE CLAIM FORM

APPROVED BY NATIONAL UNIFORM CLAIM COMMITTEE (NUCC) 02/12

Save and Print Options

1. MEDICARE (Medicare#) MEDICAID (Medicaid#) TRICARE [X] (ID#/DoD#) CHAMPVA (Member ID#) GROUP HEALTH PLAN (ID#) FECA BLK LUNG (ID#) OTHER (ID#)	1a. INSURED'S I.D. NUMBER (For Program in Item 1) 486429786
2. PATIENT'S NAME (Last Name, First Name, Middle Initial) COOK BARBARA	3. PATIENT'S BIRTH DATE 06 18 1972 SEX M [ ] F [X]	4. INSURED'S NAME (Last Name, First Name, Middle Initial) COOK CHRISTOPHER
5. PATIENT'S ADDRESS (No., Street) 8742 FAIRVIEW RD	6. PATIENT RELATIONSHIP TO INSURED Self [ ] Spouse [X] Child [ ] Other [ ]	7. INSURED'S ADDRESS (No., Street)

CITY: DALLAS STATE: TX
8. RESERVED FOR NUCC USE
CITY STATE

ZIP CODE: 12345 TELEPHONE (Include Area Code) (999) 555-3457
ZIP CODE: 12345 TELEPHONE (Include Area Code) ( )

9. OTHER INSURED'S NAME (Last Name, First Name, Middle Initial)
10. IS PATIENT'S CONDITION RELATED TO:
11. INSURED'S POLICY GROUP OR FECA NUMBER

a. OTHER INSURED'S POLICY OR GROUP NUMBER
a. EMPLOYMENT? (Current or Previous) YES [ ] NO [X]
a. INSURED'S DATE OF BIRTH 05 05 1971 SEX M [X] F [ ]

b. RESERVED FOR NUCC USE
b. AUTO ACCIDENT? YES [ ] NO [X] PLACE (State)
b. OTHER CLAIM ID (Designated by NUCC)

c. RESERVED FOR NUCC USE
c. OTHER ACCIDENT? YES [ ] NO [X]
c. INSURANCE PLAN NAME OR PROGRAM NAME TRICARE

d. INSURANCE PLAN NAME OR PROGRAM NAME
10d. CLAIM CODES (Designated by NUCC)
d. IS THERE ANOTHER HEALTH BENEFIT PLAN? YES [ ] NO [X] If yes, complete items 9, 9a, and 9d.

READ BACK OF FORM BEFORE COMPLETING & SIGNING THIS FORM.
12. PATIENT'S OR AUTHORIZED PERSON'S SIGNATURE I authorize the release of any medical or other information necessary to process this claim. I also request payment of government benefits either to myself or to the party who accepts assignment below.
SIGNED SIGNATURE ON FILE DATE

13. INSURED'S OR AUTHORIZED PERSON'S SIGNATURE I authorize payment of medical benefits to the undersigned physician or supplier for services described below.
SIGNED SIGNATURE ON FILE

14. DATE OF CURRENT ILLNESS, INJURY, or PREGNANCY (LMP) 08 21 XX QUAL.
15. OTHER DATE QUAL. MM DD YY
16. DATES PATIENT UNABLE TO WORK IN CURRENT OCCUPATION FROM TO

17. NAME OF REFERRING PROVIDER OR OTHER SOURCE 17a. 17b. NPI
18. HOSPITALIZATION DATES RELATED TO CURRENT SERVICES FROM TO

19. ADDITIONAL CLAIM INFORMATION (Designated by NUCC)
20. OUTSIDE LAB? YES [ ] NO [X] $ CHARGES

21. DIAGNOSIS OR NATURE OF ILLNESS OR INJURY Relate A-L to service line below (24E) ICD Ind.
A. J11.1 B. C. D.
E. F. G. H.
I. J. K. L.
22. RESUBMISSION CODE ORIGINAL REF. NO.
23. PRIOR AUTHORIZATION NUMBER

24. A. DATE(S) OF SERVICE From MM DD YY To MM DD YY	B. PLACE OF SERVICE	C. EMG	D. PROCEDURES, SERVICES, OR SUPPLIES CPT/HCPCS MODIFIER	E. DIAGNOSIS POINTER	F. $ CHARGES	G. DAYS OR UNITS	H. EPSDT Family Plan	I. ID. QUAL.	J. RENDERING PROVIDER ID. #
1 08 21 XX 08 21 XX	11		99213	A	85 00	1		NPI	7536982014
2								NPI	
3								NPI	
4								NPI	
5								NPI	
6								NPI	

25. FEDERAL TAX I.D. NUMBER 239872767 SSN [ ] EIN [X]
26. PATIENT'S ACCOUNT NO. COOBA
27. ACCEPT ASSIGNMENT? YES [X] NO [ ]
28. TOTAL CHARGE $ 85 00
29. AMOUNT PAID $ 16 00
30. Rsvd. for NUCC Use

31. SIGNATURE OF PHYSICIAN OR SUPPLIER INCLUDING DEGREES OR CREDENTIALS (I certify that the statements on the reverse apply to this bill and are made a part thereof.)
SIGNED SIGNATURE ON FILE XXXXXXXX DATE

32. SERVICE FACILITY LOCATION INFORMATION
CHARLES H BORDEN MD 980 FREDERICK RD DALLAS TX 12345
a. 7536982014 b.

33. BILLING PROVIDER INFO & PH # (555) 5551234
CHARLES H BORDEN MD 980 FREDERICK RD DALLAS TX 12345
a. 7536982014 b.

NUCC Instruction Manual available at: www.nucc.org **PLEASE PRINT OR TYPE** APPROVED OMB-0938-1197 FORM 1500 (02-12)

Figure 14.3 A completed CMS-1500 claim form for TRICARE.

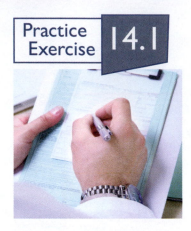

Practice Exercise 14.1

Fill out a CMS-1500 form based on the information given here. To complete this exercise, copy the CMS-1500 form provided in Appendix D or download the form from MyHealthProfessionsKit or MyHealthProfessionsLab, which accompany this text.

Physician Information:	Charles H. Borden, M.D.
	980 NE 24th St
	Silver Springs, FL 12345
Phone:	899-555-2276
EIN:	22-9872767
Professional License:	FL2056
TRICARE PIN:	9856471
NPI:	7536982014

Patient Information:	Barbara Cook
	8742 SW 17th Ave
	Ocala, FL 12345
	999-555-3457
DOB:	06/18/1972
Social Security number:	885-26-3341
Patient Account:	COOBA
Status:	Married
Sex:	Female

Patient's Insurance Information: TRICARE

Spouse's Information:	Christopher F. Cook
	P.O. Box 5431
	Fort Dix, NJ 12345
	555-124-8947
DOB:	05/05/1971
Insured's (Sponsor)	
Social Security number:	603-87-9521
Today's Date	
CC:	Influenza with Bronchitis
DX:	ICD-10-CM (J11.1)
99213 Established Patient:	Problem-focused history and examination, straightforward decision making $85.00, DX: ICD-10-CM (J11.1)

Accepting assignment

Confidential and Sensitive Information

Claims examiners who review claims for sensitive and confidential information stamp Confidential on the face of each claim form containing such information. The claim is treated as a confidential situation throughout the claims adjudication process. The examiner stamps both the envelope being mailed to the beneficiary and the provided return envelope Confidential when a claim is returned for additional information or because an incorrect claim form was used. **PGBA** employees do not provide information to parents or guardians of minors or persons who are unable to make healthcare decisions for themselves when the services are related to the following diagnoses:

- Alcoholism
- Abortion
- Drug abuse
- Venereal disease
- HIV

Chapter Summary

- In January 1994, TRICARE became the new title for CHAMPUS. Individuals can choose from five different TRICARE health plans: (1) TRICARE Standard, a fee-for-service, cost-sharing option; (2) TRICARE Prime, an HMO option; (3) TRICARE Prime Remote (TPR), another HMO option; (4) TRICARE Extra, a PPO option; or (5) TRICARE Senior Prime (aka TRICARE for Life, TFL), a program for Medicare-eligible beneficiaries age 65 and older.
- Only certified providers, that is, those who have passed a licensing credentialing process, can be authorized by TRICARE.
- Physicians submit claims to TRICARE using the CMS-1500 form. Hospitals and other inpatient facilities submit claims on the UB-04 (CMS-1450) claim form. The mailing address for claims varies depending on the provider's geographic location.
- Professional and institutional TRICARE claims must be submitted within 30 days from the date of service, or inpatient discharge date, but no later than 1 year from the date of service or discharge.

Chapter Review

True/False

Identify the statement as true (T) or false (F).

_____ **1.** A nonavailability statement in the TRICARE program excuses the beneficiary from paying the cost share.

_____ **2.** In the TRICARE and CHAMPVA programs, cost share has the same meaning as coinsurance.

_____ **3.** The TRICARE program serves families of veterans with 100% service-related disability.

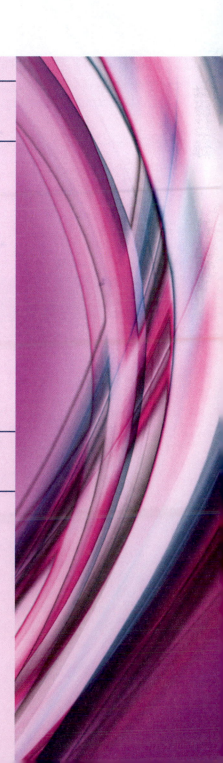

_____ 4. TRICARE participating provider charges generally follow the Medicare Fee Schedule.

_____ 5. It is not necessary to complete all form locators on the CMS-1500 form when completing a TRICARE claim.

Multiple Choice

Identify the letter of the choice that best completes the statement or answers the question.

_____ 1. The TRICARE program that offers fee-for-service coverage is:
   a. TRICARE Standard.   c. TRICARE Extra.
   b. TRICARE Prime.   d. none of the above.

_____ 2. The TRICARE program that offers an alternative managed care plan to TRICARE Prime with no enrollment fee is:
   a. TRICARE Standard.   c. CHAMPUS.
   b. TRICARE Extra.   d. CHAMPVA.

_____ 3. TRICARE Standard is a:
   a. fee-for-service plan.
   b. capitated plan.
   c. managed care organization.
   d. program for children of veterans.

_____ 4. A service that is not covered under TRICARE Standard is:
   a. chiropractic care.
   b. cosmetic surgery.
   c. routine physical examinations.
   d. all of the above.

_____ 5. Professional and institutional TRICARE claims must be submitted to PGBA within how many days from the date of service, or inpatient discharge date?
   a. 60 days   c. 120 days
   b. 30 days   d. 180 days

Completion

Complete each sentence or statement.

1. The _____ manager is the provider who coordinates care of TRICARE beneficiaries.

2. The worldwide database of TRICARE and CHAMPVA beneficiaries is _____.

3. The TRICARE fiscal year begins _____ and ends _____.

4. An online claims submission program provided by PGBA is called _____.

5. A TRICARE beneficiary who lives within a certain distance of a military hospital must file a (n) _____ before entering a civilian hospital for inpatient non-emergency care.

6. TRICARE physician charges are filed using the _____ claim form.

7. Paper claims for CHAMPVA are submitted to the _____ department of the VA Health Administration Center.

8. All enrollees in TRICARE _____ must be enrolled in Medicare Parts A and B.

9. TRICARE _____ require enrollment.

10. Active duty service members who are not near sources of military care qualify for _____.

Resources

TRICARE—U.S. Department of Defense Military Health System
www.tricare.mil/tma/default.aspx

TRICARE—Military: Explanation of Benefits
www.tricare.mil/eob

TRICARE—Provider Handbook PDF
https://www.hnfs.com/content/dam/hnfs/tn/prov/resources/pdf/2016_2017_TRICARE_Provider_Handbook.pdf

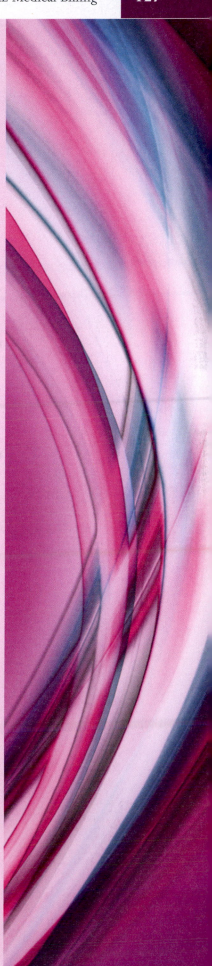

15 Explanation of Benefits and Payment Adjudication

16 Refunds, Follow-Up, and Appeals

Receivables are the strength and stability of any growing or established practice. Accounts receivables include monies owed to a practice by both payers and patients. Chapter 15 presents a thorough understanding of the Explanation of Benefits (EOB) and the Electronic Remittance Advice (ERA). With this information in hand, the medical office specialist can post payment, apply write-offs, and bill patients correctly. With a clear understanding of these documents, the medical office specialist will be able to resolve any payment issues with the payer, adjust patients' accounts, and collect balances due from patients.

In the medical office facility, it is not uncommon for the medical office specialist to receive denial notices from insurance carriers. Therefore, it is important for the medical office specialist to be familiar with medical records, verification of benefits forms, precertification/preauthorization/referral requirements, and the appeals process for each insurance carrier with which the provider contracts. Chapter 16 provides the student with the knowledge required to submit additional clinical and other pertinent information to an insurance carrier to overturn a denied or downcoded claim by the payer.

Professional Vignette

My name is Carolina Calhoun, and I recently graduated with my diploma in medical insurance billing and coding. I had previously worked as a manager in retail, but needed to find a new career direction because of a disability with my voice. A family member who works in medical coding suggested this field to me. I've always been interested in the medical field, so I jumped at the opportunity.

I enjoyed all aspects of my education and became really inspired by all the challenges that Medicare and other insurances present. For my externship, I worked in a hospital lab performing insurance verification and following up on denied claims. Thousands of claims were being denied because of improper diagnoses. I called the offices of the physicians who had ordered the lab tests to get more appropriate diagnoses. For example, they may have ordered a PSA test but indicated the patient's chronic diabetes as the diagnosis, rather than the immediate problem that gave rise to the PSA. I had to obtain the correct diagnosis and resubmit the claim.

I have been actively involved in the local chapter of a national coder's association, and I hope to start a chapter closer to my home. Now that I'm done with school, I am preparing for my certification exam and looking for permanent employment in my new field. I hope to be very successful in my new career.

Chapter Objectives

After reading this chapter, the student should be able to:

1. Define the steps for filing a medical claim.

2. Understand the importance of the Explanation of Benefits and Electronic Remittance Advice forms.

3. Calculate accurate payment by a carrier or third-party payer.

4. Make adjustments to patient accounts.

5. Review reason codes.

Key Terms

adjudication
adjustment
allowed charges
appeal
balance billing
capitation plan
charge-based fees
conversion factor
coordination of benefits (COB)
Electronic Remittance Advice (ERA)
excluded services
Explanation of Benefits (EOB)

Geographic Practice Cost Index (GPCI)
lifetime maximum
manual review
Medicare conversion factor (MCF)
Medicare Fee Schedule (MFS)
nationally uniform relative value
out-of-pocket expenses
pending claim
per member per month (PMPM)

reason codes
relative value unit (RVU)
remark codes
resource-based fees
resource-based relative value scale (RBRVS)
retention schedule
turnaround time
usual, customary, and reasonable (UCR)
withhold
write-offs

CPT-4 codes in this chapter are from the CPT-4 2017 code set. CPT® is a registered trademark of the American Medical Association.

**Explanation
of Benefits
and Payment
Adjudication**

Henry, the billing supervisor, noticed that Gloria, the biller responsible for sending out patient statements, had charged several patients for the balance that insurance had not paid. In discussing this with Gloria, Henry realized that she hadn't been properly trained regarding balance billing. He explained that in most managed care plans, the difference between the amount billed and the amount allowed by the insurer was to be entered as an adjustment and not billed to the patient.

Questions

1. What should be done regarding the patients who were incorrectly sent a statement?

2. How could Henry have prevented this error from occurring?

3. Is balance billing allowed in non–managed care plans?

Understanding the Explanation of Benefits (EOB) or the remittance advice supplied by the payer allows the medical office specialist to post payments, apply **write-offs**, and bill patients correctly. The adjustment reason codes on an EOB/ERA inform the medical office specialist about the reason for the denial, the amount due from the patient, incorrect coding, and so on. With a clear understanding of this remittance, the medical office specialist will be able to resolve any payment issues with the payer, adjust patient accounts, and collect balances due from patients. In this manner, the accounts receivable will show a true reflection of balances owed the practice, which will affect the collection process. Accounts receivable represent monies owed to a provider by insurance carriers or the patient/insured. These payments are applied to the patient's account to reduce the overall balance due. The medical office specialist is trained in communicating with patients to help resolve billing issues, such as amounts of copayments and collecting for deductibles. Accounts receivables are the strength and stability of any growing practice.

Steps for Filing a Medical Claim

An **Explanation of Benefits (EOB)** is a notification form sent from the insurance carrier to the patient and the healthcare provider after an insurance claim has been processed. The provider will receive an EOB if the claim is submitted by paper; however, if the claim is submitted electronically the provider will receive an **ERA (electronic remittance advice)**. If the provider has not accepted assignment, the payment may be sent directly to the patient. The form states the status of the claim—that is, whether it is paid, pending, rejected, or denied. The EOB received by the patient states that it is not a bill. Before an EOB is received, the medical office specialist is responsible for completing many steps, including the following:

1. Obtaining a correct and complete patient information form
2. Verifying patient insurance benefits
3. Obtaining signatures on the proper forms (release of information and assignment of benefits)
4. Accurate data entry of all information
5. Preparing encounter forms
6. Preparing sign-in sheets
7. Posting (entering into the computer) charges and diagnoses, as noted on the encounter form
8. Submitting a "clean claim"

Rejected or delayed insurance claims are expensive for the medical facility because resubmitting a claim means that work is repeated. Dealing with insurance claims that a third-party payer denies, downcodes, or requests more information on ultimately affects the financial status of the practice. Practices are successful if their **turnaround time** (the amount of time it takes for the insurance carrier to process the claim) falls within a reasonable period, depending on the payer. A continuing cash flow results in a successful practice.

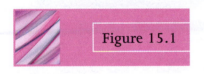

Figure 15.1 Locators on the CMS-1500 claim form that are gathered during the patient registration process.

In reality, gathering the information required on a medical claim begins when the patient first enters the physician's office or hospital. Data used to complete form locators 1 through 14 on the CMS-1500 and form locators 8–11, 50, 58–62, and 65 on the UB-04 are collected during patient registration (Figures 15.1 and 15.2). The patient's proof of insurance and identification information are photocopied (Figure 15.3) or

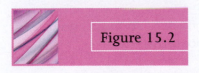

Figure 15.2 Locators on the UB-04 claim form that are gathered during the patient registration process.

Example: United States passport

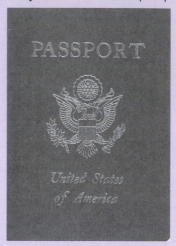

Example: Insurance carrier ID card

URHealthInsurance

Account   **12344567**
Issuer (80844)

ID: **555678899 01**
Name: **Jane Smith**
Coverage Effective Date: 01/01/2016

PCP: **James Smith**

PCP Phone: 555-214-3400

Network
Copays:
PCP Visit $15
Specialist $15
Hospital ER $50
Urgent Care $50

WWW.URHEALTH.COM

You may be asked to present this card when you receive care. The card does not guarantee coverage. You must comply with all terms and conditions of the plan. Willful misuse of this card is considered fraud.

IN AN EMERGENCY: Seek care immediately. Go directly to the nearest emergency facility or call 911. If you have selected a PCP, call your PCP (or have someone call for you) as soon as possible for further assistance and directions on follow-up care. When possible, you should call your PCP within 48 hours.

Claims: P.O. Box 5498, Albany, TN 42514-7000

Member Services: 800-555-6222   Mental Health/Substance Abuse: 800-555-6333

Back of Insurance card

Kindness Healthcare

Options PPO
Effective 01/01/16

PAID Prescriptions LLC
RX Bin 610000 UHEALTH

ANDREW SMITH
Member # 123-45-6789

WORKPLACE, INC.

Group # 500000
COPAY: Office Visit $10 ER $50
   Rx $10Gn/$15Br/$25NF

Electronic Claims Payer ID 90000   MTH

Call toll-free 800-555-0123 for Member Services

Kindness Healthcare

ADM. CERT	PLAN DBC	PRE-CERT
8888888 Identification No.		**DC000** Group
JASON BREEN Member Name		
A1234525 Physician Number		**01/11/59** Member Date of Birth
CATHERINE FRANK, M.D. Physician Name		
PS $10 ER $25 UC $10 IPO Di Copay Rider Information		

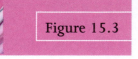

Figure 15.3   Photocopy the patient's proof of insurance and identification information (samples are only representations and not actual health insurance cards).

scanned. Signatures are required as policies and procedures are explained to the patient. It is the medical office specialist's responsibility to see that all patient, guarantor, and insurance information is in order and that all forms are completed before the patient is seen by the physician.

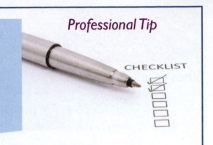

During the patient's care, all procedures and tests are documented on an encounter form or electronically. The physician will document the diagnosis after the visit or after test results have been received. All data are then integrated onto the claim form. The claim form is submitted to the carrier for payment.

Claims Process

The insurance carrier's decision regarding whether or not to pay a claim is called adjudication. **Adjudication** is the act of processing a claim that consists of edits, review, and determination (Figure 15.4). Once the insurance carrier receives a claim from the physician or healthcare facility, it is processed. The initial review of each claim consists of automated reviews by the payer's front-end claims processing system that screen the basic data on the claim form. The claim is edited to check for billing errors (such as a policy I.D. number missing, patient's name, or place of service code). Claims with errors or simple mistakes are rejected, and the payer transmits instructions to the provider to correct errors and/or omissions and to rebill the service. The medical insurance specialist should respond to such a request as quickly as possible by supplying the correct information and, if necessary, submitting a clean claim that is accepted by the payer for processing. If problems result from the automated review, the claim is suspended and set aside for review. A claim examiner will check that the diagnosis and CPT codes are linked when reviewing claims. The diagnosis and procedures are reviewed to be sure the treatment was medically necessary, which means appropriate for the diagnosis. Medical review examiners are part of the third-party payer's staff, and they verify the medical necessity of providers' reported procedures.

The claim may be denied if the reported procedure does not match the diagnosis code. The examiner determines if the claim is payable, and a payment decision is made. The claims examiner then pays, denies, or partially pays the claim. A claim that is removed from a payer's automated processing system is sent for **manual review**. When a claim is pulled for manual review, the provider may be asked to submit clinical documentation to support the claim. The carrier then makes a determination to pay the claim (or not) and provides an EOB/ERA to the provider and the insured.

To use an extreme example, suppose the codes on the insurance claim form indicate the patient has a broken arm and the treatment given was removal of the tonsils. Because removing the tonsils is not a medically necessary treatment for a broken arm, the claim would be denied. If the patient were instead treated with a cast for the broken arm, it would suit the diagnosis and would be considered medically necessary.

A carrier will downcode a claim if it is determined to not be medically necessary at the level reported. Downcoding is also referred to as medical necessity reduction. After the claim has gone through the adjudication process and a claim has been downcoded or denied, an **appeal** may be submitted to the insurance carrier by participating

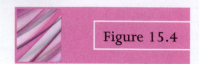

Figure 15.4

Steps of adjudication.

1. Insurance carrier receives insurance claim form. Data elements are checked by payer's front-end claims processing system. Paper claims are date-stamped and entered into payer's computer system by data entry or scanning.
2. First items checked are patient's name, plan number, service code, valid diagnosis code, date of service, patient sex in relation to gender-specific procedure code (refer to patient information form).
3. Claim is rejected and payer transmits instructions to provider to correct errors and/or omissions to rebill for services.
4. Additional edits are applied by payer's computer system such as patient eligibility for benefits, time limits for filing claims, preauthorization or referral required, duplicate dates of service.
5. Procedure codes are compared with the patient's policy schedule of benefits to see whether the reported services are covered.
6. Procedure codes and diagnostic codes are compared to see whether services were medically necessary.
7. Claim is suspended if problems results from the automated review and set aside for manual review.
8. ERA sent to provider. The remittance advice includes the amount the policy covers for each service, generally called the allowed charge or allowable charge, which is determined according to the policy's guidelines.
9. If the patient or insured must pay a deductible and/or coinsurance, *that amount is subtracted from the allowed charge.*
10. The remainder is the amount due to the provider.
11. An EOB is sent to the policyholder and an EOB or ERA is sent to the provider. Even if no benefit or payment is due from the insurance carrier, an EOB/ERA is sent out.

Special note: Completion of this process may be delayed by errors on the insurance claim form. Incomplete or inaccurate insurance claim forms are retained and a request is sent asking for additional information. Payment is withheld until problems are resolved.

providers (PARs). The person requesting an appeal is referred to as the *claimant*. These claims need to be reviewed and appealed for reconsideration. The appeals process is done in writing and may include documents such as operative reports or X-rays to aid in determining medical necessity. The medical office specialist must evaluate the claim to see if the claim needs resubmitting or if an appeal letter must be written to appeal a claim. If a carrier has continued to deny all of the practice's appeal requests, the provider can file a request to the state insurance commissioner for assistance. The state insurance commissioner has regulatory control over insurance carriers and will assist in insurance appeals or disputes.

Any precautions that can be taken when submitting claims to carriers should be taken to ensure that claims are not denied because of medical necessity reduction. If a claim is denied because of lack of medical necessity, the provider must refund any payment made on the claim by the payer and the patient.

Denials are a challenge for healthcare providers because of the loss of revenue, which includes lost resources and time. Healthcare providers work diligently to improve the management of medical necessity denials. The priority here is to prevent a denial from ever occurring by proving that the procedure or treatment is medically necessary. The medical office specialist who is posting payments needs to be aware of downcoding by the payer and take appropriate action.

Determining the Fees

Providers use different methods to determine their fee structure (the amount charged for each procedure performed). As stated by the American Medical Association (AMA), "Physicians have the right to establish their fees at a level which they believe fairly reflects the costs of providing a service and the value of the professional judgment." Two main methods are used for determining fees: charged-based and resource-based fee structures.

Charge-Based Fee Structure

Charge-based fees are the fees that many providers charge for similar services. To set their fees, providers begin with an analysis of their procedure codes. To determine if their fees are in range with other providers of the same specialty, they may research a nationwide fee database. This information may be purchased by the provider to ascertain how fees compare to national averages. The database is divided into categories to indicate fees that are 25%, 50%, 75%, and 90% higher based on fees charged throughout the United States. A provider can decide if his usual fees should be at the high, low, or midpoint range.

Resource-Based Fee Structures

Resource-based fees are based on the following three factors:

1. How difficult it is for the provider to perform the procedure (work)
2. How much office overhead the procedure involves (practice expense)
3. The relative risk that the procedure presents to the patient and the provider (malpractice)

Third-party payers also establish the amount they will reimburse providers. Each payer will determine the **usual, customary, and reasonable (UCR)** fee they feel should be charged by the provider by determining the percentage of the published fee in the national database that they will pay.

History of the Resource-Based Relative Value Scale

Because of rapidly rising expenditures in the Medicare program, in December 1985, Harvard University conducted a national study; it submitted the final report in 1988. Previously, Medicare payments had been based on a Medicare-developed "reasonable fee schedule" that used historical charges. The Omnibus Budget Reconciliation Act (OBRA) of 1989 enacted a physician payment schedule based on a **resource-based relative value scale (RBRVS)**. This law called for the reasonable fee schedule to be gradually replaced by the RBRVS payment system because it fairly represented the resources used to perform the procedure or service.

On January 1, 1992, Medicare implemented the RBRVS system as the payment system to be used. The RBRVS replaced Medicare's 25-year-old "customary, prevailing, and reasonable" (CPR) charge system. This was the most sweeping and far-reaching change to the Medicare Part B payment system to date. In brief, RBRVS ranks physician services by assigning each a relative value. It replaced providers' consensus on fees—the historical charges—with a relative value based on resources.

The RBRVS System

A **relative value unit (RVU)** is a unit of measurement assigned to a medical service based on the relative skill and time required to perform it. The RBRVS system is composed of three elements measured in RVUs:

1. **Nationally uniform relative value:** This value is based on the following three cost elements:

- *Provider's work:* the physician's individual effort (the largest cost element), which accounts for 52% of the total relative value for each service. The initial physician work RVUs were based on the results of the Harvard University study. The factors used to determine physician work include the time it takes to perform the service, the technical skill and physical effort, the required mental effort and judgment, and the stress due to the potential risk to the patient. The physician's work relative values are updated each year to account for changes in medical practice. Also, the legislation enacting the RBRVS requires the Centers for Medicare and Medicaid Services (CMS) to review the whole scale at least every 5 years.
- *Practice expense:* the practice costs associated with delivering a physician service (overhead). The practice expense component of the RBRVS accounts for an average of 44% of the total relative value for each service. Until recently, practice expense RVUs were based on a formula using average Medicare-approved charges from 1991 (the year before the RBRVS was implemented) and the proportion of each specialty's revenue that is attributable to practice expenses. However, in January 1999, CMS began a transition to resource-based practice expense RVUs for each CPT code that differs based on the site of service. In 2002, the resource-based practice expenses were fully transitioned.
- *Professional liability insurance:* the professional liability insurance premium costs (malpractice). On January 1, 2000, CMS implemented the resource-based professional liability insurance (PLI) relative value units. The PLI component of the RBRVS accounts for an *average* of 4% of the total relative value for each service. The CMS began reviewing appropriate PLI relative values. With this implementation and final transition of the resource-based practice expense relative units on January 1, 2002, all components of the RBRVS became resource based.

To understand the uniform relative value, one must look at each value separately and place a measurement on it. For example, for each $1.00 of services, the work accounts for x amount, the PE (practice expense) accounts for y amount, and the malpractice accounts for z amount, to equal the total of $1.00. A family practitioner who charges for a flu shot produces relative values that are much lower than those of a cardiac surgeon who performs open heart surgery. For each value, the number will be placed according to the provider's work performed, the cost to practice, and the cost of the malpractice insurance or liability risk to the patient.

2. **Geographic Practice Cost Index (GPCI):** This value is the number that is multiplied by each RVU to show the cost element for each value in that specific geographical location. Used by Medicare in its RBRVS payment systems, GPCIs are designed to represent the relative costs coupled with physician work, practice, and malpractice expenses in a Medicare area compared with the national average relative costs. However, in 1989, the OBRA mandated that 25% of a physician's work payment be adjusted according to geographic earnings differences. The remaining 75% of the physician's work payment is to be the same for all areas. For example, it would cost more for work, for practice overhead, and for malpractice insurance in Manhattan, NY, than in Lexington, KY. Under current law, changes in GPCIs do not impact total Medicare expenditures. Instead, GPCIs redistribute payments among Medicare payment localities.

3. Nationally uniform conversion factor: A **conversion factor** is a numerical factor (dollar amount) used to multiply or divide a quantity when converting from one system of units to another. This conversion factor is determined annually by the legislature and published in the *Federal Register*. It is used by Medicare to make adjustments according to the changes in the cost of living index. The **Medicare conversion factor (MCF)** is a national value that converts the total RVUs into payment amounts for the purpose of reimbursing physicians for services provided. The conversion factor is updated every year by CMS and published in the *Federal Register*.

The Medicare Conversion Factor

The Medicare conversion factor is a factor that converts geographically adjusted number of relative value units (RVUs) for each service provided in the Medicare physician payment schedule into a dollar payment amount. The initial Medicare conversion factor was set at $31.001 in 1992. Conversion factor updates are based on three factors:

- The Medicare economic
- Expenditure target "performance adjustment"
- Miscellaneous adjustments including those for "budget neutrality"

The Medicare Conversion Factor to be used for physician payments as of January 1, 2017 is $35.8887.

Determining the Medicare Fee

The relative value of each unit is multiplied by GPCIs for each Medicare locality and then translated into a dollar amount by an annually adjusted conversion factor. The **Medicare Fee Schedule (MFS)** is based on RBRVS fees. Therefore, the fees are based on the federal government's data regarding what each service costs.

When calculating the allowed Medicare fee for a physician, the formula is as follows:

1. Determine the procedure code for the service (CPT).
2. Use the RVUs for work, practice expense, and malpractice.
3. Use the GPCI for work, practice expense, and malpractice.
4. Multiply each RVU by each GPCI.
5. Add the three adjusted totals.
6. Multiply the total sum by the conversion factor.

The following practice exercise will help the student determine the Medicare-allowed fees for the procedures listed. The relative values are also listed with the GPCI.

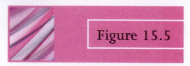

Figure 15.5

Example of how to determine the Medicare allowed fee for procedure code 99203 for a physician in Dallas, Texas.

	RVU		GPCI	
WORK	1.018	×	1.018 =	1.036324
PRACTICE EXPENSE	1.009	×	1.009 =	1.018081
MALPRACTICE	+0.772	×	0.772 =	0.595984
TOTAL				2.650389

2.650389 × 35.8887 = 95.1190157043 = $95.12

Figure 15.5 demonstrates the calculations for procedure code 99203 using the locale of Dallas, Texas, with a 2017 conversion factor of $35.8887.

To complete Practice Exercise 15.1, determine the Medicare-allowed fee for the geographical areas listed by using the GPCIs and conversion factors from Figures 15.6 and 15.7.

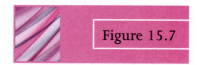

Figure 15.6

GPCIs and conversion factors.

Geographic Location	Work GPCI	Practice Expense GPCI	Malpractice Expense GPCI
Dallas, TX	1.018	1.009	0.772
Houston, TX	1.019	1.006	0.955
Ft. Worth, TX	1.005	0.995	0.772

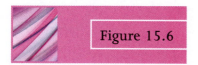

Figure 15.7

Procedure codes and conversion factors.

CPT Description	Work RVU	Practice RVU	Malpractice RVU
99203 Office outpatient/new	1.018	1.009	0.772
99213 Office outpatient/established	0.97	0.40	0.07
23500 Treat clavicle fracture	2.21	3.73	0.39

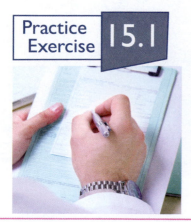

Practice Exercise 15.1

Determine the Medicare-allowed fees for the procedures listed. Use the 2017 conversion factor of $35.8887.

	Dallas	Houston	Fort Worth
99203:	95.12		
99213:			
23500:			

Other payers (insurance carriers) are switching to the resource-based fees rather than the charge-based fees that represented the providers' consensus on fees/charges. Debate surrounds the use of resource-based fees because physicians' malpractice insurance has increased so dramatically in the past few years. The increase in malpractice insurance is one of the reasons why some providers are no longer able to practice medicine. The specialists who are affected the most are obstetricians and gynecologists and orthopedic surgeons. If the RVU for malpractice were increased to accommodate the cost increase in the insurance, physicians' fees would greatly increase. In President George W. Bush's State of the Union address in 2003, he asked Congress to put into law medical liability reform. This would help alleviate the high malpractice bills. In 2005 and 2006, President Bush pushed this issue, but the legislation failed to pass both houses of Congress. At the same time, states were busily engaged in tort reform directed at medical malpractice cases. During the first half of 2005, over 60 bills were passed and signed into law in 31 states. Reform efforts are still being discussed and reviewed at the state level.

The medical office specialist must be aware of and become familiar with payers' reimbursement calculations in order to review an EOB/ERA to determine if the payment amount is correct.

Allowed Charges

Allowed charges refer to the maximum allowed amounts for covered charges. Some payers refer to this as the *maximum allowed fee, allowed amount,* or *allowable charge.* This is the amount the payer will pay the provider for her service. An allowed charge also includes the amount that the patient will pay. The provider's usual charge for the procedure or service may be higher, equal to, or lower than the allowed charge.

> ### Example
>
> The allowed amount is $100.00, but within that allowed amount the patient is responsible for 20% and the payer is responsible for 80%, equaling 100% of the allowed amount.
>
> Consider another example in which the allowed amount is $100.00. The payer will pay $75.00 of the allowed and the patient's copay is $25.00. Again, the two payments equal 100% of the allowed amount.

The allowed amount a provider receives from the third-party payer depends on whether the provider is participating or not participating in the payer's plan. Participating providers agree by contract to accept the third-party payer's allowed charge.

If a provider is a PAR with the payer, she agrees to the fees and the rules that stipulate that the provider may not bill a patient for the part of the charge that the payer did not pay.

When an allowed charge has been set, the carrier never pays more than this amount to the provider. If the provider's usual charge is less than the insurance carrier's allowed charge, the carrier will pay the lower of the two. The payment is *always* based on the lower of the two, whether it is the provider's usual charge or the allowed charge. Figure 15.8 illustrates that a provider always should review his usual charges annually to receive the highest reimbursement.

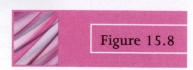

Figure 15.8

A provider should always review usual charges annually to receive the highest reimbursement.

Provider A usual charge $200.00   Allowed amount/payer pays: $150.00

Provider B usual charge $125.00   Allowed amount $150.00/payer pays: $125.00

As the medical office specialist can see, Provider B lost $25.00 because his usual charge was too low.

A non-PAR provider will only receive the allowed charge from the third-party payer and may bill the balance to the patient.

Payers' Policies

Figure 15.9 provides an example of an allowed charge for a provider who is participating with Medicare. Under Medicare Part B, reimbursement to a PAR provider will pay the physician 80% of the allowed amount *after the calendar year deductible has been satisfied.* The patient is responsible for 20%, which is her coinsurance.

A payer's policy has an allowed charge for each procedure. In Figure 15.10, the plan pays 100% of the provider's usual charges—*up to the maximum allowed by the payer.*

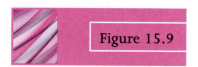

Figure 15.9

Example of an allowed charge for a provider who is participating with Medicare.

The physician charges	$300
Allowed amount	$275
	$25 (provider"s write-off)
Allowed amount	$275
Medicare deductible	−$183.00 (subtract 2017 deductible)
	$92.00

$92.00 × 80% = $73.60 Medicare pays to provider

$92.00 × 20% = $18.40 + $183.00 (deductible) = $201.40 (total patient responsibility)

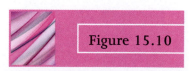

Figure 15.10

In this example, the plan pays 100% of the provider's usual charges, up to the maximum allowed by the payer.

Provider A—Participating

Provider's usual charge	$2,000.00
Policy pays its allowed charge	$1,500.00
Provider writes off the difference between the usual charge and the allowed amount	$500.00

Provider B—Nonparticipating

Provider's usual charge	$2,000.00
Policy pays its allowed charge	$1,500.00
Provider bills the patient for the difference between the usual and allowed charge.	$500.00
Provider B has no write-off.	

Provider A—Participating

Usual charge	$2,000.00
Allowed charge	$1,500.00
Policy pays 80% of the allowed charge	$1,200.00
Patient responsible for the 20% of the allowed charge	$300.00
Provider writes off the difference between the usual and allowed charge	$500.00

Figure 15.11

The patient is only responsible for the coinsurance of the maximum allowed charge if the provider is a PAR provider.

Provider B—Nonparticipating

Usual charge	$2,000.00
Allowed charge	$1,500.00
Policy pays 80% of the allowed charge	$1,200.00
Patient responsible for 20% of the allowed charge ($300.00) and the difference between the usual and allowed charge ($500.00)	$800.00
Provider B has no write-off.	

Figure 15.12

If the provider is a non-PAR provider, the patient is responsible for the difference between the provider's usual charge and the maximum allowed charge.

When a patient has a policy that requires coinsurance payments and the payer has a maximum allowed charge for each procedure, the patient is only responsible for the coinsurance of the maximum allowed charge if the provider is a PAR provider (Figure 15.11). If the provider is a non-PAR provider (Figure 15.12), the patient again is responsible for the difference between the provider's usual charge and the maximum allowed charge.

Calculate the financial responsibility of the patient, the amount the carrier will pay, and the amount the provider must write off.

Practice Exercise 15.2

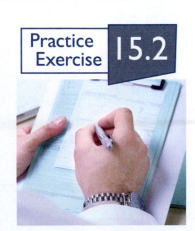

1. Debbie Ducktails was seen in Dr. Musk's office today for knee pain. Total charges are $315.00. Allowed amount is $175.00. Benefits pay at 70%.

   Usual charge _____

   Allowed charge _____

   Policy pays _____ of the allowed charge, which is _____. Patient is responsible for _____ of the allowed charge, which is _____. Provider writes off the difference between the usual and allowed charge: _____.

   _____   _____   _____
   Patient's responsibility   Write-off   Carrier pays

(Continued)

Practice Exercise 15.2

(Continued)

2. Kate Baird was seen in the doctor's office today for an ingrown toenail. Total charges are $200. Allowed amount is $135.00. Kate is subject to a deductible of $100.00. Once this is met, her benefits pay at 75%.

Usual charge   _____

Allowed charge   _____

Deductible   _____

Policy pays _____ of the allowed charge, which is _____. Patient is responsible for _____ of the allowed charge, which is _____. Provider writes off the difference between the usual and allowed charge: _____.

_____	_____	_____
Patient's responsibility	Write-off	Carrier pays

3. Sue Smith is being seen in Dr. Sampson's office today for ear piercing. Total charges are $200.00. This fee is not covered by her insurance company.

Usual charge   _____

Allowed charge   _____

Deductible   _____

Policy pays _____ of the allowed charge, which is _____. Patient is responsible for _____ of the allowed charge, which is _____. Provider writes off the difference between the usual and allowed charge: _____.

_____	_____	_____
Patient's responsibility	Write-off	Carrier pays

4. Kalvin Combs is having outpatient surgery at the Baylor Medical Center. Kalvin is on an indemnity plan. Total charges are $1,489.32. He is subject to a $250.00 deductible. Once the deductible is met, benefits pay at 80%.

Usual charge   _____

Allowed charge   _____

Deductible   _____

Policy pays _____ of the allowed charge, which is _____. Patient is responsible for _____ of the allowed charge, which is _____. Provider writes off the difference between the usual and allowed charge: _____.

_____	_____	_____
Patient's responsibility	Write-off	Carrier pays

Calculate the financial responsibility of the patient, the amount the carrier will pay, and the amount the provider must write off.

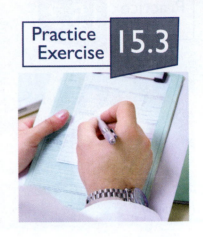

1. Annie Bates was seen in the doctor's office today for sinusitis. She is subject to her annual deductible of $150.00. Once her deductible is met, she must pay a copayment of $20.00. Today's total billed charges are $215.00. The allowed amount is $175.00.

   Usual charge   _____

   Allowed charge   _____

   Deductible   _____

   Policy pays _____ of the allowed charge, which is _____. Patient is responsible for the _____ of the allowed charge, which is _____. Provider writes off the difference between the usual and allowed charge: _____.

   _____   _____   _____
   Patient's responsibility   Write-off   Carrier pays

2. Jessica Woods was seen in the office today for an allergic reaction to Allegra. She is subject to a $500.00 deductible, and today's charges total $217.00. Total allowed amount is $125.00.

   Usual charge   _____

   Allowed charge   _____

   Deductible   _____

   Policy pays _____ of the allowed charge, which is _____. Patient is responsible for _____ of the allowed charge, which is _____. Provider writes off the difference between the usual and allowed charge: _____.

   _____   _____   _____
   Patient's responsibility   Write-off   Carrier pays

3. Melissa Jackson had outpatient surgery at Taylor Medical Center. Total charges are $3,895.56. Allowed amount is $2,956.18. Melissa is subject to a $500.00 deductible, and her rate of benefit is 90%.

   Usual charge   _____

   Allowed charge   _____

   Deductible   _____

   Policy pays _____ of the allowed charge, which is _____. Patient is responsible for _____ of the allowed charge, which is _____. Provider writes off the difference between the usual and allowed charge: _____.

   _____   _____   _____
   Patient's responsibility   Write-off   Carrier pays

(Continued)

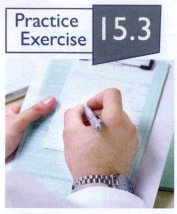

Practice Exercise 15.3

(*Continued*)

4. Sara Tipping is seen in Dr. Smith's office today for hyperthyroidism. She is subject to a $20.00 copayment. Total charges are $85.00. Allowed amount is $65.00. Dr. Smith referred her for some lab work to be done at Ballard Laboratory; total lab charges are $175.00. Allowed amount is $125.00. These lab charges are subject to her deductible of $100.00 and are paid at the 80% rate of benefit.

Usual charge   _____

Allowed charge   _____

Deductible   _____

Policy pays _____ of the allowed charge, which is _____. Patient is responsible for _____ of the allowed charge, which is _____. Provider writes off the difference between the usual and allowed charge: _____.

_____   _____   _____
Patient's responsibility   Write-off   Carrier pays

Practice Exercise 15.4

Calculate the financial responsibility of the patient, the amount the carrier will pay, and the amount the provider must write off.

1. Jill Self was seen in Dr. Dancing's office today for the flu. She is subject to a $20.00 copayment. Total charges are $175.00. Allowed amount is $125.00.

Usual charge   _____

Allowed charge   _____

Policy pays _____ of the allowed charge, which is _____. Patient is responsible for the _____ of the allowed charge, which is _____. Provider writes off the difference between the usual and allowed charge: _____.

_____   _____   _____
Patient's responsibility   Write-off   Carrier pays

2. Tanya Taylor had outpatient surgery at Baylor Medical Center. Total charges are $726.25. Allowed amount is $558.16. She is subject to a $250.00 deductible. Once her deductible is met, benefits are paid at 80%.

Usual charge   _____

Allowed charge   _____

Deductible   _____

Policy pays _____ of the allowed charge, which is _____. Patient is responsible for _____ of the allowed

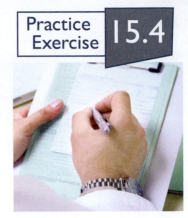

(Continued)

charge, which is _____. Provider writes off the difference between the usual and allowed charge: _____.

| _____ | _____ | _____ |
| Patient's responsibility | Write-off | Carrier pays |

3. Angie Grant was having outpatient lab work done at the Duncan Laboratory facility. Total charges were $576.00. (This is an indemnity plan, so it is a fee-for-service plan.) Angie is subject to a $250.00 deductible. Once this is met, her benefits pay at 80%.

Usual charge _____

Allowed charge _____

Deductible _____

Policy pays _____ of the allowed charge, which is _____. Patient is responsible for _____ of the allowed charge, which is _____. Provider writes off the difference between the usual and allowed charge:_____.

| _____ | _____ | _____ |
| Patient's responsibility | Write-off | Carrier pays |

4. Patricia Pegus is having a chest X-ray done at the Diagnostic Center in Dallas. Patricia is on an indemnity plan. Total charges today are $175.00. She is subject to a $100.00 deductible, and her benefits pay at 90%.

Usual charge _____

Allowed charge _____

Deductible _____

Policy pays _____ of the allowed charge, which is _____. Patient is responsible for _____ of the allowed charge, which is _____. Provider writes off the difference between the usual and allowed charge: _____.

| _____ | _____ | _____ |
| Patient's responsibility | Write-off | Carrier pays |

Capitation

When a provider enters into a **capitation plan** or contract with a carrier, the provider agrees to treat a number of members in that plan. The carrier in turn agrees to pay that provider based on a designated fee each month for each member in that plan. This is referred to as a **per member per month (PMPM)** fee. The member enrollment can change monthly. The payer sends the provider a list of the members at the beginning of the month with a check to pay for care for those members whether they are treated or not. The physician's incentive is to render as few services as possible in one sitting while still providing excellent medical care. The term *cap rate* means *capitation rate*. During the course of the year, some payers hold back or withhold a percentage of the provider's payment to pay or offset any additional costs that may be incurred for referrals, hospital admissions, or other services provided by the plan. At the end of the year, any **withhold** not used is distributed to providers as a bonus.

Consider this example of a capitation plan: A payer is negotiating with a physiatrist for physical therapy for its members. A list of procedures will be agreed on for services rendered under this contract. The payer sets a dollar amount for each member for physical therapy services listed. At the beginning of each month, the provider receives x dollars for the members enrolled—whether they are seen or not.

> ### Example
>
> For physical therapy, the provider would receive $30.00 for each member. The total members enrolled for the month equals 100. Therefore, the provider would receive $3,000.00 at the beginning of each month.

Value-based Reimbursement

Value-based Reimbursement is shifting the revenue mix and causing providers to change the way they bill for care. Instead of the provider being paid by the number of visits and tests they order, their payments are based on the value of care they deliver. In 2016, value-based payment contracts are in their infancy. The Medicare Shared Savings Program is the most well-known and standardized example. Medicare continues to reimburse providers on a fee-for-service basis, but at the end of the year shared saving bonuses are calculated. There are challenges calculating quality measures that include quality performance for each population of patients and to measure performance on a continuous basis.

Calculations of Patient Charges

The medical office specialist will determine the patient's charges at the time of service so he will know the dollar amount to collect from the patient. The employer may offer only one insurance plan for the employee, so the patient doesn't have a choice in the type of coverage she has. If choices are given, the insured has chosen her insurance policy according to the deductible, copays, coinsurance, and excluded services. Depending on the medical plan, the insured may be required to make four types of payments: deductibles, copayments, coinsurance, and payments for excluded services. The medical office specialist will be able to estimate what needs to be paid at the time of service after verifying the insured's insurance plan benefits.

Deductible

Many payers require policyholders or the insured to pay a certain amount of covered expenses to the provider before the insurance benefits begin. This amount is called the *deductible*. The reason it is called a deductible is because the payer deducts this specific amount from any charges billed before paying the bill.

> ### Example
>
> A new patient is seen in a physician's office, and the charge is $250.00. The patient's deductible is $200.00. When the medical office specialist sends a claim for $250.00, the payer deducts the $200.00 and pays according to the contract on the $50.00 only.

Some plans have individual deductibles, which must be met by each individual listed on the policy. Family deductibles are the combined amount for all individuals listed on the plan. The policy may state that a family deductible refers to at least three individuals. For the family deductible to be met, the total for all individuals listed on the policy must be met before the plan will pay for benefits.

Individual and family deductibles are a fixed dollar amount and are set by the insurance carrier. This information is stated in the insured's policy. One individual member of a family can meet a family deductible. When a deductible is required, it must be met before benefits from the carrier begin. The deductibles, copayments, and coinsurance that patients are required to pay are referred to as **out-of-pocket expenses**. Deductibles are set per calendar year. For example, each January the deductible amount is reset and must be satisfied (met) before insurance benefits pay out. It is not unusual for an annual deductible to be as high as $2,000.00 to $5,000.00.

Maximum out-of-pocket expenses are determined by the payer and listed in the insured's policy. The payer will reimburse services at 100% once the maximum out-of-pocket expenses have been met for the year. The policy may state, for example, that services will be paid at 100% after a $2,500.00 maximum out-of-pocket limit has been met within the year. This benefit protects the insured from extreme financial losses because of high medical bills.

The **lifetime maximum** benefit specified in an insurance policy is different from out-of-pocket expenses because once the stated maximum has been met for a lifetime, no more benefits will be paid. The maximum benefit should be questioned at the time the medical office specialist verifies the patient's insurance. New healthcare reform eliminated annual and lifetime limits on healthcare coverage in insurance policies beginning on September 23, 2010.

Copayments

A medical insurance plan may require a copay to be paid at the time of service. The copay is a set amount that may be printed on the insurance card. If it is not, the medical specialist should retrieve the information electronically or manually from the payer. An example would be the following:

OV $15.00 (copay for office visit)
SP $35.00 (copay for specialist visit)
ER $100.00 (copay for emergency room visit)

Coinsurance

Many payers require coinsurance payments, which are a percentage of the contracted allowable charge. For example: Medicare pays 80% of the MFS (Medicare Fee Schedule) to a participating provider after the deductible is met. The patient is responsible for 20% (which is the coinsurance amount), the deductible if it has not been met, and the copay if it applies to the type of service.

Excluded Services

Excluded services are procedures or office visits that are not covered by the insurance carrier as defined in its policy. A medical insurance contract will usually state the medical services it does not cover. The physician's office may provide care for services that are not covered under a patient's policy. In this case, the patient is expected to pay at the time service is rendered. The medical office specialist is responsible for advising the patient about nonpayment before these services are rendered to discuss payment

Table 15.1	Common Benefits under Various Plans					
Plan Types		Deductible	Copay	Coinsurance	Out of Pocket	Coinsurance Post–Out of Pocket
PPO (Managed Care)						
Office: PAR		—	$20.00[a]	—	—	—
Office: Non-PAR[b]		$250.00	—	30%	—	—
Outpatient and Inpatient: PAR[b]		$250.00	—	20%	$1,500.00	0%
Outpatient and Inpatient: Non-PAR		$250.00	—	30%	$2,500.00	0%
HMO (Managed Care)						
Office: PAR to PCP		—	$20.00[a]	—	—	
Office: Non-PAR to PCP[c]		—	—	—	—	—
Outpatient (referred by PCP)[b]			$50.00	0%		
Inpatient (referred by PCP)[b]			$100.00	0%		
Indemnity (not managed care)[d]		$250.00		20%	$1,500.00	0%

[a]Covers office visits and any lab or X-rays done in physician's office.
[b]Precertification required.
[c]All services must be authorized by primary care provider (PCP) or no benefits are available.
[d]No discounts on indemnity plans unless negotiated with the provider. UCR applies for charges billed.

options. With some payers, such as Medicare, the medical office specialist must have the patient sign a form stating that he is responsible for the non-covered service. Table 15.1 shows procedures that may not be covered under certain types of managed care plans. Because employers customize some plans offered to their employees, it is recommended that the patient's benefits always be verified.

Practice Exercise 15.5

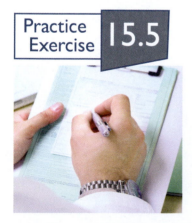

Using the information provided in the following table, calculate the patients' payment amounts.

CPT Code	Provider's Charge	Adjustment	Allowed Amount
99212	$66.00	$12.00	$54.00
93040	44.00	8.00	36.00
99201	88.00	26.00	62.00
99204	108.00	33.00	75.00
97032	45.00	16.00	29.00
97110	45.00	16.00	29.00
99213	90.00	38.00	52.00
73630	88.00	16.00	72.00

1. Patient 1 charges 99213, 73630, and 97110. No deductible applies. Plan pays at 80/20.

    Payer payment to provider _____

    Coinsurance _____

    Discount amount _____

Practice Exercise **15.5**

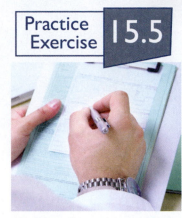

(Continued)

2. Patient 2 charges 99212 and 73630. Deductible of $100.00 applies. Plan pays at 80/20.

   Payer payment to provider _____

   Coinsurance _____

   Discount amount _____

3. Patient 3 charges 93040 and 97032. Deductible of $100.00 applies. Plan pays at 90/10.

   Payer payment to provider _____

   Coinsurance _____

   Discount amount _____

4. Patient 4 charge 99201. Copay of $20.00 applies. Plan pays at 100% after copay.

   Payer payment to provider _____

   Copayment _____

   Discount amount _____

5. Patient 5 charge 99204. Copay of $25.00 applies. Plan pays 100% after copay.

   Payer payment to provider _____

   Copayment _____

   Discount amount _____

Balance Billing

Balance billing is the act of billing a patient for any dollar amount left after the insurance carrier has paid and any copayment has been met. Whether a provider can balance the bill depends on the payer's rules. This is why it is important for medical office specialists to know the rules of their payers, especially the payers with whom they have negotiated contracts. Patients may be responsible for the amount of the usual charge that exceeds the payer's allowed charge.

Non-PAR providers can demand payment in full from the patient rather than waiting for the insurance carrier to process claims based on the UCR amount offered by healthcare plans. Because this affects the non-contracted, non-network providers, the billed charges are the full responsibility of the patient. Although the patient may have insurance coverage, when the patient is treated by a non-PAR provider, the provider can charge her usual fee. The patient will be reimbursed by the payer according to the payer's allowed fees. Under an indemnity plan, the billed amount is subject to UCR fees. The amount denied or reduced can be balance billed to the patient. Because the provider has no contract with the carrier, there are no rules binding the provider to write off any amount of the patient's account.

Processing an Explanation of Benefits

An EOB states the status of a claim—whether it is paid, pending, rejected, or denied. The medical office specialist must review all EOBs and apply payment information to the patient's account.

An explanation will not always be accompanied by payment, but it will state the status of the claim. The claim may be pending waiting for additional information. A **pending claim** is one that is received but not processed by the carrier because additional information is needed or there is an error. The EOB/ERA lists the patient, dates of services, types of service, and the charges filed on the insurance claim form. The EOB/ERA also describes how the amount of the benefit payment was determined. If claim forms were filed for more than one patient with the same insurance carrier at the same time, the provider's EOB/ERA may include information on more than one patient.

The format and contents of each EOB/ERA vary based on the benefit plan and the services provided. No universal form for explaining benefits is available. It has been a point of debate that all providers are required to use the CMS-1500 and the UB-04 standardized forms, yet carriers can customize their EOBs in any way. Terminology is also different on various EOBs/ERAs. For example, some EOBs/ERAs show the "Allowed Amount or Charge" and some EOBs/ERAs read "Deducted Amount." The medical office specialist will eventually become accustomed to the carriers with whom the provider contracts, but he should always review all EOBs/ERAs carefully before entering data.

However, many terms and categories are common to all carriers. Insurance carriers often use codes on the EOB to refer to these terms or situations. These codes are called **reason codes** and **remark codes**. Usually these codes are explained on the face or back of the EOB/ERA. If one line at a time is read, the descriptions and calculations for each patient are easily understood. An EOB/ERA contains three sections that explain how a claim was processed:

- *Service Information.* Identifies the provider (hospital or other facility, doctor, specialist, or clinic), dates of service, and charges from the provider.
- *Coverage Determination.* Summarizes the total deductions, charges not covered by the plan, and the amount the patient may owe the provider.
- *Benefit Payment Information.* Indicates who was paid, how much, and when.

Information on an EOB/ERA

The following information appears on an EOB/ERA:

1. Account name: company name
2. Date the EOB/ERA statement was finalized
3. Member's or insured's name and I.D. number
4. Patient's identification number as it appears on the I.D. card
5. Number assigned to the claim
6. Name of the person who received the service (the patient)
7. Provider's name
8. Service description column, which indicates:
   Dates of the services provided (DOS)
   Procedures performed (CPT codes)
   Total charge for each procedure
   The portion of the bill not covered by the plan
   The contractual allowed amount
   Patient's copay
   Patient's deductible or non-covered procedures or amounts
   Patient's coinsurance

9. Total payment to the provider

10. The total amount that is the patient's responsibility to the provider for services.

Practice Exercises 15.6, 15.7, and 15.8 provide examples of information shown on an EOB/ERA. Complete the tables using the payment information given.

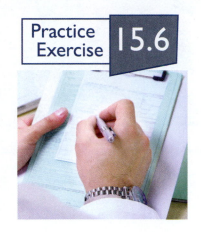

Practice Exercise 15.6

Complete the table and fill in the blanks using the payment information provided.

Physician Charges	Allowed Amounts	Insurance Pays	Deductible
$ 88.00	$66.00	80%	$150.00*
120.00	99.00		
90.00	81.00		

	Charge	Adjustment	Allowed	Deductible	Copay	Insurance Pays	Coinsurance
	$	$	$	$	$	$	$
	$	$	$	$	$	$	$
TOTALS	$	$	$	$	$	$	$

*Deductible not met.

BALANCE DUE FROM PATIENT:

Patient's Deductible: $_____

Patient's Coinsurance: $_____

TOTAL INSURANCE PAYMENT: $_____

TOTAL PHYSICIAN WRITE-OFF: $_____

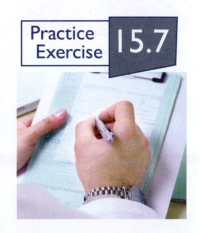

Practice Exercise 15.7

Complete the table and fill in the blanks using the payment information provided.

Physician Charges	Allowed Amounts	Insurance Pays	Deductible
$2,000.00	85%	70%	$200.00*

	Charge	Adjustment	Allowed	Deductible	Copay	Insurance Pays	Coinsurance
	$	$	$	$	$	$	$
	$	$	$	$	$	$	$
TOTALS	$	$	$	$	$	$	$

*$45.00 of deductible has been met.

BALANCE DUE FROM PATIENT:

Patient's Deductible: $_____

Patient's Coinsurance: $_____

TOTAL INSURANCE PAYMENT: $_____

TOTAL PROVIDER WRITE-OFF: $_____

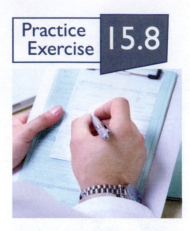

Practice Exercise 15.8

Complete the table and fill in the blanks using the payment information provided.

Physician Charges	Allowed Amounts	Insurance Pays	Deductible
$3,875.00	85%	90%	$250.00*

	Charge	Adjustment	Allowed	Deductible	Copay	Insurance Pays	Coinsurance
	$	$	$	$	$	$	$
	$	$	$	$	$	$	$
TOTALS	$	$	$	$	$	$	$

*Deductible has not been met.

BALANCE DUE FROM PATIENT:

Patient's Deductible: $_____

Patient's Coinsurance: $_____

TOTAL INSURANCE PAYMENT: $_____

TOTAL PROVIDER WRITE-OFF: $_____

After receiving an EOB/ERA and posting payments to patients' accounts, the medical office specialist must follow up on unpaid claims. Follow-up can be done online or by making telephone calls. Figures 15.13, 15.14, 15.15, and 15.16 are ERAs showing the status of claims. Insurance companies have specific time frames, called a *claim turnaround time* (and specified in the provider's contract), in which a claim will be processed once it is received.

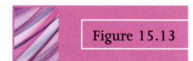

Figure 15.13

Sample ERA showing status of rejected claims.

Title: Rejected Claims Report

Purpose: To let the submitter know which claims were rejected and the reason (sometimes, very cryptic) for the rejection.

Comment: None

03/02/16 --

REJECTED CLAIMS for NAME OF DOCTOR M.D.—03/02/16

PATIENT	DATA in ERROR	DESCRIPTION
922387	97118	PROCCD INVALID FOR PAYER USE HCPC

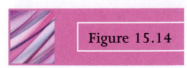

Figure 15.14

Sample ERA showing status of settled claims.

Title: Claims Settlement Report

Purpose: To let the submitter know which claims were settled (not necessarily paid) by the insurance company.

Comment: Some insurance companies will return this report, not all.

03/02/16 --

CLAIM SETTLEMENT for NAME OF DOCTOR M.D.—03/02/16

COMPLETED: EXPENSES INCURRED PRIOR TO COVERAGE

| PATIENT STATEMENT DATES | | | | TOTAL AMOUNT | |
	FROM	THRU	PAYER	CHARGES	PAID
911851	06/25/16–07/02/16		METROPOLITAN LIFE	$599.00	0.00
911879	08/13/16–08/18/16		METROPOLITAN LIFE	560.00	0.00

COMPLETED: PAYMENT MADE ACCORDING TO PLAN PROVISIONS

| PATIENT STATEMENT DATES | | | | TOTAL AMOUNT | |
	FROM	THRU	PAYER	CHARGES	PAID
917914	10/27/16–10/27/16		CIGNA	$274.00	0.00
917914	10/27/16–10/27/16		CIGNA	274.00	0.00
917922	10/29/16–10/31/16		CIGNA	560.00	0.00
917922	10/29/16–10/31/16		CIGNA	560.00	0.00
917922	10/29/16–10/31/16		CIGNA	560.00	0.00
917922	10/29/16–10/31/16		CIGNA	560.00	0.00
917922	10/29/16–10/31/16		CIGNA	560.00	0.00
917922	10/29/16–10/31/16		CIGNA	560.00	0.00
917922	10/29/16–10/31/16		CIGNA	560.00	0.00
917922	10/29/16–10/31/16		CIGNA	560.00	0.00
917894	09/29/16–09/29/16		CIGNA	274.00	0.00
917894	09/29/16–09/29/16		CIGNA	274.00	0.00
917922	11/04/16–11/06/16		CIGNA	553.00	0.00
917922	11/04/16–11/06/16		CIGNA	553.00	0.00
917922	11/04/16–11/06/16		CIGNA	553.00	0.00
917922	11/04/16–11/06/16		CIGNA	553.00	0.00

COMPLETED: NO PAYMENT WILL BE MADE FOR THIS CLAIM

| PATIENT STATEMENT DATES | | | | TOTAL AMOUNT | |
	FROM	THRU	PAYER	CHARGES	PAID
911851	06/25/16–07/02/16		METROPOLITAN LIFE	$599.00	0.00
911851	07/02/16–07/02/16		METROPOLITAN LIFE	371.00	0.00
911879	08/13/16–08/18/16		METROPOLITAN LIFE	560.00	0.00

Figure 15.14

(*Continued*)

Title: Zero Payment Report

Purpose: From insurance company to submitter. Claims that were fully processed and for which no payment will be made.

Comment: None

03/02/16 --

ZERO PAYMENT CLAIMS for NAME OF DOCTOR M.D.—03/02/16

Figure 15.15

Sample ERA showing status of claims for which no payment is forthcoming.

(*Continued*)

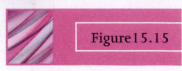

Figure15.15

(Continued)

CLAIM STATUS MESSAGE—COMPLETED: EXPENSES INCURRED
PRIOR TO COVERAGE

PATIENT NAME	CONTROL NUMBER	STATEMENT DATES FROM THRU	TOTAL CHARGES
E LIU	911851	06/25/16–07/02/16	$599.00

Payer: METROPOLITAN LIFE (714) 555-2500

E LIU	911879	08/13/16–08/18/16	560.00

Payer: METROPOLITAN LIFE (714) 555-2500

CLAIM STATUS MESSAGE—COMPLETED: NO PAYMENT WILL BE MADE
FOR THIS CLAIM

PATIENT NAME	CONTROL NUMBER	STATEMENT DATES FROM THRU	TOTAL CHARGES
E LIU	911851	06/25/16–07/02/16	$599.00

Payer: METROPOLITAN LIFE (714) 555-2500

E LIU	911851	07/02/16–07/02/16	371.00

Payer: METROPOLITAN LIFE (714) 555-2500

E LIU	911879	08/13/16–08/18/16	560.00

Payer: METROPOLITAN LIFE (714) 555-2500

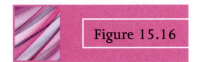

Figure 15.16

Medicare remittance allowance.

Title: Medicare Remittance Advice

Purpose: To let the submitter know the disposition of Medicare claims.

Comment: Contact Medicare for an explanation of the codes.

06-18-16 MEDICARE CLAIMS SUBMITTED FOR DR. "Name of Provider"

06-18-2016 MEDICARE Remittance Advice for "Medicare Provider Number"

DEL DOTTO, EVA M	BILLED	ALLOWED	DED.	COINS	PROV-PD	MC-ADJUST
04-16-16 21 1 99291	$250.00	$207.41	$41.48	$165.93	$ 42.59	CO42
04-17-16 21 1 99232	66.84	58.12	11.62	46.50	8.72	CO42
04-18-16 21 1 99232	66.84	58.12	11.62	46.50	8.72	CO42
CLAIM TOTALS:	383.68	323.65	64.72	258.93	60.03	

TRASVINA, CARMEN P	BILLED	ALLOWED	DED.	COINS	PROV-PD	MC-ADJUST
02-20-16 11 1 99205	157.68				157.68	CO16
CLAIM TOTALS:	157.68				157.68	

FIGLIETTI, JOSEPH S	BILLED	ALLOWED	DED.	COINS	PROV-PD	MC-ADJUST
04-16-16 11 1 95117	26.13	22.72	4.54		3.41	PR42
CLAIM TOTALS:	26.13	22.72	4.54	3.41		

WADE, DAVID M	BILLED	ALLOWED	DED.	COINS	PROV-PD	MC-ADJUST
04-15-16 11 1 99213	49.71	45.89	9.18		3.82	PR42
CLAIM TOTALS:	49.71	45.89	9.18	3.82		

TOSCHI, DAVID R	BILLED	ALLOWED	DED.	COINS	PROV-PD	MC-ADJUST
04-13-16 11 1 95117	26.13	22.72	4.54		3.41	PR42
04-13-16 11 1 9921325	49.71	45.89		9.18	3.82	PR42
CLAIM TOTALS:	75.84	68.61		13.72	7.23	

SINGLETON, IRENE M	BILLED	ALLOWED	DED.	COINS	PROV-PD	MC-ADJUST
04-13-16 11 1 99213	$ 49.71	45.89	9.18		3.82	PR42
CLAIM TOTALS:	49.71	45.89	9.18	3.82		

NELSON, MIRIAM	BILLED	ALLOWED	DED.	COINS	PROV-PD	MC-ADJUST
01-16-16 11 1 9921425	74.23			74.23		CO18
01-16-16 11 1 94060	76.92			76.92		PR50
01-16-16 11 1 90724	4.76			4.76		COB18
01-16-16 11 2 J1040	11.34			11.34		CO18
01-16-16 11 2 J1040	11.34			11.34		CO18
CLAIM TOTALS:	178.59			178.59		

BROWER, JOHN R	BILLED	ALLOWED	DED.	COINS	PROV-PD	MC-ADJUST
05-25-16 11 1 99213	49.71			49.71		CO18
05-25-16 11 2 J1040	11.34			11.34		CO18
05-25-16 11 2 J1040	11.34			11.34		CO18
05-25-16 11 2 J2010	6.52			6.52		CO18
CLAIM TOTALS:	78.91			78.91		

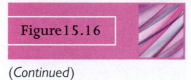

Figure 15.16

(Continued)

To apply your knowledge of EOBs and the method of calculating provider write-offs and patient financial responsibilities, complete Practice Exercises 15.9, 15.10. 15.11, and 15.12.

Complete the following EOB.

EXPLANATION OF BENEFITS

Today's Date

Payer's Name and Address

Aetna Insurance Company
P.O. Box 15999
New York, NY 12345

Provider's Name and Address

J. D. Mallard, M.D.
1933 East Beltway Road
Shreveport, LA 12345

Practice Exercise 15.9

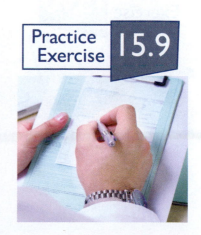

(Continued)

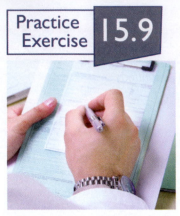

Practice Exercise 15.9

(Continued)

This statement covers payments for the following patient(s):
Claim Detail Section (If there are numbers in the "REMARKS" column, see the Remarks section for explanation.)

Patient Name: Hughes, Patsy   **Patient Account Number:** Hugan0
Patient I.D. Number: **Insured's Name:** Andrew Hughes
Group Number: 55216
Provider Name: J. D. Mallard, M.D.   **Inventory Number:** 44562   **Claim Control Number:** 28971

Service Date(s)	Procedure	Charges	Adjustment	Allowed	Copay	Deduct/Not Covered	Coins	Paid Amt.	Provider Paid/Remarks
02/16/2016	97039	$50.00	$	$49.00	$0.00	$	$	80%	
02/16/2016	97024	65.00	65.00		0.00	00.00			
02/19/2016	97039	50.00		50.00	0.00			80%	
02/21/2016	97039	50.00		50.00		50.00		80%	03
TOTALS									

BALANCE DUE FROM PATIENT:
PT'S DED/NOT COV $_____
PT'S COINS. $_____
031 Met Maximum Limit

PAYMENT SUMMARY SECTION (TOTALS)

Charges	Adjustment	Allowed	Copay	Deduct/Not Covered	Coins	Total Paid

Remarks: 031–Met Maximum Limit

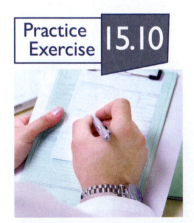

Practice Exercise 15.10

Complete the following EOB.

EXPLANATION OF BENEFITS

Today's Date

Payer's Name and Address

Aetna Insurance Company
P.O. Box 15999
New York, NY 12345

Provider's Name and Address

J. D. Mallard, M.D.
1933 Highpoint Dr.
Boise, ID 12345

This statement covers payments for the following patient(s):
Claim Detail Section (If there are numbers in the "REMARKS" column, see the Remarks section for explanation.)

Patient Name: Hughes, Patsy   **Patient Account Number:** Hugan0
Patient I.D. Number: **Insured's Name:** Andrew Hughes
Group Number: 55216
Provider Name: J. D. Mallard, M.D.   **Inventory Number:** 44562   **Claim Control Number:** 28971

Service Date(s)	Procedure	Charges	Adjustment	Allowed	Copay	Deduct/Not Covered	Coins	Paid Amt.	Provider Paid/Remarks
01/02/2016	65430	$1,500.00	$	$1,200.00	$0.00	$300.00	$	80%	
TOTALS									

BALANCE DUE FROM PATIENT: PT'S DED/NOT COV $_____
                               PT'S COINS. $_____

PAYMENT SUMMARY SECTION (TOTALS)

Charges	Adjustment	Allowed	Copay	Deduct/Not Covered	Coins	Total Paid

Remarks:

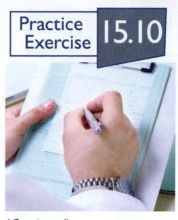

Practice Exercise **15.10**

(Continued)

Complete the following EOB.

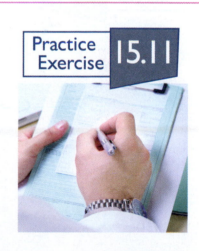

Practice Exercise **15.11**

EXPLANATION OF BENEFITS

Today's Date

Payer's Name and Address

Aetna Insurance Company
P.O. Box 15999
New York, NY 12345

Provider's Name and Address

J. D. Mallard, M.D.
1933 N. Broadway Blvd.
Las Vegas, NV 12345

This statement covers payments for the following patient(s):
Claim Detail Section (If there are numbers in the "REMARKS" column, see the Remarks Section for explanation.)

Patient Name: Hughes, Patsy   **Patient Account Number:** Hugan0
Patient I.D. Number: **Insured's Name:** Andrew Hughes
Group Number: 55216
Provider Name: J. D. Mallard, M.D.   **Inventory Number:** 44562   **Claim Control Number:** 28971

(Continued)

Practice Exercise 15.11

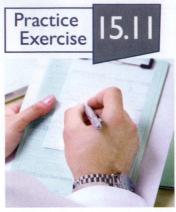

(Continued)

Service Date(s)	Procedure	Charges	Adjustment	Allowed	Copay	Deduct/Not Covered	Coins	Paid Amt.	Provider Paid/Remarks
04/09/2016	99213	$100.00	$	$ 78.00	$25.00	$0.00	$0.00	80%	
04/09/2016	80048	150.00	$	100.00				80%	
04/09/2016	71020	78.00		56.00				80%	
TOTALS									

BALANCE DUE FROM PATIENT: PT'S DED/NOT COV $_____

PT'S COINS. $_____

PAYMENT SUMMARY SECTION (TOTALS)

Charges	Adjustment	Allowed	Copay	Deduct/Not Covered	Coins	Total Paid

Remarks:

Practice Exercise 15.12

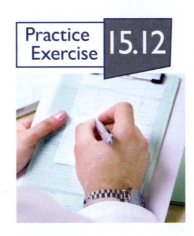

Complete the following EOB.

EXPLANATION OF BENEFITS

Today's Date

Payer's Name and Address

Aetna Insurance Company
P.O. Box 15999
New York, NY 12345

Provider's Name and Address

J. D. Mallard, M.D.
1933 W. Sepulveda
North Hills, CA 12345

This statement covers payments for the following patient(s):
Claim Detail Section (If there are numbers in the "REMARKS" column, see the Remarks section for explanation.)

Patient Name: Hughes, Patsy   **Patient Account Number:** Hugan0
Patient I.D. Number: **Insured's Name:** Andrew Hughes
Group Number: 55216
Provider Name: J. D. Mallard, M.D.   **Inventory Number:** 44562   **Claim Control Number:** 28971

Service Date(s)	Procedure	Charges	Adjustment	Allowed	Copay	Deduct/Not Covered	Coins	Paid Amt.	Provider Paid/Remarks
05/02/2016	72149	$1,300.00	$	$950.00	$0.00	$500.00	$	80%	
05/02/2016	94010	325.00		245.00	0.00			80%	
05/02/2016	99214	150.00		125.00	0.00			80%	
TOTALS									

BALANCE DUE FROM PATIENT: PT'S DED/NOT COV $_____
                                 PT'S COINS. $_____

PAYMENT SUMMARY SECTION (TOTALS)

Charges	Adjustment	Allowed	Copay	Deduct/Not Covered	Coins	Total Paid

Remarks:

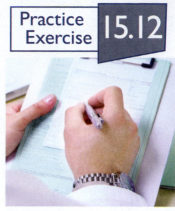

Practice Exercise 15.12

(Continued)

Reviewing Claims Information

When the EOB/ERA is received at the physician's office, the medical office specialist reviews it, checks all calculations, and makes sure that all charges submitted were processed and that the amounts paid are correct. If an error is found with the EOB, the medical office specialist must research the interoffice information first. For example, the medical office specialist should verify that the health insurance claim numbers and patient's name and date of birth were entered correctly. The medical office specialist should also review the original superbill to verify that all CPT codes, charges, and diagnoses were entered correctly. If all of those items are correct, the medical office specialist should review the medical record to confirm that the documentation matches the procedures billed. If the facility has processed the claim correctly, a request for review of the claim must be filed with the carrier.

If a claim is denied, downcoded, or partially paid after the medical office specialist has reviewed it and confirmed that all billing and documentation provided to the carrier were correct, an appeal must be filed with the payer for consideration of claim adjudication.

EOBs/ERAs are also used as evidence of payments when another insurance company needs such information to administer **coordination of benefits (COB)**. When benefits are coordinated with another insurance carrier, the primary EOB/ERA will be copied and forwarded to the secondary payer with the claim. The secondary payer will know what amount was paid by the primary insurance carrier and what is its responsibility. The goal is to provide the necessary information primarily through an EOB/ERA to help recipients understand the claim and to make sure that proper reimbursement is received by the provider

After reviewing the EOB/ERA, the medical office specialist records EOB/ERA and payment information in the insurance log, either electronically or manually. After a payment transaction has been entered into a patient's account, an adjustment should be made if required. Each transaction entry should relate to the procedure or service billed. The medical office specialist bills any remaining balance to the patients, if appropriate, and then files the EOBs/ERAs that have been paid by that insurance carrier. This file should be available for review at any time. EOB/ERA statements are to be kept according to state retention schedule requirements, in the event questions arise as to how claims were handled and paid. A **retention schedule** dictates how long patient records are to be kept and stored. This determination is based on state regulations and federal laws, such as Medicare laws.

Adjustments to Patient Accounts

An **adjustment** is a positive or negative change to a patient's account balance. Corrections, changes, and write-offs to patients' accounts are made by means of adjustments to the existing transactions. The medical office specialist will also adjust a patient's bill as a result of any discounts given. If the provider is a PAR provider, the difference between the billed amount (the provider's UCR fee) and the allowed amount is adjusted from the amount the patient owes. After posting the payment to the specific date and procedure, the adjustment should be made in the same way. This is referred to as per line item posting.

Processing Reimbursement Information

Four steps are to be followed when an EOB/ERA is received from an insurance carrier:

1. Enter the date when the EOB/ERA and any accompanying reimbursement are received.
2. Compare the EOB/ERA with the claim filed. Check dates of services, types of services, and charges to be sure all items were included on the EOB/ERA.
3. Check the accuracy of mathematical calculations.
4. Determine the amounts of any write-offs or adjustments to the patient's account that may be required. Also note whether a balance is due from the patient, or whether a refund is due the patient or insurance carrier. For example, if a patient paid for a service in advance and it was reimbursed by the carrier or if the patient or insurance carrier overpaid on an account, then a refund is due.

Confirming Amount Paid, Making Adjustments, and Determining Amount Due from Patient

To confirm the amount paid by the payer, to determine any needed adjustments or write-offs, and to determine the amount due from the patient or to be refunded to the patient, follow the steps in Figure 15.17.

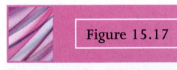

Figure 15.17

Steps for confirming what was paid by the carrier, determining any needed adjustment or write-off, and determining the amount due from the patient or to be refunded to the patient.

STEP 1

Billed Amount	$400.00
Allowed Amount	−$200.00
	−$100.00
$200.00	Write-Off
$100.00	"New" Allowed Amount

STEP 2

Allowed Amount $200.00

Minus deductible or copay (if no deductible go to Step 3)

STEP 3

"New" Allowed Amount × 70%, 80%, or 90% (whichever is the correct coinsurance percentage)

For example: $100.00
× .70
$70.00 paid by carrier to provider

STEP 4

"New" Allowed Amount × percentage of coinsurance (%) and/or copay plus deductible = **Patient's Responsibility**

Now it is time to put all your knowledge together by completing Practice Exercises 15.13, 15.14, and 15.15. Using the physician charge, allowed amount, amount insurance pays, and deductible amount, complete the EOB/ERA and fill in the missing information in the blanks for each exercise. In Practice Exercises 15.16, 15.17, 15.18, and 15.19, review the EOB and fill in the missing information in the blanks.

Practice Exercise 15.13

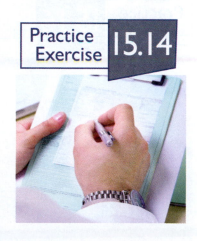

Complete the following EOB and fill in the blanks.

Physician Charges	Allowed Amounts	Insurance Pays	Deductible
$200.00	$169.43	90%	0.00
25.00	23.69		

	Charge	Adjustment	Allowed	Deductible	Copay	Insurance Pays	Coinsurance
	$	$	$	$	$	$	$
	$	$	$	$	$	$	$
TOTALS	$	$	$	$	$	$	$

BALANCE DUE FROM PATIENT:

Patient's Deductible: $_____

Patient's Coinsurance: $_____

TOTAL INSURANCE PAYMENT: $_____

TOTAL PHYSICIAN WRITE-OFF: $_____

Practice Exercise 15.14

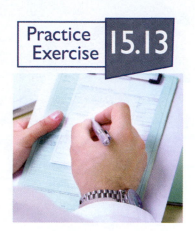

Complete the EOB and fill in the blanks below.

Physician Charges	Allowed Amounts	Insurance Pays	Deductible
$1,750.00	$1,750.00	95%	$150.00*
925.00	925.00		
400.00	400.00		
108.00	108.00		

	Charge	Adjustment	Allowed	Deductible	Copay	Insurance Pays	Coinsurance
	$	$	$	$	$	$	$
	$	$	$	$	$	$	$
	$	$	$	$	$	$	$
	$	$	$	$	$	$	$
TOTALS	$	$	$	$	$	$	$

*Deductible not met.

BALANCE DUE FROM PATIENT:

Patient's Deductible: $_____

Patient's Coinsurance: $_____

TOTAL INSURANCE PAYMENT: $_____

TOTAL PHYSICIAN WRITE-OFF: $_____

Practice Exercise 15.15

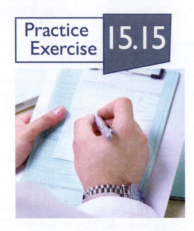

Complete the EOB and fill in the blanks below.

Physician Charges	Allowed Amounts	Insurance Pays	Deductible
$1,650.00	$123.70	95%	$250.00*
1,650.00	412.50		

	Charge	Adjustment	Allowed	Deductible	Copay	Insurance Pays	Coinsurance
	$	$	$	$	$	$	$
	$	$	$	$	$	$	$
TOTALS	$	$	$	$	$	$	$

*Deductible not met.

BALANCE DUE FROM PATIENT:

Patient's Deductible: $_____

Patient's Coinsurance: $_____

TOTAL INSURANCE PAYMENT: $_____

TOTAL PHYSICIAN WRITE-OFF: $_____

Practice Exercise 15.16

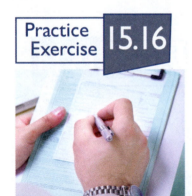

Review the EOB, then fill in the missing information in the blanks that follow the EOB.

Insured/Patient's name:

Health Insurance Company
800-555-7777
501 W. Michigan
Milwaukee, WI 12345

Explanation of Benefits   Health Insurance, Inc.

Insured's Name: Betty White
Insured I.D./Social Security number: 232-33-2222
Policy:
Claim Number: TI-4107081-001-1-01-13
Control Number: 204466533
Date: 02/14/17

The following is an Explanation of Benefits for your Medical Coverage:

Patient: Pam White   **Patient I.D./Social Security number:** 633-33-3333
Provider Name: Medical Center Subsidiary   **Patient Account Number:** 96604599

Service Code	Service Description	Service Date(s)	Provider Charge	Allowed Amount	Discount Amount	Not Covered	Deductible	Copay	Pay Amt.	Remarks	Amount Paid
	Hosp Exp	12/16/16	$5,363.50	$3,261.10	$2,102.40				100%	0054	$3,261.10
			$5,363.50	$3,261.10	$2,102.40						$3,261.10
TOTALS											

Remarks:
0054 PPO-Preferred Provider benefits applied. Your provider has agreed to the negotiated rate in accordance with the Private Healthcare Systems provider agreement. You should not be billed for this amount.

Payment Summary

Payment Sent To:	Medical Center Subsidiary
Payment Amount:	$3,261.10
Payment Date:	02/14/17
Patient's Portion:	$0.00

Total Payment Summary

Payment(s) Sent to:	Medical Center Subsidiary
Total Payment Amount:	$3,261.10
Payment Date:	02/14/17

*TOTAL PATIENT PORTION: $0.00

(Continued)

Insurance company name: _____

Patient's name: _____

Patient's I.D: _____

Provider's name: _____

Date of service: _____

Total charge: _____

Procedure(s): _____

Copay: _____

Deductible: _____

Coinsurance due from patient: _____

Allowed amount: _____

Discount amount: _____

Non-covered items: _____

Rate of benefit (%): _____

Amount paid: _____

Remarks: _____

Outcome: ■ Bill patient balance
           ■ Appeal
           ■ Call carrier
           ■ Claim paid in full

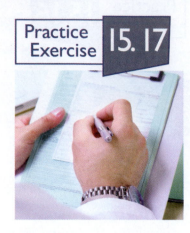

Practice Exercise **15.17**

Review the EOB, then fill in the missing information in the blanks that follow the EOB.

PROVIDER CLAIM SUMMARY

Claims processed by Medical Care
A Division of Allied Health Corp.
P.O. Box 6644
Carrollton, Georgia 12345
Toll Free (800) 555-0287

DATE: 01/30/16
PROVIDER NUMBER: 0000K223
CHECK NUMBER: 034324
TAX IDENTIFICATION NUMBER: 001223456

SURGICAL ASSOCIATES OF Washington
4001 9TH STREET
Seattle WA 12345

PATIENT: **Joe Smith**
PERF PRV: **0000000000000080430S**   IDENTIFICATION NUMBER: **555-66-4444**
CLAIM NUMBER: **0000227050697800X**   PATIENT NUMBER: **79625C0G4**   CLAIM TYPE: **MCP**

FROM/TO DATES	PROC PS* TS**	CODE	AMOUNT BILLED	CONTRACT ALLOWABLE	SERVICES NOT COVERED	DEDUCTIONS/ OTHER INELIGIBLE	AMOUNT PAID
01/02–01/02/16	**03 T**	**93880**	**$550.00**	**$190.13**	**$359.87 (1)**	**$0.00**	**$190.13**
			$550.00	$190.13	$359.87	$0.00	$190.00

AMOUNT PAID TO PROVIDER FOR THIS CLAIM: $190.13
DEDUCTIONS/OTHER INELIGIBLE

TOTAL SERVICES NOT COVERED: $359.87
PATIENT'S SHARE: $ 0.00

Insurance company name: _____

Patient's name: _____

Patient's I.D.: _____

Provider's name: _____

Date of service: _____

Total charge: _____

Procedure(s): _____

Copay: _____

Deductible: _____

Coinsurance due from patient: _____

Allowed amount: _____

Discount amount: _____

Non-covered items: _____

Rate of benefit (%): _____

Amount paid: _____

Remarks: _____

Outcome: ■ Bill patient balance
   ■ Appeal
   ■ Call carrier
   ■ Claim paid in full

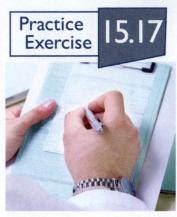

PATIENT: **Kelly Jones**
PERF PRV: **0000000000000080430S**   IDENTIFICATION NUMBER: **444-55-6666**
CLAIM NUMBER: **0000227050697810X**   PATIENT NUMBER: **79625C0G5**   CLAIM TYPE: **MCP**

FROM/TO DATES	PROC PS* TS**	CODE	AMOUNT BILLED	CONTRACT ALLOWABLE	SERVICES NOT COVERED	DEDUCTIONS/ OTHER INELIGIBLE	AMOUNT PAID
01/02–01/02/16		93880	$162.00	$41.30	$120.70	$0.00	$41.30
			$162.00	$41.30	$120.70	$0.00	$41.30

AMOUNT PAID TO PROVIDER FOR THIS CLAIM: $41.30
DEDUCTIONS/OTHER INELIGIBLE

                    TOTAL SERVICES NOT COVERED: $120.70
                    PATIENT'S SHARE: $ 0.00

Insurance company name: _____

Patient's name: _____

Patient's I.D.: _____

Provider's name: _____

Date of service: _____

Total charge: _____

Procedure(s): _____

Copay: _____

Deductible: _____

Coinsurance due from patient: _____

Allowed amount: _____

Discount amount: _____

Non-covered items: _____

Rate of benefit (%): _____

Amount paid: _____

Remarks: _____

Outcome: ■ Bill patient balance
   ■ Appeal
   ■ Call carrier
   ■ Claim paid in full

(Continued)

(Continued)

Practice Exercise 15.17

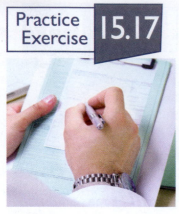

(Continued)

PATIENT: **Mary Young**
PERF PRV: **0000000000000080430S**   IDENTIFICATION NUMBER: **454-55-5555**
CLAIM NUMBER: **0000227050697820X**   PATIENT NUMBER: **79625C0C6**   CLAIM TYPE: **MCP**

FROM/TO DATES	PROC PS* TS** CODE	AMOUNT BILLED	CONTRACT ALLOWABLE	SERVICES NOT COVERED	DEDUCTIONS/ OTHER INELIGIBLE	AMOUNT PAID
01/01–01/02/16	99203	$170.00	$128.00	$42.00 (1)	$10.00	$118.00
	72100	$188.00	$150.00	$38.00 (1)	$ 0.00	$150.00
		$ 358.00	$ 278.00	$ 80.00	$ 10.00	$268.00

AMOUNT PAID TO PROVIDER FOR THIS CLAIM: $268.00
DEDUCTIONS/OTHER INELIGIBLE $10.00

TOTAL SERVICES NOT COVERED: $80.00
PATIENT'S SHARE: $10.00

PROVIDER CLAIMS AMOUNT SUMMARY

NUMBER OF CLAIMS: 3   AMOUNT PAID TO SUBSCRIBER: $0.0   AMOUNT BILLED: $1,070.00
AMOUNT PAID TO PROVIDER: $499.43   AMOUNT OVER MAXIMUM
ALLOWANCE: $560.57
RECOUPMENT AMOUNT: $0.00   AMOUNT OF SERVICES NOT
COVERED: $560.57
NET AMOUNT PAID TO PROVIDER: $499.43   AMOUNT PREVIOUSLY PAID: $0.00

(1) Contractual adjustment of billed amount

Insurance company name: _____

Patient's name: _____

Patient's ID: _____

Provider's name: _____

Date of service: _____

Total charge: _____

Procedure(s): _____

Copay: _____

Deductible: _____

Coinsurance due from patient: _____

Allowed amount: _____

Discount amount: _____

Non-covered items: _____

Rate of benefit (%): _____

Amount paid: _____

Remarks: _____

Outcome: ■ Bill patient balance
     ■ Appeal
     ■ Call carrier
     ■ Claim paid in full

Review the EOB, then fill in the missing information in the blanks that follow the EOB. Do not treat each claim individually; instead, total the amounts from the individual claims to arrive at the correct answers.

EXPLANATION OF PAYMENTS
American Insurance Company
P.O. Box 123456
Any Town, NC 12345
800-555-6543

Date: 05/10/2016 Page 1 of 3

Allied Medical Center
1933 E. Frankford Rd. Suite 110
Liberty Township, OH 12345

VENDOR NUMBER: 0012CK
PROVIDER NUMBER: 85702B

PATIENT NAME: MARY DEAN   PATIENT NUMBER: DEAMA
SUBSCRIBER: MARY DEAN   GROUP NUMBER: H9852   MEMBER NUMBER: 8523697401-01

CLAIM NUMBER: 01 011905 037 04

BGDAT	ENDDAT	SVCCOD	MD	UNITS	BILLED	ALLOWED	NOT-COVD	PREPAID	COP/DED	EP1	EP2	EP3
021016	021016	99215		I	$237.00	$141.46	$0.00	$0.00	$20.00	001		
021016	021016	82270		I	$ 27.00	$ 4.54	$0.00	$0.00	$ 0.00	001		

BILLED	ALLOWED	NOT-COVD	DISCOUNT	PREPAID	WITHHOLD	COP/DED	COB	PAID
$264.00	$146.00	$0.00	$0.00	$0.00	$0.00	$20.00	$0.00	$126.00

PATIENT NAME: JOHN SMITH   PATIENT NUMBER: SMIJO
SUBSCRIBER: JOHN SMITH   GROUP NUMBER: 85230   MEMBER NUMBER: 321654753-00

CLAIM NUMBER: 01 011907 038 20

BGDAT	ENDDAT	SVCCOD	MD	UNITS	BILLED	ALLOWED	NOT-COVD	PREPAID	COP/DED	EP1	EP2	EP3
032116	032116	99213		I	$102.00	$62.78	$0.00	$0.00	$20.00	001		

BILLED	ALLOWED	NOT-COVD	DISCOUNT	PREPAID	WITHHOLD	COP/DED	COB	PAID
$102.00	$62.78	$0.00	$0.00	$0.00	$0.00	$20.00	$0.00	$42.78

PATIENT NAME: JANE DOE   PATIENT NUMBER: DOEJA
SUBSCRIBER: MARK DOE   GROUP NUMBER: 85230   MEMBER NUMBER: 741582569-03

CLAIM NUMBER: 01 012105 035 74

BGDAT	ENDDAT	SVCCOD	MD	UNITS	BILLED	ALLOWED	NOT-COVD	PREPAID	COP/DED	EP1	EP2	EP3
032116	032116	99213		I	$102.00	$62.78	$0.00	$0.00	$20.00	001		

BILLED	ALLOWED	NOT-COVD	DISCOUNT	PREPAID	WITHHOLD	COP/DED	COB	PAID
$102.00	$62.78	$0.00	$0.00	$0.00	$0.00	$25.00	$0.00	$37.78

PATIENT NAME: SHARON ALEXANDER   PATIENT NUMBER: ALESH
SUBSCRIBER: ELLEN ALEXANDER   GROUP NUMBER: 98732   MEMBER NUMBER: 654820069-04

CLAIM NUMBER: 01 011905 037 15

BGDAT	ENDDAT	SVCCOD	MD	UNITS	BILLED	ALLOWED	NOT-COVD	PREPAID	COP/DED	EP1	EP2	EP3
021016	021016	99211		I	$56.00	$25.64	$0.00	$0.00	$12.82	001		
021016	021016	36415		I	$26.00	$3.00	$0.00	$0.00	$ 0.00	001		

BILLED	ALLOWED	NOT-COVD	DISCOUNT	PREPAID	WITHHOLD	COP/DED	COB	PAID
$82.00	$28.64	$0.00	$0.00	$0.00	$0.00	$12.82	$0.00	$15.82

(Continued)

Practice Exercise 15.18

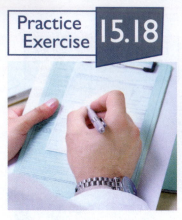

(*Continued*)

EXPLANATION OF PAYMENTS
American Insurance Company
P.O. Box 123456
Any Town, NC 12345
800-555-6543

Date: 05/10/2016 Page 2 of 3

VENDOR NUMBER: 0012CK
PROVIDER NUMBER: 85702B

PROVIDER TOTALS:

BILLED	ALLOWED	NOT-COVD	DISCOUNT	PREPAID	WITHHOLD	COP/DED	COB	PAID
$550.00	$300.20	$0.00	$0.00	$0.00	$0.00	$77.82	$0.00	$222.38

EXPLANATION OF PAYMENTS
American Insurance Company
P.O. Box 123456
Any Town, NC 12345
800-555-6543

Date: 05/10/2016 Page 3 of 3

VENDOR NUMBER: 0012CK
PROVIDER NUMBER: 85702B

PATIENT NAME: SHANNON BURG   PATIENT NUMBER: BURSH
SUBSCRIBER: SHANNON BURG   GROUP NUMBER: 63250   MEMBER NUMBER: 002586317-00

CLAIM NUMBER: 01 011210 038 60

BGDAT	ENDDAT	SVCCOD	MD	UNITS	BILLED	ALLOWED	NOT-COVD	PREPAID	COP/DED	EP1	EP2	EP3
032516	032516	99213		1	$102.00	$62.78	$0.00	$0.00	$20.00	001		

BILLED	ALLOWED	NOT-COVD	DISCOUNT	PREPAID	WITHHOLD	COP/DED	COB	PAID
$102.00	$62.78	$0.00	$0.00	$0.00	$0.00	$20.00	$0.00	$42.78

PATIENT NAME: LUCY LANGE   PATIENT NUMBER: LANLU
SUBSCRIBER: LUCY LANGE   GROUP NUMBER: 63250   MEMBER NUMBER: 54608712300

CLAIM NUMBER: 01 011907 612 14

BGDAT	ENDDAT	SVCCOD	MD	UNITS	BILLED	ALLOWED	NOT-COVD	PREPAID	COP/DED	EP1	EP2	EP3
032116	032116	99213		1	$102.00	$62.78	$0.00	$0.00	$20.00	001		

BILLED	ALLOWED	NOT-COVD	DISCOUNT	PREPAID	WITHHOLD	COP/DED	COB	PAID
$102.00	$62.78	$0.00	$0.00	$0.00	$0.00	$20.00	$0.00	$42.78

PATIENT NAME: BRUCE MONTANIO   PATIENT NUMBER: MONBR
SUBSCRIBER: TINA MONTANIO   GROUP NUMBER: 85230   MEMBER NUMBER: 098143276-05

CLAIM NUMBER: 01 012105 074 61

BGDAT	ENDDAT	SVCCOD	MD	UNITS	BILLED	ALLOWED	NOT-COVD	PREPAID	COP/DED	EP1	EP2	EP3
032116	032116	99213		1	$102.00	$62.78	$0.00	$0.00	$20.00	001		

BILLED	ALLOWED	NOT-COVD	DISCOUNT	PREPAID	WITHHOLD	COP/DED	COB	PAID
$102.00	$62.78	$0.00	$0.00	$0.00	$0.00	$20.00	$0.00	$42.78

PROVIDER TOTALS:

BILLED	ALLOWED	NOT-COVD	DISCOUNT	PREPAID	WITHHOLD	COP/DED	COB	PAID
$306.00	$188.34	$0.00	$0.00	$0.00	$0.00	$60.00	$0.00	$128.34

VENDOR TOTALS:

BILLED	ALLOWED	NOT-COVD	DISCOUNT	PREPAID	WITHHOLD	COP/DED	COB	PAID
$856.00	$488.54	$0.00	$0.00	$0.00	$0.00	$137.82	$0.00	$350.72

CHECK#—00525441284   DATE—5/10/2016   AMOUNT—$350.72

EXPLANATION OF PAYMENT CODES:

001   SERVICES PROVIDED ARE COVERED UP TO AN ALLOWED
       AMOUNT. BECAUSE THIS AMOUNT HAS BEEN PAID, NO
       ADDITIONAL PAYMENT CAN BE MADE.

TOTALS ONLY

Insurance company name: _____

Patient's name: N/A _____

Patient's I.D.: N/A _____

Provider's name: _____

Date of services: N/A _____

Total charges: _____

Procedure(s): N/A _____

Total copay: _____

Total deductibles: _____

Total coinsurance due from patients: _____

Total allowed amount: _____

Total discount amount: _____

Total non-covered items: _____

Rate of benefit (%): N/A _____

Total amount paid to provider: _____

Remarks: _____

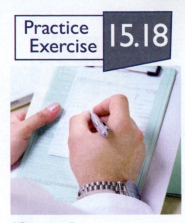

(*Continued*)

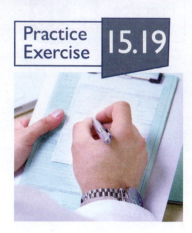

Practice Exercise 15.19

Review the EOB; then fill in the missing information in the blanks that follow the EOB.

Insurance Company of America
P. O. Box 3564-1
Any Town, AZ 12345
800-555-1634

CLAIM NUMBER	CHECK NUMBER
10268785-04	Nock895016

CHECK DATE	CHECK AMOUNT
11/09/2016	0.00

ALLIED MEDICAL CENTER
1933 E. Mulberry Dr., STE 110
Fargo, ND 12345

Insurance Company of America   **EXPLANATION OF BENEFITS**

RETAIN FOR YOUR RECORDS

Date(s) of Service: 10/13/2016–10/13/2016   Check Date: 11/09/2016
Patient: Jeff Staubach   Check Number: nock895016
Insured: Jeff Staubach   Check Amount:
Patient Account #: 3265   Group: United Peoples Employer   Group # 00025
Provider: Allied Medical Center   Contract Name: American Health Network   Claim #: 10268725

Service Code	Service Description	Service Date(s)	Provider Charge	Allowed Amount	Discount Amount	Not Covered	Deductible	Copay	Pay Amt.	Remarks	Amount Paid
99214	Office visit	10/13/16	$148.00			$148.00				ab	
TOTALS			$148.00			$148.00					

Remarks
ab   This claim was previously processed.

THIS IS NOT A BILL.

Insurance company name: _____

Patient's name: _____

Patient's I.D.: _____

Provider's name: _____

Date of service: _____

Total charge: _____

Procedure(s): _____

Copay: _____

Deductible: _____

Coinsurance due from patient: _____

Allowed amount: _____

Discount amount: _____

Non-covered items: _____

Rate of benefit (%): _____

Amount paid: _____

Remarks: _____

Outcome: ■ Bill patient balance
           ■ Appeal
           ■ Call carrier
           ■ Claim paid in full

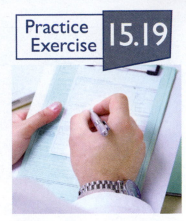

Practice Exercise 15.19

(Continued)

After completing the exercises in this chapter, the medical office specialist is able to review an EOB or ERA and determine what corrections, changes, and write-offs to the patient's account, if any, are necessary, and if the patient is responsible for a portion of the balance due. Many times the patient is confused about how to read the EOB and cannot understand why a balance is due. Often it is the responsibility of the medical office specialist to explain to the patient why a balance is owed. The following exercise will assist the medical office specialist to discuss the EOB with the patient and explain to the patient her financial responsibility. The medical office specialist should begin by explaining to the patient the purpose of the EOB, as in the following example:

Example

Medical Office Specialist: When reading the EOB the doctor or hospital is known as the "provider" because services have been provided to you, the "member." The Explanation of Benefits (EOB) is a form or report that provides details and results of how the insurance company processed the claim. It is *not* a bill. It accompanies the payment sent by the insurance company to the provider in order for the provider to know what adjustments must be made to the balance and what the patient's financial responsibility is. The EOB outlines several things:

- What services and procedures were performed
- The physician's regular charge
- The charge amount allowed by the patient's policy, which may be less than the physician's regular charge
- Any balance that must be "written off" because of the difference between the physician's regular charge and the allowed amount
- Any copay or deductible, which is the amount the patient has to pay based on the policy
- Any remarks codes or special explanations regarding payment

Figures 15.18 and 15.19 are EOBs received on a patient who has Medicare and a secondary (supplemental) policy through Blue Cross and Blue Shield of Iowa. Using the two EOBs, practice reviewing and explaining to a patient why the patient owes a balance of $33.25.

Medicare Summary Notice

John K. Doe
123 Anywhere
Your City, FL 11111

CUSTOMER SERVICE INFORMATION

Your Medicare Number: 111-11-1111A

If you have questions, write or call:
Medicare (#12345)
555 Medicare Blvd., Suite 200
Medicare Building
Medicare, USA XXXXX-XXXX

Call: 1-800-MEDICARE (1-800-633-4227)
Ask for Doctor Services
TTY for Hearing Impaired: 1-877-486-2048

This is a summary of claims processed from 11/16/2016 through 11/30/2016

PART B MEDICAL INSURANCE - UNASSIGNED CLAIMS

Dates of Service	Service Provided	Amount Charged	Medicare Approved	Medicare Paid You	You May Be Billed	See Notes Section
Claim number 01-0001-011-022 FL						
Mayo Clinic Jacksonville, 4500 San Pablo Road						
Jacksonville, FL 32224						
A Doctor M.D.						
11/14/16	Sample (99999)	$109.25	$95.00	$76.00	$109.25	

SAMPLE

THIS IS NOT A BILL - Keep this notice for your records.

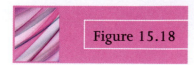

Figure 15.18   Sample Medicare Explanation of Benefits (primary)

URHealthInsurance
Identification Number: 112345678

Explanation of Health Care Benefits
Medicare Supplement

Page 1

Claim Number: 112111002222

Provider Number: 88899

Provider Name: Western Clinic

JOHN DOE
123 Washington Blvd,
Your City, USA
12345

This is not a bill. It is a statement showing how we applied your URHealthInsurance coverage to claims submitted to us. If you have a question, please detach the top of this form and send it to us with a letter or call: 888-555-5555 TOLL FREE. Customer Service is available to answer calls Mon. - Fri. 8:00 a.m.-4:00 p.m.

From	Through	SER-VICE CODE	Charge		Medicare Approved		Medicare Benefit Amount		Wellmark Benefit Amount		Notes	Claim Summary
11/15	11/30/16	36	109	25	95	00	76	00	19	00		Total Charges Submitted
												109.25
												Medicare Approved
												95.00
												Medicare Benefit Amount
												76.00
												Noncovered Services
												33.25
												Amount You Owe*
												33.25
												Wellmark Benefit Amount For This Claim
This is not a bill and you should not send us money. However, if you have not paid for the service shown here, you may owe the provider. You may want to keep this statement for your records.												19.00

Notes

SAMPLE

*This is the amount you owe the provider indicated above. If you already paid this provider, please disregard this amount.

Identification Number 112345678	Group Number 00001001-333	Claim Number 112111002222	Account Number 88888
Claim Received 12/15/16	Claim Processed 1/15/17	Provider Name Western Clinic	Patient Name JOHN DOE

If you have a question regarding this Explanation of Health Care Benefits, call: 800/555/8884 TOLL FREE

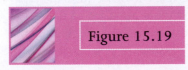
Figure 15.19   Sample Explanation of Benefits from secondary (supplemental) insurance carrier.

Methods of Receiving Funds

Various methods are available for carriers to remit funds to providers. These methods include check by mail, electronic funds transfer, and lockbox services.

Check by Mail

The carrier mails directly to the provider a check attached to an EOB. One or several patients can be listed on the EOB/ERA and a single check attached for all fees paid.

Electronic Funds Transfer

Electronic funds transfer (EFT) is used by participating providers and carriers. Providers can now have checks deposited directly into the provider's bank account, whereas in the past they would have been mailed along with an EOB. When a provider electronically files a claim, he will receive an ERA. If the provider submits a paper claim, he will receive an EOB. The ERA/EOB shows dollar amounts paid to the provider along with the amount of the patient's financial responsibility. This helps in controlling accounts receivables. The advantages of using EFTs are that funds are immediately available and the transfer is less costly than check deposits.

Lockbox Services

A lockbox service is one that is provided by a bank for accounting purposes to help control account receivables. To obtain this service, the provider must have an account with the bank.

A lockbox service helps control receivables by collecting and depositing customer payments faster. To remain competitive in today's environment, many practices look for opportunities to streamline their operations. A lockbox service does this by:

- Saving time and money while improving cash flow.
- Ensuring high-quality processing of the practice's receivables.
- Employing an aggressive mail pickup schedule.

With a lockbox service, carriers and patients remit payment to a unique zip code designated only for lockbox mail. The bank's couriers pick up the payments directly from the post office. Lockbox mail is processed and deposited to the practice's account the same day. All payment information is forwarded to the practice. The bank will:

- Make copies of all checks.
- Deposit checks into the practice's account.
- Provide a record of all deposits and totals.
- Forward receipt of all deposits with documentation.

The bank will gather all EOBs, patients' statements (that were returned with checks), and any other documentation that was attached to the check and forward it to the practice. When the practice receives the EOBs and documentation of deposit from the lockbox, the office insurance specialist should do the following:

- Add up the copies of the checks and the deposit total to ensure they match.
- Add up the EOBs to ensure that the total equals the insurance company's check.
- If everything adds up, then begin to post the EOBs. The office insurance specialist should consider "batching" the EOBs if there are a lot of them. (To "batch" means to choose a certain amount to post, for example, $1,000.00 per batch [enter the amount in the Batch account], instead of posting all EOBs at

once.) When finished with that batch, the amount should be checked to ensure that it is correct. Batching makes it easier to control posting errors because there are fewer amounts to recheck.

■ When all postings have been completed, an activities report or "day sheet" should be run for the one day only and verified that it matches the total deposit amount reported by the bank.

If there is an error in the amount the bank deposited compared with the amount totaled by the medical office specialist, the bank should be called and the error found and corrected. Any errors found, who was called, and how they were corrected should always be documented on the posting sheet.

Chapter Summary

■ An explanation of benefits (EOB/ERA) is a notification form sent from the insurance carrier to the patient and the healthcare provider (if the provider accepted assignment) after an insurance claim has been processed.

■ The EOB/ERA lists the patient, dates of services, types of service, and the charges filed on the insurance claim form. The EOB/ERA also describes the way the amount of the benefit payment was determined.

■ The Medicare Fee Schedule (MFS) is based on the RBRVS fees. Therefore, the fees are based on the federal government's data of what each service costs.

■ Allowed charges refer to the maximum allowed amount for a covered charge. Some payers refer to this as the maximum allowed fee, allowed amount, or allowable charge. This is the amount the payer will pay the provider for her services.

■ Depending on the medical plan, the insured may be required to make four types of payments: deductibles, copayments, coinsurance, and payments for excluded services. These are referred to as out-of-pocket expenses. The medical office specialist will know exactly what the insured needs to pay at the time of service after verifying the insured's insurance plan benefits.

■ The medical office specialist must be aware of and become familiar with payers' reimbursement calculations and payment methods in order to review an EOB/ERA to determine if the payment amount is correct. Various methods are available for carriers to remit funds to providers. These methods include check by mail, electronic funds transfer, and lockbox services.

Chapter Review

True/False

Identify the statement as true (T) or false (F).

_____ **1.** The allowed charge is the amount that a third-party payer will pay for a particular procedure when the patient has coinsurance.

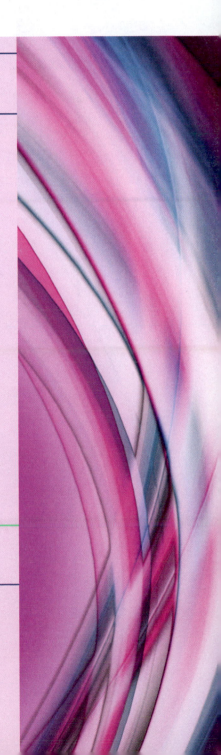

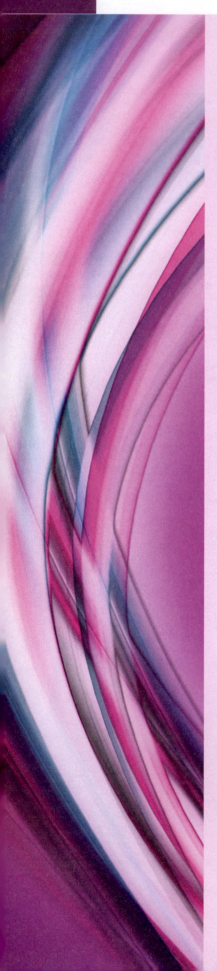

_____ **2.** Accounts receivable include monies owed to a practice by both payers and patients.

_____ **3.** An adjustment is a negative or positive change to an account balance.

_____ **4.** The claim turnaround time is the period between the patient's encounter and the transmission of the resulting claim.

_____ **5.** A payer may downcode a procedure it determines was not medically necessary at the level reported.

_____ **6.** A medical review is part of the provider's staff responsibilities.

_____ **7.** The determination of a claim refers to the payer's decision regarding payment.

_____ **8.** When a payer's ERA is received, the medical office specialist checks that the amount paid matches the expected payments.

_____ **9.** When a family deductible is required, it must be met before benefits from the payer begin.

_____ **10.** Under a plan with an individual deductible, the deductible amount can be met by the combination of payments from all family members.

_____ **11.** Posting the payment to the specific date of service and each CPT code, and then following the same procedure for posting an adjustment, is referred to as per line item posting.

_____ **12.** The provider "withhold" required by some managed care plans may be repaid to the physician.

_____ **13.** The advantages of using EFTs are that funds are immediately available and the transfer is less costly than check deposits.

Multiple Choice

Identify the letter of the choice that best completes the statement or answers the question.

_____ **1.** The three parts of an RBRVS fee are:
   a. uniform value, GPCI, and conversion factor.
   b. usual, customary, and reasonable charges.
   c. usual charges, GPCI, and conversion factor.
   d. none of the above.

_____ **2.** The purpose of the GPCI is to account for:
   a. regional differences in costs.
   b. changes in the cost-of-living index.
   c. differences in relative work values.
   d. none of the above.

_____ **3.** Which of the following payment methods is the newest?
   a. UCR
   b. RVS
   c. RBRVS
   d. GPCI

_____ **4.** Which of the following payment methods is the basis for Medicare's fees?
   a. UCR
   b. RVS
   c. RBRVS
   d. GPCI

_____ **5.** The Medicare conversion factor is set:
   a. twice a year.
   b. once each year.
   c. semiannually.
   d. each decade.

_____ **6.** Which answer correctly lists the main method(s) payers use to determine their fee structure?
   a. Allowed charges
   b. Allowed charges, contracted fee schedule, and capitation
   c. Contracted fee schedule and capitation
   d. Capitation and retrospective payments

_____ **7.** The Medicare-allowed charge for a procedure is $80.00. What amount does the participating provider receive from Medicare and what amount from the patient?
   a. $64.00/$16.00
   b. $60.00/$20.00
   c. $40.00/$40.00
   d. $80.00/$0.00

_____ **8.** The Medicare-allowed charge for a procedure is $150.00, and a PAR provider's usual charge is $200.00. What amount must the provider write off?
   a. $150.00
   b. $100.00
   c. $50.00
   d. $30.00

_____ **9.** The deductibles, coinsurance, and copayments patients pay are called their:
   a. excluded services.
   b. out-of-pocket expenses.
   c. capitation rate.
   d. maximum benefit limit.

_____ **10.** If a non-PAR provider's usual fee is $600.00, the allowed amount is $300.00, and balance billing is permitted, what amount is written off?
   a. $150.00
   b. $480.00
   c. $300.00
   d. $0.00

_____ **11.** A payer's automated claim edits may result in claim denial because of:
   a. lack of eligibility for a reported service.
   b. lack of medical necessity.
   c. lack of required preauthorization.
   d. all of the above.

_____ **12.** A claim that is removed from a payer's automated processing system is sent for:
   a. adjudication.
   b. manual review.
   c. utilization review.
   d. none of the above.

_____ 13. If a provider has accepted assignment, the payer sends the ERA or EOB to:

a. the provider.   c. the billing service.

b. the patient.   d. the carrier.

_____ 14. The payer's decision regarding whether to pay a claim is called:

a. determination.   c. evaluation.

b. adjudication.   d. utilization.

_____ 15. After the claim has gone through the adjudication process and a claim has been downcoded or denied, the medical office specialist may submit to the insurance carrier:

a. a letter of appeal.

b. the patient's medical records.

c. the provider's dictation.

d. additional insurance information.

Completion

Complete each sentence or statement.

1. An initial review of each claim consists of _____ who/that screen the basic data on the claim form.

2. Although adjudication varies somewhat depending on the payer's policies, the essential steps—edits, reviews, and _____—are universal.

3. A claim examiner reviews the claim to check if the _____ and _____ are linked.

4. Downcoding is also called _____.

5. A(n) _____ is an amount that an insured must pay to the provider before the insurance benefits begin.

6. Under the formula for calculating a Medicare fee for a procedure, the sum of the adjusted totals for work, practice expense, and malpractice are multiplied by a(n) _____.

7. If a participating provider's usual charge is higher than the allowed amount, the provider must _____ the difference between the two charges.

8. Medical insurance plans require patients to pay for all _____ services.

9. Following a payment _____, the payer either pays, denies, or partially pays the claim.

10. A payer may downcode a claim if the reported procedure does not match the reported _____.

11. Corrections, changes, and write-offs to patients' account are made with _____ to the existing transactions.

12. If a carrier has continued to deny all of the practice's appeal requests, the provider can file a request to the _____ for assistance.

Resources

https://www.premera.com/wa/member/manage-my-account/explanation-of-benefits/
How to read your EOB. Click on the Resources & Tools link; then click on the Understanding Your Explanation of Benefits (EOB) link at the bottom of the page.

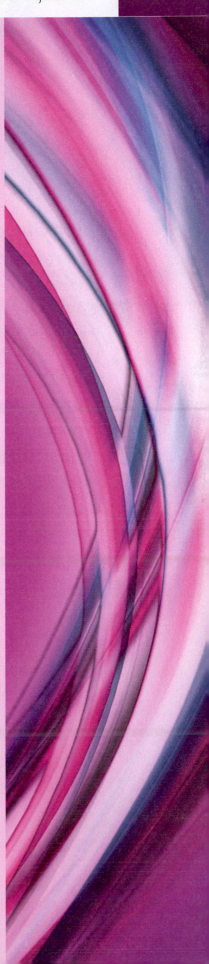

Chapter 16 / Refunds, Follow-Up, and Appeals

Chapter Objectives

After reading this chapter, the student should be able to:

1. Understand reimbursement follow-up.
2. Know the common problems and solutions for denied or delayed payments.
3. Use problem-solving and communication skills to answer patients' questions about claims.
4. Format medical records with proper documentation.
5. Understand the appeals process and register a formal appeal.
6. Understand ERISA rules and regulations.
7. Write letters of appeal on denied claims.
8. Understand refund guidelines.
9. Rebill insurance claims.
10. Discuss the three levels of Medicare appeals.
11. Calculate and issue refunds.

Key Terms

administrative law judge (ALJ) hearing	Act (ERISA) of 1974	qualified independent contractors (QICs)
documentation	follow-up	redetermination
Employee Retirement Income Security	insurance commissioner	SOAP format
	peer review	

CPT-4 codes in this chapter are from the CPT-4 2017 code set. CPT® is a registered trademark of the American Medical Association.

ICD-10-CM codes in this chapter are from the ICD-10-CM 2017 Draft code set from the Department of Health and Human Services, Centers for Disease Control and Prevention.

Case Study

Refunds, Follow-Up, and Appeals

As a new accounts receivable specialist, Amy has been given a list of denied claims to work with. One of those claims was denied because of a primary diagnosis of obesity. Amy believes that the claim will be paid if the primary code of obesity is switched with the secondary code of migraine headaches. She approaches her manager with this information. Her manager explains that it is not possible to change the order of the codes, and that if they did it would be considered insurance fraud. She informs Amy that an appeal may reverse the denial with proper documentation.

Questions

1. Why would a claim be denied because of an obesity code?
2. Why can't the order of the codes be changed by the billing office if it will provide payment?
3. What kind of documentation may be needed for such an appeal?

As discussed in Chapter 15, an *appeal* is the submission of additional clinical and other pertinent information to an insurance carrier to overturn a denied or downcoded claim by the payer.

The majority of a provider's income is generated through insurance billing. In a perfect world, the provider would be paid promptly and fully for all claims submitted. Knowing that nothing is perfect, however, the medical office specialist will receive denial notices from the insurance carriers. What to do with the denial and balance on the patient's account is vitally important. If the practice feels that the charges should be paid by the carrier, the medical office specialist must appeal the carrier's decision to deny all or parts of the claim. Some denials by the insurance carrier simply require **follow-up** and can be conducted over the telephone, whereas others may require a written appeal. Either way, the medical office specialist must be familiar with medical records, verification of benefits forms, precertification, preauthorization, and referral requirements, as well as the appeals process for each insurance carrier with whom the provider contracts.

Electronically Filing Claims

A clearinghouse is a company that will accept all claims and electronically forward them to the insurance payers for processing. They also have edits in place to check for errors in claims to help avoid delays in collecting payments. When setting up a clearinghouse, all insurance companies have their own payer ID number for filing electronic claims. There are two kinds of claims filed electronically:

- Institutional claim, which is a UB04
- Professional claim, which is a CMS-1500

The benefit of filing a claim electronically is monitoring rejections. A rejected claim is an electronically submitted claim that cannot be processed due to missing or invalid information. Each claim submitted electronically has to pass the payer's editing process, which screens certain items on the claim that are required for proper adjudication. In addition, paper billing can take up to 45 days for processing, while electronic claims will be processed in 7 to 21 business days.

Claims Rejection Follow-Up

One of the critical goals of a medical office specialist is to prepare claims that will be approved and paid by insurance carriers. Another is to help ensure *prompt* reimbursement of charges. What steps can the medical office specialist take to avoid claim rejection and to speed correct reimbursement from carriers and patients?

Regardless of the method of reimbursement, insurance claims must be monitored until payments are received. When payments are late or made incorrectly, the medical

The following are some reasons for contacting the insurance carrier:

1. A letter from the insurance carrier states that a claim is being investigated. This might be due to workers' compensation situations, or other reasons. After a period of 30 days, however, follow-up should be done by phone or letter.
2. An unclear denial of payment is received.
3. An incorrect payment is received.
4. Reimbursement is received with no indication of the amount of the allowed charge or how much is the patient's responsibility.
5. Reimbursement is received for an unknown patient. For example, a payment is assigned to Jamie Nussbaum, who is not a patient on record. When the carrier is called, the medical office specialist discovers that Jamie Nussbaum's policy covers Michael Lambert, a patient recently seen by the physician.

Figure 16.1

Some reasons to inquire about an insurance claim.

office specialist must follow up. Frequently, reimbursement follow-up is as simple as calling the insurance carrier to ask for help. Most insurance carriers have staff members whose primary duty is to answer questions about the status of claims. Figure 16.1 lists some of the reasons why a medical office specialist would inquire about an outstanding claim.

Rebilling

Some providers automatically rebill every 30 days if they have not heard from an insurance company. If the insurance company has a website to check the status of a claim, the medical office specialist should check the status of the claim online. If the status states, "No claim received" or "Not on file," then resubmitting the claim will be handled like a first-time submission. Before rebilling, however, the medical office specialist should be aware of the terms of his provider's managed care contract regarding turnaround times.

If a provider decides to resubmit claims every 30 days, some payers may think this is duplicate billing. The procedure for rebilling paper claims is to reprint the claim from the computer and write "Second Billing" in black letters at the top. This lets the insurance carrier know that it is not a duplicate claim and that payment is delinquent. If the insurance carrier has already communicated with the patient, it will send the provider a record of that information in response to the second billing. For example, the notice might read, "Paid to patient," "Applied to deductible," or "Not a covered benefit." Table 16.1 lists other reasons why the medical office specialist may need to rebill a claim.

The carrier may ask for rebilling in these situations:

- The wrong diagnosis codes or procedure codes were submitted. (One wrong number can mean denial of benefits!)
- Information is incomplete or missing (e.g., no policy number or no accident date).
- The charges, units, and costs do not total properly.

Occasionally, second billings are rejected as duplicates, which is why a medical office specialist must be careful with second billings. Some carriers may perceive

Table 16.1	Reasons to Rebill
A mistake has been made in billing.	For example, during a patient's physical examination, the physician discovers an ear infection. Ear infections are covered by the patient's insurance, but physicals are not. However, the physician noted the physical but forgot to mark the ear problem on the superbill. When this error is discovered, the insurance carrier is notified. Providers no longer write the word "corrected" on CMS-1500 paper form on a corrected claim submission. Claims need to contain the correct billing code to identify when a claim is being submitted to correct or void a claim that has been previously processed. Electronic claims are resubmitted with a billing code 7 (claim frequency type code) for a replacement/correction, or a code 8 to void a prior claim. When correcting a paper claim complete box 22 (resubmission code) to include a 7 (replacement/correction) or code 8 (void).
Charges must be detailed to receive maximum reimbursement.	When an EOB is examined, discrepancies between the amount billed and the amount paid should be analyzed. For example, assume that, per the contract, a physician should be reimbursed for actual laboratory charges. The physician charges the patient $25.00 for a stool culture, but the contractual allowed for laboratory costs for the culture were $20.00. Because the carrier's payment was for $16.00, there is probably an error. The carrier should have reimbursed the physician for the allowed amount of $20.00. In this case, a copy of the bill received from the laboratory should be sent to the insurance carrier for reimbursement of $4.00, the difference between the actual charge of $20.00 and the payment of $16.00 that was received.
A claim was overlooked by the provider's office.	This can happen when a patient undergoes a series of visits or treatments. For example, Marshall Williams gets a weekly allergy injection. He received 10 injections, but somehow claims were submitted for only 8. The 2 missing injections can still be billed. Also, a corrected claim can be sent with a request for an adjustment.

"aggressive billing techniques" as fraudulent billing. When sending claims electronically, it is very easy to resubmit all outstanding claims. However, the carrier may have just adjudicated the original claim for payment such that when a second billing is received, it may also be adjudicated for payment, resulting in the carrier overpaying on the service. Third-party payers may feel that this duplication has been done deliberately and may decide to conduct an audit. An *audit* is the process of examining and verifying claims and supporting documents submitted by a physician or medical facility.

If a claim is outstanding, instead of automatically resubmitting it the medical office specialist can call the carrier or view the status on the payer's website to investigate the problem. Participating providers usually have been provided with a personal I.D. number (PIN) so they can access third-party websites and check the status of claims immediately.

Denied or Delayed Payments

The carrier might deny or delay payment for many reasons. The following are some common problems and their solutions. Note that most of the listed denial reasons could have been avoided if eligibility and benefits had been validated prior to service or admission.

The claim is not for a covered contract benefit. Bill the patient, making a note of the insurance information directly on the patient's bill so that the patient knows the reason for the bill. (Medicare patients must have signed an ABN (advance beneficiary notice) prior to treatment. If an ABN was not signed, the provider will have to write off the balance to bad debt. The patient cannot be billed.)

The patient's coverage has been canceled. Bill the patient, making a note of the insurance information directly on the patient's bill. If the medical office specialist verified benefits before the visit, an appeal may be in order.

Workers' compensation (WC) is involved, and the case is still under consideration. Call the employer and ask for the WC case number and the address to which the claim should be submitted. If the employer cannot give you a case number, ask if there is a Notice of Contest. Notify the patient to follow up on the claim with an ombudsman or get a denial of the claim to attach to the health insurance claim form that will be sent to the patient's personal insurance plan.

The carrier believes that coordination of benefits should be done and has requested information about another carrier. The claim will not be processed until the provider provides the information. Call the patient. Explain to the patient what the insurance carrier is requesting and inform the patient that he will be responsible for paying the bill if the insurance carrier does not receive the requested information in a timely manner. (You may need to explain timely filing deadlines.)

The insurance company considers the physician's procedure experimental. A new procedure requiring an unlisted procedure code should always have an explanation of the procedure and proof of medical necessity attached to the original claim. Call the carrier to discuss the necessity of the procedure. If the procedure is still denied, an appeal letter explaining the procedure may need to be sent or a request made for a peer review. Ultimately, the provider may need to bill the patient.

The person responsible—either the physician or the patient—did not obtain preauthorization for a procedure or for hospitalization. Review the payer's contract. Some contracts impose a sanction for failure to secure preauthorization. If there are reasons why this was not done, a letter of appeal should be written. If authorization was obtained, provide the carrier with the authorization number. It is very difficult to receive authorization after treatment or hospital admission has occurred.

The physician provided services before the patient's health insurance contract went into effect. Bill the patient. A notation such as "No insurance coverage at date of service" should be marked on the bill.

The carrier asks for additional information. Send the carrier the requested information. Follow up as needed after 15 days.

When payment is denied, the insurance carrier notifies both the provider and the patient. The medical office specialist should follow up with a call or letter to the patient explaining what action is being taken. In cases of canceled coverage, the patient is responsible for the bill. Any specific written correspondence received from the insurance carrier should be filed with the patient's records. If the patient has questions, the information from the insurance carrier may help to resolve them.

Answering Patients' Questions about Claims

Often, patients need a go-between, an objective third party who is not emotionally involved. A medical office specialist with expertise and objectivity can build goodwill for the provider's office by using problem-solving and communication skills to fulfill this role. The first step toward answering patients' inquiries about claims is to find out exactly what the problem is. Find out from the patient whether she has done any of the following:

- Called the insurance carrier
- Talked to the company's employee representative
- Reviewed the policy

Often, the answer is no. The patient may not understand the insurance policy or may be confused about the rules of the managed care organization (MCO).

Patients typically get upset when they receive large bills or an incorrect payment, or when payment is delayed. Even though the complaints are with the insurance carrier, the medical office specialist is the patients' advocate. Helping solve insurance problems can soothe angry, worried patients. Sometimes the problem is just a misunderstanding because the patient does not know the right questions to ask, does not understand the answers, or is unaware that benefits have changed. In other situations, the patient may accuse the office staff of billing incorrectly. In such cases, try to listen carefully for the facts without letting feelings interfere.

If the patient has already called the insurance carrier but is still upset or confused, the medical office specialist should call the insurance carrier again and listen carefully to the explanation. The patient may have been too stressed to understand it. Explaining the solution again to the patient may help clear up misunderstandings.

The following are some techniques to use when explaining insurance issues to patients:

- Volunteer to explain. Speak slowly and calmly.
- Use simple language. Try to omit insurance jargon.
- Explain more than once when necessary.
- Ask the patient "Do you understand?" or say "Perhaps I can explain that better."
- Remember that patients are under stress. Use respect and care.

Claim Rejection Appeal

An appeal is the submission of additional clinical and other pertinent information to an insurance carrier to overturn a denied or downcoded claim by the payer. It is a formal way of asking the insurance carrier to reconsider its decision regarding a claim. An example of when a medical office specialist will submit an appeal is when an incorrect payment is received. First, the carrier's representative should be contacted. The carrier may have made a mistake and not entered the code that was submitted, which requires an adjustment to the Explanation of Benefits (EOB). Figures 16.2, 16.3, and 16.4 are sample EOBs that list rejected or denied claims. Sometimes, instead of a routine error, the provider considers the carrier's reimbursement for services inadequate or incorrect. In either case, a claim rejection can be appealed.

An appeal is used in the following cases:

- The physician did not file for preauthorization in a timely manner because of unusual circumstances.
- The physician receives what is believed to be inadequate reimbursement for surgery or a complicated procedure.
- A patient has unusual circumstances that affect medical treatment.

Figure 16.2

Sample Explanation of Benefits showing denied claim.

Medi PPO
P.O. Box 8525
Garland, TX 12345-0000

Family Medicine Associates of Pennsylvania
3251 Jennifer Lane # 936
Avella, PA 15312

Beneficiaries: 1-800-555-2832
Providers: 1-800-555-2833
Page 1 of 1
EOB Number: 15878563214

For Participating Physicians and Facilities Only—If your practice has a change of address and/or telephone number please contact Medi online at: www.medi.com/providerehealthoffice/

SUMMARY OF CLAIM

Provider Number: T5478921
Patient Account Number: Tayho0
Patient Name: Hope Taylor
Insured Name: James Taylor
Sponsor Number: 511-64-5140
Claim Number: 200354 48 9144478

Provider:	Service Dates	Pos	Proc	Mod No Type	Billed	Allowed	Code
Elaine Hamm	10/15–10/15/16	11	97010	01	$ 40.00	$0.00	282
	10/15–10/15/16	11	97012	01	$100.00	$0.00	282
	10/15–10/15/16	11	97035	02	$120.00	$0.00	282
TOTAL					$260.00	$0.00	

Other Ins. Allowed	Other Ins. Paid	Reduction Days	Reduction Amount	Paid by Patient
$0.00	$00.00	0	$0.00	$0.00

Deduct	Cost-share/Copayment	Total Payable	Interest Paid	Net Payment
$0.0	$0.00	$0.00	$0.00	$0.00

Remarks:
Code 282: Not covered; due to automobile accident, submit to auto carrier

********************************Voucher Summary*********************************

TOTAL PAYABLE
$0.0

NET PAYMENT
$0.00

For example, consider the case in which a medical office specialist filed a claim for a child who was chronically ill. When the child began choking at home, his parents called an ambulance. The ambulance took the child to his physician's hospital, which was 5 miles farther than the nearest facility. The insurance carrier denied payment, stating that the ambulance was not necessary. In addition, the carrier felt that the ambulance should have gone to the nearest facility. To press payment for this claim, the physician wrote an appeal letter to the insurance carrier detailing the child's special problems that made it necessary to call an ambulance. This letter included the child's medical information from birth. The physician also explained what was done in the ambulance and why it was necessary for him to treat the child, rather than a physician in the closer emergency room.

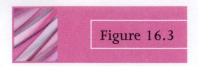

Figure 16.3

Sample Explanation of Benefits showing denied claims.

Health Care Insurance
504 Explorer Way
Milwaukee, WI 12345
800-555-7777

Explanation of Benefits   Health Care

Our Customer Service Dept. is available
Monday–Friday, between the hours of
7:30 am and 6:00 pm (CT) at 800-555-7666

Insured Name: Mike Zamora
Insured I.D./Social Security number: 214-55-1711
Policy: 531AA14788
Claim Number: TI-4107081-001-1-01-13
Control Number: 204466533
Date: 06/25/16

Summary of Benefits

Patient: Maggie Zamora   **Patient ID/Social Security number:** 214-55-1711
Provider Name: Medical Center Subsidiary   **Patient Account Number:** 789624599

Service Code	Service Description	Service Date(s)	Provider Charge	Allowed Amount	Discount Amount	Not Covered	Deductible	Copay	Pay Amt.	Remarks	Amount Paid
96000	Motion analysis	06/16/16	$165.00							0023	$00.00

TOTALS

Remarks

0023   This plan does not cover services rendered that are not considered medically necessary

Peer Review

If, after an appeal, the insurance carrier denies what the physician considers fair compensation for services, the physician may request a peer review. (In responding to an appeal, the insurance carrier sometimes sends a claim for peer review as a matter of routine.) A peer review is usually the physician's last attempt to resolve the problem after all other communications have been exhausted. In a **peer review**, an objective, unbiased group of physicians determines what payment is adequate for services provided. If the physician requests the peer review and it is determined that the procedures were not medically necessary, the physician is responsible for paying for the peer review.

State Insurance Commissioner

Each state's **insurance commissioner** heads the regulatory government agency for the insurance industry and serves as a liaison between the patient and the carrier, and between the physician and carrier. The medical office specialist should contact this agency if multiple appeals fail. The physician, carrier, or patient may appeal to the insurance commissioner if any of the three feel unfairly treated.

For example, suppose two insurance carriers cannot determine who the primary carrier is and as a result the physician has not been paid. The physician can write to the insurance commissioner on behalf of the patient to request resolution of the problem.

Claims processed by
Medical Care
A Division of Allied Health Corp
NUMBER: 0000K223
P.O. Box 6644
Kingston, New York 12402-6644
Toll Free (800) 555-0287

Date:
PROVIDER: 001223456
CHECK NUMBER: 034324
TAX IDENTIFICATION NUMBER: BV458796

Figure 16.4

Sample Explanation of Benefits showing denied claims.

Surgical Associates of New York
4001 9th Street
Kingston, New York 12402

PATIENT: Joe Pendergrass
PERF PRV: 0000000000000080430S
CLAIM NUMBER: 0000227050697800X

IDENTIFICATION NUMBER: 555-66-4444
PATIENT NUMBER: 79625C0G4

CLAIM TYPE: MCP

FROM/TO DATES	PROC PS*	CODE	AMOUNT BILLED	CONTRACT ALLOWABLE	SERVICES NOT COVERED	DEDUCTIONS/OTHER INELIGIBLE	AMOUNT PAID
01/02–01/02/16	11	99212	$50.00	$23.00	$50.00 (4)	$0.00	$0.00
			$50.00	$23.00	$50.00	$0.00	$0.00

AMOUNT PAID TO PROVIDER FOR THIS CLAIM: $0.00
DEDUCTIONS/OTHER INELIGIBLE

TOTAL SERVICES NOT COVERED: $50.00
PATIENT'S SHARE: $ 0.00

PATIENT: Kelly McIntire
PERF PRV: 0000000000000080430S
CLAIM Number: 0000227050697810X

IDENTIFICATION Number: 444-55-6666
PATIENT Number: 79625C0G5

CLAIM TYPE: MCP

FROM/TO DATES	PROC PS*	CODE	AMOUNT BILLED	CONTRACT ALLOWABLE	SERVICES NOT COVERED	DEDUCTIONS/OTHER INELIGIBLE	AMOUNT PAID
01/02–01/02/16	11	99214	$62.00	$29.00	$62.00 (5)	$0.00	$00.00
			$62.00	$29.00	$62.00	$0.00	$00.00

AMOUNT PAID TO PROVIDER FOR THIS CLAIM: $00.00
DEDUCTIONS/OTHER INELIGIBLE

TOTAL SERVICES NOT COVERED: $62.00
PATIENT'S SHARE: $62.00

PATIENT: Ben Bates
PERF PRV: 0000000000000080430S
CLAIM NUMBER: 0000227050697820X

IDENTIFICATION Number: 454-55-5555
PATIENT Number: 79625C0C6

CLAIM TYPE: MCP

FROM/TO DATES	PROC PS*	CODE	AMOUNT BILLED	CONTRACT ALLOWABLE	SERVICES NOT COVERED	DEDUCTIONS/OTHER INELIGIBLE	AMOUNT PAID
01/01–01/02/16	11	99386	$125.00	$90.00	$125.00 (6)	$0.00	$00.00
		72100	$188.00	$110.00	$188.00 (6)	$0.00	$00.00
			$313.00	$200.00	$313.00	$0.00	$00.00

AMOUNT PAID TO PROVIDER FOR THIS CLAIM: $0.00
DEDUCTIONS/OTHER INELIGIBLE $0.00

TOTAL SERVICES NOT COVERED: $313.00
PATIENT'S SHARE: $313.00

- -

PROVIDER CLAIMS AMOUNT SUMMARY

NUMBER OF CLAIMS:	3		AMOUNT PAID TO SUBSCRIBER:	$ 0.00
AMOUNT BILLED:	**$425.00**		**AMOUNT PAID TO PROVIDER:**	**$00.00**
AMOUNT OVER MAXIMUM ALLOWANCE:	$173.00		RECOUPMENT AMOUNT:	$ 0.00
AMOUNT OF SERVICES NOT COVERED:	$252.00		NET AMOUNT PAID TO PROVIDER:	$00.00
AMOUNT PREVIOUSLY PAID:	$ 0.00			

(4) Services rendered after termination date of coverage.
(5) This plan does not cover pre-existing conditions.
(6) Only one (1) physical exam is covered for every 24-month period.

First, the insurance commissioner formally notifies each party involved and asks each to present the documents that apply to the case. The commissioner then looks at all the facts and makes an impartial decision.

Carrier Audits

When a physician contracts to participate in a specific network with a particular insurance company, the company has the right to audit, or review, the physician's billing practices. Sometimes carriers audit selected providers because they provide extraordinary or very specialized services. Other audits are conducted in cases where fraud or other misrepresentation of services is suspected.

The insurance carrier will notify the provider before an audit is conducted. The dates and the types of records that will be audited are specified ahead of time. For example, the carrier may review billing practices or completeness of medical records. The role of the medical office specialist is to make sure the records are available, complete, and signed by the physician. To avoid problems, the medical office specialist should:

- Make sure that each claim is complete and that each diagnosis matches the services provided.
- Be as specific as possible when choosing diagnoses and modifiers for procedure codes.
- Make sure all patients' medical records are complete; check to see if everything involved in each patient's care has been documented.

Documentation

Documentation is defined as the chronological recording of pertinent facts and observations regarding a patient's health status in a logical sequence. The structure of the medical record must be consistent, and the information must be recorded in a format that allows the physician to access it easily and quickly. Documentation helps in making a proper diagnosis and formulating a sound therapeutic plan. For those who work with a patient, it provides a means to understand quickly the patient's history and current medical status. Documentation promotes continuity of care among physicians and other healthcare providers. The medical record is also a collection of information that may be useful for research and education. It is also important to maintain a record of all the treatments received by a patient to reflect what has been reported to third-party payers. Consistently, the CPT and ICD-10-CM codes reported to payers should reflect the documentation in the medical record. An unwritten rule states that "If it was not documented, it was not done; if it was not done, it cannot be reported or billed." A properly documented medical record provides the legal means of verifying care. Millions of dollars are paid in malpractice cases annually because the care was good but the medical record was not.

Documentation Guidelines

Medical record documentation is required to record pertinent facts, findings, and observations about an individual's health history, including past and present illnesses, examinations, tests, treatments, and outcomes. The medical record chronologically documents the care of the patient and is an important element contributing to high-quality care. An appropriately documented medical record can reduce many of the problems associated with claims processing and, if necessary, may serve as legal documents to verify the care provided. Because payers have a contractual obligation to enrollees, they may require reasonable documentation that services are consistent with the insurance coverage provided. They may request information to validate the following:

- The site of service
- The medical necessity and appropriateness of the diagnostic and/or therapeutic services provided
- That services provided have been accurately reported

SOAP Record-Keeping Format

The method of documentation most widely used by physicians is the **SOAP format**. SOAP stands for Subjective, Objective, Assessment, and Plan. The SOAP record-keeping format is taught in medical schools and can be adapted to the evaluation and management section of the CPT-4 book. With the SOAP format, the patient's treatment is recorded in an organized and consistent sequence. Otherwise, the physician may not document important components of the Evaluation and Management (E/M) procedure codes. The SOAP format can be described as follows:

S: *Subjective* (E/M history): the chief complaint or the reason for the medical encounter. Generally includes the history of the present illness (HPI) and a review of systems. This is usually information the patient tells the doctor. The subjective format also includes past, family, and/or social history.

O: *Objective* (E/M examination): the physical examination of the patient, including vital signs, height, weight, and blood pressure.

A: *Assessment* (E/M decision making): the doctor's diagnosis at the time of the encounter or a documenting of the impression if a diagnosis cannot be made.

P: *Plan* (E/M recommended treatment): a documenting of recommended treatment, testing ordered or other workup contemplated, new medications or adjustments of medications, therapies, and planned surgical procedures.

Necessity of Appeals

At times, during the posting of the EOB or Electronic Remittance Advice (ERA), a decision has to be made about the necessity of an appeal. Submitting an appeal is very different from submitting a new claim or following up on an outstanding claim because an appeal involves extra time and manpower. Additional information must be supplied, and detailed clinical information that may involve the physician might also be requested by the carrier.

The appeals process involves a lot of administrative work for the medical office specialist and other staff members. Because the appeals process is time consuming, it is often not done properly or consistently. Rather than appeal, some facilities make it easy on themselves by submitting a statement to the patient. Consider the example of a college student who went to her gynecologist for the insertion of an IUD. The medical office specialist called to verify benefits and was given the information that the procedure was covered along with the allowed amount. After the procedure was performed and the claim was filed, the claim was denied as a non-covered service. The verification was completed correctly, but the carrier's representative had misquoted. The patient was sent a statement to pay the full amount. The misrepresentation placed a financial burden on the patient who was not able to pay the $700.00 now due.

It is the belief of the authors that all appeals efforts should be made by the provider before expecting the patient to pay for these services.

Registering a Formal Appeal

If the decision is made to go ahead with an appeal, the first step is to know and follow the appeals policy of the payer. For example, the medical office specialist must register the appeal in a timely manner, because there is often a cutoff date for doing so. Most practices learn about the appeals policies of the major plans they work with by referring to physician administrative manuals, contracts, and newsletters. Plan representatives may also be contacted to learn about specific policies. Be aware that some plans are instituting paperless review procedures, which will decrease the time spent gathering and documenting detailed information.

The next step is for the medical office specialist to differentiate between denials of total charges and disallowances. Disallowances represent partial payment on claims because they are above the maximum allowable fee. Every practice should have a policy for determining when to appeal a disallowance. Some practices set a dollar amount limit, such as $50.00 to $200.00, depending on the specialty, beyond which an appeal will be registered with the plan. Some practices set a percentage, such as 20% of the billed charge. When a specific policy is in place regarding disallowance limits, the staff does not have to check with a supervisor before registering an appeal. Appeals are automatic and consistent. Standard form letters are used to appeal disallowances when working with a plan that does not accept verbal requests. When appealing disallowances resulting from low maximum allowable fees (MAFs), the medical office specialist should include data regarding what other plans pay for the same CPT code if the plan being appealed to is a much lower payer than others for this code. Phrases such as "Medicare allows $1,636.00, Medicaid allows $1,233.00, XYZ plan allows $2,100.00, and your MAF is $1,088.00" may be used.

A practice may want to appeal a claim for many other reasons, but unfortunately some of these reasons are not easy to identify and file. This is especially true when claims are denied because the payer feels a certain procedure is excluded from coverage or that medical necessity was not proven. Regardless of the specific reason, a standard opening for an appeal letter can be developed. All that is left to do, then, is to insert the special explanations and attach the clinical information.

The Appeals Process

No matter how clean claims are, some denials or partial payments always will need to be appealed. The two types of appeals are written and telephone appeals. The circumstances of each claim will determine which appeal process is necessary. It is best practice to direct initial appeals letters to the claims examiner. Some examples follow of simple appeals that can be handled by phone and/or fax:

■ The insurance company has denied the claim because information—for example, secondary payer information—was requested from the patient and never received. Sometimes the patient will contact the insurance company and respond by phone. Once the insurance company has the correct information, the claim can be processed.

■ A claim is denied because accident details are not available. An E code should be used when submitting an accident claim along with a CPT code. In the case of an auto accident, the medical office specialist may also receive a request to submit a police report. If the insurance company requests the police report, the medical office specialist can usually fax it. The same applies to the operative report for surgery and office notes.

■ An insurance company might routinely deny coverage for well-person care for a patient. This can be appealed by phone also. Simply ask the insurance representative to review the policy documentation.

■ A claim might be denied because a modifier was used in a multiple procedure that the insurance company decided to bundle. Bundling occurs when multiple services are performed. Every insurance company has a list that they refer to which enables them to list procedures as inclusive to another procedure, as explained in the following example.

Example

A patient with a headache comes in for an office visit. While being examined, the patient asks the doctor to look at his toe as long as he is there. The doctor discovers an ingrown toenail and performs minor surgery. A modifier is used to establish that a distinct and separate procedure was performed. The claims examiner disregards the modifier and denies the office visit as global. The medical office specialist should try to get the claim reconsidered by phone, requesting that the claim be paid and stating that the reason can be backed up with documentation. The medical office specialist should offer to fax the documentation.

The decision has been made to appeal the following situations. Which ones can be appealed by telephone, and which would be appealed in writing? Please use a T for a telephone appeal and a W for a written appeal.

Practice Exercise 16.1

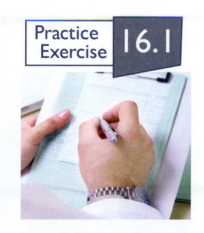

1. Diagnosis does not match procedure. _____

2. Insurance company is requesting accident details on a 3-year-old. _____

3. Services were not authorized. _____

4. Services were not medically necessary. _____

5. Services were previously paid. _____

6. Multiple surgical procedures were lumped and paid under primary procedure even though modifiers were used. _____

7. Radiology charges for a precertified surgery were performed by a contracted provider paid as out of network. _____

8. Lab charges for an inpatient precertified stay were applied toward the out-of-network deductible. _____

Table 16.2	Reason Codes That Require a Formal Appeal		
100	Services payable at 100%	DUP	Duplicate (previously processed)*
19	Dependent over age 19	ELIG	Pending eligibility
21	Dependent over age 21	ERR	Claim processing error or adjustment
1yr	Limited to one per year*	EXP	Experimental service not covered*
2ND	COB secondary payment	FUD	Included in surgical package*
3yr	Allowed once in 3 years*	INFO	Pending additional information
6MO	Allowed once in 6 months*	MAX	Maximum benefits paid
80%	Service(s) payable at 80%	MED	Not medically necessary*
ADD	Need additional information	N/C	Non-covered services*
ADM	Administrative adjustment	NER	Non-covered emergency services*
AOP	Approved out-of-plan	NOA	No answer to inquiry
AVE	Authorized number of visits exceeded*	NOD	No ordering doctor listed
BE	Billing error*	NPD	Nonparticipating doctor
BOI	Bill other insurance	NPP	Nonparticipating provider
CAP	Capitated services*	NREF	No referral or unauthorized*
CMC	Contractual maximum charge	PCI	Patient convenience item not covered*
COB	Possible COB involved	PRE	Before effective date
COS	Cosmetic service not covered*	TNR	Not related to diagnosis*
DNC	Dental service not covered*	UA	No authorization number; do not bill patient*

Appeals in writing may be required, as when a claim is denied as not medically necessary or the carrier has misquoted benefits. Sometimes billed procedures are missed, and it is not uncommon, even though the insurance company made the mistake, to be asked to submit a written appeal. One very important thing to remember is that most managed care companies set deadlines for filing an appeal; therefore, the medical office specialist must know the contents of the contract with the carrier regarding the appeals process and deadlines.

Reason Codes That Require a Formal Appeal

In Table 16.2, reasons marked with an asterisk require a formal appeal to be initiated by the practice whenever it suspects the claim was not adjudicated properly by the insurance plan. In addition to those occasions listed in Table 16.2, many others may require a special explanation when registering a formal appeal.

Employee Retirement Income Security Act of 1974

The **Employee Retirement Income Security Act (ERISA) of 1974** protects the interests of participants and their beneficiaries who depend on benefits from private employee benefit plans. ERISA sets standards for administering these plans, including a requirement that financial and other information be disclosed to plan participants and beneficiaries and requirements for the processing of claims for benefits under the plan.

Although some employee benefit plans are not covered by ERISA (such as church or government plans), the insured and provider have certain rights if a claim is denied. Contact the plan administrator regarding filing a claim and appeal. Self-funded plans are subject to ERISA and U.S. Department of Labor regulations. Seek assistance from the U.S. Department of Labor:

> U.S. Department of Labor
> Division of Technical Assistance and Inquiries
> 200 Constitution Ave.
> Washington, DC 20210
> (202) 219-8776

The medical office specialist should be aware of what insurance plans fall under ERISA. I.D. cards for ERISA plans are marked in different ways by different payers.

Waiting Period for an ERISA Claim

Within 90 days after an ERISA claim has been filed, the insurance plan must respond as to whether the claim will be paid or whether additional information is needed. If additional information is requested, the plan must specify why and the day by which the plan expects to render a final decision. If no response is received within the 90-day period, the claim is considered denied. Explanation is required for a denied claim.

Appeal to ERISA

The plan administrator must inform the provider how to submit a denied ERISA claim for a fair and full review. The provider has at least 60 days to appeal. Some plans allow more time, but again this is determined according to each individual plan. If review of the appeal is going to take longer than 60 days, the insured must be notified in writing of the delay. A decision on the appeal must be made within 120 days.

Medical office specialists should separate the EOBs that are from administrators for a self-insured employer from all other carriers so the specialists' time is spent appealing in the correct format. These claims and appeals fall under federal guidelines and are not mandated by the state insurance commissioner.

Medicare Appeals

In the mid-2000s, the government made significant structural and procedural changes in the existing Medicare appeals process. The three levels of appeals are discussed next: redetermination, the second level of appeal, and the third level of appeal.

Redetermination

A provider has 120 days to file a request for a Medicare review, also known as a **redetermination**, with a Medicare carrier. A Medicare redetermination is the first level of appeal for physician claims. The law stipulates that Medicare carriers must process redeterminations within 30 days.

Second Level of Appeal

The second level of the appeals process is handled by **qualified independent contractors (QICs)** who process "reconsiderations" of carriers' initial determinations and redeterminations. As a result of the recent changes, appellants now have easier access to this second level of appeal because the $100.00 threshold for the amount in question was removed. Physicians can also expect a quicker turnaround on these second-level appeals than in the past because QICs must now process their reconsiderations within 30 days. Physicians essentially have 6 months to file a second-level appeal.

Third Level of Appeal and Beyond

The third level of appeal is an **administrative law judge (ALJ) hearing**, and physicians have 60 days to file an appeal with an ALJ. In order to request a hearing by an ALJ, the amount remaining in controversy must meet the threshold requirement. The threshold amount is recalculated each year and is subject to change. For 2016 calendar year, the amount in controversy threshold is $150. For 2017 calendar year, the amount is $160. ALJs have 90 days in which to make a decision. Thus, physicians should have an easier time than in the past getting an ALJ hearing, if needed, and they should receive a quicker decision in most cases.

The levels of appeal beyond the ALJ are the Departmental Appeals Board and federal district courts. Appeals of physicians' claims rarely reach either of these levels. There have been no major changes in the process for these stages, except that there is now a 90-day time limit on decisions at the Departmental Appeals Board level; previously, there was no time limit on these decisions.

Medicare Part B has found that the number one reason an appeal is returned is for an invalid signature or lack of an acceptable one. Acceptable signatures on appeals are as follows:

- Actual signature by the provider or authorized employee
- A rubber-stamped signature of provider or authorized employee
- Signature of provider signed and initialed by an authorized employee
- Signature on the review request (A signature on just the operative report or claim form is unacceptable.)

When requesting a redetermination or filing an appeal with Medicare, the Medicare redetermination request form shown in Appendix D must be used.

Appeal Letters

Many appeal letters can be standardized, with the medical office specialist then inserting specific details and providing necessary information and documentation. Sometimes, however, the specific situation calls for an original letter. To strengthen an appeal, court rulings can and should be used in appeal letters. Returning to our earlier example of the college student whose claim was rejected, Figures 16.5 and 16.6 are examples of two appeal letters regarding the denial of payment for insertion of an IUD. The letter in Figure 16.5 does not include court rulings and is not as effective as the

Allied Medical Center
1933 E. Frankford Rd. #110
Yucaipa, CA 92399

Dear Claims Examiner,

I am writing to you in regard to a claim submitted for Tessa Kirk for services provided by Dr. Stewart on June 12, 2016. The charges total $700.00.

This claim was sent to ABC Insurance Company, which has since denied the charges. The reason given for the denial is that insertion of an IUD isn't covered by her health insurance plan. However, I called the customer service number listed on the back of her insurance card and was told that it would be a covered expense.

On June 9, 2016, I called and spoke with Phyllis Rose and asked about benefits for an IUD. She not only told me that it was a covered service, but she also quoted me the payment benefits and assured me that it would be paid. I feel that Dr. Stewart should not be penalized for receiving incorrect information from your insurance company. I was using the customer service number provided on the back of the insurance plan and I believe that the insurance company should be held accountable for what is quoted over the phone. Furthermore, had we known the service was not covered, we would have notified the patient in advance of that and would have given her the opportunity to make payment arrangements or not to have the procedure.

Please review this letter and reconsider the charges you have previously denied. Thank you for your time and assistance in this matter.

Sincerely,

Linda Baldwin
Medical Office Specialist

Figure 16.5

Sample appeal letter regarding denial of payment for insertion of an IUD. It does not include court rulings.

one in Figure 16.6, which does include court rulings. Note also that Figure 16.6 is more formal and includes more details about the patient, such as the policy number. This, too, helps its effectiveness.

It is important for the medical office specialist to research and share information regarding the federal and state laws that affect the provider's claim submission and appeals process. We discussed earlier the importance of medical necessity and the fact that this is a reason many claims are denied. Figures 16.7 and 16.8 are examples of appeal letters that deal with denial because of medical necessity.

Closing Words

Note the similarities among the appeal letters in Figure 16.5, Figure 16.6, and Figure 16.7. They (1) provide a specific description of the charges being appealed; (2) identify the names of people contacted at the insurance company with the

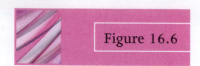

Figure 16.6

Sample appeal letter regarding the denial of payment for insertion of an IUD. It does include court rulings.

Allied Medical Center
1933 E. Frankford Rd. #110
Yucaipa, CA 92399

July 20, 2016
Attn: Director of Claims
ABC Insurance Company
2246 Midway Road, #110
Phoenix, AZ 12345

Re: Tessa Kirk
Policy: 455-29-2020
Insured: Tessa Kirk
Treatment Date: June 12, 2016
Amount: $700.00

Dear Director of Claims:

The above-referenced claim was denied despite the fact that verification of benefits and/or preauthorization of care was obtained from your company on June 9, 2016. Please be advised that our facility relies on information received from your company regarding coverage. We extended treatment in good faith based on the expectation of payment. Further, state courts have held that insurers are liable for misrepresentations made during coverage verification. In *Hermann Hospital v. National Standard Insurance Company*, 776 SW 2nd 249, the Court of Appeals of Texas ruled that coverage misrepresentations could be construed as both negligent and fraudulent. In rendering this decision, the court wrote:

"Hospital and other healthcare providers must, and do, rely on the insurance carriers' representations of coverage in making their decision regarding admission of potential patients. If insurance coverage and benefits cannot be verified, or no coverage exists, the medical provider can then make alternative financial arrangements. To insulate the insurance carriers from liability leaves the medical care provider without recourse against the party causing it damage, if it acted in reliance on the representation of coverage."

Therefore, we request your review of the denial in light of the information obtained by your company at the time treatment was rendered.

Sincerely,

Dee Phillips
Medical Office Specialist

dates the conversations took place; (3) provide concise explanations of what is being requested, either a re-verification of the policy requirements or asking for an exception to the rules; in either case, a strong argument defining the position of the letter writer is stated precisely; and (4) explain clearly the anticipated result anticipated by the letter writer.

Figure 16.7

Sample appeal letter dealing with denial because of medical necessity.

Allied Medical Center
1933 E. Frankford Rd. #110
Yucaipa, CA 92399

Dear Mr. Hess,

We have received the explanation of benefits for a patient, Mr. Robert Crawford. However, we believe the charges totaling $480.00 for February 25, 2016 through March 14, 2016 have been considered incorrectly.

The EOB states that the March 15th charge of $80.00 is not a medical necessity. When I spoke to you at the claims center earlier this week, your explanation of the denial was because the patient is not homebound and the insurance company believes the visit was for patient convenience and not medically necessary.

In reviewing the nurse's notes for each skilled nursing visit, medical necessity appears to have been established. The March 15th visit should not have been denied. A new infusion therapy was started on that date and the patient required instruction on drug administration.

Skilled nursing visits are a medical necessity to follow up on how well the patient is learning and, indeed, errors in the patient's technique were discovered. Throughout the therapy, the patient was fatigued, weak, and felt sick. The patient also felt overwhelmed with the therapies, requiring further instruction and reinforcement. The results of not having skilled nursing visits could lead to further complications, such as not following the drug schedule or performing inaccurate drug administration.

It appears that a review of the nurse's notes would support the medical necessity of the nursing charges. Please reconsider the denied portion of the charges and issue a payment to Value Home Care in the amount of $80.00.

Sincerely,

Bill Ingram
Collections Manager, Value Home Care

Appeals and Customer Service

Many providers view appealing denied medical claims as an unwanted, but necessary, function of back-end collections. An aggressive appeals program in a provider's office can also be a tremendous bonus to the practice's reputation for extending exemplary customer service.

Most patients recognize that a medical provider is going above the call of duty when the provider attempts to overturn an unfair claim denial for the patient. To the patient, already beset with a medical malady, any assistance in dealing with complicated insurance issues is greatly appreciated. Further, a successful appeal letter that relieves the patient of a possible financial burden will be something the patient is sure to discuss with friends, neighbors, and mere acquaintances—all prospects for growing clientele.

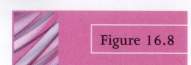

Figure 16.8

Sample appeal letter for dealing with denial because of medical necessity.

Allied Medical Center
1933 E. Frankford Rd. #110
Yucaipa, CA 92399

April 20, 2016
Attn: Director of Claims
ABC Insurance Company
2246 Midway Road #110
Phoenix, AZ 12345

Re: Mr. Robert Crawford
Policy: 636-33-459
Insured: Robert Crawford
Treatment Dates: February 25, 2016–March 14, 2016
Amount: $80.00

Dear Director of Claims:

It is our understanding that this claim was denied pursuant to your decision that the care was not medically necessary.

The Explanation of Benefits did not give adequate information to establish the accuracy of this decision. Therefore, please provide the following information to support the denial of benefits for this treatment.

Please furnish the name and credentials of the insurance representative who reviewed the treatment records. Also, please provide an outline of the specific records reviewed and a description of any records that would be necessary in order to approve the treatment.

Further, we would appreciate copies of any expert medical opinions that have been secured by your company with regard to treatments of this nature and its efficacy so that the treating physician may respond to its applicability to this patient's condition.

Thank you for your assistance.

Sincerely,

Dee Phillips
Medical Office Specialist

Ways to reinforce this positive aspect of appealing denied claims include the following:

- In an appeal letter, refer to the patient by name, rather than using the generic term *patient*. For example, state "Mr. Brown was treated in our office on May 5," rather than "This patient was treated. . . ."
- Send a copy of the appeal letter to the patient. Put a "cc:" notation at the bottom of the original so the patient will know that the carrier is being advised that the patient should be advised of all communications.
- When sending the copy of the appeal letter to the patient, include a brief cover letter explaining that the appeal was filed as a courtesy to the patient.

Ask the patient to also appeal the denial, inviting her to use any information in your letter that supports the request for payment. Give the patient the name of your insurance representative who might be able to answer questions about medical appeals.

■ Advise the patient of his alternatives. The provider might want to keep literature in the office from the state's Department of Insurance, Labor Department information, or business cards of companies and law firms that offer appeal assistance.

■ Finally, and most important, phone the patient when an appeal letter is sent.

Appeals Require Perseverance and Attitude

In appealing denied insurance claims, you need to have the mind-set that it is the insurance carrier's burden to prove that the claim has been processed correctly and that any ambiguities in the coverage terms were construed in the insured's favor. A strong mind-set will also give you the perseverance necessary to continue to appeal a claim the insurer strongly defends.

Attitude is more important than facts because the right attitude will help you persuade the insurance carrier to look at the facts differently. The initial appeal should be addressed to the appeals department.

Many claims are overturned after a single appeal letter. However, you should persist with filing appeals until you get a satisfactory answer. When you do not receive an adequate response to your appeal from the appeals committee, it is imperative that you continue to appeal.

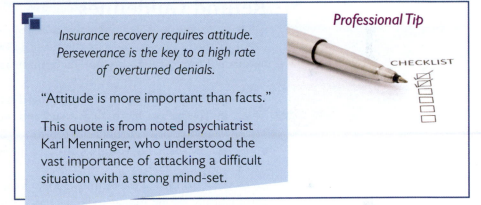

Professional Tip

Insurance recovery requires attitude. Perseverance is the key to a high rate of overturned denials.

"Attitude is more important than facts."

This quote is from noted psychiatrist Karl Menninger, who understood the vast importance of attacking a difficult situation with a strong mind-set.

CHECKLIST

Persistence is often the key to overturning a denied claim. Many carriers overturn as many appeals during the second and third appeals as on the first appeal. It is crucial to keep the appeal active, even after the initial denial. In fact, statistics released from major insurance carriers indicate that about 25% of appeals are overturned on the first appeal and another 25% are overturned on the second appeal.

If you believe payment is indicated by the policy terms, continue to appeal the claim. See the next section for information on keeping your appeal alive.

Do Not Settle for "Denial Upheld"

As noted, appealing denied insurance claims requires perseverance. You may find that the claims department is not reviewing your carefully researched and strongly worded appeal adequately. In such instances, you can redirect your appeal to someone in a better position to review and respond to the information you have cited. Consider sending your appeal to one of the following:

■ *Carrier legal counsel.* If you have cited regulatory information, you can request a review and written response from the legal department.

■ *Carrier president.* If your appeal involves a possible breach of claim processing procedures, ask the president or other senior management official to respond.

- *Department of Labor.* If the insurance is self-funded, file a complaint with the Department of Labor. Send a copy of the complaint to the insurer.
- *Employer.* The employer will have an appeals committee if the group is self-insured.
- *Department of Insurance.* File a formal complaint with your state's Department of Insurance if you are unable to get a satisfactory response. Send a copy of the complaint to the insurer.
- *State medical association.* Many medical associations now have a complaint review process and will assist you with resolving denied insurance claims.

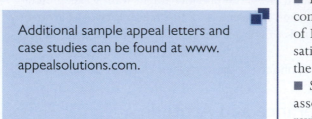

Professional Tip

CHECKLIST

Additional sample appeal letters and case studies can be found at www.appealsolutions.com.

Refund Guidelines

Credit balances and refunds are the result of overpayments by the patient or insurance company. Overpayments are not uncommon and can occur for various reasons:

- The patient pays in excess of her financial responsibility.
- The patient has both primary and secondary insurance. Both insurance companies pay as primary in error.
- The insurance company makes a duplicate payment on a previously paid claim.

A good portion of the refund process is accomplished using common sense. Do not automatically refund money to an insurance carrier just because it has requested money back. Research must first be completed. The medical office specialist must know what type of plan is involved and whether prompt payment rules apply.

Make sure the EOB/ERA request for a refund clearly states why a refund is warranted. If the insurance carrier states coverage was canceled before or not in effect on the date services were performed, check to see if a verification of benefits (VOB) form is on file for that date of service. If a VOB form is on file for that date of service, appeal the refund request by citing the information given on the VOB. If the insurance carrier states a refund is due because of overpayment on the patient's account, check the carrier contract and fee schedule to see if that is the case.

If the insurance carrier states other insurance should have paid first (coordination of benefits), research the other insurance coverage. If this is true, refund the money. If it is not, appeal the refund request. If the insurance carrier has paid twice for the same date of service and is requesting a refund, check the first EOB/ERA to see that it was posted to the correct date of service. If it was, refund the overpayment amount. If it was not, the first EOB/ERA should be posted correctly and an appeal should be sent to the insurance carrier.

If a patient is requesting a refund because of a prepayment made for a service, you will first need to research the patient account to ensure that the patient has no other outstanding balance (i.e., from an earlier date of service). If the patient does have an outstanding balance, apply the money appropriately and refund the difference. If there is no other outstanding balance, the patient should be sent the entire refund amount.

A patient may have a secondary insurance policy that will pay his copayment amount due on the primary insurance policy. If the patient paid his copay at the time of service and both insurance companies have paid their shares—the second policy having

Practice Exercise **16.2**

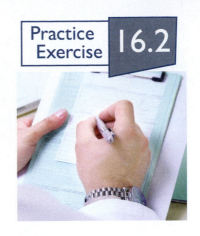

Read the following scenarios. On a separate sheet of paper, explain what steps you would take to handle each situation. If you believe an appeal is necessary, explain why, write the appeal letter, and explain what you would attach to the appeal letter. If you believe a patient bill is necessary, create a patient bill. If you feel more research into the case is needed, explain what research should be done. Please make up an insurance address, provider address, and the patient's address, policy number, and claim number. Use your imagination with the scenarios.

1. Jane Shadrack saw Dr. Eugene A. Brady on July 8, 2016. She complained of severe headaches, blurred vision, and disorientation. Dr. Brady diagnosed her with migraine headaches. The claim was denied by her insurance carrier, Aetna, stating that her treatment was not medically necessary. Ms. Shadrack's medical records show she was in serious need of medical care.

2. Bobbie Montgomery, age 12, saw Dr. Eugene A. Brady on September 21, 2016. A claim was submitted to his father's insurance carrier, Great West Life, on September 24. Great West Life has sent Dr. Brady an EOB stating that coordination of benefits should be observed and is being researched.

3. Shannon Macaroni was seen by Dr. Eugene A. Brady as an emergency patient on October 5 at 9:00 p.m. because she had a stick in her right eye. A claim was submitted on October 8 and denied for no prior authorization number.

4. Dr. Eugene A. Brady performed surgery on Lois Buttons's index finger on August 15. The claim was submitted to Aetna and denied as an experimental procedure.

covered the primary copay amount—then the patient may be entitled to a refund. Again, check the patient account for any outstanding balances. If there is a balance, apply the copay amount to that balance and refund the difference if any. If there is no outstanding balance, refund the entire copay amount to the patient.

Usually, the accounting department or office manager must approve all refunds. If a refund is warranted, print out the patient's financial record for the appropriate date of service, attach a copy of the EOB or ERA/refund request and any research you completed, and give it to the accounting department or office manager.

Although there is no way to completely avoid credit balances, policies can be put in place to keep them at a minimum. Whatever the reasons for the overpayment, make sure that the reason for the credit balance is identified and do not issue a refund unless requested by the carrier. The reason to wait for a request by the carrier is the carrier may withhold funds from another claim to address the refund.

The medical office specialist's goal should always be to keep accounts as clean as possible. To issue a refund, the medical office specialist must first go into the computer transaction screen. Any time financial information is entered to alter an account balance, a transaction is being performed. To issue a refund to an insurance company, the medical office specialist makes an adjustment to the balance of patient's accounts. A negative adjustment will increase the balance, whereas a positive adjustment will decrease it. To issue a refund, use a positive adjustment. Entering a positive adjustment code will offset the credit. After the adjustment codes have been entered, the medical office specialist documents the patient's account, explaining the reason for the refund. When an insurance company has requested a refund for an overpayment, it should be examined as soon as possible. If the carrier does not receive the refund or an appeal, the carrier has the right to automatically recoup payments from any current payment due on adjudicated claims before it is ever actually issued. The insurance company does this simply by flagging the provider's I.D. number, showing that the provider owes a refund. This should be avoided at all costs. All government health plans can also do automatic recoupments without notice. Automatic recoupments can become an accounting nightmare. The insurance company will recoup money from any payment going out of its office to the provider, whether this is the account where the overpayment occurred or not. Therefore, adjustments will have to be made to several accounts depending on the amount of money the insurance company has recouped.

Avoid Excessive Overpayments

Patients' copayments are to be verified with the insurance carrier prior to or at the time of service if at all possible. As companies renew their coverage each year, sometimes the deductibles and copays change. The patient may not have her new card when she comes into the office. Therefore, every effort must be made to verify copays with the carrier. Best practice is to verify all benefits prior to date of service. If the card is asking for a $25.00 copay and the patient states that her copay has changed and it is now $10.00, take the patient's word for it. It is good customer service to do so—the patient usually knows what her copay is. A bill can be sent later if it is incorrect, which is preferable to risk losing a patient and having to issue a refund later.

The deductible should be requested up front if the services are being rendered before the patient has met his deductible. Also, if the procedure is not covered by the insurance plan, the charged amount should be requested before the services are provided. For some services, the copays and deductibles are not applicable. For example, a routine well-person visit may not apply to the deductible. Always verify with the insurance carrier or the managed care organization (MCO).

Guidelines for Insurance Overpayments and Refund Requests

The American Medical Association and its staff receive questions daily from medical offices about payer requests for refunds. The following general information will help the medical office specialist properly assess most refund requests:

Self-funded employer ERISA plans. Time limits are based on individual contractual agreements. Nothing prevents carriers from automatically recouping refunds from current or future payments, regardless of whether the physician is contracted or noncontracted.

Medicare overpayments. In general, there is no defined time limit after which Medicare may not ask for money back. Automatic recoupments from current and/or future payments are permitted. For Medicare beneficiaries, the provider who is not participating and not accepting assignment can only charge a *limiting charge*. A Medicare Limiting Charge form is a request for a refund to the patient by Medicare. This form can be found in Appendix D. The form states to the patient that the provider has been informed of the overcharge.

Medicaid overpayments. In general, Medicaid may request refunds for up to 5 years. Depending on the circumstances, this time frame can be exceeded.

Civil Practice and Remedies Code §16.004. In rare situations where no contract language governs refunds, the statute of limitations is 4 years (excluding government programs).

Preauthorization. For all payer types, preauthorization pertains only to medical necessity and is never a guarantee of payment.

Wrongful retention. A physician should never retain any amount truly not owed to the practice. Wrongful retention of an overpayment is called *conversion* and is illegal. If the practice did not perform the service(s), or if the reimbursement is clearly more than the plan owes, the practice should return the overpayment.

Practice Exercises

Take the time now to complete Practice Exercises 16.3, 16.4, 16.5, and 16.6 to gain experience working with situations in which refunds are required.

Review the following claim information and (1) complete a CMS-1500, (2) apply refund calculations, and (3) then fill in the missing information in the blanks provided.

Practice Exercise 16.3

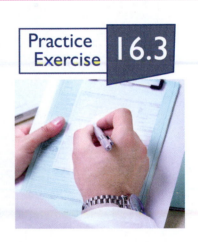

Patient:	Sandra Brown	**DOB:**	09/06/1975
Address:	1658 N. Lovers Lane	**Ins Co:**	Aetna
	Wichita, KS 67214		P.O. Box 1399,
			Topeka, KS 67210
Phone Number:	316-555-8288	**I.D. Number:**	581144448
Employer:	Central Market	**Group Number:**	1274
	Highland Park Village		
	Wichita, KS 67214		

Patient is seen for first time. Reason for visit is sore throat and fever. She is the insured and has selected your doctor, Dr. Mallard, as her PCP. Refer to the following physician information.

Physician Name:	Mallard and Associates, P.A.
	J. D. Mallard, M.D.
License Number:	KS54308
Address:	19333 Forrest Haven
	Wichita, KS 67214
Phone Number:	316-555-5040

Group Identification Numbers:

Group PIN:	M23548711
Group NPI:	7777788888
Referring Physician:	William F. Bonner, M.D.

(Continued)

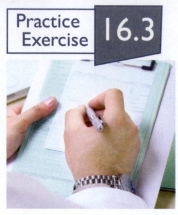

Practice Exercise 16.3

(Continued)

Dr. William F. Bonner Identification Numbers

NPI: 1111199999

Dr. J. D. Mallard Identification Numbers

EIN: 72-5727222
NPI: 8888877777
DX: 487.1   ICD-10
Office visit   99204 $180.00
Strep Test   87081 $ 54.00

Sandra paid $234.00 up front because she has a $250.00 deductible and is not sure whether or not it has been met.

You receive an EOB 30 days after submitting a paper claim. The insurance company allowed $125.00 of the visit and $20.00 of the lab charges. All allowable charges were applied to the deductible. Enter payments on account as well as any contractual write-offs.

1. Is there a credit on this account? _____

2. If so, how much? _____

3. What type of adjustment should be entered? _____

4. Is a refund due? _____

5. If so, how much? _____

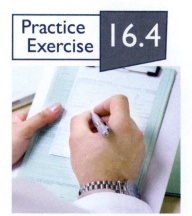

Practice Exercise 16.4

Review the following claim information and (1) complete a CMS-1500, (2) apply refund calculations, and (3) then fill in the missing information in the blanks provided.

Patient: Elizabeth O'Connor   **DOB:** 04/08/1982
I.D. Number: 625148544   **Employer:** CVS Pharmacy
Group Number: 11158
Address: 1900 Lemon Lane
                     Birmingham, AL 35283
Phone Number: 214-555-1589
Ins Co: United Healthcare
                     P.O. Box 1014
                     Birmingham, AL 35283

Elizabeth was seen today for scoliosis. She is the insured and has selected Dr. Mallard as her PCP. Refer to Practice Exercise 16.3 for physician information.

Diagnosis code: 737.30 (ICD-10) M41.9

Office visit	99214	$65.00
	97260	$30.00

Elizabeth made a payment of $47.00 for her services today. Her deductible has been met for the year.

You receive an EOB 30 days after submitting a paper claim. The insurance company allowed $55.00 of the visit and $20.00 of the second charge. The rate of benefit is 80%.

1. Is there a credit on this account? _____

2. If so, how much? _____

3. What type of adjustment should be entered? _____

4. Is a refund due? _____

5. If so, how much? _____

Practice Exercise 16.4

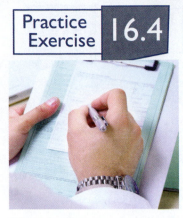

(Continued)

Review the following claim information and (1) complete a CMS-1500, (2) apply refund calculations, and (3) then fill in the missing information in the blanks provided.

Practice Exercise 16.5

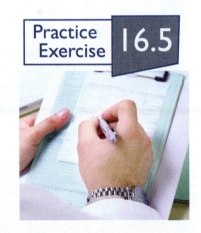

Patient:	Norbert Blake	**DOB:** 05/07/1984
I.D. Number:	514258522	**Employer:** Lizis Chicken
Group Number:	58999	
Address:	1721 Elm Street	
	Denver, CO 80023	
Phone Number:	972-414-8544	
Ins Co:	Cigna Health Care	
	P.O. Box 99874	
	Denver, CO 80023	

Norbert was seen today for injury to his hand. He is the insured and has selected Dr. Mallard as his PCP. Refer to Practice Exercise 16.3 for physician information.

Diagnosis code: 959.4 (ICD-10) S69.80XA

Office visit	99213	$60.00
X-ray	73130	$45.00

Norbert made a payment of $32.00 for his services today. His deductible has been met for the year.

(Continued)

Practice Exercise 16.5

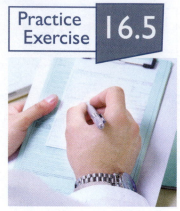

You receive an EOB 30 days after submitting a paper claim. The insurance company allowed $53.00 of the visit and $33.00 of the X-ray charge. The rate of benefit is 70%.

1. Is there a credit on this account? _____

2. If so, how much? _____

3. What type of adjustment should be entered? _____

4. Is a refund due? _____

5. If so, how much? _____

(Continued)

Practice Exercise 16.6

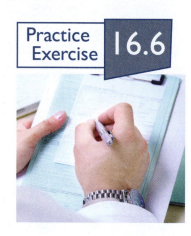

Review the following claim information and (1) complete a CMS-1500, (2) apply refund calculations, and (3) then fill in the missing information in the blanks provided.

Patient: Hanna Hill   **DOB:** 02/04/75
I.D. Number: 411-65-8744   **Employer:** Tony's Beauty Supply
Group Number: 15555
Address: 1818 High Beach Dr.
             Barrigada, Guam 96921
Phone Number: 939-939-8244
Ins Co: All Health Care
            P.O. Box 23803
            Barrigada, Guam 96921

Hanna was seen today for an upper respiratory infection. She is the insured and has selected Dr. Mallard as her PCP. Refer to Practice Exercise 16.3 for physician information.

Diagnosis code: 465.9 (ICD-10) J06.9

Office visit	99213	$60.00
X-ray	71040	$50.00
Lab	81000	$11.00

Hanna made a payment of $35.00 for her services today. Her deductible has been met for the year.

You receive an EOB 30 days after submitting a paper claim. The insurance company allowed $53.00 of the visit, $35.00 of the X-ray charge, and $9.00 on the lab. The rate of benefit is 90%.

1. Is there a credit on this account? _____

2. If so, how much? _____

3. What type of adjustment should be entered? _____

4. Is a refund due? _____

5. If so, how much? _____

Figure 16.9 is an example of a letter refusing a refund request from an insurance carrier. Each state has its own laws and regulations regarding refunds. The medical office specialist can contact his local medical association, attorney general, or state insurance board for state and local information regarding refund guidelines.

Figure 16.9

Example of a letter refusing a refund request from an insurance carrier.

Allied Medical Center
1933 E. Frankford Rd. #110
Carrollton, TX 12345

February 10, 2016
Aetna Healthcare
OSR Department
P. O. Box 45987
Nashville, TN 12345

Re: Patient Name
Policy Number: 0000000000
Claim Number: 0000000000

Dear Sirs:

On behalf of Allied Medical Center, I am writing to notify you of our refusal to comply with your refund request on the referenced member. Attached for your review is a copy of your letter requesting a refund.

Texas courts have already decided on this issue and have ruled in favor of the providers. If 180 days have lapsed from the day payment was received, no refund is due. Your request for payment is past this deadline. Insurers are not entitled to restitution for an overpayment that resulted solely from the insurer's mistake. Instead, the courts have stated that the medical provider is an innocent party and that the party who created the situation (the insurer) leading to the loss must bear the loss. Refer to the cases of *Lincoln National Life Insurance Co v. Brown Schools, Inc.*, 787 SW 2nd 411, and *Lincoln National v. Rittman*, 79 SW 2nd 791.

Furthermore, "The Retention of Insurance Overpayments by Health Care Providers," 30 So. Tex. L. 387-395, concluded the following on the subject: "Overpayments or payments otherwise mistakenly made by an insurer may be retained by the healthcare provider who is innocent, acts in good faith without prior knowledge of the mistake, and makes no misrepresentation to the insurer, provided the amount retained relates only to the amount actually due for services rendered."

Please correct your records on this case and contact me should you have any questions.

Sincerely,

Melissa Haverty
Practice Manager
cc: Texas Medical Association

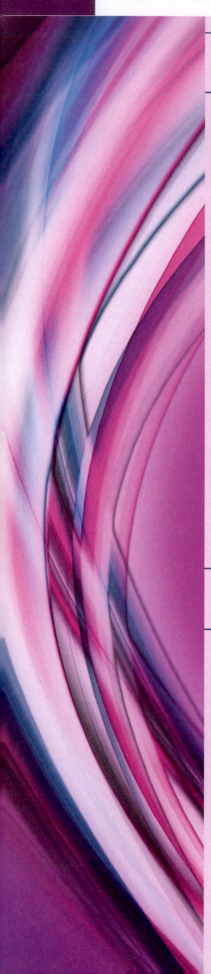

Chapter Summary

- Insurance claims that a third-party payer denies, downcodes, or requests more information on ultimately affect the financial status of the practice.
- A claim appeal is a request for a review of reimbursements. It is a formal way of asking the insurance carrier to reconsider its decision regarding a claim.
- The structure of the medical record must be consistent, and the information must be recorded in a format that allows the physician to access it easily and quickly. Documentation helps in making a proper diagnosis and formulating a sound therapeutic plan.
- When a physician contracts to participate in a specific network with a particular insurance company, the company has the right to audit or review the physician's billing practices or completeness of medical records.
- The method of documentation most widely used by physicians is the SOAP (Subjective, Objective, Assessment, Plan) format for record keeping.
- The medical office specialist should differentiate between denials of total charges and disallowances. Disallowances represent partial payment on claims because they are above the maximum allowable fee. Denials are the case when no payment is forthcoming because payment is denied.
- Self-funded plans are subject to ERISA and U.S. Department of Labor regulations. The MSO should contact the plan administrator regarding filing an ERISA claim and appeal.
- The three levels of Medicare appeals include redetermination, the processing of reconsiderations of carriers' initial determinations and redeterminations by qualified independent contractors (QICs), and administrative law judge (ALJ) hearings.
- Credit balances and refunds are a result of an overpayment by the patient or insurance company. Overpayments are not uncommon.

Chapter Review

True/False

Identify the statement as true (T) or false (F).

_____ **1.** Some appeals may be conducted over the telephone, whereas others may require a written appeal.

_____ **2.** If a payer has rejected all of the appeals on a claim, the claimant may take the case to the state's insurance commissioner.

_____ **3.** The Medicare program provides four levels of appeals.

_____ **4.** The SOAP format is used when calling insurance companies to verify benefits.

_____ **5.** When a third-party payer issues a refund request in writing, the practice should issue a refund within 24 hours.

_____ **6.** ERISA stands for Employee Retirement Income Security Act (of 1974).

_____ **7.** The office of each state's insurance commissioner is the regulatory agency for the insurance industry and serves as a liaison between the patient and the provider.

_____ **8.** Regardless of the method of reimbursement, insurance claims must be monitored until payments are received.

Multiple Choice

Identify the letter of the choice that best completes the statement or answers the question.

_____ **1.** The government department you should go to if multiple appeals to an MCO fail is:
   a. the Department of Health.
   b. the CMS.
   c. the state department of insurance/insurance commissioner.
   d. HIPAA.

_____ **2.** What percentage of denied claims are overturned on the first appeal?
   a. 25%   c. 30%
   b. 15%   d. 45%

_____ **3.** If your first appeal is denied, it is appropriate to:
   a. write a second appeal.
   b. forward the denial with a bill for the unpaid portions to the patient.
   c. call the carrier and complain.
   d. do all of the above.

_____ **4.** It is best to direct initial appeal letters to:
   a. the appeals department.
   b. the customer service representative.
   c. the claims examiner.
   d. the president of the insurance company.

_____ **5.** The method of documentation most widely used by physicians is the:
   a. RVU format.   c. ERA format.
   b. SOAP format.   d. HIPAA format.

_____ **6.** What percentage of denied claims are overturned on the second appeal?
   a. 35%   c. 20%
   b. 25%   d. 60%

_____ **7.** Appealing denied insurance claims requires:
   a. a college degree in mental health.
   b. perseverance.
   c. knowledge in preventative medicine.
   d. none of the above.

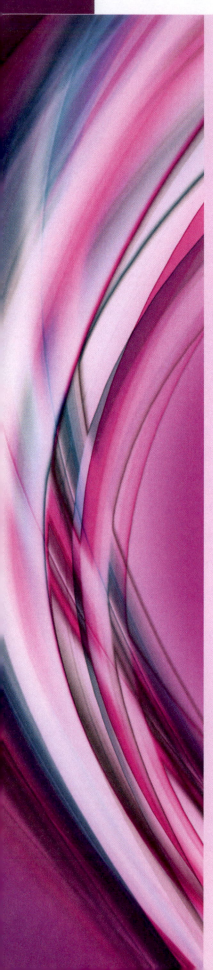

_____ **8.** Medicare Part B states that the number one reason an appeal is returned is because:

    a. it is beyond the time limit.

    b. it is invalid or there is no acceptable signature.

    c. the benefit plan is not covered by ERISA.

    d. a modifier was not used.

Matching

Choose the best word or phrase that matches the definition.

a. audit	e. documentation
b. peer review	f. administrative law judge (ALJ) hearing
c. claim appeal	g. insurance commissioner
d. SOAP	

_____ **1.** Third level of Medicare appeal

_____ **2.** Chronological recording of pertinent facts and observations regarding a patient's health status in a logical sequence

_____ **3.** A written request for a review of reimbursements

_____ **4.** An objective, unbiased group of physicians who determine what payment is adequate for services provided

_____ **5.** The regulatory agency for the insurance industry; serves as a liaison between the patient and the carrier

_____ **6.** A method of documentation most widely used by physicians for record keeping

_____ **7.** A process of examining and verifying claims and supporting documents submitted by a physician or medical facility

For Additional Practice

Review the following case study and determine the necessary action to be taken.

Mary Johnson saw Dr. Nichols today for a well-woman exam. Total charges are $185.00. Mary has two insurance companies:

Primary Insurance	**Secondary Insurance**
BCBS	Cigna Health Care
Copay: $25.00	Deductible: $200.00 (already met)
100% benefit after copay	80% benefit after deductible
Allowed amount: $150.00	Allowed amount: $125.00

Both claims were submitted at the same time in error.

Money collected from the patient: $0.00

1. How much money did Dr. Nichols receive?

2. How much should BCBS have paid?

3. How much should Cigna have paid?

4. How much is this claim overpaid?

5. Who overpaid on this claim?

6. How could this situation have been avoided?

Resources

Aetna

www.aetna.com

Under "Health Care Professionals," a provider can access newsletters that provide information regarding processing of claims and how to appeal denied claims.

Claims Resolution for Healthcare Providers

www.appealsolutions.com

Provides examples of free appeal letters.

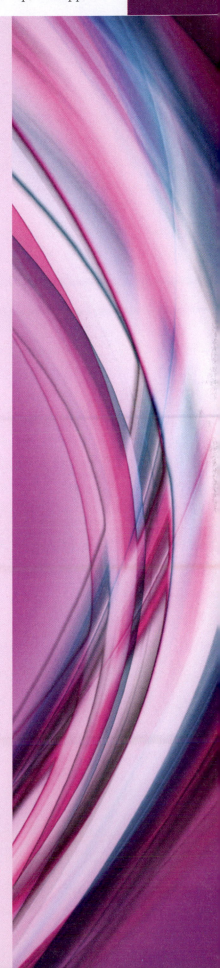

Section VII / Injured Employee Medical Claims

17 Workers' Compensation

Workers' compensation is a state-regulated insurance program that pays medical bills and some lost wages for employees who are injured on the job or who have work-related diseases or illnesses. It was developed to benefit both the injured employee and the employer. Chapter 17 presents the student with in-depth knowledge of federal and state workers' compensation programs and how to file workers' compensation insurance claims.

Professional Vignette

My name is Valarie B. Clement, CMA (AAMA). I worked as a medical biller and coder for 18 years before beginning my current teaching career. My first introduction to medical billing and coding was when I worked for a medical laboratory. The medical coder was getting married and the practice needed someone to learn her position while she was on leave. I gladly volunteered as it was an opportunity to learn something new. Looking up, now ICD-10, and CPT codes was fascinating to me. I never realized just how many there were. Although I learned a lot about medical coding I recognized that I needed to go back to school to fully understand the process.

Shortly after completing my studies, I was hired by a family physician to do his billing. I was as shocked as he was to find a file cabinet full of rejected claims. These claims had been billed but rejected for various reasons. Some were rejected for simply needing an insured's I.D. number. Time was of the essence in getting these claims processed, as many were close to filing time limits. I went right to work on correcting or providing additional information then resubmitting the claims for payment. Within 45 days, 95% of the claims were paid or transferred to patients for their responsible amounts. The physician was so pleased with my results that he gave me a nice bonus for my hard work and determination. I had found a career that I fully enjoyed and that challenged me on a routine basis.

I have learned that the key to successful medical collections is to be persistent and knowledgeable. I have had a long and successful career in the medical field both as a certified medical assistant and as a professional medical biller and coder. Today, I have the privilege of teaching students at Everest Institute about medical billing and coding while still working part time as a professional medical billing consultant.

Chapter 17 / Workers' Compensation

Chapter Objectives

After reading this chapter, the student should be able to:

1. Understand the history of workers' compensation.

2. Distinguish between federal workers' compensation and state workers' compensation.

3. List the classifications of a work-related injury.

4. Know injured workers' responsibilities and rights.

5. Understand the responsibilities of the treating doctor/physician of record.

6. Understand the role of an ombudsman in assisting with claims.

7. Know the four types of workers' compensation benefits.

8. Discuss the different types of disability.

9. Accurately complete a CMS-1500 form for a workers' compensation claim.

10. Determine the workers' compensation fee based on the Medicare Fee Schedule.

Key Terms

Admission of Liability
burial benefits
death benefits
designated doctor
disability
disability compensation
    programs
District of Columbia
    Workers'
    Compensation Act

Employer's First Report
    of Injury or Illness
Energy Employees
    Occupational Illness
    Compensation
    Program Act (EEOICP)
Federal Coal Mine Health
    and Safety Act
(Black Lung Benefits
    Reform Act)

Federal Employees'
    Compensation Act
    (FECA)
final report
fraud indicators
impairment
impairment income
    benefits
impairment rating
income benefits

CPT-4 codes in this chapter are from the CPT-4 2017 code set. CPT® is a registered trademark of the American Medical Association.

independent review organization (IRO)	occupational diseases and illnesses	physician of record
lifetime income benefits	Occupational Safety and Health Act	Social Security Disability Insurance (SSDI)
Longshore and Harbor Workers' Compensation Act (LHWCA)	Occupational Safety and Health Administration (OSHA)	treating doctor
		Veteran's Disability Compensation
maximum medical improvement (MMI)	Office of Workers' Compensation Programs (OWCP)	Veteran's Disability Pension Benefits
medical benefits		vocational rehabilitation
Notice of Contest	ombudsmen	Work Status Report

Case Study

Workers' Compensation

Julie, the front desk assistant, is speaking with Paula regarding a patient who just left the office. He has a workers' compensation claim involving an injury he suffered on the job. Julie feels that the patient shouldn't be allowed the claim because she thought he seemed fine when he was at the desk. She felt that he may be faking his injury. Paula explained that it was up to the doctor to decide the type and level of injury incurred by the patient, not Julie. The office manager overheard part of the conversation and told Julie that she was not to make such comments about a patient because there was no way for her to know the whole story.

Questions

1. Would you consider Julie's statements unprofessional?
2. Do you believe that Julie's attitude toward the patient would be obvious if she felt this strongly about the issue? How could her body language be indicative of her viewpoint?
3. Do you think the office manager should take more steps to educate Julie on workers' compensation claims?

Workers' compensation was developed to benefit both the injured employee and the employer. Before the availability of workers' compensation insurance, injured workers and families of workers killed on the job had to pursue legal action against the employer to attempt to receive compensation for the injury or death. For the court case to be successful, the injured worker had to prove that her employer was negligent. As you can imagine, the cases were difficult to prove and often took years to settle.

History of Workers' Compensation

By the late 1800s, the idea of compensating injured workers from an insurance fund to which employers would contribute had gained a foothold in the United States. A few states tried to establish such compensation programs, but organized labor successfully opposed the concept because it was not intended as a preventive measure but rather more as a humanitarian measure. That is, the general level of compensation insurance premiums was so low that it did not encourage employers to adopt safer work environments to eliminate the causes of accidents.

In 1908, Congress passed a limited workers' compensation law for federal employees. Encouraged by this example, several states tried to enact workers' compensation laws. Maryland and New York were the first. Courts later overturned both laws because they believed that mandatory government-administered workers' compensation programs denied employers their property rights without due process of law. To ease the objections, most states enacted laws that allowed employers to choose whether or not to participate in the state's workers' compensation program. In 1911, Wisconsin became the first state to successfully establish a workers' compensation program. By 1947, the tide had turned and almost all states *required* employers to purchase workers' compensation insurance. Texas is the only state that currently allows any private employer to choose whether or not to provide workers' compensation, although public employees and employers who enter into a building or construction contract with a government entity must provide workers' compensation coverage. In other states, such as Arkansas, Florida, and Mississippi, it is not required if the company has less than or equal to three or four employees. Some states have a state funded program such as New Mexico.

Today we are seeing other states pushing to "opt out." In 2014, the Oklahoma Option was established, allowing qualified employers to elect to be exempt from the state's Workers' Compensation system. Oklahoma law provides for employer to choose between a reformed "administrative" Workers' Compensation system and an "Option" to provide benefits outside of the Workers' Compensation system for all on-the-job injuries. The Option combines attractive elements from successful Workers' Compensation programs and Texas Nonsubscription.

Helping employees receive compensation for workplace injuries was a good start. However, as stated previously, the generally small premium for the policy did not encourage employers to improve the workplace conditions that led to accidents and illnesses in the first place. Therefore, the **Occupational Safety and Health Act** was signed into law on December 29, 1970. This act gave the federal government the authority to set and enforce safety and health standards for most U.S. employers. If covered businesses do not meet the standards set by the act, they are subject to large fines. If an employee feels that his work environment is unhealthy or unsafe, he may file a complaint directly with the **Occupational Safety and Health Administration (OSHA)**, which was created by the act. The types of employers not regulated by that act include churches, independent contractors, and federal employees.

Federal Workers' Compensation Programs

Civilian employees of federal agencies are covered for work-related injuries and illnesses under various programs administered by the **Office of Workers' Compensation Programs (OWCP)**, which is part of the U.S. Department of Labor. The following programs are administered by the OWCP:

- The **Federal Employees' Compensation Act (FECA)**. This act provides workers' compensation benefits to millions of civilian employees of the United States, members of the Peace Corps, and AmeriCorps VISTA volunteers.
- The **Federal Coal Mine Health and Safety Act** (also called the **Black Lung Benefits Reform Act**). This act provides benefits to current coal mine employees as well as monthly payments to surviving dependents of deceased workers.
- The **District of Columbia Workers' Compensation Act**. This act provides benefits for any employee performing work (or who did perform work—for deceased/disabled workers) on a regular (i.e., not short-term or temporary) basis in the District of Columbia. Until 1982, any job-related injuries were covered under the Longshore and Harbor Workers' Compensation Act (see next entry).
- The **Longshore and Harbor Workers' Compensation Act (LHWCA)**. This act covers maritime workers injured or killed on navigable waters of the United States, employees working on adjoining piers, docks, and terminals, plus some other special groups. Compensation under this act is paid through policies provided by private insurers or employers who are self-insured.
- The **Energy Employees Occupational Illness Compensation Program Act (EEOICP)**. The newest program administered by OWCP, this act provides benefits to eligible and former employees of the U.S. Department of Energy, its contractors and subcontractors, and/or to certain survivors of such individuals.

State Workers' Compensation Plans

Each state has its own statutes that govern workers' compensation, and each administers its own workers' compensation program. There are three major components to workers' compensation:

- *Medical expense*—the cost for hospitals, doctors, medical treatment, and so on. Some programs permit the injured worker to select a medical provider of her own choice. Some states have a closed panel system that requires an employee to seek medical attention from a medical provider chosen by the employer or the employer's insurance company.

■ *Disability pay*—either temporary while the employee is getting back to normal, or permanent if the employee will never fully recover. The amount varies, but it can be as high as one-half to two-thirds of the individual's normal pay.

■ *Vocational rehabilitation*—if an employee's injury renders him unable to perform the usual duties of his occupation, he may need retraining so that he can enter into a new trade or business. Also, he may need physical therapy to get his normal strength back.

Employers can obtain workers' compensation insurance policies through a private insurance carrier or a state workers' compensation fund, or they may self-insure if they meet specific criteria. Most employers purchase policies through private insurance companies. If they use a state workers' compensation fund, the employer pays premiums into the fund and claims are paid out of it. Most states require an employer who chooses to self-insure to obtain authorization from the state. When an employer self-insures, money is set aside in a special fund that can only be used to pay workers' compensation claims. The employer pays for workers' compensation; no money is taken from an employee's pay.

Employers must file proof of their workers' compensation insurance with the state Workers' Compensation Board. The employer must also post a Notice of Workers' Compensation Coverage in a place where all employees will see it. The notice must state the name, address, and telephone number of the company's workers' compensation insurance administrator.

Overview of Covered Injuries, Illnesses, and Benefits

Workers' compensation pays medical bills and some lost wages for employees who are injured on the job or who have work-related diseases or illnesses. With workers' compensation insurance, the compensation is paid in one of two possible ways:

■ In the form of wage replacement (usually at about two-thirds salary) for the period of total disability

■ In the form of lump-sum payments for any residual permanent partial disability

Injuries do not have to take place on the job site. They may occur during the performance of duties on behalf of the company, such as driving to the store to purchase office supplies. Taking a fall in the company parking lot is also covered under workers' compensation.

A **Notice of Contest** is given to the employee if the employer denies a workers' compensation claim. An **Admission of Liability** is the acknowledgment to the employee of a successful workers' compensation claim.

Each state determines the types of injuries that will be covered under workers' compensation. In general, an injury, accident, or illness is covered under the following circumstances:

■ It occurs during the course of employment.
■ It arises out of employment.

- It occurs by accident.
- It results in personal injury or death.

Examples of compensable injuries include the following:

- Falls in the company parking lot
- Injuries/accidents that occur on the employee's "personal time," such as in the restroom or lunchroom at work
- Back injuries because of required heavy lifting on the job or from a fall
- Repetitive motion/stress injuries, such as carpal tunnel syndrome (not all states consider carpal tunnel syndrome an on-the-job injury)

An injured worker may not receive benefits for a generally covered injury in the following circumstances:

- The injury occurred while the worker was intoxicated.
- The worker injured herself intentionally or while unlawfully attempting to injure someone else.
- The worker was injured by another person for personal reasons.
- The worker was injured while voluntarily participating in an off-work activity.
- The worker was injured by an act of God.
- The injury occurred during horseplay.
- The worker failed to use safety equipment or failed to obey safety procedures.
- The worker is also receiving Social Security disability benefits.
- The worker is also a recipient of unemployment insurance.
- The worker receives an employer-paid pension or disability benefit.

Occupational Diseases and Illnesses

Occupational diseases and illnesses (also called nontraumatic injuries/illnesses) are health problems that result from exposure to a workplace health hazard, such as dust, gases, fumes, radiation, repetitive motions, and loud noises. These illnesses may come on rapidly or develop over time, such as with carpal tunnel syndrome.

Work-Related Injury Classifications

Work-related injuries are divided into the following five categories:

1. Injury without disability
2. Injury with temporary disability
3. Injury with permanent disability
4. Injury requiring vocational rehabilitation
5. Injury resulting in death

Injury without Disability

This category describes an employee who is injured on the job, requires treatment, and is able to return to work within several days. The medical expenses will be fully taken care of by workers' compensation if the injury is deemed compensable.

Injury with Temporary Disability

This category describes an employee who is injured on the job, requires treatment, but is not able to return to work within several days. Not only will all medical expenses be paid by workers' compensation (if deemed compensable), but also the employee will receive compensation for lost wages.

Injury with Permanent Disability

This category describes an employee who is injured on the job, requires treatment, is not able to return to work, and is not expected to be able to perform his regular job in the future. This employee usually has been on temporary disability for some time and is still unable to return to work. All medical expenses are paid by workers' compensation and the employee will receive compensation for lost wages.

Injury Requiring Vocational Rehabilitation

An employee in this category has been injured on the job, requires treatment, and is unable to return to work without vocational rehabilitation. **Vocational rehabilitation** is the retraining of the employee so she can return to the workforce. Because of the injury or illness, the employee may not be able to perform the same job duties as before and so would be trained to perform another job.

Injury Resulting in Death

In this category, the employee dies as a result of an on-the-job injury. Death benefits are paid to the worker's survivors.

Injured Worker Responsibilities and Rights

The injured worker has the right to receive medical care that is necessary to treat the work-related injury or illness. The injured worker has the right to an initial choice of doctor (called the **treating doctor** or **physician of record**), with some limitations:

- If a covered employer contracts with an insurance carrier that establishes or contracts with a certified managed care network, the employer's employees will be required to obtain medical care for their work-related injuries through the network if the employees live within the network service area. However, the insurance carrier will be liable for approved out-of-network referred care, emergency care, and healthcare for an employee who does not live in the network service area.

- An injured employee who lives in the network service area may choose a treating doctor from the list of doctors maintained by the network. If an injured employee does not make an initial choice within 14 days, the network will assign a treating doctor to the injured employee. An injured employee who does not live within the network's service area would continue to choose a treating doctor from the Approved Doctor's List (ADL). However, an injured employee may be liable for medical care that is related to the compensable injury if that employee is required to seek care within a network and that employee sees a non-network provider without network approval.

- If an injured employee is dissatisfied with his initial choice of treating doctor, the injured employee is entitled to select another treating doctor from the network's list of doctors. A network cannot deny an injured employee's initial request to change treating doctors. However, any subsequent requests by an injured employee to change treating doctors are subject to network approval.

- An injured employee may request that her primary care provider (PCP) under a group health maintenance organization (HMO) plan also serve as her treating doctor if the PCP agrees to abide by the network requirements.
- The injured worker has the responsibility to tell his employer of a work-related injury or illness within a specific number of days.

The injured worker has the responsibility to tell the treating physician of record how she was injured and if she believes the injury to be work related. The worker should tell the doctor about the injury or illness and whether it may be work related before receiving medical treatment. An injured worker may not sue her employer after receiving workers' compensation benefits.

Treating Doctor's Responsibilities

If an injured worker has a managed care plan as his personal insurance and would like to see his PCP for a workers' compensation–related injury or illness, the inured employee must check with the state where their claim is filed. Some states require that an injured worker be seen by a doctor chosen by the employer or the employer's workers' compensation insurance carrier. Other states allow injured workers to choose any doctor within a network, and admission to the network is determined by the state, the employer, or the employer's insurance company. Rules also vary for whether they can choose a doctor for the initial treatment visit as compared to continuing treatment for an industrially related condition. If a patient schedules an appointment and discloses they are being seen for a worker's compensation injury, the medical office specialist must check interoffice policies on treating such patients.

The treating doctor (physician of record) is responsible for treating the injured worker's condition and determining the worker's **impairment rating**. The treating doctor will need to distinguish if the patient is impaired or disabled. Determination and rating guidelines are not universal but many providers, workers' compensation systems, and insurance companies use the sixth edition of *Guides to the Evaluation of Permanent Impairment* published by American Medical Association (AMA; sixth edition, January 2008, reprinted 2012). At that time, the provider determines the patient's impairment. According to the AMA guidelines, **impairment** is the permanent physical damage to a worker's body from a work-related injury or illness. A doctor will determine whether the worker has any permanent physical damage and will assign an impairment rating. If it is determined by the treating doctor that the patient is impaired, she will also determine the **maximum medical improvement (MMI)**, which is the earliest of the point in time that an injured worker's injury or illness has improved as much as it is likely to improve. **Disability** is described as "activity limitations and/or participation restrictions in an individual with a health condition, disorder, or disease." Social Security Disability (SSD) defines disability as "the inability to engage in any substantial, gainful activity by reason of any medically determinable physical or mental impairment(s), which can be expected to result in death or which has lasted or can be expected to last for a continuous period of not less than 12 months."

The treating doctor will also determine a return-to-work date. After the initial visit with the injured worker, the treating doctor is required to file a Work Status Report. A **Work Status Report** is a state form that is used for transmission of information among the employer, employee, insurance carrier, and treating doctor. It provides the employer and insurance carrier with information on the employee's limitations in performing her job responsibilities. The treating doctor is also required to file a new

Work Status Report (sometimes referred to as a *progress report* or *supplemental report*) with the employer's workers' compensation insurance carrier if there is a substantial change to the injured worker's condition that might affect the worker's disability status or return-to-work date or when required by state rules and regulations. Any time the injured worker is seen by the treating doctor, a Work Status Report must be sent in with the insurance claim.

The treating doctor will file a **final report** when the injured worker is released from medical care. This report affirms that the worker is fit to return to work and resume normal job responsibilities.

If an injured worker disagrees with the treating doctor's findings (i.e., the percentage of disability or maximum medical improvement), the worker may contact the insurance carrier and/or the state's workers' compensation office. The worker will be referred to a **designated doctor**. A designated doctor is an impartial doctor who helps resolve workers' compensation claim disputes about maximum medical improvement and impairment ratings. The designated doctor may be chosen by agreement between the injured worker and the insurance company. If the injured worker and the insurance company cannot agree, the designated doctor is chosen by the state's Department of Insurance for Workers' Compensation.

Selecting a Designated Doctor and Scheduling an Appointment

When the state Workers' Compensation (WC) Department receives notice about a dispute, it will select a designated doctor from a list of approved doctors; make an appointment with the designated doctor for the worker; and send the worker and the insurance carrier a written notice with the date, time, and location of the appointment.

The WC Department will not select a doctor who has already examined the worker; it will instead attempt to select a doctor licensed by the same medical board as the worker's treating doctor.

The worker and the insurance company may agree on a different designated doctor. If the two sides agree on a different designated doctor, the insurance company will inform the WC Department of the agreement and the name of the doctor both sides agreed on; make an appointment with the doctor for the worker; and tell the worker and the department the date, time, and location of the appointment. If the appointment is canceled by the patient, the medical office specialist must contact the WC Department.

An injured worker may reschedule the appointment with the designated doctor if necessary.

Communicating with the Designated Doctor

An injured worker may talk with the designated doctor to reschedule an appointment or to discuss the worker's medical condition. However, once the doctor has examined the worker, the worker may not contact the doctor directly. All communication with the designated doctor must go through the workers' compensation office handling the claim. No one else involved in the dispute may contact the designated doctor directly at any time. Because of this, it is suggested that the designated doctor use a color-coded paper medical record or flag an electronic medical record to indicate that it is strictly for an Independent Medical Examination (IME). That way, if a patient calls with questions after the appointment, the medical office specialist will know not to release information to anyone.

What the Designated Doctor Will Do

The designated doctor will do the following:

- Review medical information from the treating doctor and other doctors who have treated the worker for the work-related injury or illness
- Examine, test, and evaluate the parts of the worker's body affected by the injury or illness
- Determine if the worker has reached maximum medical improvement and, if so, when
- Give the worker an impairment rating if the worker has reached maximum medical improvement
- Submit an IME report, including a narrative report and documentation of the impairment rating, to the WC Department. The doctor may determine the impairment rating using the American Medical Association's *Guides to the Evaluation of Permanent Impairment*.

Disputing the Designated Doctor's Findings

The injured worker or the insurance company may dispute the designated doctor's findings. To dispute the designated doctor's findings, call the state's Workers Compensation Department. Workers compensation systems are established by statutes in each state.

If the worker and the insurance company agree on the designated doctor, the WC Department is required by law to accept the impairment rating the designated doctor assigned. Otherwise, the WC Department must accept the maximum medical improvement date and the impairment rating the designated doctor assigned unless stronger medical evidence clearly indicates that another date or rating is more appropriate.

Disputing Maximum Medical Improvement or Impairment Rating

The injured worker or insurance company may dispute the maximum medical improvement date or the impairment rating a doctor assigned the worker. The worker will be required to see a designated doctor to resolve the dispute.

Ombudsmen

If the injured worker needs assistance with his workers' compensation claim, a Workers' Compensation Department of Insurance ombudsman can help. **Ombudsmen** are division employees that can help the worker with his claim, at no charge, once a proceeding has been scheduled. The injured worker may ask for help from an ombudsman if she has not hired an attorney to represent her and does not have any other type of representation.

Ombudsmen can do the following:

- Give the injured worker information to help make decisions
- Communicate with employers, insurance companies, and healthcare providers on the worker's behalf

- Show how to gather and prepare facts and evidence for dispute resolution proceedings
- Help present facts and evidence at dispute resolution proceedings
- Help the injured worker ask questions of witnesses and raise questions about evidence at dispute resolution proceedings
- Give information about how to appeal a dispute resolution decision

Note, however, that ombudsmen are not attorneys and so they may not give legal advice, make any decisions for the injured worker, or sign agreements or forms on the worker's behalf.

Practice Exercise 17.1

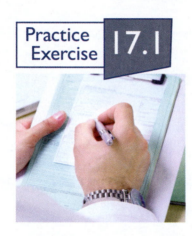

Indicate which of the following scenarios would qualify for workers' compensation benefits and which would not by circling the appropriate answer.

1. Mary drove to the office supply store to buy supplies for the office as instructed by her boss. On her way back to the office, she stopped at the post office to mail her tax return. While exiting her car at the post office, her skirt got caught in her car door. As a result, Mary fell down and landed on her left knee, which immediately became swollen and painful. Mary found it quite difficult to walk.

   WC covered   Not WC covered

2. Theo slipped and bruised his tailbone in the employee lunchroom because of a mess a co-worker left on the floor.

   WC covered   Not WC covered

3. Louis and Robert work in a warehouse. When the supervisor is not nearby, they often goof around on skateboards or roller skates. One day, Robert and Louis were racing each other on skateboards from one end of the warehouse to the other. Louis wasn't paying close attention to where he was going and slammed into a handcart filled with empty wooden pallets. The handcart was not supposed to be in that part of the warehouse; another employee had left it there before going on break. Louis took a fall, spilled all the pallets, and broke his arm.

   WC covered   Not WC covered

4. Nicholas was encouraged by his fellow employees to play on the softball team sponsored by their employer. Participation on the team is voluntary, but his co-workers pressured him to play. He joined the team and enjoyed the camaraderie and spirit of his co-workers. All was going well until one day he slid into second base and sprained his ankle.

   WC covered   Not WC covered

5. Cynthia and her co-worker Monica play practical jokes on each other all the time. One day while Cynthia was sneaking away from Monica's cubicle after smearing everything in sight with petroleum jelly, she tripped on a rip in the carpet that all of the employees had been complaining about

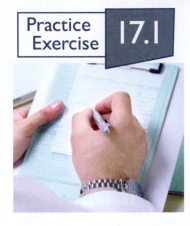

for the past month. Because the rip in the carpet had not been fixed, Cynthia fell and landed on her wrist, spraining it.

WC covered   Not WC covered

6. On a day when the wind was gusting up to 50 miles per hour, Norma Jean was blown into a light pole in the company parking lot while trying to get to her car to leave for the day. She bruised her left hip and sprained vertebrae in her neck.

WC covered   Not WC covered

7. Scott has a data entry position and has served his company well for the past 3 years. One day he told his supervisor that his hands and wrists ached and that sometimes he felt pain that radiated up his arm to his shoulder.

WC covered   Not WC covered

8. Betty returned to work after a doctor's appointment. She stated to her supervisor that she had to have back surgery for a slipped disk. She told her supervisor that she probably would not have had this problem if she had not fallen off the ladder 2 years ago while replacing light bulbs in the employee lounge. That was the first time Betty's supervisor had heard about the fall from the ladder, and there was no mention of it in Betty's employee file.

WC covered   Not WC covered

(Continued)

Types of Workers' Compensation Benefits

The four types of workers' compensation benefits—medical, income, death, and burial—are discussed next.

Medical Benefits

Medical benefits pay for any medical care that is reasonable and necessary to treat a work-related injury or illness. The employer's workers' compensation insurance company pays medical benefits directly to the doctor or healthcare provider who treated the injured worker.

Amount of Medical Benefits

Medical benefits pay only for the treatment of work-related injuries and illnesses. They do not pay for the treatment of other injuries or illnesses, even if the treatment was provided at the same time as the treatment for the work-related injury. A doctor or healthcare provider may not bill an injured worker for treating a work-related injury or illness, but she may bill the worker for treating other injuries or illnesses.

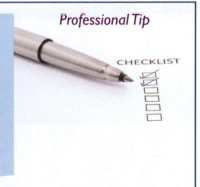

Professional Tip

Workers' compensation is administered on a state-by-state basis, with a state governing board overseeing varying public/private combinations of workers' compensation systems. A medical office specialist who processes workers' compensation claims must be familiar with legislation of the state in which the injury occurred.

CHECKLIST

When Medical Benefits Begin and End

Injured workers may receive reasonable and necessary medical care immediately after onset of the injury or illness. The worker may choose a doctor, but the doctor must be on a list of doctors approved by the workers' compensation department. Except in an emergency, the injured worker's treating doctor must approve all medical care for an injury or illness.

An injured worker may receive medical care that is reasonable and necessary to treat a work-related injury or illness without any specific time limit.

Income Benefits

Income benefits replace a portion of any wages a worker loses because of a work-related injury or illness. The following are the three types of income benefits:

1. Temporary income benefits
2. Impairment income benefits
3. Lifetime income benefits

Income benefits may not exceed a maximum weekly amount. Temporary income benefits, impairment income benefits, and lifetime income benefits also are subject to a minimum amount.

Temporary Income Benefits

An injured worker may get **temporary income benefits** if the injury or illness causes the worker to lose some or all income.

Temporary income benefits end at the earlier of the following:

- The date the worker reaches maximum medical improvement (MMI), which is when the work-related injury or illness has improved as much as it is going to improve.
- The date the worker is again physically able to earn the average weekly wage

Impairment Income Benefits

An injured worker may get **impairment income benefits** if the worker has a permanent impairment from a work-related injury or illness.

Lifetime Income Benefits

Certain work-related injuries may result in a condition for which the injured person is entitled to income benefits for his lifetime. **Lifetime income benefits** may be paid if the worker incurs any of the following:

- Total and permanent loss of sight in both eyes
- Loss of both feet at or above the ankle
- Loss of both hands at or above the wrist
- Loss of one foot at or above the ankle and the loss of one hand, at or above the wrist
- An injury to the spine that results in permanent and complete paralysis of both arms
- Both legs, or one arm and one leg
- A physically traumatic injury to the brain resulting in incurable insanity or imbecility
- Third-degree burns that cover at least 40% of the body and require grafting
- Third-degree burns covering the majority of either both hands or one hand and the face

Death and Burial Benefits

Death benefits can replace a portion of lost family income for the eligible family members of workers killed on the job and can pay for some of the deceased worker's funeral expenses. **Burial benefits** are paid to the person who paid the deceased worker's burial expenses.

Eligible Beneficiaries

A spouse is eligible to receive death benefits for life unless she or he remarries. If there are minor children, the benefit is divided between the spouse and the minor children. One-half is paid to the spouse and the other half is divided equally among the children. If the spouse remarries, the entire benefit will be divided equally among the minor children who are eligible for benefits.

Eligible children can receive death benefits until age 18, or until age 25 if enrolled as a full-time student in an accredited college. If there is more than one minor child, as a child loses eligibility, the benefits are redistributed among the other eligible children.

Benefits and Compensation Termination

Temporary partial and temporary permanent disability benefits may be terminated when one of the following occurs:

- The injured worker is released from treatment by her treating doctor and is authorized to return to her regular job.
- The injured worker has returned to work.
- The injured worker has been offered a different job by his employer and has either accepted (returning to work) or has rejected the job offer.
- The injured worker has exhausted the maximum workers' compensation benefits for the injury or illness.
- The injured worker does not cooperate with requests for a medical examination that will determine the type and duration of the disability and the relationship of the injury to the patient's condition.
- The worker has died. However, death benefits will be paid to the worker's survivors.

Disability Compensation Programs

Disability compensation programs reimburse a covered individual for lost wages that occur because of a disability that prevents the individual from working. Disability programs do not pay for medical treatment. Unlike with workers' compensation benefits, the injury does not have to be work related to qualify for lost wages benefits. Some employers offer disability insurance to employees, but they are not required to do so. Individuals may purchase their own disability policy.

Many individuals who are covered by employer disability programs or private policies are also eligible for government-sponsored programs, such as Social Security Disability Insurance or the veteran's compensation programs (discussed next). If the individual is eligible for benefits under a government program, the employer-sponsored or private disability policy would supplement the government program's coverage. This means that the government program would pay first, followed by the other policy if applicable.

Types of Government Disability Policies

Various types of government disability policies are available:

- **Veteran's Disability Compensation** is a benefit paid to a veteran because of injuries or diseases that happened while on active duty, or were made worse by active military service.
- **Veteran's Disability Pension Benefits** is a benefit paid to wartime veterans with limited income who are no longer able to work.
- **Social Security Disability Insurance (SSDI)** pays benefits to people who cannot work because they have a medical condition that is expected to last at least 1 year (12 months) or result in death. Federal law requires this very strict definition of disability. Although some programs give money to people with partial disability or short-term disability, SSDI does not. SSDI is funded by workers' payroll deductions—as a result of the Federal Insurance Contribution Act (FICA)—and matching employer contributions.

In general, to receive disability benefits, a person must meet certain requirements. These include the following:

- Recipients must be employed or self-employed individuals with disabilities who are under age 65 and have paid Social Security taxes for a minimum number of calendar year quarters. The number of quarters worked varies depending on the age of the individual.
- Recipients must be disabled before the age of 22 and have a parent receiving Social Security benefits who retires, becomes disabled, or dies.
- Recipients must be employees who are blind or whose vision cannot be corrected to better than 20/200 in their better eye, or if their visual field is 20 degrees or less in their better eye. The blind employee also must have worked long enough in a job that she paid Social Security taxes.

Certain family members of a worker with a disability may qualify for benefits based on the worker's work history:

- Worker's spouse, if the spouse is 62 or older
- Worker's spouse, at any age if caring for a child of the worker with a disability who is younger than age 16 or has a disability
- The worker's unmarried child, including an adopted child, or, in some cases, a stepchild or grandchild, who is under age 18, or under age 19 if in elementary or secondary school full time
- The worker's unmarried child, age 18 or older, if the child has a disability that started before age 22 and meets the definition of disability for adults

After submitting an application for SSDI, the approval process can take from 3 to 5 months. If the application is approved, the first Social Security disability benefits will be paid for the sixth full month after the date the disability began (meaning there is a 5-month waiting period).

> ## Example
>
> If the state agency decides the disability began on January 15, the first disability benefit will be paid for the month of July. Social Security benefits are paid in the month following the month for which they are due, so the worker with the disability will receive her July benefit in August. The amount of the monthly disability benefit is based on the worker's average lifetime earnings.

Supplemental Security Income (SSI) is another type of federal income supplement program funded by general tax revenues (not Social Security taxes). It is designed to help the elderly, people who are blind or have disabilities, and those who have little or no income (i.e., are eligible for welfare). It provides cash to meet basic needs for food, clothing, and shelter.

Whether a person is eligible to receive SSI depends on his income and what he owns. Also, to receive SSI, the individual must live in the United States or the Northern Mariana Islands and be a U.S. citizen or national. In some cases, noncitizen residents can qualify for SSI.

Verifying Insurance Benefits

As with any patient, before treating a patient with a workers' compensation injury (except in emergency cases), it is necessary to verify insurance information and benefits provided by the worker's compensation insurance company (or self-insured employer). The medical office specialist should obtain the injured worker's employer information before the appointment. A call to the employer will confirm whether or not the employer carries workers' compensation insurance and whether or not the employer has filed an **Employer's First Report of Injury or Illness** form. The medical office specialist should also ask for a workers' compensation case number at this time if it is available.

As soon as the employer has completed and sent the Employer's First Report of Injury or Illness form to the insurance carrier, the carrier will assign a case number for the injured worker. If the employer has not filed an Employer's First Report of Injury or Illness form, the medical office specialist will not be able to obtain a case number. This is the first indication that there may be some trouble regarding insurance payment. A workers' compensation claim will not be paid by the carrier if there is no case number. If the form has not been filed or the employer does not carry workers' compensation insurance, you must request the patient's personal health insurance information because this is the insurance company to whom you will end up submitting claims.

Preauthorization

Preauthorization is prospective approval of healthcare based solely on medical necessity. Preauthorization is obtained from an insurance carrier by the requester or injured worker before the health care is provided.

Requirements for the Preauthorization Request

The requester (the healthcare provider or designated representative, including office staff or a referral healthcare provider/facility, who requests preauthorization, concurrent review, or voluntary certification) or the injured worker must request preauthorization from the insurance carrier via the carrier's designated phone line, fax line, or email address. Preauthorization must be obtained before the healthcare is rendered. Healthcare for an emergency does not require preauthorization.

Filing Insurance Claims

Universal claim forms CMS-1500 and UB-04 are used to file workers' compensation insurance claims. The completion of the forms for a workers' compensation claim, however, differs from submitting a standard medical insurance claim. For example, the patient's (injured worker's) signature is not required on the form, and payment will automatically be sent directly to the medical provider. The billed amount for services rendered is calculated using the Medicare Fee Schedule (MFS) for the procedure and multiplying that amount by a certain amount designated by the state insurance commissioner. If the employer is contracted though a managed care organization, the physician's usual fee is billed and the carrier indicates the monetary contractual adjustments (write-offs) on the Explanation of Benefits (EOB) or Electronic Remittance Advice (ERA). The medical office specialist makes the adjustments to the patient's account after the EOB or ERA is received. Additional information for calculating the fees for service is covered later in this chapter.

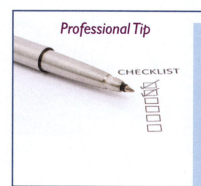

Professional Tip

CHECKLIST

An updated treating doctor's Work Status Report is sent in with every claim that is submitted. If this is not done, the carrier will assume the injured worker has reached maximum medical improvement and will cease paying for future claims on the reported injury.

Completing the CMS-1500 for Workers' Compensation Claims

Detailed instructions for completing the CMS-1500 claim form are given in Chapter 11; details about the UB-04 claim form are given in Chapter 12. Here, we discuss the specific form locators on the CMS-1500 that are different when submitting a workers' compensation claim. Note that workers' compensation claims procedures vary from state to state.

Form Locator 1: Type of Insurance   Check the "Other" or FECA Black Lung box.

Form Locator 1a: Insured's I.D. Number   Enter the employee I.D. number.

Form Locator 4: Insured's Name   Enter the insured employer's local name. This is the employer at the time of the injury.

Form Locator 5: Patient's Address   If required by a payer to report a telephone number, do not use a hyphen or space as a separator within the telephone number.

Form Locator 7: Insured's Address   Enter the insured employer's current business address, including city, state, zip code. "Insured's Telephone" does not exist in 5010A1. The NUCC recommends that the phone number not be reported. Phone extensions are not supported.

Form Locator 10: Is Patient's Condition Related To? Check the "YES" box in Part A to indicate that this is an employment-related condition.

Form Locator 10d: The original reference number must be entered in Box 22 when submitting a bill that is a duplicate or an appeal. NOTE: Do not use condition codes when submitted a revised or corrected workers' compensation bill.

Form Locator 11b: Other Claim ID Required if known. Enter the claim number assigned by the payer.

Form Locator 11c: Insurance Plan Name or Program Name Enter Workers' Compensation Insurance plan name.

Form Locators 12 and 13: Patient's/Insured's or Authorized Person's Signature Leave blank. No signature is required for workers' compensation claims.

Form Locator 14: Date of Current: Illness, Injury, Pregnancy Enter date of injury or occupational illness.

Form Locator 16: Dates Patient Unable to Work in Current Occupation Enter dates patient is unable to work in current occupation.

Form Locator 18: Hospitalization Dates Related to Current Services Enter the dates of hospitalization related to the injury or the occupational illness.

Form Locator 19: Additional Claim Information Required based on Jurisdictional Workers' Compensation Guidelines

Form Locator 33: Billing Provider Information and Phone Number Enter the billing name of the provider/supplier, including complete address, city, state, zip code, and telephone number. The PIN (personal identification number) for a workers' compensation claim is the provider's license number with the state in front of it or a specific identification number from the WC Department.

Independent Review Organizations

If a health insurer or HMO refuses to pay for a treatment because it considers the treatment medically unnecessary or inappropriate, the injured worker or the treating doctor may be able to have an **independent review organization (IRO)** review the decision. An IRO review is a system for final administrative review of the medical necessity and appropriateness of healthcare services provided or proposed to patients. The IRO's decision is binding on the healthcare plan, which pays for the review. An independent review is available in either of the following circumstances:

- The employer's plan or its utilization review agent (URA) determines that a treatment that has been recommended, but not yet performed, is medically unnecessary or inappropriate.
- The employer's plan or its URA determines that an ongoing treatment is medically unnecessary or inappropriate.

A healthcare plan must base its denial on written screening criteria established and updated with involvement by practicing physicians and other providers. The injured worker, the worker's representative, or the injured worker's treating doctor may request an independent review. Only the injured worker or the worker's legal guardian, however, may sign a medical records release form.

HEALTH INSURANCE CLAIM FORM

APPROVED BY NATIONAL UNIFORM CLAIM COMMITTEE (NUCC) 02/12

AETNA FL
20 FOREST AVENUE
TALLAHASSEE FL 12345

PICA		PICA

1. MEDICARE ☐ MEDICAID ☐ TRICARE ☐ CHAMPVA ☐ GROUP HEALTH PLAN ☐ FECA BLK LUNG ☐ OTHER ☒ | 1a. INSURED'S I.D. NUMBER 0888 (For Program in Item 1)

2. PATIENT'S NAME (Last Name, First Name, Middle Initial)
HILL, HANNA

3. PATIENT'S BIRTH DATE 04 25 1940 SEX M ☐ F ☒

4. INSURED'S NAME (Last Name, First Name, Middle Initial)
DELTA GLASS , INC.

5. PATIENT'S ADDRESS (No., Street)
346 AUSTIN BOULEVARD

6. PATIENT RELATIONSHIP TO INSURED
Self ☒ Spouse ☐ Child ☐ Other ☐

7. INSURED'S ADDRESS (No., Street)
3000 MAIN STREET

CITY THOMASVILLE STATE GA

8. RESERVED FOR NUCC USE

CITY THOMASVILLE STATE GA

ZIP CODE 12345 TELEPHONE (Include Area Code) (972) 5550087

ZIP CODE 12345 TELEPHONE (Include Area Code) (214) 5551245

9. OTHER INSURED'S NAME (Last Name, First Name, Middle Initial)

10. IS PATIENT'S CONDITION RELATED TO:

11. INSURED'S POLICY GROUP OR FECA NUMBER
PP-AA-45899

a. OTHER INSURED'S POLICY OR GROUP NUMBER

a. EMPLOYMENT? (Current or Previous) ☒ YES ☐ NO

a. INSURED'S DATE OF BIRTH 04 25 1940 SEX M ☐ F ☒

b. RESERVED FOR NUCC USE

b. AUTO ACCIDENT? ☐ YES ☒ NO PLACE (State)

b. OTHER CLAIM ID (Designated by NUCC)

c. RESERVED FOR NUCC USE

c. OTHER ACCIDENT? ☐ YES ☒ NO

c. INSURANCE PLAN NAME OR PROGRAM NAME
AETNA FL

d. INSURANCE PLAN NAME OR PROGRAM NAME

10d. CLAIM CODES (Designated by NUCC)

d. IS THERE ANOTHER HEALTH BENEFIT PLAN? ☐ YES ☒ NO If yes, complete items 9, 9a, and 9d.

READ BACK OF FORM BEFORE COMPLETING & SIGNING THIS FORM.

12. PATIENT'S OR AUTHORIZED PERSON'S SIGNATURE I authorize the release of any medical or other information necessary to process this claim. I also request payment of government benefits either to myself or to the party who accepts assignment below.

SIGNED _____ DATE _____

13. INSURED'S OR AUTHORIZED PERSON'S SIGNATURE I authorize payment of medical benefits to the undersigned physician or supplier for services described below.

SIGNED _____

14. DATE OF CURRENT ILLNESS, INJURY, or PREGNANCY (LMP) 10 05 2016 QUAL.

15. OTHER DATE QUAL. MM DD YY

16. DATES PATIENT UNABLE TO WORK IN CURRENT OCCUPATION FROM TO

17. NAME OF REFERRING PROVIDER OR OTHER SOURCE
17a.
17b. NPI

18. HOSPITALIZATION DATES RELATED TO CURRENT SERVICES FROM TO

19. ADDITIONAL CLAIM INFORMATION (Designated by NUCC)

20. OUTSIDE LAB? ☐ YES ☒ NO $ CHARGES

21. DIAGNOSIS OR NATURE OF ILLNESS OR INJURY Relate A-L to service line below (24E) ICD Ind. 0

A. G5602 B. C. D.
E. F. G. H.
I. J. K. L.

22. RESUBMISSION CODE ORIGINAL REF. NO.

23. PRIOR AUTHORIZATION NUMBER

24. A. DATE(S) OF SERVICE From To						B. PLACE OF SERVICE	C. EMG	D. PROCEDURES, SERVICES, OR SUPPLIES (Explain Unusual Circumstances) CPT/HCPCS MODIFIER	E. DIAGNOSIS POINTER	F. $ CHARGES	G. DAYS OR UNITS	H. EPSDT Family Plan	I. ID QUAL	J. RENDERING PROVIDER ID. #
MM	DD	YY	MM	DD	YY									
10	05	16	10	05	16	11		99202	A	98 00	1		NPI	ZZ1521 7539600218
													NPI	ZZ1521 7539600218
													NPI	ZZ1521 7539600218
													NPI	ZZ1521 7539600218
													NPI	ZZ1521 7539600218
													NPI	ZZ1521 7539600218

25. FEDERAL TAX I.D. NUMBER 248927677 SSN EIN ☒

26. PATIENT'S ACCOUNT NO. 12345

27. ACCEPT ASSIGNMENT? ☒ YES ☐ NO

28. TOTAL CHARGE $ 98 00

29. AMOUNT PAID $

30. Rsvd for NUCC Use

31. SIGNATURE OF PHYSICIAN OR SUPPLIER INCLUDING DEGREES OR CREDENTIALS (I certify that the statements on the reverse apply to this bill and are made a part thereof.)
CHARLES H. HESS MD

32. SERVICE FACILITY LOCATION INFORMATION
CHARLES H. HESS M.D.
980 FREDERICK ROAD
JOHNSOON CITY TN 12345
a. 7539600218 b. ZZ1521

33. BILLING PROVIDER INFO & PH # (899) 5552276
CHARLES H. HESS M.D.
980 FREDERICK ROAD
JOHNSOON CITY TN 12345
a. 7539600218 b. ZZ1521

SIGNED _____ DATE _____

NUCC Instruction Manual available at: www.nucc.org

PLEASE PRINT OR TYPE

APPROVED OMB-0938-1197 FORM 1500 (02-12)

Figure 17.1 Sample of a completed Workers Compensation CMS 1500.

In most cases, the injured worker must use the healthcare plan's internal appeal process before requesting an IRO review. The injured worker can bypass the appeal process, however, if the worker or treating doctor believes the injured worker's condition is life threatening.

An independent review is not available in the following circumstances:

- The employer's WC healthcare plan refuses to pay for a service the plan does not cover, such as cosmetic surgery.
- The injured worker has already received treatment and the plan then determines that the treatment was not medically necessary or appropriate.
- The employer's healthcare plan is not subject to the law related to the IRO process. For example, Medicaid and Medicare, including Medicare HMO healthcare plans, are not required to participate in the IRO process. Other healthcare plans may not be subject to the IRO process. The medical office assistant should contact the healthcare plan to find out if it participates in the IRO process.

If the IRO process is not available, the injured worker, the worker's treating doctor, or another provider may file a complaint or appeal regarding the denial of healthcare or the denial of payment for healthcare already performed.

How to Obtain an Independent Review

If the employer's WC healthcare plan participates in the IRO process and denies a treatment because it regards the treatment as medically unnecessary or inappropriate, the plan must provide the injured worker with the necessary form for requesting an appeal and an independent review. If the injured worker wants an independent review, she must complete the form and return it to the health plan or URA.

Professional Tip

The healthcare plan or the URA must give the injured worker the independent review request form again after denying an appeal.

CHECKLIST

The IRO Decision

The WC insurer or HMO must pay for a treatment if the IRO decides the care is medically necessary or appropriate. The IRO will provide the injured worker and treating doctor with a notice of its decision that includes the clinical basis for the decision, the screening criteria used to make the decision, a list of qualifications of the IRO staff who reviewed the case, and a statement certifying that the IRO has no conflict of interest involving the insurer, HMO, or URA.

Medical Records

Workers' compensation medical records are to be kept separate from a patient's regular medical records. If a previously established patient is being seen for a workers' compensation–related case, make sure not to mix the two medical records. A workers' compensation chart is made for the specific injury only. If a provider is still using paper charts, it is suggested that the medical office use color-coded charts for workers' compensation cases. Color-coded charts are an immediate indication that the case is for workers' compensation and that specific information should be collected from the patient, including a copy of the patient's state driver's license or state identification card and Social Security card. Another reason to keep workers' compensation files separate from a patient's regular medical records is because workers' compensation claim information is not subject to the same confidentiality rules or laws as private medical records. In most states, carriers, claims adjusters, and employers are allowed unrestricted access to workers' compensation medical records but not private/regular medical records. The financial information (transactions) relating to a workers' compensation case should be kept separate as well.

Fraud

Workers' compensation fraud costs millions of dollars each year. Employers, employees, insurance carriers, and consumers pay the cost of fraud in lost jobs and profit, lower wages and benefits, and higher costs for services and premiums.

The Workers' Compensation Commission's Office of Investigations works with numerous special investigation units to deter fraud by assisting in the prosecution of those who commit fraud. These units include state and federal law enforcement, other regulatory agencies, and insurance carrier special investigation units.

Investigations often lead to prosecution and recovery of money gained through fraudulent schemes. Fraud can be committed by employers, employees, healthcare providers, attorneys, insurance agents, and others.

Fraud occurs when a person knowingly or intentionally conceals, misrepresents, or makes a false statement to either deny or obtain workers' compensation benefits or insurance coverage, or to otherwise profit from the deceit. The key to conviction is proving in court that the misrepresentation or concealment occurred knowingly or intentionally. Premium fraud and benefit fraud are the most common types of workers' compensation fraud. Premium fraud is usually committed by an employer who misrepresents the amount of payroll or classification of employees, or who attempts to avoid a higher insurance risk modifier by transferring employees to a new business entity rated as a lower risk category.

Benefit fraud is usually committed by:

- A worker who works full time at an unreported job and draws benefits when he is supposed to be unable to work, or when a worker fakes an injury.
- A healthcare provider or attorney who assists the worker in fraudulent schemes, or participates in double billing or billing for services not provided.

Fraud indicators do not mean fraud has occurred, but they may require a closer review of the claim or application. Employer fraud indicators include but are not limited to the following:

- Classification codes not consistent with duties normally associated with the employer's type of business—for example, a construction company that reports mainly clerical classifications
- Much larger premium paid for the previous year's policy
- Small payroll reported by a large company or employee leasing company
- Frequent addition and cancellation of coverage, especially if several business entities appear to be owned or controlled by the same person or group

Employee fraud indicators include but are not limited to the following:

- Injuries that have no witness other than the worker
- Injuries occurring late Friday or early Monday
- Injuries not reported until a week or more after they occur
- Injuries occurring before a strike or holiday, or in anticipation of a layoff or termination

- Injuries occurring where the worker would not usually work
- Injuries not usually occurring in the particular job description—for example, an administrative assistant injured while lifting a heavy object
- Worker observed in activities inconsistent with the reported injury
- Worker history of workers' compensation claims
- Conflicting diagnoses from subsequent treating doctors
- Any evidence of working elsewhere while drawing benefits

Attorney and healthcare provider fraud indicators include the following:

- Submission of bills or Explanation of Benefits forms for services that seem unnecessary or fictitious
- Submission of boilerplate medical reports, or reports that are merely copies of previously submitted reports
- Treatment dates on holidays for nonemergency situations
- Bills from a healthcare provider or attorney that present an unreasonable amount or hours per day
- Complaints from the worker that the attorney is "never" available although the attorney files fee affidavits for services
- Attorney relationship with a healthcare provider that appears to be a partnership in handling workers' compensation claims

Penalties

If an investigation establishes criminal fraud, the local district attorney may begin prosecution. Workers' compensation fraud involving amounts of $1,500.00 or more in benefits or premiums is a felony punishable by fines, orders for restitution, and imprisonment. If the amount is below $1,500.00, the action is a Class A misdemeanor punishable by fines, orders for restitution, and imprisonment.

Medical Provider Fraud

Fraud by medical providers can evolve as the nature of medical care changes over time. Outright fraud occurs when providers bill for treatments that never occur or were blatantly unnecessary. Some of the newer forms of medical provider fraud include specialists and other treatment providers giving kickbacks to referring physicians and provider upcoding, in which the provider's charges exceed the scheduled amount. Fraud also occurs when providers shift from the less expensive, all-inclusive patient report to supplemental reports, which add evaluations as a charge and thus incur separate charges.

Medical provider fraud schemes include the following:

- *Creative billing:* billing for services not performed
- *Self-referrals:* medical providers inappropriately referring a patient to a clinic or laboratory in which the provider has an interest
- *Upcoding:* billing for a more expensive treatment than the one performed
- *Unbundling:* performing a single service but billing it as a series of separate procedures
- *Product switching:* a pharmacy or other provider billing for one type of product but dispensing a cheaper version, such as a generic drug

According to the National Council on Compensation, "The increased use of managed care for workers' compensation, as well as for other insurance lines, is bringing new twists to old schemes." Managed care creates more opportunities for fraud because of the financial relationships and incentives among players. Newer forms of fraud and abuse occurring under managed care arrangements include the following:

- *Underutilization:* doctors receiving a fixed fee per patient but not providing a sufficient level of treatment
- *Overutilization:* ordering unnecessary treatments or tests to justify higher patient fees in a new contract year
- *Kickbacks:* offering incentives for patient referrals
- *Internal fraud:* providers colluding with the medical plan or insurance company to defraud the employer through a number of schemes

Calculating Reimbursements

When the insured employer's insurance policy is not a managed care plan, the fees for services must be calculated using the Medicare Fee Schedule (MFS) and multiplying the MFS fees by a certain percentage that is determined by each individual state. Conveniently, the MFS can be found on the Internet. Each state contracts with a carrier to administrate Medicare and Medicaid claims. These are called Medicare Administrative Contractors (MACs). For example, Novitas Solutions contracts with the states of Arkansas, Colorado, New Mexico, Oklahoma, Texas, Louisiana, and Mississippi. Each carrier may have a website to provide information on workers' compensation claims. The Novitas Solutions website (www.novitas-solutions.com) has each CPT code listed along with its MFS amount.

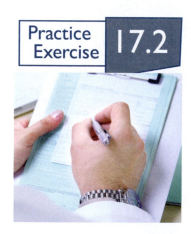

Practice Exercise 17.2

To determine the fee, use the Novitas Solutions website for the state of Texas and a multiple of 125%. Fill in each box in the following grid. Specifics about each procedure code are listed below the grid.

CPT Code	Dallas County 2016		Dallas County 2016		Dallas County 2016	
	MFS	WC	MFS	WC	MFS	WC
95861						
95907						
95909						
99201						
99202						
99203						
99204						

Workers' Compensation Fees

95861	Needle Electromyography: 2 extremities with or without paraspinal areas
95907	Nerve conduction, amplitude, latency, velocity study (each nerve); motor without F wave
95909	Sensory
99201	New Patient Outpatient O.V. problem-focused history, problem-focused exam, and straightforward medical decision making
99202	New Patient Outpatient O.V. expanded problem-focused history, expanded problem-focused examination, and straightforward medical decision making
99203	New Patient detailed history, detailed examination, and medical decision making of low complexity
99204	New Patient comprehensive history, comprehensive examination, and medical decision making of moderate complexity

Practice Exercise 17.2

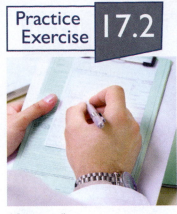

(Continued)

Use the information provided to prepare a workers' compensation claim.

Practice Exercise 17.3

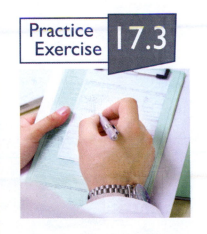

Physician Information:

Name:	Dennis J. Bonner, M.D.
Address:	980 Frederick Road Thomasville, GA 12345
Phone:	800-555-5000
Employer I.D. Number:	57-5562147
License Number:	GA 5529
NPI:	7536982100

Patient Information Form:

Name:	Kennedy Moore
Birth Date:	April 25, 1944
Phone:	972-555-0087
Address:	346 Austin Boulevard, Thomasville, GA 12345
Sex:	Female
Status:	Married
Social Security number:	968-44-9876
Insurance Carrier:	Aetna FL
Insurance Carrier Address:	20 Forester Avenue, Tallahassee, FL 12345
Phone:	555-443-3987
Insurance Group Number:	AR 187267-T
Insurance I.D./Policy Number:	66543
Employer:	Datamatic Inc., 644 San Juan Street, Thomasville, GA 12345
Phone:	214-555-8674
WC Case Number:	0856

(Continued)

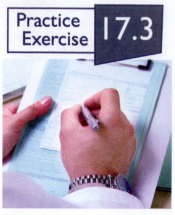

Practice Exercise 17.3

(*Continued*)

Please note that the employer is self-insured.

Patient's Encounter Form:

Date: Use today's date

Patient Encounter Information:

CC: Patient presents complaining of numbness and tingling in the left hand. She states that her job description is data entry.

Patient presents for evaluation of left hand numbness intermittently for the past 3 weeks.

Dx: Carpal tunnel syndrome, ICD-10 (G56.02)

Service and Charges: 99203—Office visit; for the evaluation and management of a new patient, which includes a detailed history, detailed examination, and medical decision of low complexity.

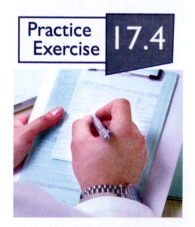

Practice Exercise 17.4

Use the information provided to prepare a workers' compensation claim.

Physician Information: Charles H. Hess, M.D., 980 Frederick Road, Johnson City, TN 12345

Phone: 899-555-2276
EIN: 22-9872767
Professional License: TX2056
NPI: 1471236545

Patient Information: Catherine Daley, 346 Highpoint Drive, Johnson City, TN 12345

                                           999-555-0756
DOB: 04/25/1969
Social Security number: 968-34-0025
Status: Married
Sex: Female

Patient's Insurance Information: BC/BS
I.D./Policy Number 2543097
Gr Number 08632
1123 Riverwalk, Nashville,
TN 12345 800-555-1123

Practice Exercise 17.4

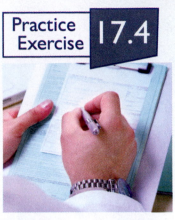

(Continued)

Employer's Information: Coca-Cola Corp.,
6345 Harvey Drive,
Johnson City,
TN 12345 998-555-6785

Employer Insurance Carrier: Aetna TX
I.D./Policy Number 0231
Gr Number 55111
20 Forest Drive, Nashville,
TN 12345

Phone: 972-555-0050
Reason for Visit: Injured at work
Workers' Compensation Case Number: 81526

Use today's date.

Patient Encounter Information:

CC: Patient presents with low back pain.
"Patient states that she slipped on a
wet floor two days ago, which had
recently been cleaned, and landed on
her back and has been unable to go to
work."

DX: Lumbar Sprain,
ICD-10 (S33.5XXA)

List of fees for services for Catherine Daley:
Listed below are our UCR fees:

- 99202 NP Office Visit Problem-focused history and examination, straightforward decision making, $100.00
- 95861 Needle Electromyography 2 extremities, $250.00
- 95907 Nerve Conduction (each nerve) motor (6x), $75.00 each nerve
- 95909 Nerve Conduction (each nerve) sensory (3x), $60.00 each nerve

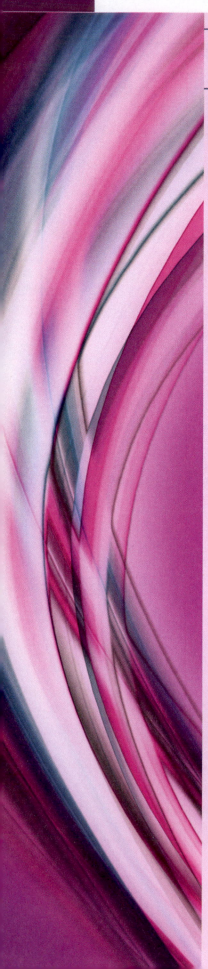

Chapter Summary

- All states with mandatory workers' compensation provide two types of workers' compensation coverage. One pays the medical expenses that resulted from the work-related injury or illness, and the other pays the employee's lost wages while she is unable to work.

- Civilian employees of federal agencies are covered for work-related injuries and illnesses under various programs administered by the Office of Workers' Compensation Programs.

- Workers' compensation benefits pay only for the treatment of work-related injuries and illnesses. They do not pay for the treatment of other injuries or illnesses, even if the treatment was provided at the same time as the treatment for the work-related injury.

- The medical office specialist must have knowledge of covered and non-covered workers' compensation services.

- Work-related injuries are divided into the following five categories:
  - Injury without disability
  - Injury with temporary disability
  - Injury with permanent disability
  - Injury requiring vocational rehabilitation
  - Injury resulting in death

- The injured worker has the right to receive medical care that is necessary to treat the work-related injury or illness.

- The injured worker has the responsibility to tell his employer of a work-related injury or illness within a specific number of days of the injury or on realizing the illness/nontraumatic injury may be the result of his employment.

- The treating doctor (physician of record) is responsible for treating the injured worker's condition, determining whether the worker has any permanent physical damage, and determining the worker's impairment rating. The treating doctor will also determine a return-to-work date and is required to file a Work Status Report.

- The four types of workers' compensation benefits are medical, income, death, and burial.

- Medical providers send their insurance claims directly to the employer's workers' compensation insurance carrier, and the carrier pays them directly. The fees for services are limited to the established state fees or the managed care network's fees.

- Universal claim forms CMS-1500 and UB-04 are used to file workers' compensation insurance paper claims. The completion of the forms for a workers' compensation claim differs from submitting a standard medical insurance claim.

- A provider waives any right to payment unless a medical bill is submitted to the insurance carrier within a specific amount of days after the date of service. The insurance carrier, in turn, must pay, reduce, deny, or determine to audit the claim within a specific number of days after receipt of the claim.

- If a health insurer or HMO refuses to pay for a treatment because it considers the treatment medically unnecessary or inappropriate, the injured worker/treating doctor may be able to have an independent review organization (IRO) review the decision.

- Fraud can be committed by the employee, employer, and/or provider. The medical office specialist should be aware of all the ways a provider and patient can conduct fraud.

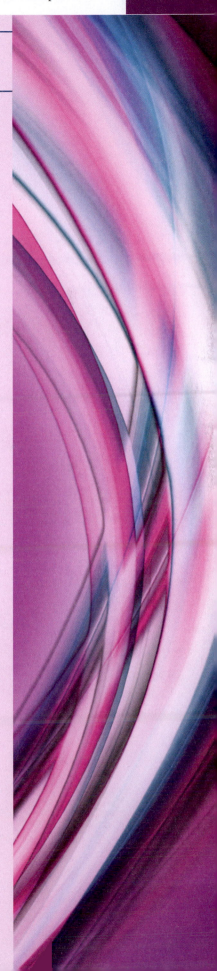

Chapter Review

True/False

Identify the statement as true (T) or false (F).

_____ **1.** MMI stands for major medical income.

_____ **2.** Disability compensation programs reimburse the insured only when a work-related injury causes the person to lose income.

_____ **3.** The Admission of Liability and the Notice of Contest determinations both find the employer liable in a workers' compensation case.

_____ **4.** An occupational disease or illness is caused by some factor in the work environment that exists over a period of time.

_____ **5.** Under workers' compensation regulations, the treating doctor is the provider who prepares the final report.

_____ **6.** FECA is the abbreviation for Federal Employees' Compensation Act.

_____ **7.** Employees who are injured on the job must be diagnosed by an approved provider as having a physical or mental impairment that results in loss of income.

_____ **8.** Disability compensation programs do not pay medical benefits.

_____ **9.** OSHA is the abbreviation for Occupational Safety and Hazard Administration.

_____ **10.** Vocational rehabilitation is not covered by workers' compensation plans.

_____ **11.** The employer sends in the First Report of Injury or Illness in a workers' compensation case.

_____ **12.** The fees for workers' compensation cases are based on the UCR fee.

_____ **13.** Any employee can purchase a disability plan.

_____ **14.** IME is an abbreviation for Individual Medical Examination.

Multiple Choice

Identify the letter of the choice that best completes the statement or answers the question.

_____ **1.** After discharging a workers' compensation patient, the provider must file a(n):
a. First Report of Injury.
b. First Report of Illness.
c. Admission of Liability.
d. Final report.

_____ **2.** When a provider initially examines a workers' compensation patient, what document must be filed with the state?
   a. Final report
   b. Admission of Liability
   c. Work Status Report
   d. Vocational report

_____ **3.** Social Security Disability Insurance provides compensation for lost wages to individuals who:
   a. are qualified for welfare programs.
   b. have contributed to Social Security.
   c. Either a or b.
   d. Neither a nor b.

_____ **4.** Supplemental Security Income provides financial assistance to individuals who:
   a. are qualified for welfare programs.
   b. have contributed to Social Security.
   c. Either a or b.
   d. Neither a nor b.

_____ **5.** What information is required in form locator 1a when preparing a workers' compensation claim?
   a. Patient's name
   b. Patient's Social Security number
   c. Employer's name
   d. Insured's I.D. number

_____ **6.** Workers' compensation fees are based on what fee schedule and a percentage?
   a. Aetna
   b. State insurance fees
   c. Medicare
   d. Medicaid

_____ **7.** What form locators are left blank on a CMS-1500 claim form for a workers' compensation claim?
   a. Form locators 4 and 5
   b. Form locators 12 and 13
   c. Form locators 32 and 33
   d. Form locators 25 and 26

Completion

Complete each sentence or statement.

1. _____ is the permanent physical damage to a worker's body from a work-related injury or illness.

2. The Federal Employees' Compensation Act provides _____ insurance for civilian employees of the federal government.

3. In the workers' compensation classification of injuries, _____ injury occurs when a worker is injured on the job and cannot resume work within several days of receiving treatment.

4. In the workers' compensation classification of injuries, _____ injury occurs when a worker is injured on the job, is unable to resume work, and is not expected to be able to return to the regular job in the future.

5. In the workers' compensation classification of injuries, an injury requiring _____ occurs when a worker is injured on the job and cannot resume work without retraining.

6. When a person knowingly or intentionally conceals, misrepresents, or makes a false statement to either deny or obtain workers' compensation benefits or insurance coverage, or otherwise profit from the deceit, this action is called _____.

7. Carpal tunnel syndrome is an example of a(n) _____ illness.

8. _____ describes the degree of permanent damage done to a worker's body as a whole.

9. An injured worker may not receive benefits if _____.

10. MMI is the abbreviation for _____.

11. Workers' compensation bills need to be submitted with a(n) _____.

Resources

U.S. Department of Labor—Office of Workers' Compensation Programs
www.dol.gov/dol/topic/workcomp

U.S. Department of Labor—Occupational Health &; Safety Administration (OSHA)
www.osha.gov

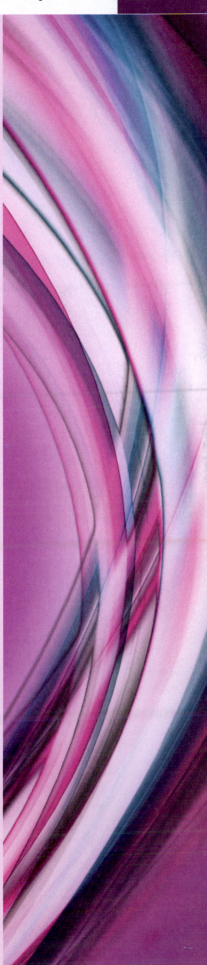

Completing the CMS-1500 Form for Physician Outpatient Billing

The case studies in this appendix are provided for additional practice in completing the CMS-1500 claim form for physician outpatient billing. Your objective is to accurately complete a CMS-1500 claim form for each case study by applying what you have learned in this text. Patient demographics and a brief case history are provided. Complete the cases based on the following criteria. All patients have release of information and assignment of benefit signatures on file. All providers are participating and accept assignment. The group practice is the billing entity. The national transition to NPI numbers is complete, and legacy PINs of individual payers are no longer used. The 2017 ICD-10-CM and CPT codes are used. For the cases in this appendix, the student should provide the ICD-10-CM code(s) on the claim forms. For other exercises in the textbook, the student is asked to provide the ICD-10-CM code(s). Use eight-digit dates for birthdates. Use six-digit dates for all other dates. Enter all street names using standard postal abbreviations, even if they are spelled out on the source documents. To complete each case study, copy the CMS-1500 form provided in Appendix D or download it from the MyHealthProfessionsKit or MyHealthProfessionsLab, which accompany this text. Refer to the Capital City Medical Fee Schedule on page 615 to determine the correct fees. For a list of abbreviations used in these case studies and their meanings, also refer to the MyHealthProfessionsKit or MyHealthProfessionsLab.

CASE STUDIES

Primary Payer

Case	Patient	Primary Payer
A-1	Dennis Hurst	Medicaid
A-2	Tamara Jackson	Blue Cross Blue Shield
A-3	Zeb Nickles	Medicaid
A-4	Connie Aven	Health America
A-5	Celeste Donegan	Aetna
A-6	Carlos Clemenza	Blue Cross Blue Shield
A-7	Guy Colich	Aetna
A-8	Klaus Davies	Blue Cross Blue Shield
A-9	Matilda Vogel	TRICARE
A-10	Isaac Houston	Advantage Compensation Insurance (workers' compensation)

Primary/Secondary Payer

Case	Patient	Primary Payer/Secondary Payer
A-11	Kenneth Sung	Medicare/Medicaid
A-12	Viola Harrison	Medicare/Medicaid
A-13	Quaylord Quigley	Medicare/Medicaid
A-14	Winifred Myers	Medicare/Aetna (Retiree)
A-15	Stella Jaworski	Medicare/Medicaid
A-16	Murphy Bromley	Medicare/Blue Cross Blue Shield (Medigap)
A-17	Gus Powers	Medicare/Aetna (Retiree)
A-18	Kimber Acosta	Aetna/Medicare (MSP)
A-19	Chester Fields	Medicare/Blue Cross Blue Shield (Medigap)
A-20	Gertrude Huckle	Medicare/Health America (Retiree)

Capital City Medical—123 Unknown Boulevard, Capital City, NY 12345-2222, (555) 555-1234

Phil Wells, M.D., Mannie Mends, M.D., Bette R. Soone, M.D.

Patient Information Form

Tax ID: 75-0246810

Group NPI: 1513171216

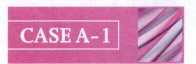

CASE A-1

Patient Information:

Name: (Last, First) Hurst, Dennis   ☒ Male   ☐ Female   Birth Date: 10/21/1992

Address: 347 Fern St, Capital City, NY 12345   Phone: (555)555-6337

Social Security Number: 723-58-3742   Full-Time Student: ☐ Yes   ☒ No

Marital Status: ☒ Single   ☐ Married   ☐ Divorced   ☐ Other

Employment:

Employer: _____ Phone: ( ) _____

Address: _____

Condition Related to: ☐ Auto Accident   ☐ Employment   ☐ Other Accident

Date of Accident: _____ State _____

Emergency Contact: _____ Phone: ( ) _____

Primary Insurance: Medicaid   Phone: ( ) _____

Address: 4875 Capital Blvd, Capital City, NY 12345

Insurance Policyholder's Name: Same   ☐ M   ☐ F   DOB: _____

Address: Same

Phone: _____   Relationship to Insured: ☒ Self ☐ Spouse ☐ Child ☐ Other

Employer: McDinkles   Phone: (555) 555-1597

Employer's Address: 7563 W. Washington St, Capital City, NY 12345

Policy/I.D. No: 0000652381139 Group No: ___ Percent Covered: ___%, Copay Amt: $5.00

Secondary Insurance: _____ Phone: ( ) _____

Address: _____

Insurance Policyholder's Name: _____ ☐ M ☐ F DOB: _____

Address: _____

Phone: _____ Relationship to Insured: ☐ Self ☐ Spouse ☐ Child ☐ Other

Employer: _____ Phone: ( ) _____

Employer's Address: _____

Policy/I.D. No: _____ Group No: _____ Percent Covered: _____%, Copay Amt: $ _____

Reason for Visit: Stitches infected from recent surgery for the removal of a ganglion cyst

Known Allergies: _____

Were you referred here? If so, by whom?: Dr. Eva N. Good, Internal Medicine, NPI: 8976453201

CASE A-1
SOAP

06/27/20XX
Assignment of Benefits: Y
Signature on File: Y
Referring Physician: Y

S: Dennis Hurst presents for complications of infected sutures postoperative.

O: Pt. had a ganglion cyst removed from his left hand on 6/25/XX. Mother concerned that the sutures are infected. On exam, there is noted infection at the site. This infection is localized. T: 99.9°F.

A: 1. Infected sutures postoperative—ICD-10 (T81.4XXA)

2. Status postsurgery—ICD-10 (Z98.89)

3. Ganglion cyst—ICD-10 (M67.40)

P: 1. Start on oral antibiotic for 10 days.

2. Keep area clean and dry.

3. Call office if condition worsens.

4. Return in 1 week for suture removal.

_____

Mannie Mends, M.D.

General Surgeon

NPI: 0123456789

Medicaid PIN: 5324896

Date of service:	06/27/XX			Waiver? ☐				
Patient name:	Dennis Hurst			Insurance:				
				Subscriber name:				
Address:	347 Fern St			Group #:			Previous balance:	
	Capital City, NY 12345			Copay:			Today's charges:	
Phone:	555-555-6337			Account #:			Today's payment: check#	
DOB:	10/21/1992	Age:	Sex:	Physician name:			Balance due:	

RANK	Office visit	New	Est	RANK	Office procedures			RANK	Laboratory		
	Minimal		99211		Anoscopy		46600		Venipuncture		36415
X	Problem focused	99201	99212		Audiometry		92551		Blood glucose, monitoring device		82962
	Expanded problem focused	99202	99213		Cerumen removal		69210		Blood glucose, visual dipstick		82948
	Detailed	99203	99214		Colposcopy		57452		CBC, w/ auto differential		85025
	Comprehensive	99204	99215		Colposcopy w/biopsy		57455		CBC, w/o auto differential		85027
	Comprehensive (new patient)	99205			ECG, w/interpretation		93000		Cholesterol		82465
	Significant, separate service	-25	-25		ECG, rhythm strip		93040		Hemoccult, guaiac		82270
	Well visit	**New**	**Est**		Endometrial biopsy		58100		Hemoccult, immunoassay		82274
	< 1 y	99381	99391		Flexible sigmoidoscopy		45330		Hemoglobin A1C		85018
	1-4 y	99382	99392		Flexible sigmoidoscopy w/biopsy		45331		Lipid panel		80061
	5-11 y	99383	99393		Fracture care, cast/splint		29____		Liver panel		80076
	12-17 y	99384	99394		Site:				KOH prep (skin, hair, nails)		87220
	18-39 y	99385	99395		Nebulizer		94640		Metabolic panel, basic		80048
	40-64 y	99386	99396		Nebulizer demo		94664		Metabolic panel, comprehensive		80053
	65 y +	99387	99397		Spirometry		94010		Mononucleosis		86308
	Medicare preventive services				Spirometry, pre and post		94060		Pregnancy, blood		84703
	Pap		Q0091		Tympanometry		92567		Pregnancy, urine		81025
	Pelvic & breast		G0101		Vasectomy		55250		Renal panel		80069
	Prostate/PSA		G0103		**Skin procedures**		**Units**		Sedimentation rate		85651
	Tobacco counseling/3-10 min		99406		Burn care, initial	16000			Strep, rapid		86403
	Tobacco counseling/>10 min		99407		Foreign body, skin, simple	10120			Strep culture		87081
	Welcome to Medicare exam		G0344		Foreign body, skin, complex	10121			Strep A		87880
	ECG w/Welcome to Medicare exam		G0366		I&D, abscess	10060			TB		86580
	Flexible sigmoidoscopy		G0104		I&D, hematoma/seroma	10140			UA, complete, non-automated		81000
	Hemoccult, guaiac		G0107		Laceration repair, simple	120____			UA, w/o micro, non-automated		81002
	Flu shot		G0008		Site: _____ Size: _____				UA, w/ micro, non-automated		81003
	Pneumonia shot		G0009		Laceration repair, layered	120____			Urine colony count		87086
	Consultation/preop clearance				Site: _____ Size: _____				Urine culture, presumptive		87088
	Expanded problem focused		99242		Lesion, biopsy, one	11100			Wet mount/KOH		87210
	Detailed		99243		Lesion, biopsy, each add'l	11101			**Vaccines**		
	Comprehensive/mod complexity		99244		Lesion, destruct., benign, 1-14	17110			DT, <7 y		90702
	Comprehensive/high complexity		99245		Lesion, destruct., premal., single	17000			DTP		90701
	Other services				Lesion, destruct., premal., ea. add'l	17003			DtaP, <7 y		90700
	After posted hours		99050		Lesion, excision, benign	114____			Flu, 6-35 months		90657
	Evening/weekend appointment		99051		Site: _____ Size: _____				Flu, 3 y +		90658
	Home health certification		G0180		Lesion, excision, malignant	116____			Hep A, adult		90632
	Home health recertification		G0179		Site: _____ Size: _____				Hep A, ped/adol, 2 dose		90633
	Post-op follow-up		99024		Lesion, paring/cutting, one	11055			Hep B, adult		90746
	Prolonged/30-74 min		99354		Lesion, paring/cutting, 2-4	11056			Hep B, ped/adol 3 dose		90744
	Special reports/forms		99080		Lesion, shave	113____			Hep B-Hib		90748
	Disability/Workers comp		99455		Site: _____ Size: _____				Hib, 4 dose		90645
	Radiology				Nail removal, partial	11730			HPV		90649
					Nail removal, w/matrix	11750			IPV		90713
					Skin tag, 1-15	11200			MMR		90707
	Diagnoses				**Medications**		**Units**		Pneumonia, >2 y		90732
1	T81.4XXA				Ampicillin, up to 500mg	J0290			Pneumonia conjugate, <5 y		90669
2	Z98.89				B-12, up to 1,000 mcg	J3420			Td, >7 y		90718
3	M67.40				Epinephrine, up to 1ml	J0170			Varicella		90716
4					Kenalog, 10mg	J3301			**Immunizations & Injections**		**Units**
Next office visit					Lidocaine, 10mg	J2001			Allergen, one	95115	
Recheck	Prev	PRN	____ D W M Y		Normal saline, 1000cc	J7030			Allergen, multiple	95117	
Instructions:					Phenergan, up to 50mg	J2550			Imm admin, one	90471	
					Progesterone, 150mg	J1055			Imm admin, each add'l	90472	
					Rocephin, 250mg	J0696			Imm admin, intranasal, one	90473	
					Testosterone, 200mg	J1080			Imm admin, intranasal, each add'l	90474	
Referral					Tigan, up to 200 mg	J3250			Injection, joint, small	20600	
To:					Toradol, 15mg	J1885			Injection, joint, intermediate	20605	
Instructions:					**Miscellaneous services**				Injection, joint, major	20610	
									Injection, ther/proph/diag	90772	
									Injection, trigger point	20552	
Physician signature								**Supplies**		
X _____										

CASE A-1 ENCOUNTER FORM

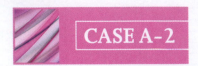

CASE A-2

Capital City Medical—123 Unknown Boulevard, Capital City, NY 12345-2222, (555) 555-1234
Phil Wells, M.D., Mannie Mends, M.D., Bette R. Soone, M.D.

Patient Information Form
Tax ID: 75-0246810
Group NPI: 1513171216

Patient Information:

Name: (Last, First) Jackson, Tamara   ❑ Male   ❑ Female   Birth Date: 07/16/1988
Address: 41 Acorn Dr, Capital City, NY 12345   Phone: (555) 555-7650
Social Security Number: 201-19-4399   Full-Time Student: ❑ Yes   ☒ No
Marital Status: ❑ Single   ☒ Married   ❑ Divorced   ❑ Other

Employment:

Employer: Capital City Hospital   Phone: (555) 555-1516
Address: One Quality Care Way, Capital City, NY 12345
Condition Related to: ❑ Auto Accident   ❑ Employment   ❑ Other Accident
Date of Accident: _____ State _____
Emergency Contact: _____   Phone: ( ) _____

Primary Insurance: Blue Cross Blue Shield   Phone: ( ) _____

Address: 379 Blue Plaza, Capital City, NY 12345
Insurance Policyholder's Name: Same   ❑ M   ❑ F   DOB: _____
Address: _____
Phone: _____   Relationship to Insured: ☒ Self   ❑ Spouse   ❑ Child   ❑ Other
Employer: _____   Phone: _____
Employer's Address: _____
Policy/I.D. No: YYZ401528821 Group No: 20639 Percent Covered: _____, Copay Amt: $25.00

Secondary Insurance: _____   Phone: ( ) _____

Address: _____
Insurance Policyholder's Name: _____   ❑ M   ❑ F   DOB: _____
Address: _____
Phone: _____   Relationship to Insured: ❑ Self   ❑ Spouse   ❑ Child   ❑ Other
Employer: _____   Phone: ( ) _____
Employer's Address: _____
Policy/I.D. No: Group No: Percent Covered: %, Copay Amt: $

Reason for Visit: My period is about 2 weeks late
Known Allergies: _____
Were you referred here? If so, by whom? _____

07/19/20XX
Assignment of Benefits: Y
Signature on File: Y
Referring Physician: N

CASE A-2 SOAP

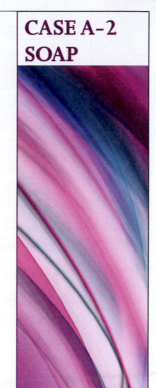

S: Tamara Jackson is a new patient who complains of a missed menses × 2 weeks. She has an irregular cycle. She also says that an OTC urine pregnancy test was positive yesterday.

O: Pt. denies any birth control methods. She is married and has a zero pregnancy history. Nausea is present. Denies vomiting. Says she has lost 12 lbs. in the past 2 weeks. Menses began at age 14. Pregnancy test today.

A: 1. Irregular menstrual cycle—ICD-10 (N92.6)

   2. Abnormal weight loss—ICD-10 (R63.4)

P: 1. Serum pregnancy test today.

   2. Will call pt. with results.

_____

Bette R. Soone, M.D.

Obstetrics/Gynecology

NPI: 0987654321

PIN: 654321

Date of service:	07/19/XX		Waiver? ☐		
Patient name:	Tamra Jackson		Insurance:		
			Subscriber name:		
Address:	41 Acorn Dr		Group #:		Previous balance:
	Capital City, NY 12345		Copay:		Today's charges:
Phone:	555-555-7650		Account #:		Today's payment: check#
DOB:	10/21/1992 Age: Sex:		Physician name:		Balance due:

RANK	Office visit	New	Est
	Minimal		99211
	Problem focused	99201	99212
X	Expanded problem focused	99202	99213
	Detailed	99203	99214
	Comprehensive	99204	99215
	Comprehensive (new patient)	99205	
	Significant, separate service	-25	-25
	Well visit	**New**	**Est**
	< 1 y	99381	99391
	1-4 y	99382	99392
	5-11 y	99383	99393
	12-17 y	99384	99394
	18-39 y	99385	99395
	40-64 y	99386	99396
	65 y +	99387	99397
	Medicare preventive services		
	Pap		Q0091
	Pelvic & breast		G0101
	Prostate/PSA		G0103
	Tobacco counseling/3-10 min		99406
	Tobacco counseling/>10 min		99407
	Welcome to Medicare exam		G0344
	ECG w/Welcome to Medicare exam		G0366
	Flexible sigmoidoscopy		G0104
	Hemoccult, guaiac		G0107
	Flu shot		G0008
	Pneumonia shot		G0009
	Consultation/preop clearance		
	Expanded problem focused		99242
	Detailed		99243
	Comprehensive/mod complexity		99244
	Comprehensive/high complexity		99245
	Other services		
	After posted hours		99050
	Evening/weekend appointment		99051
	Home health certification		G0180
	Home health recertification		G0179
	Post-op follow-up		99024
	Prolonged/30-74 min		99354
	Special reports/forms		99080
	Disability/Workers comp		99455
	Radiology		

RANK	Office procedures		
	Anoscopy		46600
	Audiometry		92551
	Cerumen removal		69210
	Colposcopy		57452
	Colposcopy w/biopsy		57455
	ECG, w/interpretation		93000
	ECG, rhythm strip		93040
	Endometrial biopsy		58100
	Flexible sigmoidoscopy		45330
	Flexible sigmoidoscopy w/biopsy		45331
	Fracture care, cast/splint		29____
	Site: ____		
	Nebulizer		94640
	Nebulizer demo		94664
	Spirometry		94010
	Spirometry, pre and post		94060
	Tympanometry		92567
	Vasectomy		55250
	Skin procedures		**Units**
	Burn care, initial	16000	
	Foreign body, skin, simple	10120	
	Foreign body, skin, complex	10121	
	I&D, abscess	10060	
	I&D, hematoma/seroma	10140	
	Laceration repair, simple	120____	
	Site: ____ Size: ____		
	Laceration repair, layered	120____	
	Site: ____ Size: ____		
	Lesion, biopsy, one	11100	
	Lesion, biopsy, each add'l	11101	
	Lesion, destruct., benign, 1-14	17110	
	Lesion, destruct., premal., single	17000	
	Lesion, destruct., premal., ea. add'l	17003	
	Lesion, excision, benign	114____	
	Site: ____ Size: ____		
	Lesion, excision, malignant	116____	
	Site: ____ Size: ____		
	Lesion, paring/cutting, one	11055	
	Lesion, paring/cutting, 2-4	11056	
	Lesion, shave	113____	
	Site: ____ Size: ____		
	Nail removal, partial	11730	
	Nail removal, w/matrix	11750	
	Skin tag, 1-15	11200	
	Medications		**Units**
	Ampicillin, up to 500mg	J0290	
	B-12, up to 1,000 mcg	J3420	
	Epinephrine, up to 1ml	J0170	
	Kenalog, 10mg	J3301	
	Lidocaine, 10mg	J2001	
	Normal saline, 1000cc	J7030	
	Phenergan, up to 50mg	J2550	
	Progesterone, 150mg	J1055	
	Rocephin, 250mg	J0696	
	Testosterone, 200mg	J1080	
	Tigan, up to 200 mg	J3250	
	Toradol, 15mg	J1885	
	Miscellaneous services		

RANK	Laboratory		
X	Venipuncture		36415
	Blood glucose, monitoring device		82962
	Blood glucose, visual dipstick		82948
	CBC, w/ auto differential		85025
	CBC, w/o auto differential		85027
	Cholesterol		82465
	Hemoccult, guaiac		82270
	Hemoccult, immunoassay		82274
	Hemoglobin A1C		85018
	Lipid panel		80061
	Liver panel		80076
	KOH prep (skin, hair, nails)		87220
	Metabolic panel, basic		80048
	Metabolic panel, comprehensive		80053
	Mononucleosis		86308
X	Pregnancy, blood		84703
	Pregnancy, urine		81025
	Renal panel		80069
	Sedimentation rate		85651
	Strep, rapid		86403
	Strep culture		87081
	Strep A		87880
	TB		86580
	UA, complete, non-automated		81000
	UA, w/o micro, non-automated		81002
	UA, w/ micro, non-automated		81003
	Urine colony count		87086
	Urine culture, presumptive		87088
	Wet mount/KOH		87210
	Vaccines		
	DT, <7 y		90702
	DTP		90701
	DtaP, <7 y		90700
	Flu, 6-35 months		90657
	Flu, 3 y +		90658
	Hep A, adult		90632
	Hep A, ped/adol, 2 dose		90633
	Hep B, adult		90746
	Hep B, ped/adol 3 dose		90744
	Hep B-Hib		90748
	Hib, 4 dose		90645
	HPV		90649
	IPV		90713
	MMR		90707
	Pneumonia, >2 y		90732
	Pneumonia conjugate, <5 y		90669
	Td, >7 y		90718
	Varicella		90716
	Immunizations & Injections		**Units**
	Allergen, one	95115	
	Allergen, multiple	95117	
	Imm admin, one	90471	
	Imm admin, each add'l	90472	
	Imm admin, intranasal, one	90473	
	Imm admin, intranasal, each add'l	90474	
	Injection, joint, small	20600	
	Injection, joint, intermediate	20605	
	Injection, joint, major	20610	
	Injection, ther/proph/diag	90772	
	Injection, trigger point	20552	
	Supplies		

	Diagnoses		
1	N92.6		
2	R63.4		
3			
4			

Next office visit							
Recheck	Prev	PRN	____	D	W	M	Y
Instructions:							

Referral

To:

Instructions:

Physician signature

X _____

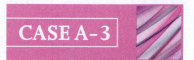

Capital City Medical—123 Unknown Boulevard, Capital City, NY 12345-2222, (555) 555-1234
Phil Wells, M.D., Mannie Mends, M.D., Bette R. Soone, M.D.

Patient Information Form
Tax ID: 75-0246810
Group NPI: 1513171216

Patient Information:

Name: (Last, First) Nickles, Zeb   ☒ Male   ☐ Female   Birth Date: 01/14/1966

Address: 409 Elm St, Capital City, NY 12345   Phone: (555)555-0123

Social Security Number: 251-89-3485   Full-Time Student: ☐ Yes   ☒ No

Marital Status: ☐ Single   ☒ Married   ☐ Divorced   ☐ Other

Employment:

Employer: Calver and Associates, Esq.   Phone: (555) 555-0123

Address: 4702 Hillman Ave., Suite 201, Township, NY 12345

Condition Related to: ☐ Auto Accident   ☐ Employment   ☐ Other Accident

Date of Accident: _____ State _____

Emergency Contact: _____   Phone: ( ) _____

Primary Insurance: Medicaid   Phone: ( ) _____

Address: 4875 Capital City Blvd, Capital City, NY 12345

Insurance Policyholder's Name: Same   ☐ M   ☐ F   DOB: _____

Address: _____

Phone: _____   Relationship to Insured: ☒ Self ☐ Spouse ☐ Child ☐ Other

Employer: _____   Phone: _____

Employer's Address: _____

Policy/I.D. No: 94099483171 Group No: ___ Percent Covered: ___%, Copay Amt: $20.00

Secondary Insurance: _____   Phone: ( ) _____

Address: _____

Insurance Policyholder's Name: _____   ☐ M ☐ F DOB: _____

Address: _____

Phone: _____   Relationship to Insured: ☐ Self ☐ Spouse ☐ Child ☐ Other

Employer: _____   Phone: ( ) _____

Employer's Address: _____

Policy/I.D. No: _____   Group No: _____   Percent Covered: _____%, Copay Amt: $

Reason for Visit: My face hurts, my nose is draining, and I have been sneezing

Known Allergies: _____

Were you referred here? If so, by whom?: _____

CASE A-3 SOAP

07/16/20XX
Assignment of Benefits: Y
Signature on File: Y
Referring Physician: N

S: Zeb Nickles presents today with complaints of facial pressure, nasal drainage, and sneezing.

O: Respiratory tract reveals postnasal drip, edema, and yellowish-green mucus.

A: 1. Acute sinusitis—ICD-10 (J01.90)

   2. Acute rhinitis—ICD-10 (J00)

P: 1. Z-Pak.

   2. Nasonex 1 spray each nostril once daily.

   3. Return p.r.n.

_____

Phil Wells, M.D.

Family Practice

NPI: 1234567890

Medicaid PIN: 5324896

Date of service:	07/16/XX	Waiver? ☐	
Patient name:	Zeb Nickles	Insurance:	
		Subscriber name:	
Address:	409 Elm St Township, NY 12345	Group #:	Previous balance:
		Copay:	Today's charges:
Phone:	555-555-0123	Account #:	Today's payment: check#
DOB:	01/14/1966 Age: Sex:	Physician name:	Balance due:

RANK	Office visit	New	Est
	Minimal		99211
X	Problem focused	99201	99212
	Expanded problem focused	99202	99213
	Detailed	99203	99214
	Comprehensive	99204	99215
	Comprehensive (new patient)	99205	
	Significant, separate service	-25	-25
	Well visit	**New**	**Est**
	< 1 y	99381	99391
	1-4 y	99382	99392
	5-11 y	99383	99393
	12-17 y	99384	99394
	18-39 y	99385	99395
	40-64 y	99386	99396
	65 y +	99387	99397
	Medicare preventive services		
	Pap		Q0091
	Pelvic & breast		G0101
	Prostate/PSA		G0103
	Tobacco counseling/3-10 min		99406
	Tobacco counseling/>10 min		99407
	Welcome to Medicare exam		G0344
	ECG w/Welcome to Medicare exam		G0366
	Flexible sigmoidoscopy		G0104
	Hemoccult, guaiac		G0107
	Flu shot		G0008
	Pneumonia shot		G0009
	Consultation/preop clearance		
	Expanded problem focused		99242
	Detailed		99243
	Comprehensive/mod complexity		99244
	Comprehensive/high complexity		99245
	Other services		
	After posted hours		99050
	Evening/weekend appointment		99051
	Home health certification		G0180
	Home health recertification		G0179
	Post-op follow-up		99024
	Prolonged/30-74 min		99354
	Special reports/forms		99080
	Disability/Workers comp		99455
	Radiology		

RANK	Office procedures		
	Anoscopy		46600
	Audiometry		92551
	Cerumen removal		69210
	Colposcopy		57452
	Colposcopy w/biopsy		57455
	ECG, w/interpretation		93000
	ECG, rhythm strip		93040
	Endometrial biopsy		58100
	Flexible sigmoidoscopy		45330
	Flexible sigmoidoscopy w/biopsy		45331
	Fracture care, cast/splint	29_____	
	Site: _____		
	Nebulizer		94640
	Nebulizer demo		94664
	Spirometry		94010
	Spirometry, pre and post		94060
	Tympanometry		92567
	Vasectomy		55250
	Skin procedures		**Units**
	Burn care, initial	16000	
	Foreign body, skin, simple	10120	
	Foreign body, skin, complex	10121	
	I&D, abscess	10060	
	I&D, hematoma/seroma	10140	
	Laceration repair, simple	120___	
	Site: _____ Size: _____		
	Laceration repair, layered	120___	
	Site: _____ Size: _____		
	Lesion, biopsy, one	11100	
	Lesion, biopsy, each add'l	11101	
	Lesion, destruct., benign, 1-14	17110	
	Lesion, destruct., premal., single	17000	
	Lesion, destruct., premal., ea. add'l	17003	
	Lesion, excision, benign	114___	
	Site: _____ Size: _____		
	Lesion, excision, malignant	116___	
	Site: _____ Size: _____		
	Lesion, paring/cutting, one	11055	
	Lesion, paring/cutting, 2-4	11056	
	Lesion, shave	113___	
	Site: _____ Size: _____		
	Nail removal, partial	11730	
	Nail removal, w/matrix	11750	
	Skin tag, 1-15	11200	

RANK	Laboratory	
	Venipuncture	36415
	Blood glucose, monitoring device	82962
	Blood glucose, visual dipstick	82948
	CBC, w/ auto differential	85025
	CBC, w/o auto differential	85027
	Cholesterol	82465
	Hemoccult, guaiac	82270
	Hemoccult, immunoassay	82274
	Hemoglobin A1C	85018
	Lipid panel	80061
	Liver panel	80076
	KOH prep (skin, hair, nails)	87220
	Metabolic panel, basic	80048
	Metabolic panel, comprehensive	80053
	Mononucleosis	86308
	Pregnancy, blood	84703
	Pregnancy, urine	81025
	Renal panel	80069
	Sedimentation rate	85651
	Strep, rapid	86403
	Strep culture	87081
	Strep A	87880
	TB	86580
	UA, complete, non-automated	81000
	UA, w/o micro, non-automated	81002
	UA, w/ micro, non-automated	81003
	Urine colony count	87086
	Urine culture, presumptive	87088
	Wet mount/KOH	87210
	Vaccines	
	DT, <7 y	90702
	DTP	90701
	DtaP, <7 y	90700
	Flu, 6-35 months	90657
	Flu, 3 y +	90658
	Hep A, adult	90632
	Hep A, ped/adol, 2 dose	90633
	Hep B, adult	90746
	Hep B, ped/adol 3 dose	90744
	Hep B-Hib	90748
	Hib, 4 dose	90645
	HPV	90649
	IPV	90713
	MMR	90707
	Pneumonia, >2 y	90732
	Pneumonia conjugate, <5 y	90669
	Td, >7 y	90718
	Varicella	90716

Diagnoses	
1	J01.90
2	J00
3	
4	

Medications		Units
Ampicillin, up to 500mg	J0290	
B-12, up to 1,000 mcg	J3420	
Epinephrine, up to 1ml	J0170	
Kenalog, 10mg	J3301	
Lidocaine, 10mg	J2001	
Normal saline, 1000cc	J7030	
Phenergan, up to 50mg	J2550	
Progesterone, 150mg	J1055	
Rocephin, 250mg	J0696	
Testosterone, 200mg	J1080	
Tigan, up to 200 mg	J3250	
Toradol, 15mg	J1885	
Miscellaneous services		

Immunizations & Injections		Units
Allergen, one	95115	
Allergen, multiple	95117	
Imm admin, one	90471	
Imm admin, each add'l	90472	
Imm admin, intranasal, one	90473	
Imm admin, intranasal, each add'l	90474	
Injection, joint, small	20600	
Injection, joint, intermediate	20605	
Injection, joint, major	20610	
Injection, ther/proph/diag	90772	
Injection, trigger point	20552	
Supplies		

Next office visit

Recheck	Prev	PRN	_____	D W M Y

Instructions:

Referral

To:

Instructions:

Physician signature

X _____

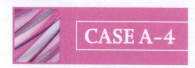

CASE A-4

Capital City Medical—123 Unknown Boulevard, Capital City, NY 12345-2222, (555) 555-1234

Phil Wells, M.D., Mannie Mends, M.D., Bette R. Soone, M.D.

Patient Information Form
Tax ID: 75-0246810
Group NPI: 1513171216

Patient Information:

Name: (Last, First) Aven, Connie   ☒ Male   ❑ Female   Birth Date: 01/28/1984

Address: 55 Buckeye Dr, Capital City, NY 12345   Phone: (555) 555-3165

Social Security Number: 309-14-7286   Full-Time Student: ❑ Yes   ☒ No

Marital Status: ❑ Single   ☒ Married   ❑ Divorced   ❑ Other

Employment:

Employer: Swellsville Fireworks International   Phone: (555) 555-2200

Address: 1019 Kaboom Rd, Township, NY 12345

Condition Related to: ❑ Auto Accident   ❑ Employment   ❑ Other Accident

Date of Accident: _____ State _____

Emergency Contact: _____   Phone: ( ) _____

Primary Insurance: Health America   Phone: ( ) _____

Address: 2031 Healthica Center, Capital City, NY 12345

Insurance Policyholder's Name: Marc Aven   ☒ M   ❑ F   DOB: 08/18/1983

Address: _____ Same

Phone: _____   Relationship to Insured: ☒ Self ❑ Spouse ❑ Child ❑ Other

Employer: Computer Training Academy   Phone: (555) 555-8852

Employer's Address: 10 Parkway Center, Capital City, NY 12345

Policy/I.D. No: 7325185 Group No: 01429 Percent Covered: ____%, Copay Amt: $15.00

Secondary Insurance: _____   Phone: ( ) _____

Address: _____

Insurance Policyholder's Name: _____   ❑ M ❑ F DOB: _____

Address: _____

Phone: _____ Relationship to Insured: ❑ Self ❑ Spouse ❑ Child ❑ Other

Employer: _____   Phone: ( ) _____

Employer's Address: _____

Policy/I.D. No: _____   Group No: _____   Percent Covered: _____%, Copay Amt: $

Reason for Visit: I am having pain in my right eye, and it is swollen

Known Allergies: _____

Were you referred here? If so, by whom?: _____

12/01/20XX

Assignment of Benefits: Y

Signature on File: Y

Referring Physician: N

CASE A-4
SOAP

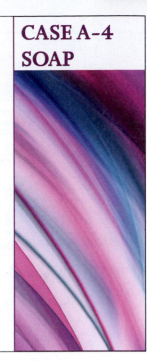

S: Connie Aven presents in the office for a painful and swollen right eye.

O: Pt. denies any injury to the eye. She doesn't have any seasonal allergies. On exam, the right eye is infected. She can barely open it.

A: 1. Conjunctivitis, right eye—ICD-10 (H10.33)

P: 1. Ophthalmic ointment 1 drop q 6 h.

   2. Return as needed.

_____

Phil Wells, M.D.

Family Practice

NPI: 1234567890

PIN: 822093

Date of service:	12/01/XX		Waiver? ☐		
Patient name: Connie Aven			Insurance:		
			Subscriber name:		
Address: 55 Buckeye Dr Capital City, NY 12345			Group #:		Previous balance:
			Copay:		Today's charges:
Phone: 555-555-3165			Account #:		Today's payment: check#
DOB: 01/14/1966 Age: Sex:			Physician name:		Balance due:

RANK	Office visit	New	Est
	Minimal		99211
X	Problem focused	99201	99212
	Expanded problem focused	99202	99213
	Detailed	99203	99214
	Comprehensive	99204	99215
	Comprehensive (new patient)	99205	
	Significant, separate service	-25	-25
	Well visit	**New**	**Est**
	< 1 y	99381	99391
	1-4 y	99382	99392
	5-11 y	99383	99393
	12-17 y	99384	99394
	18-39 y	99385	99395
	40-64 y	99386	99396
	65 y +	99387	99397
	Medicare preventive services		
	Pap		Q0091
	Pelvic & breast		G0101
	Prostate/PSA		G0103
	Tobacco counseling/3-10 min		99406
	Tobacco counseling/>10 min		99407
	Welcome to Medicare exam		G0344
	ECG w/Welcome to Medicare exam		G0366
	Flexible sigmoidoscopy		G0104
	Hemoccult, guaiac		G0107
	Flu shot		G0008
	Pneumonia shot		G0009
	Consultation/preop clearance		
	Expanded problem focused		99242
	Detailed		99243
	Comprehensive/mod complexity		99244
	Comprehensive/high complexity		99245
	Other services		
	After posted hours		99050
	Evening/weekend appointment		99051
	Home health certification		G0180
	Home health recertification		G0179
	Post-op follow-up		99024
	Prolonged/30-74 min		99354
	Special reports/forms		99080
	Disability/Workers comp		99455
	Radiology		

RANK	Office procedures		
	Anoscopy		46600
	Audiometry		92551
	Cerumen removal		69210
	Colposcopy		57452
	Colposcopy w/biopsy		57455
	ECG, w/interpretation		93000
	ECG, rhythm strip		93040
	Endometrial biopsy		58100
	Flexible sigmoidoscopy		45330
	Flexible sigmoidoscopy w/biopsy		45331
	Fracture care, cast/splint		29____
	Site: _____		
	Nebulizer		94640
	Nebulizer demo		94664
	Spirometry		94010
	Spirometry, pre and post		94060
	Tympanometry		92567
	Vasectomy		55250
	Skin procedures		**Units**
	Burn care, initial	16000	
	Foreign body, skin, simple	10120	
	Foreign body, skin, complex	10121	
	I&D, abscess	10060	
	I&D, hematoma/seroma	10140	
	Laceration repair, simple	120____	
	Site: _____ Size: ____		
	Laceration repair, layered	120____	
	Site: _____ Size: ____		
	Lesion, biopsy, one	11100	
	Lesion, biopsy, each add'l	11101	
	Lesion, destruct., benign, 1-14	17110	
	Lesion, destruct., premal., single	17000	
	Lesion, destruct., premal., ea. add'l	17003	
	Lesion, excision, benign	114____	
	Site: _____ Size: ____		
	Lesion, excision, malignant	116____	
	Site: _____ Size: ____		
	Lesion, paring/cutting, one	11055	
	Lesion, paring/cutting, 2-4	11056	
	Lesion, shave	113____	
	Site: _____ Size: ____		
	Nail removal, partial	11730	
	Nail removal, w/matrix	11750	
	Skin tag, 1-15	11200	
	Medications		**Units**
	Ampicillin, up to 500mg	J0290	
	B-12, up to 1,000 mcg	J3420	
	Epinephrine, up to 1ml	J0170	
	Kenalog, 10mg	J3301	
	Lidocaine, 10mg	J2001	
	Normal saline, 1000cc	J7030	
	Phenergan, up to 50mg	J2550	
	Progesterone, 150mg	J1055	
	Rocephin, 250mg	J0696	
	Testosterone, 200mg	J1080	
	Tigan, up to 200 mg	J3250	
	Toradol, 15mg	J1885	
	Miscellaneous services		

RANK	Laboratory	
	Venipuncture	36415
	Blood glucose, monitoring device	82962
	Blood glucose, visual dipstick	82948
	CBC, w/ auto differential	85025
	CBC, w/o auto differential	85027
	Cholesterol	82465
	Hemoccult, guaiac	82270
	Hemoccult, immunoassay	82274
	Hemoglobin A1C	85018
	Lipid panel	80061
	Liver panel	80076
	KOH prep (skin, hair, nails)	87220
	Metabolic panel, basic	80048
	Metabolic panel, comprehensive	80053
	Mononucleosis	86308
	Pregnancy, blood	84703
	Pregnancy, urine	81025
	Renal panel	80069
	Sedimentation rate	85651
	Strep, rapid	86403
	Strep culture	87081
	Strep A	87880
	TB	86580
	UA, complete, non-automated	81000
	UA, w/o micro, non-automated	81002
	UA, w/ micro, non-automated	81003
	Urine colony count	87086
	Urine culture, presumptive	87088
	Wet mount/KOH	87210
	Vaccines	
	DT, <7 y	90702
	DTP	90701
	DtaP, <7 y	90700
	Flu, 6-35 months	90657
	Flu, 3 y +	90658
	Hep A, adult	90632
	Hep A, ped/adol, 2 dose	90633
	Hep B, adult	90746
	Hep B, ped/adol 3 dose	90744
	Hep B-Hib	90748
	Hib, 4 dose	90645
	HPV	90649
	IPV	90713
	MMR	90707
	Pneumonia, >2 y	90732
	Pneumonia conjugate, <5 y	90669
	Td, >7 y	90718
	Varicella	90716

RANK	Immunizations & Injections		Units
	Allergen, one	95115	
	Allergen, multiple	95117	
	Imm admin, one	90471	
	Imm admin, each add'l	90472	
	Imm admin, intranasal, one	90473	
	Imm admin, intranasal, each add'l	90474	
	Injection, joint, small	20600	
	Injection, joint, intermediate	20605	
	Injection, joint, major	20610	
	Injection, ther/proph/diag	90772	
	Injection, trigger point	20552	
	Supplies		

	Diagnoses
1	H10.33
2	
3	
4	

Next office visit

Recheck	Prev	PRN	_____	D W M Y

Instructions:

Referral

To:

Instructions:

Physician signature

X _____

CASE A-4 ENCOUNTER FORM

Capital City Medical—123 Unknown Boulevard, Capital City, NY 12345-2222, (555) 555-1234

Phil Wells, M.D., Mannie Mends, M.D., Bette R. Soone, M.D.

Patient Information Form
Tax ID: 75-0246810
Group NPI: 1513171216

CASE A-5

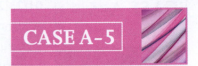

Patient Information:

Name: (Last, First) Donegan, Celeste   ☒ Male   ☐ Female   Birth Date: 12/20/1981

Address: 2829 Pine Ln, Capital City, NY 12345   Phone: (555) 555-6789

Social Security Number: 453-80-0147   Full-Time Student: ☐ Yes   ☒ No

Marital Status: ☐ Single   ☒ Married   ☐ Divorced   ☐ Other

Employment:

Employer: Drexell Business College   Phone: (555) 555-1500

Address: 2426 Clark Bldg, Township, NY 12345

Condition Related to: ☐ Auto Accident   ☐ Employment   ☐ Other Accident

Date of Accident: _____ State _____

Emergency Contact: _____   Phone: ( ) _____

Primary Insurance: Aetna   Phone: ( ) _____

Address: 1625 Healthcare Bldg, Capital City, NY 12345

Insurance Policyholder's Name: Douglas Donegan   ☒ M   ☐ F   DOB: 09/20/1981

Address: Same

Phone: _____   Relationship to Insured: ☒ Self ☐ Spouse ☐ Child ☐ Other

Employer: Number One Construction, Inc.   Phone: (555) 555-1063

Employer's Address: 1700 King Ave, Township, NY 12345

Policy/I.D. No: 4983282   Group No: 60531   Percent Covered: 90 %, Copay Amt: $__

Secondary Insurance: _____   Phone: ( ) _____

Address: _____

Insurance Policyholder's Name: _____   ☐ M   ☐ F   DOB: _____

Address: _____

Phone: _____   Relationship to Insured: ☐ Self ☐ Spouse ☐ Child ☐ Other

Employer: _____   Phone: ( ) _____

Employer's Address: _____

Policy/I.D. No: _____   Group No: _____   Percent Covered: _____ %, Copay Amt: $ _____

Reason for Visit: Yearly gynecological exam

Known Allergies: _____

Were you referred here? If so, by whom? _____

CASE A-5 SOAP

01/23/20XX

Assignment of Benefits: Y

Signature on File: Y

Referring Physician: N

S: Celeste Donegan is in office today for a gynecological exam. She presents without complaints.

O: Pelvic and abdominal exam negative. Breasts: No masses felt.

A: 1. Routine gynecological exam with pap—ICD-10 (Z01.419)

P: 1. Healthy female gynecological examination.
     2. Chlamydia screen today.
     3. Return p.r.n.

_____

Bette R. Soone, M.D.

Obstetrics/Gynecology

NPI: 0987654321

Date of service:	01/23/XX			Waiver? ☐				
Patient name:	Celeste Donegan			Insurance:				
				Subscriber name:				
Address:	2829 Pine Ln			Group #:			Previous balance:	
	Township, NY 12345			Copay:			Today's charges:	
Phone:	555-555-6789			Account #:			Today's payment: check#	
DOB:	12/20/1981	Age:	Sex:	Physician name:			Balance due:	

RANK	Office visit	New	Est	RANK	Office procedures			RANK	Laboratory	
	Minimal		99211		Anoscopy		46600	X	Venipuncture	36415
	Problem focused	99201	99212		Audiometry		92551		Blood glucose, monitoring device	82962
	Expanded problem focused	99202	99213		Cerumen removal		69210		Blood glucose, visual dipstick	82948
	Detailed	99203	99214		Colposcopy		57452		CBC, w/ auto differential	85025
	Comprehensive	99204	99215		Colposcopy w/biopsy		57455		CBC, w/o auto differential	85027
	Comprehensive (new patient)	99205			ECG, w/interpretation		93000		Cholesterol	82465
	Significant, separate service	-25	-25		ECG, rhythm strip		93040		Hemoccult, guaiac	82270
	Well visit	**New**	**Est**		Endometrial biopsy		58100		Hemoccult, immunoassay	82274
	< 1 y	99381	99391		Flexible sigmoidoscopy		45330		Hemoglobin A1C	85018
	1-4 y	99382	99392		Flexible sigmoidoscopy w/biopsy		45331		Lipid panel	80061
	5-11 y	99383	99393		Fracture care, cast/splint		29___		Liver panel	80076
	12-17 y	99384	99394		Site: _____				KOH prep (skin, hair, nails)	87220
X	18-39 y	99385	99395		Nebulizer		94640		Metabolic panel, basic	80048
	40-64 y	99386	99396		Nebulizer demo		94664		Metabolic panel, comprehensive	80053
	65 y +	99387	99397		Spirometry		94010		Mononucleosis	86308
	Medicare preventive services				Spirometry, pre and post		94060		Pregnancy, blood	84703
	Pap		Q0091		Tympanometry		92567		Pregnancy, urine	81025
	Pelvic & breast		G0101		Vasectomy		55250		Renal panel	80069
	Prostate/PSA		G0103		**Skin procedures**		**Units**		Sedimentation rate	85651
	Tobacco counseling/3-10 min		99406		Burn care, initial	16000			Strep, rapid	86403
	Tobacco counseling/>10 min		99407		Foreign body, skin, simple	10120			Strep culture	87081
	Welcome to Medicare exam		G0344		Foreign body, skin, complex	10121			Strep A	87880
	ECG w/Welcome to Medicare exam		G0366		I&D, abscess	10060			TB	86580
	Flexible sigmoidoscopy		G0104		I&D, hematoma/seroma	10140		X	UA, complete, non-automated	81000
	Hemoccult, guaiac		G0107		Laceration repair, simple	120___			UA, w/o micro, non-automated	81002
	Flu shot		G0008		Site: _____ Size: _____				UA, w/ micro, non-automated	81003
	Pneumonia shot		G0009		Laceration repair, layered	120___			Urine colony count	87086
	Consultation/preop clearance				Site: _____ Size: _____				Urine culture, presumptive	87088
	Expanded problem focused		99242		Lesion, biopsy, one	11100			Wet mount/KOH	87210
	Detailed		99243		Lesion, biopsy, each add'l	11101			**Vaccines**	
	Comprehensive/mod complexity		99244		Lesion, destruct., benign, 1-14	17110			DT, <7 y	90702
	Comprehensive/high complexity		99245		Lesion, destruct., premal., single	17000			DTP	90701
	Other services				Lesion, destruct., premal., ea. add'l	17003			DtaP, <7 y	90700
	After posted hours		99050		Lesion, excision, benign	114___			Flu, 6-35 months	90657
	Evening/weekend appointment		99051		Site: _____ Size: _____				Flu, 3 y +	90658
	Home health certification		G0180		Lesion, excision, malignant	116___			Hep A, adult	90632
	Home health recertification		G0179		Site: _____ Size: _____				Hep A, ped/adol, 2 dose	90633
	Post-op follow-up		99024		Lesion, paring/cutting, one	11055			Hep B, adult	90746
	Prolonged/30-74 min		99354		Lesion, paring/cutting, 2-4	11056			Hep B, ped/adol 3 dose	90744
	Special reports/forms		99080		Lesion, shave	113___			Hep B-Hib	90748
	Disability/Workers comp		99455		Site: _____ Size: _____				Hib, 4 dose	90645
	Radiology				Nail removal, partial	11730			HPV	90649
					Nail removal, w/matrix	11750			IPV	90713
					Skin tag, 1-15	11200			MMR	90707
	Diagnoses				**Medications**		**Units**		Pneumonia, >2 y	90732
1	H10.33				Ampicillin, up to 500mg	J0290			Pneumonia conjugate, <5 y	90669
2					B-12, up to 1,000 mcg	J3420			Td, >7 y	90718
3					Epinephrine, up to 1ml	J0170			Varicella	90716
4					Kenalog, 10mg	J3301			**Immunizations & Injections**	**Units**
	Next office visit				Lidocaine, 10mg	J2001			Allergen, one	95115
Recheck	Prev	PRN	___ D W M Y		Normal saline, 1000cc	J7030			Allergen, multiple	95117
Instructions:					Phenergan, up to 50mg	J2550			Imm admin, one	90471
					Progesterone, 150mg	J1055			Imm admin, each add'l	90472
					Rocephin, 250mg	J0696			Imm admin, intranasal, one	90473
					Testosterone, 200mg	J1080			Imm admin, intranasal, each add'l	90474
	Referral				Tigan, up to 200 mg	J3250			Injection, joint, small	20600
To:					Toradol, 15mg	J1885			Injection, joint, intermediate	20605
					Miscellaneous services				Injection, joint, major	20610
Instructions:									Injection, ther/proph/diag	90772
					Cytopathology - 88142, 88155				Injection, trigger point	20552
Physician signature					Chlamydia culture - 87110				**Supplies**	
X _____										

CASE A-5 ENCOUNTER FORM

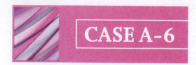

CASE A-6

Capital City Medical—123 Unknown Boulevard, Capital City, NY 12345-2222, (555) 555-1234

Phil Wells, M.D., Mannie Mends, M.D., Bette R. Soone, M.D.

Patient Information Form

Tax ID: 75-0246810

Group NPI: 1513171216

Patient Information:

Name: (Last, First) Clemenza, Carlos   ☒ Male   ☐ Female   Birth Date: 02/27/2012

Address: 33 Oak St, Capital City, NY 12345   Phone: (555) 555-4577

Social Security Number: 313-80-7422   Full-Time Student: ☐ Yes   ☒ No

Marital Status: ☒ Single   ☐ Married   ☐ Divorced   ☐ Other

Employment:

Employer: _____   Phone: ( ) _____

Address: _____

Condition Related to: ☐ Auto Accident   ☐ Employment   ☐ Other Accident

Date of Accident: _____ State _____

Emergency Contact: _____   Phone: ( ) _____

Primary Insurance: Blue Cross Blue Shield HMO   Phone: ( ) _____

Address: 379 Blue Plaza, Capital City, NY 12345

Insurance Policyholder's Name: Maria Clemenza   ☐ M   ☒ F   DOB: 06/25/1985

Address: Same

Phone: _____   Relationship to Insured: ☐ Self ☐ Spouse ☒ Child ☐ Other

Employer: Carrollton Wing Shack   Phone: (555) 555-1717

Employer's Address: 1604 State St, Capital City, NY 12345

Policy/I.D. No: YYJ885631259 Group No: 162878 Percent Covered: ___%, Copay Amt: $10.00

Secondary Insurance: _____   Phone: ( ) _____

Address: _____

Insurance Policyholder's Name: _____   ☐ M   ☐ F   DOB: _____

Address: _____

Phone: _____ Relationship to Insured: ☐ Self ☐ Spouse ☐ Child ☐ Other

Employer: _____   Phone: ( ) _____

Employer's Address: _____

Policy/I.D. No: _____ Group No: _____ Percent Covered: ____%, Copay Amt: $

Reason for Visit: Right ear pain

Known Allergies: _____

Were you referred here? If so, by whom? _____

07/16/20XX

Assignment of Benefits: Y

Signature on File: Y

Referring Physician: N

CASE A-6 SOAP

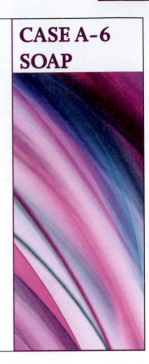

S: Carlos Clemenza presents for his well exam. His mother says he has been complaining of pain in his right ear since yesterday evening.

O: Pt. is 5 years old. His right ear is swollen, and there is minimal drainage. His left ear is unremarkable.

A: 1. Otitis media—ICD-10 (H66.90)

2. Well child exam—ICD-10 (Z00.129)

P: 1. Start Amox 1 b.i.d. × 10 days.

Phil Wells, M.D.

Family Practice

NPI: 1234567890

Date of service:	07/16XX			Waiver? ☐				
Patient name:	Carlos Clemenza			Insurance:				
				Subscriber name:				
Address:	33 Oak St			Group #:			Previous balance:	
	Capital City NY 12345			Copay:			Today's charges:	
Phone:	555-555-4577			Account #:			Today's payment: check#	
DOB:	02/27/2012 Age: Sex:			Physician name:			Balance due:	

RANK	Office visit	New	Est
	Minimal		99211
X	Problem focused	99201	99212
	Expanded problem focused	99202	99213
	Detailed	99203	99214
	Comprehensive	99204	99215
	Comprehensive (new patient)	99205	
X	Significant, separate service	-25	-25
	Well visit	**New**	**Est**
	< 1 y	99381	99391
	1-4 y	99382	99392
X	5-11 y	99383	99393
	12-17 y	99384	99394
	18-39 y	99385	99395
	40-64 y	99386	99396
	65 y +	99387	99397
	Medicare preventive services		
	Pap		Q0091
	Pelvic & breast		G0101
	Prostate/PSA		G0103
	Tobacco counseling/3-10 min		99406
	Tobacco counseling/>10 min		99407
	Welcome to Medicare exam		G0344
	ECG w/Welcome to Medicare exam		G0366
	Flexible sigmoidoscopy		G0104
	Hemoccult, guaiac		G0107
	Flu shot		G0008
	Pneumonia shot		G0009
	Consultation/preop clearance		
	Expanded problem focused		99242
	Detailed		99243
	Comprehensive/mod complexity		99244
	Comprehensive/high complexity		99245
	Other services		
	After posted hours		99050
	Evening/weekend appointment		99051
	Home health certification		G0180
	Home health recertification		G0179
	Post-op follow-up		99024
	Prolonged/30-74 min		99354
	Special reports/forms		99080
	Disability/Workers comp		99455
	Radiology		

RANK	Office procedures		
	Anoscopy		46600
	Audiometry		92551
	Cerumen removal		69210
	Colposcopy		57452
	Colposcopy w/biopsy		57455
	ECG, w/interpretation		93000
	ECG, rhythm strip		93040
	Endometrial biopsy		58100
	Flexible sigmoidoscopy		45330
	Flexible sigmoidoscopy w/biopsy		45331
	Fracture care, cast/splint		29____
	Site:		
	Nebulizer		94640
	Nebulizer demo		94664
	Spirometry		94010
	Spirometry, pre and post		94060
	Tympanometry		92567
	Vasectomy		55250
	Skin procedures		**Units**
	Burn care, initial	16000	
	Foreign body, skin, simple	10120	
	Foreign body, skin, complex	10121	
	I&D, abscess	10060	
	I&D, hematoma/seroma	10140	
	Laceration repair, simple	120___	
	Site: _____ Size: _____		
	Laceration repair, layered	120___	
	Site: _____ Size: _____		
	Lesion, biopsy, one	11100	
	Lesion, biopsy, each add'l	11101	
	Lesion, destruct., benign, 1-14	17110	
	Lesion, destruct., premal., single	17000	
	Lesion, destruct., premal., ea. add'l	17003	
	Lesion, excision, benign	114___	
	Site: _____ Size: _____		
	Lesion, excision, malignant	116___	
	Site: _____ Size: _____		
	Lesion, paring/cutting, one	11055	
	Lesion, paring/cutting, 2-4	11056	
	Lesion, shave	113___	
	Site: _____ Size: _____		
	Nail removal, partial	11730	
	Nail removal, w/matrix	11750	
	Skin tag, 1-15	11200	
	Medications		**Units**
	Ampicillin, up to 500mg	J0290	
	B-12, up to 1,000 mcg	J3420	
	Epinephrine, up to 1ml	J0170	
	Kenalog, 10mg	J3301	
	Lidocaine, 10mg	J2001	
	Normal saline, 1000cc	J7030	
	Phenergan, up to 50mg	J2550	
	Progesterone, 150mg	J1055	
	Rocephin, 250mg	J0696	
	Testosterone, 200mg	J1080	
	Tigan, up to 200 mg	J3250	
	Toradol, 15mg	J1885	
	Miscellaneous services		

RANK	Laboratory	
	Venipuncture	36415
	Blood glucose, monitoring device	82962
	Blood glucose, visual dipstick	82948
	CBC, w/ auto differential	85025
	CBC, w/o auto differential	85027
	Cholesterol	82465
	Hemoccult, guaiac	82270
	Hemoccult, immunoassay	82274
	Hemoglobin A1C	85018
	Lipid panel	80061
	Liver panel	80076
	KOH prep (skin, hair, nails)	87220
	Metabolic panel, basic	80048
	Metabolic panel, comprehensive	80053
	Mononucleosis	86308
	Pregnancy, blood	84703
	Pregnancy, urine	81025
	Renal panel	80069
	Sedimentation rate	85651
	Strep, rapid	86403
	Strep culture	87081
	Strep A	87880
	TB	86580
	UA, complete, non-automated	81000
	UA, w/o micro, non-automated	81002
	UA, w/ micro, non-automated	81003
	Urine colony count	87086
	Urine culture, presumptive	87088
	Wet mount/KOH	87210
	Vaccines	
	DT, <7 y	90702
	DTP	90701
	DtaP, <7 y	90700
	Flu, 6-35 months	90657
	Flu, 3 y +	90658
	Hep A, adult	90632
	Hep A, ped/adol, 2 dose	90633
	Hep B, adult	90746
	Hep B, ped/adol 3 dose	90744
	Hep B-Hib	90748
	Hib, 4 dose	90645
	HPV	90649
	IPV	90713
	MMR	90707
	Pneumonia, >2 y	90732
	Pneumonia conjugate, <5 y	90669
	Td, >7 y	90718
	Varicella	90716

RANK	Immunizations & Injections		Units
	Allergen, one	95115	
	Allergen, multiple	95117	
	Imm admin, one	90471	
	Imm admin, each add'l	90472	
	Imm admin, intranasal, one	90473	
	Imm admin, intranasal, each add'l	90474	
	Injection, joint, small	20600	
	Injection, joint, intermediate	20605	
	Injection, joint, major	20610	
	Injection, ther/proph/diag	90772	
	Injection, trigger point	20552	
	Supplies		

	Diagnoses
1	H66.90
2	Z00.129
3	
4	

Next office visit

Recheck	Prev	PRN	_____	D W M Y

Instructions:

Referral

To:

Instructions:

Physician signature

X _____

CASE A-6 ENCOUNTER FORM

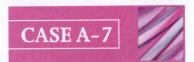

Capital City Medical—123 Unknown Boulevard, Capital City, NY 12345-2222, (555) 555-1234

Phil Wells, M.D., Mannie Mends, M.D., Bette R. Soone, M.D.

Patient Information Form

Tax ID: 75-0246810

Group NPI: 1513171216

Patient Information:

Name: (Last, First) Colich, Guy ☒ Male ☐ Female Birth Date: 04/23/1958

Address: 872 Hickory Pl, Capital City, NY 12345 Phone: (555) 555-9069

Social Security Number: 142-86-2078 Full-Time Student: ☐ Yes ☒ No

Marital Status: ☐ Single ☒ Married ☐ Divorced ☐ Other

Employment:

Employer: None Phone:

Address:

Condition Related to: ☐ Auto Accident ☐ Employment ☐ Other Accident

Date of Accident: State

Emergency Contact: Phone: ( )

Primary Insurance: Aetna Phone: ( )

Address: 1625 Healthcare Bldg, Capital City, NY 12345

Insurance Policyholder's Name: Same ☐ M ☐ F DOB:

Address:

Phone: Relationship to Insured: ☒ Self ☐ Spouse ☐ Child ☐ Other

Employer: Phone:

Employer's Address:

Policy/I.D. No: 9567305 Group No: 511669 Percent Covered: %, Copay Amt: $35.00

Secondary Insurance: Phone: ( )

Address:

Insurance Policyholder's Name: ☐ M ☐ F DOB:

Address:

Phone: Relationship to Insured: ☐ Self ☐ Spouse ☐ Child ☐ Other

Employer: Phone: ( )

Employer's Address:

Policy/I.D. No: Group No: Percent Covered: %, Copay Amt: $

Reason for Visit: I am here for a recheck on my manic depression

Known Allergies:

Were you referred here? If so, by whom?

CASE A-7 SOAP

10/07/20XX
Assignment of Benefits: Y
Signature on File: Y
Referring Physician: N

S: Guy Colich presents today for a checkup on his manic depression.

O: Pt. says that he has been taking his medicine faithfully since the last visit. Lab displays good value. Mental status is normal, alert, and oriented × 3. He has no complaints today.

A: 1. Bipolar disorder—ICD-10 (F31.9)

P: 1. Pt. is to keep psychotherapy appointment for this month.
    2. Return in 1 month for recheck on lithium level.

_____

Phil Wells, M.D.
Family Practice
NPI: 1234567890

Date of service:	10/07/XX			Waiver? ☐				
Patient name:	Guy Colich			Insurance:				
				Subscriber name:				
Address:	872 Hickory Pl			Group #:			Previous balance:	
	Capital City, NY 12345			Copay:			Today's charges:	
Phone:	555-555-9069			Account #:			Today's payment: check#	
DOB:	04/23/1958 Age: Sex:			Physician name:			Balance due:	

RANK	Office visit	New	Est
	Minimal		99211
	Problem focused	99201	99212
X	Expanded problem focused	99202	99213
	Detailed	99203	99214
	Comprehensive	99204	99215
	Comprehensive (new patient)	99205	
	Significant, separate service	-25	-25

	Well visit	New	Est
	< 1 y	99381	99391
	1-4 y	99382	99392
	5-11 y	99383	99393
	12-17 y	99384	99394
	18-39 y	99385	99395
	40-64 y	99386	99396
	65 y +	99387	99397

	Medicare preventive services	
	Pap	Q0091
	Pelvic & breast	G0101
	Prostate/PSA	G0103
	Tobacco counseling/3-10 min	99406
	Tobacco counseling/>10 min	99407
	Welcome to Medicare exam	G0344
	ECG w/Welcome to Medicare exam	G0366
	Flexible sigmoidoscopy	G0104
	Hemoccult, guaiac	G0107
	Flu shot	G0008
	Pneumonia shot	G0009

	Consultation/preop clearance	
	Expanded problem focused	99242
	Detailed	99243
	Comprehensive/mod complexity	99244
	Comprehensive/high complexity	99245

	Other services	
	After posted hours	99050
	Evening/weekend appointment	99051
	Home health certification	G0180
	Home health recertification	G0179
	Post-op follow-up	99024
	Prolonged/30-74 min	99354
	Special reports/forms	99080
	Disability/Workers comp	99455

	Radiology	

	Diagnoses
1	F31.9
2	
3	
4	

Next office visit

Recheck	Prev	PRN	_____	D	W	M	Y

Instructions:

Referral

To:

Instructions:

Physician signature

X _____

RANK	Office procedures		
	Anoscopy		46600
	Audiometry		92551
	Cerumen removal		69210
	Colposcopy		57452
	Colposcopy w/biopsy		57455
	ECG, w/interpretation		93000
	ECG, rhythm strip		93040
	Endometrial biopsy		58100
	Flexible sigmoidoscopy		45330
	Flexible sigmoidoscopy w/biopsy		45331
	Fracture care, cast/splint		29____
	Site:		
	Nebulizer		94640
	Nebulizer demo		94664
	Spirometry		94010
	Spirometry, pre and post		94060
	Tympanometry		92567
	Vasectomy		55250

	Skin procedures		Units
	Burn care, initial	16000	
	Foreign body, skin, simple	10120	
	Foreign body, skin, complex	10121	
	I&D, abscess	10060	
	I&D, hematoma/seroma	10140	
	Laceration repair, simple	120___	
	Site: ____ Size: ____		
	Laceration repair, layered	120___	
	Site: ____ Size: ____		
	Lesion, biopsy, one	11100	
	Lesion, biopsy, each add'l	11101	
	Lesion, destruct., benign, 1-14	17110	
	Lesion, destruct., premal., single	17000	
	Lesion, destruct., premal., ea. add'l	17003	
	Lesion, excision, benign	114___	
	Site: ____ Size: ____		
	Lesion, excision, malignant	116___	
	Site: ____ Size: ____		
	Lesion, paring/cutting, one	11055	
	Lesion, paring/cutting, 2-4	11056	
	Lesion, shave	113___	
	Site: ____ Size: ____		
	Nail removal, partial	11730	
	Nail removal, w/matrix	11750	
	Skin tag, 1-15	11200	

	Medications		Units
	Ampicillin, up to 500mg	J0290	
	B-12, up to 1,000 mcg	J3420	
	Epinephrine, up to 1ml	J0170	
	Kenalog, 10mg	J3301	
	Lidocaine, 10mg	J2001	
	Normal saline, 1000cc	J7030	
	Phenergan, up to 50mg	J2550	
	Progesterone, 150mg	J1055	
	Rocephin, 250mg	J0696	
	Testosterone, 200mg	J1080	
	Tigan, up to 200 mg	J3250	
	Toradol, 15mg	J1885	

	Miscellaneous services	

RANK	Laboratory	
	Venipuncture	36415
	Blood glucose, monitoring device	82962
	Blood glucose, visual dipstick	82948
	CBC, w/ auto differential	85025
	CBC, w/o auto differential	85027
	Cholesterol	82465
	Hemoccult, guaiac	82270
	Hemoccult, immunoassay	82274
	Hemoglobin A1C	85018
	Lipid panel	80061
	Liver panel	80076
	KOH prep (skin, hair, nails)	87220
	Metabolic panel, basic	80048
	Metabolic panel, comprehensive	80053
	Mononucleosis	86308
	Pregnancy, blood	84703
	Pregnancy, urine	81025
	Renal panel	80069
	Sedimentation rate	85651
	Strep, rapid	86403
	Strep culture	87081
	Strep A	87880
	TB	86580
	UA, complete, non-automated	81000
	UA, w/o micro, non-automated	81002
	UA, w/ micro, non-automated	81003
	Urine colony count	87086
	Urine culture, presumptive	87088
	Wet mount/KOH	87210

	Vaccines	
	DT, <7 y	90702
	DTP	90701
	DtaP, <7 y	90700
	Flu, 6-35 months	90657
	Flu, 3 y +	90658
	Hep A, adult	90632
	Hep A, ped/adol, 2 dose	90633
	Hep B, adult	90746
	Hep B, ped/adol 3 dose	90744
	Hep B-Hib	90748
	Hib, 4 dose	90645
	HPV	90649
	IPV	90713
	MMR	90707
	Pneumonia, >2 y	90732
	Pneumonia conjugate, <5 y	90669
	Td, >7 y	90718
	Varicella	90716

	Immunizations & Injections		Units
	Allergen, one	95115	
	Allergen, multiple	95117	
	Imm admin, one	90471	
	Imm admin, each add'l	90472	
	Imm admin, intranasal, one	90473	
	Imm admin, intranasal, each add'l	90474	
	Injection, joint, small	20600	
	Injection, joint, intermediate	20605	
	Injection, joint, major	20610	
	Injection, ther/proph/diag	90772	
	Injection, trigger point	20552	

	Supplies	

CASE A-7 ENCOUNTER FORM

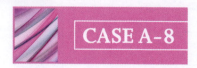

CASE A-8

Patient Information:

Name: (Last, First) Davies, Klaus   ☒ Male   ☐ Female   Birth Date: 10/24/1965

Address: 19 Willow Rd, Capital City, NY 12345   Phone: (555) 555-1276

Social Security Number: 631-03-4305   Full-Time Student: ☐ Yes   ☒ No

Marital Status: ☐ Single   ☒ Married   ☐ Divorced   ☐ Other

Employment:

Employer: Organic Food Mart   Phone: (555) 555-5619

Address: 13 Mile Blvd, Township, NY 12345

Condition Related to: ☐ Auto Accident   ☐ Employment   ☐ Other Accident

Date of Accident: _____ State _____

Emergency Contact: _____   Phone: ( ) _____

Primary Insurance: Blue Cross Blue Shield PPO   Phone: ( ) _____

Address: 379 Blue Plaza, Capital City, NY 12345

Insurance Policyholder's Name: Same _____   ☐ M   ☐ F   DOB: _____

Address: _____

Phone: _____   Relationship to Insured: ☒ Self ☐ Spouse ☐ Child ☐ Other

Employer: _____   Phone: _____

Employer's Address: _____

Policy/I.D. No: YYZ8436489 Group No: 326463 Percent Covered: __%, Copay Amt: $35.00

Secondary Insurance: _____   Phone: ( ) _____

Address: _____

Insurance Policyholder's Name: _____   ☐ M   ☐ F   DOB: _____

Address: _____

Phone: _____ Relationship to Insured: ☐ Self ☐ Spouse ☐ Child ☐ Other

Employer: _____   Phone: _____

Employer's Address: _____

Policy/I.D. No: Group No: Percent Covered: %, Copay Amt: $

Reason for Visit: Need my blood pressure and cholesterol checked today _____

Known Allergies: _____

Were you referred here? If so, by whom? _____

CASE A-8 SOAP

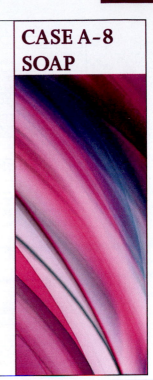

10/26/20XX
Assignment of Benefits: Y
Signature on File: Y
Referring Physician: N

S: Klaus Davies is in the office for a checkup on HTN and hypercholesterolemia.

O: Pt. denies any headaches, dizziness, or CP. Says he feels good. Vitals: P 88, R 16, BP 142/72. Review of lab shows stable numbers with total cholesterol at 222.

A: 1. HTN—ICD-10 (I10)

2. Hypercholesterolemia—ICD-10 (E78.00)

P: 1. Refill Lipitor 20 mg 1 daily, 30 × 3.

2. Repeat fasting lab in 3 months.

3. Schedule checkup in 3 months.

Phil Wells, M.D.
Family Practice
NPI: 1234567890

Date of service:	10/26/XX			Waiver? ☐		
Patient name:	Klause Davies			Insurance:		
				Subscriber name:		
Address:	19 Willow Rd			Group #:		Previous balance:
	Capital City, NY 12345			Copay:		Today's charges:
Phone:	555-555-1276			Account #:		Today's payment: check#
DOB:	10/24/1965 Age: Sex:			Physician name:		Balance due:

RANK	Office visit	New	Est
	Minimal		99211
	Problem focused	99201	99212
X	Expanded problem focused	99202	99213
	Detailed	99203	99214
	Comprehensive	99204	99215
	Comprehensive (new patient)	99205	
	Significant, separate service	-25	-25
	Well visit	**New**	**Est**
	< 1 y	99381	99391
	1-4 y	99382	99392
	5-11 y	99383	99393
	12-17 y	99384	99394
	18-39 y	99385	99395
	40-64 y	99386	99396
	65 y +	99387	99397
	Medicare preventive services		
	Pap		Q0091
	Pelvic & breast		G0101
	Prostate/PSA		G0103
	Tobacco counseling/3-10 min		99406
	Tobacco counseling/>10 min		99407
	Welcome to Medicare exam		G0344
	ECG w/Welcome to Medicare exam		G0366
	Flexible sigmoidoscopy		G0104
	Hemoccult, guaiac		G0107
	Flu shot		G0008
	Pneumonia shot		G0009
	Consultation/preop clearance		
	Expanded problem focused		99242
	Detailed		99243
	Comprehensive/mod complexity		99244
	Comprehensive/high complexity		99245
	Other services		
	After posted hours		99050
	Evening/weekend appointment		99051
	Home health certification		G0180
	Home health recertification		G0179
	Post-op follow-up		99024
	Prolonged/30-74 min		99354
	Special reports/forms		99080
	Disability/Workers comp		99455
	Radiology		

	Diagnoses
1	I10
2	E78.00
3	
4	

Next office visit

| Recheck | Prev | PRN | _____ | D | W | M | Y |

Instructions:

Referral

To:

Instructions:

Physician signature

X _____

RANK	Office procedures		
	Anoscopy		46600
	Audiometry		92551
	Cerumen removal		69210
	Colposcopy		57452
	Colposcopy w/biopsy		57455
	ECG, w/interpretation		93000
	ECG, rhythm strip		93040
	Endometrial biopsy		58100
	Flexible sigmoidoscopy		45330
	Flexible sigmoidoscopy w/biopsy		45331
	Fracture care, cast/splint		29____
	Site: _____		
	Nebulizer		94640
	Nebulizer demo		94664
	Spirometry		94010
	Spirometry, pre and post		94060
	Tympanometry		92567
	Vasectomy		55250
	Skin procedures		**Units**
	Burn care, initial	16000	
	Foreign body, skin, simple	10120	
	Foreign body, skin, complex	10121	
	I&D, abscess	10060	
	I&D, hematoma/seroma	10140	
	Laceration repair, simple	120____	
	Site: _____ Size: _____		
	Laceration repair, layered	120____	
	Site: _____ Size: _____		
	Lesion, biopsy, one	11100	
	Lesion, biopsy, each add'l	11101	
	Lesion, destruct., benign, 1-14	17110	
	Lesion, destruct., premal., single	17000	
	Lesion, destruct., premal., ea. add'l	17003	
	Lesion, excision, benign	114____	
	Site: _____ Size: _____		
	Lesion, excision, malignant	116____	
	Site: _____ Size: _____		
	Lesion, paring/cutting, one	11055	
	Lesion, paring/cutting, 2-4	11056	
	Lesion, shave	113____	
	Site: _____ Size: _____		
	Nail removal, partial	11730	
	Nail removal, w/matrix	11750	
	Skin tag, 1-15	11200	
	Medications		**Units**
	Ampicillin, up to 500mg	J0290	
	B-12, up to 1,000 mcg	J3420	
	Epinephrine, up to 1ml	J0170	
	Kenalog, 10mg	J3301	
	Lidocaine, 10mg	J2001	
	Normal saline, 1000cc	J7030	
	Phenergan, up to 50mg	J2550	
	Progesterone, 150mg	J1055	
	Rocephin, 250mg	J0696	
	Testosterone, 200mg	J1080	
	Tigan, up to 200 mg	J3250	
	Toradol, 15mg	J1885	
	Miscellaneous services		

RANK	Laboratory	
X	Venipuncture	36415
	Blood glucose, monitoring device	82962
	Blood glucose, visual dipstick	82948
X	CBC, w/ auto differential	85025
	CBC, w/o auto differential	85027
	Cholesterol	82465
	Hemoccult, guaiac	82270
	Hemoccult, immunoassay	82274
	Hemoglobin A1C	85018
X	Lipid panel	80061
X	Liver panel	80076
	KOH prep (skin, hair, nails)	87220
	Metabolic panel, basic	80048
	Metabolic panel, comprehensive	80053
	Mononucleosis	86308
	Pregnancy, blood	84703
	Pregnancy, urine	81025
	Renal panel	80069
	Sedimentation rate	85651
	Strep, rapid	86403
	Strep culture	87081
	Strep A	87880
	TB	86580
	UA, complete, non-automated	81000
	UA, w/o micro, non-automated	81002
	UA, w/ micro, non-automated	81003
	Urine colony count	87086
	Urine culture, presumptive	87088
	Wet mount/KOH	87210
	Vaccines	
	DT, <7 y	90702
	DTP	90701
	DtaP, <7 y	90700
	Flu, 6-35 months	90657
	Flu, 3 y +	90658
	Hep A, adult	90632
	Hep A, ped/adol, 2 dose	90633
	Hep B, adult	90746
	Hep B, ped/adol 3 dose	90744
	Hep B-Hib	90748
	Hib, 4 dose	90645
	HPV	90649
	IPV	90713
	MMR	90707
	Pneumonia, >2 y	90732
	Pneumonia conjugate, <5 y	90669
	Td, >7 y	90718
	Varicella	90716
	Immunizations & Injections	**Units**
	Allergen, one	95115
	Allergen, multiple	95117
	Imm admin, one	90471
	Imm admin, each add'l	90472
	Imm admin, intranasal, one	90473
	Imm admin, intranasal, each add'l	90474
	Injection, joint, small	20600
	Injection, joint, intermediate	20605
	Injection, joint, major	20610
	Injection, ther/proph/diag	90772
	Injection, trigger point	20552
	Supplies	

CASE A-8 ENCOUNTER FORM

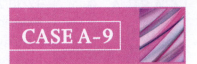

Capital City Medical—123 Unknown Boulevard, Capital City, NY 12345-2222, (555) 555-1234

Phil Wells, M.D., Mannie Mends, M.D., Bette R. Soone, M.D.

Patient Information Form

Tax ID: 75-0246810

Group NPI: 1513171216

Patient Information:

Name: (Last, First) Vogel, Matilda   ☐ Male   ☐ Female   Birth Date: 05/19/1974

Address: 431 Forrest Ave, Capital City, NY 12345   Phone: (555) 555-5634

Social Security Number: 601-51-7806   Full-Time Student: ☐ Yes   ☒ No

Marital Status: ☐ Single   ☒ Married   ☐ Divorced   ☐ Other

Employment:

Employer: Roxie's Record Den   Phone: (555) 555-9873

Address: 6446 Lockhurst Ave, Capital City, NY 12345

Condition Related to: ☐ Auto Accident   ☐ Employment   ☐ Other Accident

Date of Accident: _____ State _____

Emergency Contact: _____   Phone: ( ) _____

Primary Insurance: Tricare   Phone: ( ) _____

Address: 7594 Forces-Run Rd, Millitaryville, NY 12345

Insurance Policyholder's Name: Edward Vogel   ☒ M   ☐ F   DOB: 02/17/1979

Address: Same

Phone: _____   Relationship to Insured: ☐ Self   ☒ Spouse   ☐ Child   ☐ Other

Employer: United States Army Reserves   Phone: ( ) _____

Employer's Address: 43 S. Army Blvd, Millitaryville, NY 12345

Policy/I.D. No: 333 22 9867   Group No: ___   Percent Covered: ___%, Copay Amt: $35.00

Secondary Insurance: _____   Phone: ( ) _____

Address: _____

Insurance Policyholder's Name: _____   ☐ M   ☐ F   DOB: _____

Address: _____

Phone: _____   Relationship to Insured: ☐ Self   ☐ Spouse   ☐ Child   ☐ Other

Employer: _____   Phone: ( ) _____

Employer's Address: _____

Policy/I.D. No: _____   Group No: _____   Percent Covered: _____%, Copay Amt: $ _____

Reason for Visit: I have burning when I urinate

Known Allergies: _____

Were you referred here? If so, by whom? _____

CASE A-9 SOAP

12/30/20XX
Assignment of Benefits: Y
Signature on File: Y
Referring Physician: N

S: New patient, Matilda Vogel, is in the office for a burning sensation upon urination. She thinks it may be a vaginal yeast infection.

O: Social history negative for any promiscuity. Vulva negative for yeast. U/A with C&S ordered. Positive for WBCs.

A: 1. UTI—ICD-10 (N39.0), due to *E. coli* infection—ICD-10 (B96.21)

P: 1. Septra DS 1 q.i.d. for 7 days.

   2. Recommended cranberry juice.

_____

Bette R. Soone, M.D.
Obstetrics/Gynecology
NPI: 9876543210

Date of service:	12/30/XX				Waiver? ☐			
Patient name:	Matilda Vogel				Insurance:			
					Subscriber name:			
Address:	431 Forrest Ave Capital City NY 12345				Group #:		Previous balance:	
					Copay:		Today's charges:	
Phone:	555-555-5634				Account #:		Today's payment: check#	
DOB:	05/19/1974 Age: Sex:				Physician name:		Balance due:	

RANK	Office visit	New	Est	RANK	Office procedures		Units	RANK	Laboratory	
	Minimal		99211		Anoscopy	46600			Venipuncture	36415
	Problem focused	99201	99212 X		Audiometry	92551			Blood glucose, monitoring device	82962
	Expanded problem focused	99202	99213		Cerumen removal	69210			Blood glucose, visual dipstick	82948
X	Detailed	99203	99214		Colposcopy	57452			CBC, w/ auto differential	85025
	Comprehensive	99204	99215		Colposcopy w/biopsy	57455			CBC, w/o auto differential	85027
	Comprehensive (new patient)	99205			ECG, w/interpretation	93000			Cholesterol	82465
	Significant, separate service	-25	-25		ECG, rhythm strip	93040			Hemoccult, guaiac	82270
	Well visit	**New**	**Est**		Endometrial biopsy	58100			Hemoccult, immunoassay	82274
	< 1 y	99381	99391		Flexible sigmoidoscopy	45330			Hemoglobin A1C	85018
	1-4 y	99382	99392		Flexible sigmoidoscopy w/biopsy	45331			Lipid panel	80061
	5-11 y	99383	99393		Fracture care, cast/splint	29___			Liver panel	80076
	12-17 y	99384	99394		Site:				KOH prep (skin, hair, nails)	87220
	18-39 y	99385	99395		Nebulizer	94640			Metabolic panel, basic	80048
	40-64 y	99386	99396		Nebulizer demo	94664			Metabolic panel, comprehensive	80053
	65 y +	99387	99397		Spirometry	94010			Mononucleosis	86308
	Medicare preventive services				Spirometry, pre and post	94060			Pregnancy, blood	84703
	Pap		Q0091		Tympanometry	92567			Pregnancy, urine	81025
	Pelvic & breast		G0101		Vasectomy	55250			Renal panel	80069
	Prostate/PSA		G0103		**Skin procedures**		**Units**		Sedimentation rate	85651
	Tobacco counseling/3-10 min		99406		Burn care, initial	16000			Strep, rapid	86403
	Tobacco counseling/>10 min		99407		Foreign body, skin, simple	10120			Strep culture	87081
	Welcome to Medicare exam		G0344		Foreign body, skin, complex	10121			Strep A	87880
	ECG w/Welcome to Medicare exam		G0366		I&D, abscess	10060			TB	86580
	Flexible sigmoidoscopy		G0104		I&D, hematoma/seroma	10140		X	UA, complete, non-automated	81000
	Hemoccult, guaiac		G0107		Laceration repair, simple	120___			UA, w/o micro, non-automated	81002
	Flu shot		G0008		Site:___ Size:___				UA, w/ micro, non-automated	81003
	Pneumonia shot		G0009		Laceration repair, layered	120___			Urine colony count	87086
	Consultation/preop clearance				Site:___ Size:___			X	Urine culture, presumptive	87088
	Expanded problem focused		99242		Lesion, biopsy, one	11100			Wet mount/KOH	87210
	Detailed		99243		Lesion, biopsy, each add'l	11101			**Vaccines**	
	Comprehensive/mod complexity		99244		Lesion, destruct., benign, 1-14	17110			DT, <7 y	90702
	Comprehensive/high complexity		99245		Lesion, destruct., premal., single	17000			DTP	90701
	Other services				Lesion, destruct., premal., ea. add'l	17003			DtaP, <7 y	90700
	After posted hours		99050		Lesion, excision, benign	114___			Flu, 6-35 months	90657
	Evening/weekend appointment		99051		Site:___ Size:___				Flu, 3 y +	90658
	Home health certification		G0180		Lesion, excision, malignant	116___			Hep A, adult	90632
	Home health recertification		G0179		Site:___ Size:___				Hep A, ped/adol, 2 dose	90633
	Post-op follow-up		99024		Lesion, paring/cutting, one	11055			Hep B, adult	90746
	Prolonged/30-74 min		99354		Lesion, paring/cutting, 2-4	11056			Hep B, ped/adol 3 dose	90744
	Special reports/forms		99080		Lesion, shave	113___			Hep B-Hib	90748
	Disability/Workers comp		99455		Site:___ Size:___				Hib, 4 dose	90645
	Radiology				Nail removal, partial	11730			HPV	90649
					Nail removal, w/matrix	11750			IPV	90713
					Skin tag, 1-15	11200			MMR	90707
	Diagnoses				**Medications**		**Units**		Pneumonia, >2 y	90732
1	N39.0				Ampicillin, up to 500mg	J0290			Pneumonia conjugate, <5 y	90669
2	B96.21				B-12, up to 1,000 mcg	J3420			Td, >7 y	90718
3					Epinephrine, up to 1ml	J0170			Varicella	90716
4					Kenalog, 10mg	J3301			**Immunizations & Injections**	**Units**
	Next office visit				Lidocaine, 10mg	J2001			Allergen, one	95115
	Recheck Prev PRN ___ D W M Y				Normal saline, 1000cc	J7030			Allergen, multiple	95117
	Instructions:				Phenergan, up to 50mg	J2550			Imm admin, one	90471
					Progesterone, 150mg	J1055			Imm admin, each add'l	90472
					Rocephin, 250mg	J0696			Imm admin, intranasal, one	90473
					Testosterone, 200mg	J1080			Imm admin, intranasal, each add'l	90474
	Referral				Tigan, up to 200 mg	J3250			Injection, joint, small	20600
	To:				Toradol, 15mg	J1885			Injection, joint, intermediate	20605
	Instructions:				**Miscellaneous services**				Injection, joint, major	20610
									Injection, ther/proph/diag	90772
									Injection, trigger point	20552
	Physician signature								**Supplies**	
	X _____									

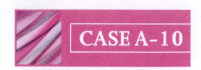

CASE A-10

Capital City Medical—123 Unknown Boulevard, Capital City, NY 12345-2222, (555) 555-1234

Phil Wells, M.D., Mannie Mends, M.D., Bette R. Soone, M.D.

Patient Information Form

Tax ID: 75-0246810

Group NPI: 1513171216

Patient Information:

Name: (Last, First) Houston, Isaac   ☒ Male   ☐ Female   Birth Date: 09/02/1961

Address: 71 Fern St, Capital City, NY 12345   Phone: (555) 555-2021

Social Security Number: 542-78-1236   Full-Time Student: ☐ Yes   ☐ No

Marital Status: ☒ Single   ☐ Married   ☐ Divorced   ☐ Other

Employment:

Employer: Mr. Construction Co.   Phone: (555) 555-6211

Address: 44 Builder's Dr, Capital City, NY 12345

Condition Related to: ☐ Auto Accident   ☒ Employment   ☐ Other Accident

Date of Accident: 05/18/20XX   State NY

Emergency Contact: _____   Phone: ( ) _____

Primary Insurance: Advantage Compensation Ins.   Phone: ( ) _____

Address: 1629 Accident Ave, Sickville NY 12345

Insurance Policyholder's Name: Mr. Construction Co.   ☐ M   ☐ F   DOB: _____

Address: See employer

Phone: _____   Relationship to Insured: ☐ Self ☐ Spouse ☐ Child ☒ Other

Employer: Mr. Construction Co.   Phone: ( ) _____

Employer's Address: See employer

Policy/I.D. No: Claim #H135246901 Group No: __ Percent Covered: __%, Copay Amt: $__

Secondary Insurance: Health America (if denied by WC)   Phone: ( ) _____

Address: 2031 Healthica Ctr, Capital City, NY 12345

Insurance Policyholder's Name: Same   ☐ M   ☐ F   DOB: _____

Address: _____

Phone: _____   Relationship to Insured: ☒ Self ☐ Spouse ☐ Child ☐ Other

Employer: _____ Phone: ( ) _____

Employer's Address: _____

Policy/I.D. No: 35643166   Group No: MRC753 Percent Covered: __%, Copay Amt: $35.00

Reason for Visit: I fell off a ladder at work and hurt my chest

Known Allergies: _____

Were you referred here? If so, by whom? _____

05/18/20XX
Assignment of Benefits: Y
Signature on File: Y
Referring Physician: N

CASE A-10 SOAP

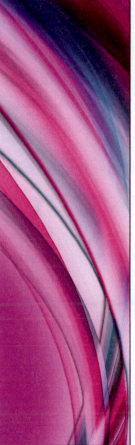

S: Isaac Houston presents today with pain in the right thoracic area. He fell off of a ladder at work today, almost 2 hours ago.

O: Pt. denies any trauma to any other body area. He does have pain during inspiration and expiration. Pt. was on a ladder putting up a shutter on a house when suddenly he lost his balance and fell to the ground. CXR shows 3 cracked ribs on the right side.

A: 1. Fracture; ribs—ICD-10 (S22.49XA)

2. Fall off of ladder—ICD-10 (W11.XXXA)

P: 1. Ibuprofen 1 b.i.d. for 15 days

2. Vicodin 1 q6h p.r.n. #20

3. Off work 3 days, then light duty

4. Please bill his workers' compensation. Info is as follows:

Advantage Compensation Ins.

1629 Accident Avenue

Sickville, NY 12345

Claim #H135246901

_____

Phil Wells, M.D.
Family Practice
NIP: 1234567890
PIN: 123456

Date of service:	05/18/XX			Waiver? ☐			
Patient name:		Isaac Houston		Insurance:			
				Subscriber name:			
Address:	731 Fern St			Group #:		Previous balance:	
	Capital City, NY 12345			Copay:		Today's charges:	
Phone:	555-555-2021			Account #:		Today's payment: check#	
DOB:	09/02/1961	Age:	Sex:	Physician name:		Balance due:	

RANK	Office visit	New	Est	RANK	Office procedures			RANK	Laboratory		
	Minimal		99211		Anoscopy		46600		Venipuncture		36415
	Problem focused	99201	99212		Audiometry		92551		Blood glucose, monitoring device		82962
X	Expanded problem focused	99202	99213		Cerumen removal		69210		Blood glucose, visual dipstick		82948
	Detailed	99203	99214		Colposcopy		57452		CBC, w/ auto differential		85025
	Comprehensive	99204	99215		Colposcopy w/biopsy		57455		CBC, w/o auto differential		85027
	Comprehensive (new patient)	99205			ECG, w/interpretation		93000		Cholesterol		82465
	Significant, separate service	-25	-25		ECG, rhythm strip		93040		Hemoccult, guaiac		82270
	Well visit	**New**	**Est**		Endometrial biopsy		58100		Hemoccult, immunoassay		82274
	< 1 y	99381	99391		Flexible sigmoidoscopy		45330		Hemoglobin A1C		85018
	1-4 y	99382	99392		Flexible sigmoidoscopy w/biopsy		45331		Lipid panel		80061
	5-11 y	99383	99393		Fracture care, cast/splint		29____		Liver panel		80076
	12-17 y	99384	99394		Site: _____				KOH prep (skin, hair, nails)		87220
	18-39 y	99385	99395		Nebulizer		94640		Metabolic panel, basic		80048
	40-64 y	99386	99396		Nebulizer demo		94664		Metabolic panel, comprehensive		80053
	65 y +	99387	99397		Spirometry		94010		Mononucleosis		86308
	Medicare preventive services				Spirometry, pre and post		94060		Pregnancy, blood		84703
	Pap		Q0091		Tympanometry		92567		Pregnancy, urine		81025
	Pelvic & breast		G0101		Vasectomy		55250		Renal panel		80069
	Prostate/PSA		G0103		**Skin procedures**		**Units**		Sedimentation rate		85651
	Tobacco counseling/3-10 min		99406		Burn care, initial	16000			Strep, rapid		86403
	Tobacco counseling/>10 min		99407		Foreign body, skin, simple	10120			Strep culture		87081
	Welcome to Medicare exam		G0344		Foreign body, skin, complex	10121			Strep A		87880
	ECG w/Welcome to Medicare exam		G0366		I&D, abscess	10060			TB		86580
	Flexible sigmoidoscopy		G0104		I&D, hematoma/seroma	10140			UA, complete, non-automated		81000
	Hemoccult, guaiac		G0107		Laceration repair, simple	120___			UA, w/o micro, non-automated		81002
	Flu shot		G0008		Site: _____ Size: _____				UA, w/ micro, non-automated		81003
	Pneumonia shot		G0009		Laceration repair, layered	120___			Urine colony count		87086
	Consultation/preop clearance				Site: _____ Size: _____				Urine culture, presumptive		87088
	Expanded problem focused		99242		Lesion, biopsy, one	11100			Wet mount/KOH		87210
	Detailed		99243		Lesion, biopsy, each add'l	11101			**Vaccines**		
	Comprehensive/mod complexity		99244		Lesion, destruct., benign, 1-14	17110			DT, <7 y		90702
	Comprehensive/high complexity		99245		Lesion, destruct., premal., single	17000			DTP		90701
	Other services				Lesion, destruct., premal., ea. add'l	17003			DtaP, <7 y		90700
	After posted hours		99050		Lesion, excision, benign	114___			Flu, 6-35 months		90657
	Evening/weekend appointment		99051		Site: _____ Size: _____				Flu, 3 y +		90658
	Home health certification		G0180		Lesion, excision, malignant	116___			Hep A, adult		90632
	Home health recertification		G0179		Site: _____ Size: _____				Hep A, ped/adol, 2 dose		90633
	Post-op follow-up		99024		Lesion, paring/cutting, one	11055			Hep B, adult		90746
	Prolonged/30-74 min		99354		Lesion, paring/cutting, 2-4	11056			Hep B, ped/adol 3 dose		90744
	Special reports/forms		99080		Lesion, shave	113___			Hep B-Hib		90748
	Disability/Workers comp		99455		Site: _____ Size: _____				Hib, 4 dose		90645
	Radiology				Nail removal, partial	11730			HPV		90649
	Chest X-ray - 71030				Nail removal, w/matrix	11750			IPV		90713
					Skin tag, 1-15	11200			MMR		90707
	Diagnoses				**Medications**		**Units**		Pneumonia, >2 y		90732
1	S22.49XA				Ampicillin, up to 500mg	J0290			Pneumonia conjugate, <5 y		90669
2	W11.XXXA				B-12, up to 1,000 mcg	J3420			Td, >7 y		90718
3					Epinephrine, up to 1ml	J0170			Varicella		90716
4					Kenalog, 10mg	J3301			**Immunizations & Injections**		**Units**

Next office visit

Recheck	Prev	PRN	_____	D W M Y

Instructions:

		Lidocaine, 10mg	J2001		Allergen, one	95115	
		Normal saline, 1000cc	J7030		Allergen, multiple	95117	
		Phenergan, up to 50mg	J2550		Imm admin, one	90471	
		Progesterone, 150mg	J1055		Imm admin, each add'l	90472	
		Rocephin, 250mg	J0696		Imm admin, intranasal, one	90473	
		Testosterone, 200mg	J1080		Imm admin, intranasal, each add'l	90474	

Referral

To:

		Tigan, up to 200 mg	J3250		Injection, joint, small	20600	
		Toradol, 15mg	J1885		Injection, joint, intermediate	20605	
		Miscellaneous services			Injection, joint, major	20610	

Instructions:

				Injection, ther/proph/diag	90772	
				Injection, trigger point	20552	

Physician signature

				Supplies	

X _____

CASE A-10 ENCOUNTER FORM

Capital City Medical—123 Unknown Boulevard, Capital City, NY 12345-2222, (555) 555-1234
Phil Wells, M.D., Mannie Mends, M.D., Bette R. Soone, M.D.

Patient Information Form
Tax ID: 75-0246810
Group NPI: 1513171216

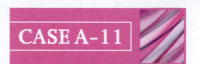

CASE A-11

Patient Information:

Name: (Last, First) Sung, Kenneth   ☒ Male   ❑ Female   Birth Date: 10/03/1930

Address: 501 Locust St, Capital City, NY 12345   Phone: (555) 555-1718

Social Security Number: 189-42-9163   Full-Time Student: ❑ Yes   ☒ No

Marital Status: ❑ Single   ☒ Married   ❑ Divorced   ❑ Other

Employment:

Employer: Retired   Phone: _____

Address: _____

Condition Related to: ❑ Auto Accident   ❑ Employment   ❑ Other Accident

Date of Accident: _____   State _____

Emergency Contact: _____   Phone: ( ) _____

Primary Insurance: Medicare   Phone: ( ) _____

Address: P.O. Box 9834, Capital City, NY 12345

Insurance Policyholder's Name: Same   ❑ M   ❑ F   DOB: _____

Address: _____

Phone: _____   Relationship to Insured: ☒ Self ❑ Spouse ❑ Child ❑ Other

Employer: _____   Phone: ( ) _____

Employer's Address: _____

Policy/I.D. No: 894362514A   Group No: __ Percent Covered: 80 %, Copay Amt: $__

Secondary Insurance: Medicaid   Phone: ( ) _____

Address: 4875 Capital Blvd, Capital City, NY 12345

Insurance Policyholder's Name: Same   ❑ M   ❑ F   DOB: _____

Address: _____

Phone: _____   Relationship to Insured: ☒ Self ❑ Spouse ❑ Child ❑ Other

Employer: _____   Phone: ( ) _____

Employer's Address: _____

Policy/I.D. No: 000684493216   Group No: ___ Percent Covered: ___%, Copay Amt: $5.00

Reason for Visit: High blood pressure and my past stroke

Known Allergies: _____

Were you referred here? If so, by whom? _____

CASE A-11 SOAP

08/11/20XX
Assignment of Benefits: Y
Signature on File: Y
Referring Physician: N

S: Kenneth Sung is seen in the office for a follow-up on HTN and an old CVA.

O: Pt. denies any complaints. ROS unremarkable. BP: 136/88. EKG normal.

A: 1. HTN, malignant—ICD-10 (I10)

   2. Old CVA—ICD-10 (Z86.79)

P: 1. Refill medicine.

   2. PT and INR today.

   3. Return in 6 months.

_____

Phil Wells, M.D.
Family Practice
NPI: 1234567890
Medicaid: 53248961

Date of service:	08/11/XX	Waiver? ☐			
Patient name: Kenneth Sung		Insurance:			
		Subscriber name:			
Address: 501 Locust St Capital City, NY 12345		Group #:		Previous balance:	
		Copay:		Today's charges:	
Phone: 555-555-1718		Account #:		Today's payment: check#	
DOB: 10/03/1930 Age: Sex:		Physician name:		Balance due:	

RANK	Office visit	New	Est	RANK	Office procedures			RANK	Laboratory	
	Minimal		99211		Anoscopy		46600	X	Venipuncture	36415
	Problem focused	99201	99212		Audiometry		92551		Blood glucose, monitoring device	82962
X	Expanded problem focused	99202	99213		Cerumen removal		69210		Blood glucose, visual dipstick	82948
	Detailed	99203	99214		Colposcopy		57452	X	CBC, w/ auto differential	85025
	Comprehensive	99204	99215		Colposcopy w/biopsy		57455		CBC, w/o auto differential	85027
	Comprehensive (new patient)	99205		X	ECG, w/interpretation		93000		Cholesterol	82465
	Significant, separate service	-25	-25		ECG, rhythm strip		93040		Hemoccult, guaiac	82270
	Well visit	**New**	**Est**		Endometrial biopsy		58100		Hemoccult, immunoassay	82274
	< 1 y	99381	99391		Flexible sigmoidoscopy		45330		Hemoglobin A1C	85018
	1-4 y	99382	99392		Flexible sigmoidoscopy w/biopsy		45331		Lipid panel	80061
	5-11 y	99383	99393		Fracture care, cast/splint		29____		Liver panel	80076
	12-17 y	99384	99394		Site: _____				KOH prep (skin, hair, nails)	87220
	18-39 y	99385	99395		Nebulizer		94640		Metabolic panel, basic	80048
	40-64 y	99386	99396		Nebulizer demo		94664	X	Metabolic panel, comprehensive	80053
	65 y +	99387	99397		Spirometry		94010		Mononucleosis	86308
	Medicare preventive services				Spirometry, pre and post		94060		Pregnancy, blood	84703
	Pap		Q0091		Tympanometry		92567		Pregnancy, urine	81025
	Pelvic & breast		G0101		Vasectomy		55250		Renal panel	80069
	Prostate/PSA		G0103		**Skin procedures**	**Units**			Sedimentation rate	85651
	Tobacco counseling/3-10 min		99406		Burn care, initial	16000			Strep, rapid	86403
	Tobacco counseling/>10 min		99407		Foreign body, skin, simple	10120			Strep culture	87081
	Welcome to Medicare exam		G0344		Foreign body, skin, complex	10121			Strep A	87880
	ECG w/Welcome to Medicare exam		G0366		I&D, abscess	10060			TB	86580
	Flexible sigmoidoscopy		G0104		I&D, hematoma/seroma	10140			UA, complete, non-automated	81000
	Hemoccult, guaiac		G0107		Laceration repair, simple	120___			UA, w/o micro, non-automated	81002
	Flu shot		G0008		Site: _____ Size: _____				UA, w/ micro, non-automated	81003
	Pneumonia shot		G0009		Laceration repair, layered	120___			Urine colony count	87086
	Consultation/preop clearance				Site: _____ Size: _____				Urine culture, presumptive	87088
	Expanded problem focused		99242		Lesion, biopsy, one	11100			Wet mount/KOH	87210
	Detailed		99243		Lesion, biopsy, each add'l	11101			**Vaccines**	
	Comprehensive/mod complexity		99244		Lesion, destruct., benign, 1-14	17110			DT, <7 y	90702
	Comprehensive/high complexity		99245		Lesion, destruct., premal., single	17000			DTP	90701
	Other services				Lesion, destruct., premal., ea. add'l	17003			DtaP, <7 y	90700
	After posted hours		99050		Lesion, excision, benign	114___			Flu, 6-35 months	90657
	Evening/weekend appointment		99051		Site: _____ Size: _____				Flu, 3 y +	90658
	Home health certification		G0180		Lesion, excision, malignant	116___			Hep A, adult	90632
	Home health recertification		G0179		Site: _____ Size: _____				Hep A, ped/adol, 2 dose	90633
	Post-op follow-up		99024		Lesion, paring/cutting, one	11055			Hep B, adult	90746
	Prolonged/30-74 min		99354		Lesion, paring/cutting, 2-4	11056			Hep B, ped/adol 3 dose	90744
	Special reports/forms		99080		Lesion, shave	113___			Hep B-Hib	90748
	Disability/Workers comp		99455		Site: _____ Size: _____				Hib, 4 dose	90645
	Radiology				Nail removal, partial	11730			HPV	90649
	Chest X-ray - 71030				Nail removal, w/matrix	11750			IPV	90713
					Skin tag, 1-15	11200			MMR	90707
	Diagnoses				**Medications**	**Units**			Pneumonia, >2 y	90732
1	I10				Ampicillin, up to 500mg	J0290			Pneumonia conjugate, <5 y	90669
2	Z86.79				B-12, up to 1,000 mcg	J3420			Td, >7 y	90718
3					Epinephrine, up to 1ml	J0170			Varicella	90716
4					Kenalog, 10mg	J3301			**Immunizations & Injections**	**Units**
	Next office visit				Lidocaine, 10mg	J2001			Allergen, one	95115
	Recheck Prev PRN _____ D W M Y				Normal saline, 1000cc	J7030			Allergen, multiple	95117
	Instructions:				Phenergan, up to 50mg	J2550			Imm admin, one	90471
					Progesterone, 150mg	J1055			Imm admin, each add'l	90472
					Rocephin, 250mg	J0696			Imm admin, intranasal, one	90473
					Testosterone, 200mg	J1080			Imm admin, intranasal, each add'l	90474
					Tigan, up to 200 mg	J3250			Injection, joint, small	20600
	Referral				Toradol, 15mg	J1885			Injection, joint, intermediate	20605
	To:				**Miscellaneous services**				Injection, joint, major	20610
	Instructions:								Injection, ther/proph/diag	90772
					Prothrombin time - 85610				Injection, trigger point	20552
	Physician signature								**Supplies**	
	X									

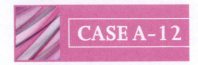

CASE A-12

Capital City Medical—123 Unknown Boulevard, Capital City, NY 12345-2222, (555) 555-1234
Phil Wells, M.D., Mannie Mends, M.D., Bette R. Soone, M.D.

Patient Information Form
Tax ID: 75-0246810
Group NPI: 1513171216

Patient Information:

Name: (Last, First) Harrison, Viola   ☐ Male   ☐ Female   Birth Date: 01/31/1935

Address: 567 Walnut St, Capital City, NY 12345   Phone: (555) 555-8641

Social Security Number: 918-49-1978   Full-Time Student: ☐ Yes   ☒ No

Marital Status: ☒ Single   ☐ Married   ☐ Divorced   ☐ Other

Employment:

Employer: Retired   Phone: ( )

Address:

Condition Related to: ☐ Auto Accident   ☐ Employment   ☐ Other Accident

Date of Accident: State

Emergency Contact: **Phone: ( )**

Primary Insurance: Medicare   Phone: ( )

Address: P.O. Box 9834, Capital City, NY 12345

Insurance Policyholder's Name: Same   ☐ M   ☐ F   DOB:

Address:

Phone: Relationship to Insured: ☒ Self ☐ Spouse ☐ Child ☐ Other

Employer: Phone: ( )

Employer's Address:

Policy/I.D. No: 881536935A   Group No: ___ Percent Covered: 80 %, Copay Amt: $___

Secondary Insurance: Medicaid   Phone: ( )

Address: 4875 Capital Blvd, Capital City, NY 12345

Insurance Policyholder's Name: Same   ☐ M   ☐ F DOB:

Address:

Phone: Relationship to Insured: ☒ Self ☐ Spouse ☐ Child ☐ Other

Employer: Phone: ( )

Employer's Address:

Policy/I.D. No: 00009916596   Group No: ___ Percent Covered: ___%, Copay Amt: $5.00

Reason for Visit: My rheumatoid arthritis

Known Allergies:

Were you referred here? If so, by whom?

05/05/20XX
Assignment of Benefits: Y
Signature on File: Y
Referring Physician: N

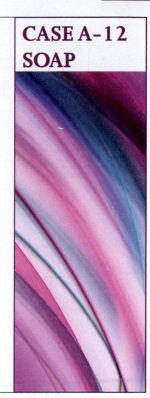

**CASE A-12
SOAP**

S: Viola Harrison is being seen today for a check on her rheumatoid arthritis.

O: ROS is unremarkable, other than what is noted in the CC. Pt. has no new progression of this disease. Lab work reviewed.

A: 1. Rheumatoid arthritis—ICD-10 (M06.9)

   2. Polyarthralgia—ICD-10 (M25.50)

P: 1. Recheck in 3 months.

   2. Gold injection at next visit.

   3. Continue Celebrex.

_____

Phil Wells, M.D.
Family Practice
NPI: 1234567890
Medicaid: 53248961

Date of service:	05/05/XX		Waiver? ☐		
Patient name:	Viola Harrison		Insurance:		
			Subscriber name:		
Address:	567 Walnut St		Group #:		Previous balance:
	Capital City, NY 12345		Copay:		Today's charges:
Phone:	555-555-8641		Account #:		Today's payment: check#
DOB:	01/31/1935 Age: Sex:		Physician name:		Balance due:

RANK	Office visit	New	Est	RANK	Office procedures			RANK	Laboratory		
	Minimal		99211		Anoscopy		46600	X	Venipuncture		36415
	Problem focused	99201	99212		Audiometry		92551		Blood glucose, monitoring device		82962
	Expanded problem focused	99202	99213		Cerumen removal		69210		Blood glucose, visual dipstick		82948
X	Detailed	99203	99214		Colposcopy		57452	X	CBC, w/ auto differential		85025
	Comprehensive	99204	99215		Colposcopy w/biopsy		57455		CBC, w/o auto differential		85027
	Comprehensive (new patient)	99205			ECG, w/interpretation		93000		Cholesterol		82465
	Significant, separate service	-25	-25		ECG, rhythm strip		93040		Hemoccult, guaiac		82270
	Well visit	**New**	**Est**		Endometrial biopsy		58100		Hemoccult, immunoassay		82274
	< 1 y	99381	99391		Flexible sigmoidoscopy		45330		Hemoglobin A1C		85018
	1-4 y	99382	99392		Flexible sigmoidoscopy w/biopsy		45331		Lipid panel		80061
	5-11 y	99383	99393		Fracture care, cast/splint		29____		Liver panel		80076
	12-17 y	99384	99394		Site: _____				KOH prep (skin, hair, nails)		87220
	18-39 y	99385	99395		Nebulizer		94640		Metabolic panel, basic		80048
	40-64 y	99386	99396		Nebulizer demo		94664	X	Metabolic panel, comprehensive		80053
	65 y +	99387	99397		Spirometry		94010		Mononucleosis		86308
	Medicare preventive services				Spirometry, pre and post		94060		Pregnancy, blood		84703
	Pap		Q0091		Tympanometry		92567		Pregnancy, urine		81025
	Pelvic & breast		G0101		Vasectomy		55250		Renal panel		80069
	Prostate/PSA		G0103		**Skin procedures**		**Units**	X	Sedimentation rate		85651
	Tobacco counseling/3-10 min		99406		Burn care, initial	16000			Strep, rapid		86403
	Tobacco counseling/>10 min		99407		Foreign body, skin, simple	10120			Strep culture		87081
	Welcome to Medicare exam		G0344		Foreign body, skin, complex	10121			Strep A		87880
	ECG w/Welcome to Medicare exam		G0366		I&D, abscess	10060			TB		86580
	Flexible sigmoidoscopy		G0104		I&D, hematoma/seroma	10140			UA, complete, non-automated		81000
	Hemoccult, guaiac		G0107		Laceration repair, simple	120____			UA, w/o micro, non-automated		81002
	Flu shot		G0008		Site: _____ Size: _____				UA, w/ micro, non-automated		81003
	Pneumonia shot		G0009		Laceration repair, layered	120____			Urine colony count		87086
	Consultation/preop clearance				Site: _____ Size: _____				Urine culture, presumptive		87088
	Expanded problem focused		99242		Lesion, biopsy, one	11100			Wet mount/KOH		87210
	Detailed		99243		Lesion, biopsy, each add'l	11101			**Vaccines**		
	Comprehensive/mod complexity		99244		Lesion, destruct., benign, 1-14	17110			DT, <7 y		90702
	Comprehensive/high complexity		99245		Lesion, destruct., premal., single	17000			DTP		90701
	Other services				Lesion, destruct., premal., ea. add'l	17003			DtaP, <7 y		90700
	After posted hours		99050		Lesion, excision, benign	114____			Flu, 6-35 months		90657
	Evening/weekend appointment		99051		Site: _____ Size: _____				Flu, 3 y +		90658
	Home health certification		G0180		Lesion, excision, malignant	116____			Hep A, adult		90632
	Home health recertification		G0179		Site: _____ Size: _____				Hep A, ped/adol, 2 dose		90633
	Post-op follow-up		99024		Lesion, paring/cutting, one	11055			Hep B, adult		90746
	Prolonged/30-74 min		99354		Lesion, paring/cutting, 2-4	11056			Hep B, ped/adol 3 dose		90744
	Special reports/forms		99080		Lesion, shave	113____			Hep B-Hib		90748
	Disability/Workers comp		99455		Site: _____ Size: _____				Hib, 4 dose		90645
	Radiology				Nail removal, partial	11730			HPV		90649
					Nail removal, w/matrix	11750			IPV		90713
					Skin tag, 1-15	11200			MMR		90707
	Diagnoses				**Medications**		**Units**		Pneumonia, >2 y		90732
1	M06.9				Ampicillin, up to 500mg	J0290			Pneumonia conjugate, <5 y		90669
2	M25.50				B-12, up to 1,000 mcg	J3420			Td, >7 y		90718
3					Epinephrine, up to 1ml	J0170			Varicella		90716
4					Kenalog, 10mg	J3301			**Immunizations & Injections**		**Units**
	Next office visit				Lidocaine, 10mg	J2001			Allergen, one	95115	
	Recheck Prev PRN _____ D W M Y				Normal saline, 1000cc	J7030			Allergen, multiple	95117	
	Instructions:				Phenergan, up to 50mg	J2550			Imm admin, one	90471	
					Progesterone, 150mg	J1055			Imm admin, each add'l	90472	
					Rocephin, 250mg	J0696			Imm admin, intranasal, one	90473	
					Testosterone, 200mg	J1080			Imm admin, intranasal, each add'l	90474	
	Referral				Tigan, up to 200 mg	J3250			Injection, joint, small	20600	
	To:				Toradol, 15mg	J1885			Injection, joint, intermediate	20605	
	Instructions:				**Miscellaneous services**				Injection, joint, major	20610	
									Injection, ther/proph/diag	90772	
									Injection, trigger point	20552	
	Physician signature								**Supplies**		
	X _____										

CASE A-12 ENCOUNTER FORM

Capital City Medical—123 Unknown Boulevard, Capital City, NY 12345-2222, (555) 555-1234

Phil Wells, M.D., Mannie Mends, M.D., Bette R. Soone, M.D.

Patient Information Form

Tax ID: 75-0246810

Group NPI: 1513171216

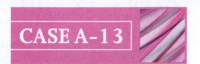

CASE A-13

Patient Information:

Name: (Last, First) Quigley, Quaylord   ☒ Male   ☐ Female   Birth Date: 06/02/1943

Address: 54 Chesnut Ave, Capital City, NY 12345   Phone: (555) 555-9123

Social Security Number: 767-40-7981   Full-Time Student: ☐ Yes   ☒ No

Marital Status: ☐ Single   ☒ Married   ☐ Divorced   ☐ Other

Employment:

Employer: Retired   Phone: ( )

Address:

Condition Related to: ☐ Auto Accident   ☐ Employment   ☒ Other Accident

Date of Accident: State

Emergency Contact: Phone: ( )

Primary Insurance: Medicare   Phone: ( )

Address: P.O. Box 9834, Capital City, NY 12345

Insurance Policyholder's Name: Same   ☐ M   ☐ F   DOB:

Address:

Phone: Relationship to Insured: ☒ Self   ☐ Spouse   ☐ Child   ☐ Other

Employer: Phone: ( )

Employer's Address:

Policy/I.D. No: 645800022A   Group No: Percent Covered: 80 %, Copay Amt: $

Secondary Insurance: Medicare   Phone: ( )

Address: 4875 Capital Blvd, Capital City, NY 12345

Insurance Policyholder's Name: Same   ☐ M   ☐ F   DOB:

Address:

Phone: Relationship to Insured: ☒ Self   ☐ Spouse   ☐ Child   ☐ Other

Employer: Phone: ( )

Employer's Address:

Policy/I.D. No: 0005486598735 Group No: Percent Covered: %, Copay Amt: $5.00

Reason for Visit: I fell off of my bike and now my back hurts

Known Allergies:

Were you referred here? If so, by whom?

CASE A-13 SOAP

11/09/20XX
Assignment of Benefits: Y
Signature on File: Y
Referring Physician: N

S: Quaylord Quigley presents today for a fall off of his bike earlier today causing him LBP.

O: On exam, there are a few scratches. No noted bruising or bleeding. Patient has pain with movement. ROM unremarkable. Pt. does have a history of HTN.

A: 1. LBP—ICD-10 (M54.5)
   2. Fall off bicycle—ICD-10 (V10.0XXA)

P: 1. X-ray of lumbar spine reveals no evidence of fracture or sprain.
   2. Ibuprofen 800 mg 1 b.i.d. p.r.n.
   3. Patient to return to office if no improvement.

_____

Phil Wells, M.D.
Family Practice
NPI: 1234567890
Medicaid: 53248961

Date of service:	11/09//XX		Waiver? ☐		
Patient name:	Quaylord Quigley		Insurance:		
			Subscriber name:		
Address:	54 Chestnut Ave		Group #:		Previous balance:
	Capital City, NY 12345		Copay:		Today's charges:
Phone:	555-555-6337		Account #:		Today's payment: check#
DOB: 06/02/1943	Age:	Sex:	Physician name:		Balance due:

RANK	Office visit	New	Est
	Minimal		99211
	Problem focused	99201	99212
X	Expanded problem focused	99202	99213
	Detailed	99203	99214
	Comprehensive	99204	99215
	Comprehensive (new patient)	99205	
	Significant, separate service	-25	-25
	Well visit	**New**	**Est**
	<1 y	99381	99391
	1-4 y	99382	99392
	5-11 y	99383	99393
	12-17 y	99384	99394
	18-39 y	99385	99395
	40-64 y	99386	99396
	65 y +	99387	99397
	Medicare preventive services		
	Pap		Q0091
	Pelvic & breast		G0101
	Prostate/PSA		G0103
	Tobacco counseling/3-10 min		99406
	Tobacco counseling/>10 min		99407
	Welcome to Medicare exam		G0344
	ECG w/Welcome to Medicare exam		G0366
	Flexible sigmoidoscopy		G0104
	Hemoccult, guaiac		G0107
	Flu shot		G0008
	Pneumonia shot		G0009
	Consultation/preop clearance		
	Expanded problem focused		99242
	Detailed		99243
	Comprehensive/mod complexity		99244
	Comprehensive/high complexity		99245
	Other services		
	After posted hours		99050
	Evening/weekend appointment		99051
	Home health certification		G0180
	Home health recertification		G0179
	Post-op follow-up		99024
	Prolonged/30-74 min		99354
	Special reports/forms		99080
	Disability/Workers comp		99455
	Radiology		
	X-ray Lumbar Spine - 72100		

RANK	Office procedures	
	Anoscopy	46600
	Audiometry	92551
	Cerumen removal	69210
	Colposcopy	57452
	Colposcopy w/biopsy	57455
	ECG, w/interpretation	93000
	ECG, rhythm strip	93040
	Endometrial biopsy	58100
	Flexible sigmoidoscopy	45330
	Flexible sigmoidoscopy w/biopsy	45331
	Fracture care, cast/splint	29____
	Site: _____	
	Nebulizer	94640
	Nebulizer demo	94664
	Spirometry	94010
	Spirometry, pre and post	94060
	Tympanometry	92567
	Vasectomy	55250

	Skin procedures		**Units**
	Burn care, initial	16000	
	Foreign body, skin, simple	10120	
	Foreign body, skin, complex	10121	
	I&D, abscess	10060	
	I&D, hematoma/seroma	10140	
	Laceration repair, simple	120___	
	Site: _____ Size: _____		
	Laceration repair, layered	120___	
	Site: _____ Size: _____		
	Lesion, biopsy, one	11100	
	Lesion, biopsy, each add'l	11101	
	Lesion, destruct., benign, 1-14	17110	
	Lesion, destruct., premal., single	17000	
	Lesion, destruct., premal., ea. add'l	17003	
	Lesion, excision, benign	114___	
	Site: _____ Size: _____		
	Lesion, excision, malignant	116___	
	Site: _____ Size: _____		
	Lesion, paring/cutting, one	11055	
	Lesion, paring/cutting, 2-4	11056	
	Lesion, shave	113___	
	Site: _____ Size: _____		
	Nail removal, partial	11730	
	Nail removal, w/matrix	11750	
	Skin tag, 1-15	11200	

	Medications		**Units**
	Ampicillin, up to 500mg	J0290	
	B-12, up to 1,000 mcg	J3420	
	Epinephrine, up to 1ml	J0170	
	Kenalog, 10mg	J3301	
	Lidocaine, 10mg	J2001	
	Normal saline, 1000cc	J7030	
	Phenergan, up to 50mg	J2550	
	Progesterone, 150mg	J1055	
	Rocephin, 250mg	J0696	
	Testosterone, 200mg	J1080	
	Tigan, up to 200 mg	J3250	
	Toradol, 15mg	J1885	
	Miscellaneous services		

	Laboratory	
	Venipuncture	36415
	Blood glucose, monitoring device	82962
	Blood glucose, visual dipstick	82948
	CBC, w/ auto differential	85025
	CBC, w/o auto differential	85027
	Cholesterol	82465
	Hemoccult, guaiac	82270
	Hemoccult, immunoassay	82274
	Hemoglobin A1C	85018
	Lipid panel	80061
	Liver panel	80076
	KOH prep (skin, hair, nails)	87220
	Metabolic panel, basic	80048
	Metabolic panel, comprehensive	80053
	Mononucleosis	86308
	Pregnancy, blood	84703
	Pregnancy, urine	81025
	Renal panel	80069
	Sedimentation rate	85651
	Strep, rapid	86403
	Strep culture	87081
	Strep A	87880
	TB	86580
	UA, complete, non-automated	81000
	UA, w/o micro, non-automated	81002
	UA, w/ micro, non-automated	81003
	Urine colony count	87086
	Urine culture, presumptive	87088
	Wet mount/KOH	87210
	Vaccines	
	DT, <7 y	90702
	DTP	90701
	DtaP, <7 y	90700
	Flu, 6-35 months	90657
	Flu, 3 y +	90658
	Hep A, adult	90632
	Hep A, ped/adol, 2 dose	90633
	Hep B, adult	90746
	Hep B, ped/adol 3 dose	90744
	Hep B-Hib	90748
	Hib, 4 dose	90645
	HPV	90649
	IPV	90713
	MMR	90707
	Pneumonia, >2 y	90732
	Pneumonia conjugate, <5 y	90669
	Td, >7 y	90718
	Varicella	90716

	Immunizations & Injections		**Units**
	Allergen, one	95115	
	Allergen, multiple	95117	
	Imm admin, one	90471	
	Imm admin, each add'l	90472	
	Imm admin, intranasal, one	90473	
	Imm admin, intranasal, each add'l	90474	
	Injection, joint, small	20600	
	Injection, joint, intermediate	20605	
	Injection, joint, major	20610	
	Injection, ther/proph/diag	90772	
	Injection, trigger point	20552	
	Supplies		

	Diagnoses
1	M54.5
2	V10.0XXA
3	
4	

Next office visit

Recheck	Prev	PRN	_____	D W M Y

Instructions:

Referral

To:

Instructions:

Physician signature

X _____

CASE A-13 ENCOUNTER FORM

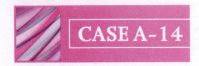

CASE A-14

Capital City Medical—123 Unknown Boulevard, Capital City, NY 12345-2222, (555) 555-1234
Phil Wells, M.D., Mannie Mends, M.D., Bette R. Soone, M.D.

Patient Information Form
Tax ID: 75-0246810
Group NPI: 1513171216

Patient Information:

Name: (Last, First) Myers, Winifred   ❑ Male   ❑ Female   Birth Date: 08/10/1936

Address: 80 Wintergreen Ave, Capital City, NY 12345   Phone: (555) 555-1984

Social Security Number: 143-22-6433   Full-Time Student: ❑ Yes   ☒ No

Marital Status: ❑ Single   ☒ Married   ❑ Divorced   ❑ Other

Employment:

Employer: Retired   Phone: ( ) _____

Address: _____

Condition Related to: ❑ Auto Accident   ❑ Employment   ❑ Other Accident

Date of Accident: _____ State _____

Emergency Contact: _____   **Phone: ( )** _____

Primary Insurance: Medicare   **Phone: ( )** _____

Address: P.O. Box 9834, Capital City, NY 12345

Insurance Policyholder's Name: Same   ❑ M ❑ F DOB: _____

Address: _____

Phone: _____   Relationship to Insured: ☒ Self ❑ Spouse ❑ Child ❑ Other

Employer: _____   Phone: ( ) _____

Employer's Address: _____

Policy/I.D. No: 115272728A   Group No: ___ Percent Covered: 80 %, Copay Amt: $___

Secondary Insurance: Aetna   **Phone: ( )** _____

Address: 1625 Healthcare Bldg, Capital City, NY 12345

Insurance Policyholder's Name: Same   ❑ M ❑ F DOB: _____

Address: _____

Phone: _____   Relationship to Insured: ☒ Self ❑ Spouse ❑ Child ❑ Other

Employer: Retired   Phone: ( ) _____

Employer's Address: _____

Policy/I.D. No: 12656489 Group No: 6896 Percent Covered: ____%, Copay Amt: $10.00

Reason for Visit: I'm having skin tags removed

Known Allergies: _____

Were you referred here? If so, by whom? _____

03/24/20XX

Assignment of Benefits: Y

Signature on File: Y

Referring Physician: N

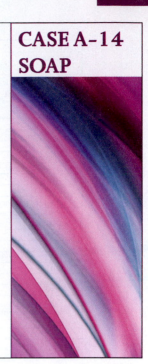

**CASE A-14
SOAP**

S: Winifred Myers (established patient) comes in today for the removal of 18 skin tags.

O: Pt. was prepped and draped in the usual fashion. Skin tags were removed successfully without any complications.

A: 1. Skin tags; congenital—ICD-10 (Q81.9)

P: 1. Keep area clean and dry.

    2. Follow up in 1 week.

_____

Mannie Mends, M.D.

General Surgeon

NPI: 0123456789

PIN: 654321

Date of service:	03/24/XX	Waiver? ☐		
Patient name:	Winifred Myers	Insurance:		
		Subscriber name:		
Address: 80 Wintergreen Ave Capital City, NY 12345		Group #:		Previous balance:
		Copay:		Today's charges:
Phone: 555-555-1984		Account #:		Today's payment: check#
DOB: 10/21/1992 Age: Sex:		Physician name:		Balance due:

RANK	Office visit	New	Est	RANK	Office procedures			RANK	Laboratory		
	Minimal		99211		Anoscopy		46600		Venipuncture		36415
	Problem focused	99201	99212		Audiometry		92551		Blood glucose, monitoring device		82962
	Expanded problem focused	99202	99213		Cerumen removal		69210		Blood glucose, visual dipstick		82948
	Detailed	99203	99214		Colposcopy		57452		CBC, w/ auto differential		85025
	Comprehensive	99204	99215		Colposcopy w/biopsy		57455		CBC, w/o auto differential		85027
	Comprehensive (new patient)	99205			ECG, w/interpretation		93000		Cholesterol		82465
	Significant, separate service	-25	-25		ECG, rhythm strip		93040		Hemoccult, guaiac		82270
	Well visit	**New**	**Est**		Endometrial biopsy		58100		Hemoccult, immunoassay		82274
	< 1 y	99381	99391		Flexible sigmoidoscopy		45330		Hemoglobin A1C		85018
	1-4 y	99382	99392		Flexible sigmoidoscopy w/biopsy		45331		Lipid panel		80061
	5-11 y	99383	99393		Fracture care, cast/splint		29____		Liver panel		80076
	12-17 y	99384	99394		Site: _____				KOH prep (skin, hair, nails)		87220
	18-39 y	99385	99395		Nebulizer		94640		Metabolic panel, basic		80048
	40-64 y	99386	99396		Nebulizer demo		94664		Metabolic panel, comprehensive		80053
	65 y +	99387	99397		Spirometry		94010		Mononucleosis		86308
	Medicare preventive services				Spirometry, pre and post		94060		Pregnancy, blood		84703
	Pap		Q0091		Tympanometry		92567		Pregnancy, urine		81025
	Pelvic & breast		G0101		Vasectomy		55250		Renal panel		80069
	Prostate/PSA		G0103		**Skin procedures**		**Units**		Sedimentation rate		85651
	Tobacco counseling/3-10 min		99406		Burn care, initial	16000			Strep, rapid		86403
	Tobacco counseling/>10 min		99407		Foreign body, skin, simple	10120			Strep culture		87081
	Welcome to Medicare exam		G0344		Foreign body, skin, complex	10121			Strep A		87880
	ECG w/Welcome to Medicare exam		G0366		I&D, abscess	10060			TB		86580
	Flexible sigmoidoscopy		G0104		I&D, hematoma/seroma	10140			UA, complete, non-automated		81000
	Hemoccult, guaiac		G0107		Laceration repair, simple	120___			UA, w/o micro, non-automated		81002
	Flu shot		G0008		Site: _____ Size: _____				UA, w/ micro, non-automated		81003
	Pneumonia shot		G0009		Laceration repair, layered	120___			Urine colony count		87086
	Consultation/preop clearance				Site: _____ Size: _____				Urine culture, presumptive		87088
	Expanded problem focused		99242		Lesion, biopsy, one	11100			Wet mount/KOH		87210
	Detailed		99243		Lesion, biopsy, each add'l	11101			**Vaccines**		
	Comprehensive/mod complexity		99244		Lesion, destruct., benign, 1-14	17110			DT, <7 y		90702
	Comprehensive/high complexity		99245		Lesion, destruct., premal., single	17000			DTP		90701
	Other services				Lesion, destruct., premal., ea. add'l	17003			DtaP, <7 y		90700
	After posted hours		99050		Lesion, excision, benign	114___			Flu, 6-35 months		90657
	Evening/weekend appointment		99051		Site: _____ Size: _____				Flu, 3 y +		90658
	Home health certification		G0180		Lesion, excision, malignant	116___			Hep A, adult		90632
	Home health recertification		G0179		Site: _____ Size: _____				Hep A, ped/adol, 2 dose		90633
	Post-op follow-up		99024		Lesion, paring/cutting, one	11055			Hep B, adult		90746
	Prolonged/30-74 min		99354		Lesion, paring/cutting, 2-4	11056			Hep B, ped/adol 3 dose		90744
	Special reports/forms		99080		Lesion, shave	113___			Hep B-Hib		90748
	Disability/Workers comp		99455		Site: _____ Size: _____				Hib, 4 dose		90645
	Radiology				Nail removal, partial	11730			HPV		90649
					Nail removal, w/matrix	11750			IPV		90713
				X	Skin tag, 1-15	11200			MMR		90707
	Diagnoses				**Medications**		**Units**		Pneumonia, >2 y		90732
1	Q81.9				Ampicillin, up to 500mg	J0290			Pneumonia conjugate, <5 y		90669
2					B-12, up to 1,000 mcg	J3420			Td, >7 y		90718
3					Epinephrine, up to 1ml	J0170			Varicella		90716
4					Kenalog, 10mg	J3301			**Immunizations & Injections**		**Units**
Next office visit					Lidocaine, 10mg	J2001			Allergen, one	95115	
Recheck Prev PRN _____ D W M Y					Normal saline, 1000cc	J7030			Allergen, multiple	95117	
Instructions:					Phenergan, up to 50mg	J2550			Imm admin, one	90471	
					Progesterone, 150mg	J1055			Imm admin, each add'l	90472	
					Rocephin, 250mg	J0696			Imm admin, intranasal, one	90473	
					Testosterone, 200mg	J1080			Imm admin, intranasal, each add'l	90474	
					Tigan, up to 200 mg	J3250			Injection, joint, small	20600	
Referral					Toradol, 15mg	J1885			Injection, joint, intermediate	20605	
To:					**Miscellaneous services**				Injection, joint, major	20610	
Instructions:									Injection, ther/proph/diag	90772	
					Ea Ad 10 Skin Lesion - 11201				Injection, trigger point	20552	
Physician signature									**Supplies**		
X _____											

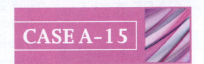

CASE A-15

Capital City Medical—123 Unknown Boulevard, Capital City, NY 12345-2222, (555) 555-1234

Phil Wells, M.D., Mannie Mends, M.D., Bette R. Soone, M.D.

Patient Information Form

Tax ID: 75-0246810

Group NPI: 1513171216

Patient Information:

Name: (Last, First) Jaworski, Stella   ☐ Male   ☐ Female   Birth Date: 04/04/1936

Address: 13 Evergreen Ave, Capital City, NY 12345   Phone: (555) 555-3456

Social Security Number: 954-24-9835   Full-Time Student: ☐ Yes   ☒ No

Marital Status: ☐ Single   ☒ Married   ☐ Divorced   ☐ Other

Employment:

Employer: Retired   Phone: ( )

Address:

Condition Related to: ☐ Auto Accident   ☐ Employment   ☐ Other Accident

Date of Accident: State

Emergency Contact: **Phone: ( )**

Primary Insurance: Medicare   **Phone: ( )**

Address: P.O. Box 9834, Capital City, NY 12345

Insurance Policyholder's Name: Joseph Jaworski   ☒ M   ☐ F   DOB: 08/18/1935

Address: Same

Phone: Relationship to Insured: ☐ Self ☒ Spouse ☐ Child ☐ Other

Employer: Retired   Phone: ( )

Employer's Address:

Policy/I.D. No: 843648901A   Group No: ___   Percent Covered: 80 %, Copay Amt: $___

Secondary Insurance: Medicaid   **Phone: ( )**

Address: 4875 Capital Blvd, Capital City, NY 12345

Insurance Policyholder's Name: Same   ☐ M   ☐ F   DOB:

Address:

Phone: Relationship to Insured: ☒ Self ☐ Spouse ☐ Child ☐ Other

Employer: Phone: ( )

Employer's Address:

Policy/I.D. No: 0015358763896 Group No: ___ Percent Covered: ___%, Copay Amt: $5.00

Reason for Visit: I have chills, a sick stomach, body aches, and I have been vomiting

Known Allergies:

Were you referred here? If so, by whom?

CASE A-15 SOAP	09/09/20XX

Assignment of Benefits: Y

Signature on File: Y

Referring Physician: N

S: Stella Jaworski presents today with complaints of N&V, chills, and her body aches.

O: On exam, pt. has fever; T 100.6°F. No diarrhea. Other systems unremarkable.

A: 1. Influenza—ICD-10 (J11.1)

P: 1. Clear liquids for the next 24 hours.

   2. Bed rest.

   3. If symptoms worsen, she is to call the office.

_____

Phil Wells, M.D.

Family Practice

NPI: 1234567890

Medicaid: 53248961

Date of service:	09/09/XX			Waiver? ☐		
Patient name:	Stella Jaworski			Insurance:		
				Subscriber name:		
Address:	13 Evergreen Ave			Group #:		Previous balance:
	Capital City, NY 12345			Copay:		Today's charges:
Phone:	555-555-3456			Account #:		Today's payment: check#
DOB:	04/04/1936 Age: Sex:			Physician name:		Balance due:

RANK	Office visit	New	Est	RANK	Office procedures			RANK	Laboratory	
	Minimal		99211		Anoscopy		46600	X	Venipuncture	36415
	Problem focused	99201	99212		Audiometry		92551		Blood glucose, monitoring device	82962
X	Expanded problem focused	99202	99213		Cerumen removal		69210		Blood glucose, visual dipstick	82948
	Detailed	99203	99214		Colposcopy		57452	X	CBC, w/ auto differential	85025
	Comprehensive	99204	99215		Colposcopy w/biopsy		57455		CBC, w/o auto differential	85027
	Comprehensive (new patient)	99205			ECG, w/interpretation		93000		Cholesterol	82465
	Significant, separate service	-25	-25		ECG, rhythm strip		93040		Hemoccult, guaiac	82270
	Well visit	**New**	**Est**		Endometrial biopsy		58100		Hemoccult, immunoassay	82274
	< 1 y	99381	99391		Flexible sigmoidoscopy		45330		Hemoglobin A1C	85018
	1-4 y	99382	99392		Flexible sigmoidoscopy w/biopsy		45331		Lipid panel	80061
	5-11 y	99383	99393		Fracture care, cast/splint		29___		Liver panel	80076
	12-17 y	99384	99394		Site: ___				KOH prep (skin, hair, nails)	87220
	18-39 y	99385	99395		Nebulizer		94640		Metabolic panel, basic	80048
	40-64 y	99386	99396		Nebulizer demo		94664		Metabolic panel, comprehensive	80053
	65 y +	99387	99397		Spirometry		94010		Mononucleosis	86308
	Medicare preventive services				Spirometry, pre and post		94060		Pregnancy, blood	84703
	Pap		Q0091		Tympanometry		92567		Pregnancy, urine	81025
	Pelvic & breast		G0101		Vasectomy		55250		Renal panel	80069
	Prostate/PSA		G0103		**Skin procedures**		**Units**		Sedimentation rate	85651
	Tobacco counseling/3-10 min		99406		Burn care, initial	16000			Strep, rapid	86403
	Tobacco counseling/>10 min		99407		Foreign body, skin, simple	10120			Strep culture	87081
	Welcome to Medicare exam		G0344		Foreign body, skin, complex	10121			Strep A	87880
	ECG w/Welcome to Medicare exam		G0366		I&D, abscess	10060			TB	86580
	Flexible sigmoidoscopy		G0104		I&D, hematoma/seroma	10140			UA, complete, non-automated	81000
	Hemoccult, guaiac		G0107		Laceration repair, simple	120___			UA, w/o micro, non-automated	81002
	Flu shot		G0008		Site: ___ Size: ___				UA, w/ micro, non-automated	81003
	Pneumonia shot		G0009		Laceration repair, layered	120___			Urine colony count	87086
	Consultation/preop clearance				Site: ___ Size: ___				Urine culture, presumptive	87088
	Expanded problem focused		99242		Lesion, biopsy, one	11100			Wet mount/KOH	87210
	Detailed		99243		Lesion, biopsy, each add'l	11101			**Vaccines**	
	Comprehensive/mod complexity		99244		Lesion, destruct., benign, 1-14	17110			DT, <7 y	90702
	Comprehensive/high complexity		99245		Lesion, destruct., premal., single	17000			DTP	90701
	Other services				Lesion, destruct., premal., ea. add'l	17003			DtaP, <7 y	90700
	After posted hours		99050		Lesion, excision, benign	114___			Flu, 6-35 months	90657
	Evening/weekend appointment		99051		Site: ___ Size: ___				Flu, 3 y +	90658
	Home health certification		G0180		Lesion, excision, malignant	116___			Hep A, adult	90632
	Home health recertification		G0179		Site: ___ Size: ___				Hep A, ped/adol, 2 dose	90633
	Post-op follow-up		99024		Lesion, paring/cutting, one	11055			Hep B, adult	90746
	Prolonged/30-74 min		99354		Lesion, paring/cutting, 2-4	11056			Hep B, ped/adol 3 dose	90744
	Special reports/forms		99080		Lesion, shave	113___			Hep B-Hib	90748
	Disability/Workers comp		99455		Site: ___ Size: ___				Hib, 4 dose	90645
	Radiology				Nail removal, partial	11730			HPV	90649
					Nail removal, w/matrix	11750			IPV	90713
					Skin tag, 1-15	11200			MMR	90707
	Diagnoses				**Medications**		**Units**		Pneumonia, >2 y	90732
1	J11.1				Ampicillin, up to 500mg	J0290			Pneumonia conjugate, <5 y	90669
2					B-12, up to 1,000 mcg	J3420			Td, >7 y	90718
3					Epinephrine, up to 1ml	J0170			Varicella	90716
4					Kenalog, 10mg	J3301			**Immunizations & Injections**		**Units**
	Next office visit				Lidocaine, 10mg	J2001			Allergen, one	95115
	Recheck Prev PRN ___ D W M Y				Normal saline, 1000cc	J7030			Allergen, multiple	95117
	Instructions:				Phenergan, up to 50mg	J2550			Imm admin, one	90471
					Progesterone, 150mg	J1055			Imm admin, each add'l	90472
					Rocephin, 250mg	J0696			Imm admin, intranasal, one	90473
					Testosterone, 200mg	J1080			Imm admin, intranasal, each add'l	90474
	Referral				Tigan, up to 200 mg	J3250			Injection, joint, small	20600
	To:				Toradol, 15mg	J1885			Injection, joint, intermediate	20605
	Instructions:				**Miscellaneous services**				Injection, joint, major	20610
									Injection, ther/proph/diag	90772
					Electrolyte Panel - 80051				Injection, trigger point	20552
	Physician signature								**Supplies**	
	X ___									

CASE A-15 ENCOUNTER FORM

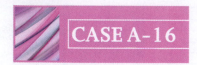

CASE A-16

Capital City Medical—123 Unknown Boulevard, Capital City, NY 12345-2222, (555) 555-1234	Patient Information Form
Phil Wells, M.D., Mannie Mends, M.D., Bette R. Soone, M.D.	Tax ID: 75-0246810 Group NPI: 1513171216

Patient Information:

Name: (Last, First) Bromley, Murphy   ☒ Male   ☐ Female   Birth Date: 09/13/1956

Address: 9 Redwood Dr, Capital City, NY 12345   Phone: (555) 555-4972

Social Security Number: 785-10-8339   Full-Time Student: ☐ Yes   ☒ No

Marital Status: ☐ Single   ☒ Married   ☐ Divorced   ☐ Other

Employment:

Employer: Retired   Phone: _____

Address: _____

Condition Related to: ☐ Auto Accident   ☐ Employment   ☐ Other Accident

Date of Accident: _____ State _____

Emergency Contact: _____   **Phone: ( )** _____

Primary Insurance: Medicare   **Phone: ( )** _____

Address: P.O. Box 9834, Capital City, NY 12345

Insurance Policyholder's Name: Same   ☐ M   ☐ F   DOB _____

Address: _____

Phone: _____   Relationship to Insured: ☒ Self ☐ Spouse ☐ Child ☐ Other

Employer: _____   Phone: ( ) _____

Employer's Address: _____

Policy/I.D. No: 481654563A   Group No: ___ Percent Covered: 80 %, Copay Amt: $ ___

Secondary Insurance: Blue Cross Blue Shield Medigap   **Phone: ( )** _____

Address: 379 Blue Plaza, Capital City, NY 12345

Insurance Policyholder's Name: Same   ☐ M   ☐ F   DOB: _____

Address: _____

Phone: _____   Relationship to Insured: ☒ Self ☐ Spouse ☐ Child ☐ Other

Employer: _____   Phone: ( ) _____

Employer's Address: _____

Policy/I.D. No: YYJ0472009 Group No: ___   Percent Covered: ___ %, Copay Amt: $

Reason for Visit: My three-month checkup on high blood pressure, migraines, and diabetes

Known Allergies: _____

Were you referred here? If so, by whom? _____

**CASE A-16
SOAP**

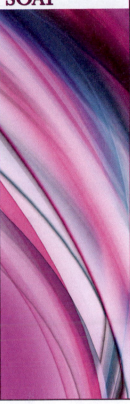

03/17/20XX
Assignment of Benefits: Y
Signature on File: Y
Referring Physician: N

S: Murphy Bromley is in the office today for a checkup on HTN, DM I, and migraine disorder.

O: Pt. is in no acute distress. BP: 152/90. He says that his diastolic pressure has been running higher than normal for the past couple of weeks. He denies any stress or increased salt intake. Migraines have been under control with medicine. Wt. is stable at 174 lbs.

A: 1. HTN—ICD-10 (I10)

2. Atypical migraines—ICD-10 (G43.009)

3. DM I—ICD-10 (E10.9)

P: 1. DC Norvasc.

2. Start Diazide 1 b.i.d.

3. Return to office for BP check around the same time every day × 4 days.

4. Refill insulin.

5. Schedule appointment for 2 months.

Phil Wells, M.D.
Family Practice
NPI: 1234567890
PIN: 358612

Date of service:	03/17/XX		Waiver? ☐	
Patient name:	Murphy Bromley		Insurance:	
			Subscriber name:	
Address:	9 Redwood Dr		Group #:	Previous balance:
	Capital City, NY 12345		Copay:	Today's charges:
Phone:	555-555-4972		Account #:	Today's payment: check#
DOB:	09/13/1956 Age: Sex:		Physician name:	Balance due:

RANK	Office visit	New	Est	RANK	Office procedures			RANK	Laboratory	
	Minimal		99211		Anoscopy		46600	X	Venipuncture	36415
	Problem focused	99201	99212		Audiometry		92551		Blood glucose, monitoring device	82962
X	Expanded problem focused	99202	99213		Cerumen removal		69210		Blood glucose, visual dipstick	82948
	Detailed	99203	99214		Colposcopy		57452	X	CBC, w/ auto differential	85025
	Comprehensive	99204	99215		Colposcopy w/biopsy		57455		CBC, w/o auto differential	85027
	Comprehensive (new patient)	99205			ECG, w/interpretation		93000		Cholesterol	82465
	Significant, separate service	-25	-25		ECG, rhythm strip		93040		Hemoccult, guaiac	82270
	Well visit	**New**	**Est**		Endometrial biopsy		58100		Hemoccult, immunoassay	82274
	< 1 y	99381	99391		Flexible sigmoidoscopy		45330		Hemoglobin A1C	85018
	1-4 y	99382	99392		Flexible sigmoidoscopy w/biopsy		45331		Lipid panel	80061
	5-11 y	99383	99393		Fracture care, cast/splint		29___		Liver panel	80076
	12-17 y	99384	99394		Site: _____				KOH prep (skin, hair, nails)	87220
	18-39 y	99385	99395		Nebulizer		94640		Metabolic panel, basic	80048
	40-64 y	99386	99396		Nebulizer demo		94664	X	Metabolic panel, comprehensive	80053
	65 y +	99387	99397		Spirometry		94010		Mononucleosis	86308
	Medicare preventive services				Spirometry, pre and post		94060		Pregnancy, blood	84703
	Pap		Q0091		Tympanometry		92567		Pregnancy, urine	81025
	Pelvic & breast		G0101		Vasectomy		55250		Renal panel	80069
	Prostate/PSA		G0103		**Skin procedures**		**Units**		Sedimentation rate	85651
	Tobacco counseling/3-10 min		99406		Burn care, initial	16000			Strep, rapid	86403
	Tobacco counseling/>10 min		99407		Foreign body, skin, simple	10120			Strep culture	87081
	Welcome to Medicare exam		G0344		Foreign body, skin, complex	10121			Strep A	87880
	ECG w/Welcome to Medicare exam		G0366		I&D, abscess	10060			TB	86580
	Flexible sigmoidoscopy		G0104		I&D, hematoma/seroma	10140			UA, complete, non-automated	81000
	Hemoccult, guaiac		G0107		Laceration repair, simple	120___			UA, w/o micro, non-automated	81002
	Flu shot		G0008		Site: _____ Size: _____				UA, w/ micro, non-automated	81003
	Pneumonia shot		G0009		Laceration repair, layered	120___			Urine colony count	87086
	Consultation/preop clearance				Site: _____ Size: _____				Urine culture, presumptive	87088
	Expanded problem focused		99242		Lesion, biopsy, one	11100			Wet mount/KOH	87210
	Detailed		99243		Lesion, biopsy, each add'l	11101			**Vaccines**	
	Comprehensive/mod complexity		99244		Lesion, destruct., benign, 1-14	17110			DT, <7 y	90702
	Comprehensive/high complexity		99245		Lesion, destruct., premal., single	17000			DTP	90701
	Other services				Lesion, destruct., premal., ea. add'l	17003			DtaP, <7 y	90700
	After posted hours		99050		Lesion, excision, benign	114___			Flu, 6-35 months	90657
	Evening/weekend appointment		99051		Site: _____ Size: _____				Flu, 3 y +	90658
	Home health certification		G0180		Lesion, excision, malignant	116___			Hep A, adult	90632
	Home health recertification		G0179		Site: _____ Size: _____				Hep A, ped/adol, 2 dose	90633
	Post-op follow-up		99024		Lesion, paring/cutting, one	11055			Hep B, adult	90746
	Prolonged/30-74 min		99354		Lesion, paring/cutting, 2-4	11056			Hep B, ped/adol 3 dose	90744
	Special reports/forms		99080		Lesion, shave	113___			Hep B-Hib	90748
	Disability/Workers comp		99455		Site: _____ Size: _____				Hib, 4 dose	90645
	Radiology				Nail removal, partial	11730			HPV	90649
					Nail removal, w/matrix	11750			IPV	90713
					Skin tag, 1-15	11200			MMR	90707
	Diagnoses				**Medications**		**Units**		Pneumonia, >2 y	90732
1	I10				Ampicillin, up to 500mg	J0290			Pneumonia conjugate, <5 y	90669
2	G43.009				B-12, up to 1,000 mcg	J3420			Td, >7 y	90718
3	E10.9				Epinephrine, up to 1ml	J0170			Varicella	90716
4					Kenalog, 10mg	J3301			**Immunizations & Injections**	**Units**
	Next office visit				Lidocaine, 10mg	J2001			Allergen, one	95115
	Recheck Prev PRN _____ D W M Y				Normal saline, 1000cc	J7030			Allergen, multiple	95117
	Instructions:				Phenergan, up to 50mg	J2550			Imm admin, one	90471
					Progesterone, 150mg	J1055			Imm admin, each add'l	90472
					Rocephin, 250mg	J0696			Imm admin, intranasal, one	90473
					Testosterone, 200mg	J1080			Imm admin, intranasal, each add'l	90474
	Referral				Tigan, up to 200 mg	J3250			Injection, joint, small	20600
	To:				Toradol, 15mg	J1885			Injection, joint, intermediate	20605
	Instructions:				**Miscellaneous services**				Injection, joint, major	20610
									Injection, ther/proph/diag	90772
									Injection, trigger point	20552
	Physician signature								**Supplies**	
	X _____									

Capital City Medical—123 Unknown Boulevard, Capital City, NY 12345-2222, (555) 555-1234

Phil Wells, M.D., Mannie Mends, M.D., Bette R. Soone, M.D.

Patient Information Form

Tax ID: 75-0246810

Group NPI: 1513171216

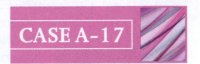

CASE A-17

Patient Information:

Name: (Last, First) <u>Powers, Gus</u>   ☒ Male   ☐ Female   Birth Date: <u>12/25/1940</u>

Address: <u>3982 Cedar St, Capital City, NY 12345</u>   Phone: <u>(555) 555-1112</u>

Social Security Number: <u>243-52-0069</u>   Full-Time Student: ☐ Yes   ☒ No

Marital Status: ☐ Single   ☐ Married   ☒ Divorced   ☐ Other

Employment:

Employer: <u>Retired</u>   Phone: ( ) _____

Address: _____

Condition Related to: ☐ Auto Accident   ☐ Employment   ☒ Other Accident

Date of Accident: _____ State _____

Emergency Contact: _____   Phone: ( ) _____

Primary Insurance: <u>Medicare</u>   Phone: ( ) _____

Address: <u>P.O Box 9834, Capital City, NY 12345</u>

Insurance Policyholder's Name: <u>Same</u>   ☐ M   ☐ F   DOB: _____

Address: _____

Phone: _____   Relationship to Insured: ☒ Self   ☐ Spouse   ☐ Child   ☐ Other

Employer: _____   Phone: ( ) _____

Employer's Address: _____

Policy/I.D. No: <u>366736530A</u>   Group No: ____   Percent Covered: <u>80</u> %, Copay Amt: $__

Secondary Insurance: <u>Aetna</u>   Phone: ( ) _____

Address: <u>1625 Healthcare Bldg, Capital City, NY 12345</u>

Insurance Policyholder's Name: <u>Same</u>   ☐ M   ☐ F   DOB: _____

Address: _____

Phone: _____   Relationship to Insured: ☒ Self   ☐ Spouse   ☐ Child   ☐ Other

Employer: <u>Retired</u>   Phone: ( ) _____

Employer's Address: _____

Policy/I.D. No: <u>0059843</u>   Group No: <u>312007</u>   Percent Covered: ____%, Copay Amt: $<u>15.00</u>

Reason for Visit: <u>I was working around the house when a nail shot into my leg</u>

Known Allergies: _____

Were you referred here? If so, by whom? _____

CASE A-17 SOAP

09/07/20XX
Assignment of Benefits: Y
Signature on File: Y
Referring Physician: N

S: New patient, Gus Powers, is seen today for a wound that occurred today in his left thigh due to a nail gun.

O: The wound penetrates only the epidermis layers without dermal involvement. This area was cleansed with hydrogen peroxide. There is no need for sutures, but tetanus needs updated.

A: 1. Wound; thigh—ICD-10 (S71.109A), due to nail gun accident—ICD-10 (W29.8XXA)

   2. Tetanus vaccination—ICD-10 (Z23)

P: 1. Pt. to keep wound clean and bandage.

   2. To return to office if redness, swelling, pus, discoloration, or fever occurs.

_____

Mannie Mends, M.D.
General Surgeon
NPI: 1234567890
PIN: 654321

Date of service:	09/07/XX		Waiver? ☐				
Patient name:	Gus Power		Insurance:				
			Subscriber name:				
Address:	3982 Cedar St		Group #:			Previous balance:	
	Township NY 12345		Copay:			Today's charges:	
Phone:	555-555-1112		Account #:			Today's payment: check#	
DOB:	12/25/1940 Age: Sex:		Physician name:			Balance due:	

RANK	Office visit	New	Est	RANK	Office procedures			RANK	Laboratory	
	Minimal		99211		Anoscopy		46600		Venipuncture	36415
	Problem focused	99201	99212		Audiometry		92551		Blood glucose, monitoring device	82962
	Expanded problem focused	99202	99213		Cerumen removal		69210		Blood glucose, visual dipstick	82948
X	Detailed	99203	99214		Colposcopy		57452		CBC, w/ auto differential	85025
	Comprehensive	99204	99215		Colposcopy w/biopsy		57455		CBC, w/o auto differential	85027
	Comprehensive (new patient)	99205			ECG, w/interpretation		93000		Cholesterol	82465
	Significant, separate service	-25	-25		ECG, rhythm strip		93040		Hemoccult, guaiac	82270
	Well visit	**New**	**Est**		Endometrial biopsy		58100		Hemoccult, immunoassay	82274
	< 1 y	99381	99391		Flexible sigmoidoscopy		45330		Hemoglobin A1C	85018
	1-4 y	99382	99392		Flexible sigmoidoscopy w/biopsy		45331		Lipid panel	80061
	5-11 y	99383	99393		Fracture care, cast/splint		29____		Liver panel	80076
	12-17 y	99384	99394		Site: _____				KOH prep (skin, hair, nails)	87220
	18-39 y	99385	99395		Nebulizer		94640		Metabolic panel, basic	80048
	40-64 y	99386	99396		Nebulizer demo		94664		Metabolic panel, comprehensive	80053
	65 y +	99387	99397		Spirometry		94010		Mononucleosis	86308
	Medicare preventive services				Spirometry, pre and post		94060		Pregnancy, blood	84703
	Pap		Q0091		Tympanometry		92567		Pregnancy, urine	81025
	Pelvic & breast		G0101		Vasectomy		55250		Renal panel	80069
	Prostate/PSA		G0103		**Skin procedures**		**Units**		Sedimentation rate	85651
	Tobacco counseling/3-10 min		99406		Burn care, initial	16000			Strep, rapid	86403
	Tobacco counseling/>10 min		99407		Foreign body, skin, simple	10120			Strep culture	87081
	Welcome to Medicare exam		G0344		Foreign body, skin, complex	10121			Strep A	87880
	ECG w/Welcome to Medicare exam		G0366		I&D, abscess	10060			TB	86580
	Flexible sigmoidoscopy		G0104		I&D, hematoma/seroma	10140			UA, complete, non-automated	81000
	Hemoccult, guaiac		G0107		Laceration repair, simple	120___			UA, w/o micro, non-automated	81002
	Flu shot		G0008		Site: _____ Size: _____				UA, w/ micro, non-automated	81003
	Pneumonia shot		G0009		Laceration repair, layered	120___			Urine colony count	87086
	Consultation/preop clearance				Site: _____ Size: _____				Urine culture, presumptive	87088
	Expanded problem focused		99242		Lesion, biopsy, one	11100			Wet mount/KOH	87210
	Detailed		99243		Lesion, biopsy, each add'l	11101			**Vaccines**	
	Comprehensive/mod complexity		99244		Lesion, destruct., benign, 1-14	17110			DT, <7 y	90702
	Comprehensive/high complexity		99245		Lesion, destruct., premal., single	17000			DTP	90701
	Other services				Lesion, destruct., premal., ea. add'l	17003			DtaP, <7 y	90700
	After posted hours		99050		Lesion, excision, benign	114___			Flu, 6-35 months	90657
	Evening/weekend appointment		99051		Site: _____ Size: _____				Flu, 3 y +	90658
	Home health certification		G0180		Lesion, excision, malignant	116___			Hep A, adult	90632
	Home health recertification		G0179		Site: _____ Size: _____				Hep A, ped/adol, 2 dose	90633
	Post-op follow-up		99024		Lesion, paring/cutting, one	11055			Hep B, adult	90746
	Prolonged/30-74 min		99354		Lesion, paring/cutting, 2-4	11056			Hep B, ped/adol 3 dose	90744
	Special reports/forms		99080		Lesion, shave	113___			Hep B-Hib	90748
	Disability/Workers comp		99455		Site: _____ Size: _____				Hib, 4 dose	90645
	Radiology				Nail removal, partial	11730			HPV	90649
					Nail removal, w/matrix	11750			IPV	90713
					Skin tag, 1-15	11200			MMR	90707
	Diagnoses				**Medications**		**Units**		Pneumonia, >2 y	90732
1	S71.109A				Ampicillin, up to 500mg	J0290			Pneumonia conjugate, <5 y	90669
2	W29.8XXA				B-12, up to 1,000 mcg	J3420			Td, >7 y	90718
3	Z23				Epinephrine, up to 1ml	J0170			Varicella	90716
4					Kenalog, 10mg	J3301			**Immunizations & Injections**	**Units**
	Next office visit				Lidocaine, 10mg	J2001			Allergen, one	95115	
	Recheck Prev PRN ____ D W M Y				Normal saline, 1000cc	J7030			Allergen, multiple	95117	
	Instructions:				Phenergan, up to 50mg	J2550		X	Imm admin, one	90471	
					Progesterone, 150mg	J1055			Imm admin, each add'l	90472	
					Rocephin, 250mg	J0696			Imm admin, intranasal, one	90473	
					Testosterone, 200mg	J1080			Imm admin, intranasal, each add'l	90474	
	Referral				Tigan, up to 200 mg	J3250			Injection, joint, small	20600	
	To:				Toradol, 15mg	J1885			Injection, joint, intermediate	20605	
					Miscellaneous services				Injection, joint, major	20610	
	Instructions:								Injection, ther/proph/diag	90772	
									Injection, trigger point	20552	
	Physician signature								**Supplies**	
									Tetanus and diptheria toxoids - 90714	
	X _____									

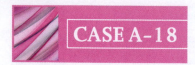

Capital City Medical—123 Unknown Boulevard, Capital City, NY 12345-2222, (555) 555-1234

Phil Wells, M.D., Mannie Mends, M.D., Bette R. Soone, M.D.

Patient Information Form

Tax ID: 75-0246810

Group NPI: 1513171216

Patient Information:

Name: (Last, First) Acosta, Kimber   ❑ Male Female   Birth Date: 08/01/1946

Address: 821 Spruce St, Capital City, NY 12345   Phone: (555) 555-5678

Social Security Number: 101-19-6205   Full-Time Student: ❑ Yes   ☒ No

Marital Status: ❑ Single   ❑ Married   ☒ Divorced   ❑ Other

Employment:

Employer: Braddock Care Home   Phone: (555) 555-2060

Address: 294 Elmhurst Way, Township, NY 12345

Condition Related to: ❑ Auto Accident   ❑ Employment   ❑ Other Accident

Date of Accident: _____ State _____

Emergency Contact: _____   **Phone: ( )** _____

Primary Insurance: Aetna   Phone: ( ) _____

Address: 1625 Healthcare Bldg, Capital City, NY 12345

Insurance Policyholder's Name: Same _____   ❑ M   ❑ F   DOB: _____

Address: _____

Phone: _____   Relationship to Insured: ☒ Self ❑ Spouse ❑ Child ❑ Other

Employer: Braddock Care Home   Phone: ( ) _____

Employer's Address: Same

Policy/I.D. No: 2054654 Group No: 201410 Percent Covered: ____%, Copay Amt: $10.00

Secondary Insurance: Medicare   Phone: ( ) _____

Address: P.O. Box 9834, Capital City, NY 12345

Insurance Policyholder's Name: Same _____   ❑ M   ❑ F   DOB: _____

Address: _____

Phone: _____   Relationship to Insured: ☒ Self ❑ Spouse ❑ Child ❑ Other

Employer: _____   Phone: ( ) _____

Employer's Address: _____

Policy/I.D. No: 856426598A Group No: ____ Percent Covered: 80 %, Copay Amt: $____

Reason for Visit: I need a physical and a check on my diabetes _____

Known Allergies: _____

Were you referred here? If so, by whom? _____

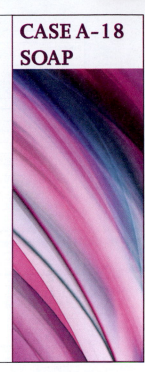

CASE A-18
SOAP

03/11/20XX
Assignment of Benefits: Y
Signature on File: Y
Referring Physician: N

S: Kimber Acosta is being seen for her annual physical.

O: ROS shows negative findings consistent with any disease process. Pt. does have DM II. Glucose, and U/A shows stable blood sugar levels.

A: 1. Annual PE—ICD-10 (Z00.00)
   2. DM II—ICD-10 (E11.9)

P: 1. Healthy female.
   2. Flu vaccine today—ICD-10 (Z23).

Phil Wells, M.D.

Family Practice

NPI: 1234567890

PIN: 654321

Date of service:	03/11/XX		Waiver? ☐	
Patient name:	Kimber Acosta		Insurance:	
			Subscriber name:	
Address:	821 Spruce St		Group #:	Previous balance:
	Township, NY 12345		Copay:	Today's charges:
Phone:	555-555-5678		Account #:	Today's payment: check#
DOB:	08/01/1946 Age: Sex:		Physician name:	Balance due:

RANK	Office visit	New	Est	RANK	Office procedures			RANK	Laboratory		
	Minimal		99211		Anoscopy		46600	X	Venipuncture		36415
	Problem focused	99201	99212		Audiometry		92551		Blood glucose, monitoring device		82962
	Expanded problem focused	99202	99213		Cerumen removal		69210		Blood glucose, visual dipstick		82948
	Detailed	99203	99214		Colposcopy		57452		CBC, w/ auto differential		85025
	Comprehensive	99204	99215		Colposcopy w/biopsy		57455		CBC, w/o auto differential		85027
	Comprehensive (new patient)	99205			ECG, w/interpretation		93000		Cholesterol		82465
	Significant, separate service	-25	-25		ECG, rhythm strip		93040		Hemoccult, guaiac		82270
	Well visit	**New**	**Est**		Endometrial biopsy		58100		Hemoccult, immunoassay		82274
	< 1 y	99381	99391		Flexible sigmoidoscopy		45330		Hemoglobin A1C		85018
	1-4 y	99382	99392		Flexible sigmoidoscopy w/biopsy		45331		Lipid panel		80061
	5-11 y	99383	99393		Fracture care, cast/splint		29____		Liver panel		80076
	12-17 y	99384	99394		Site: _____				KOH prep (skin, hair, nails)		87220
	18-39 y	99385	99395		Nebulizer		94640		Metabolic panel, basic		80048
X	40-64 y	99386	99396		Nebulizer demo		94664		Metabolic panel, comprehensive		80053
	65 y +	99387	99397		Spirometry		94010		Mononucleosis		86308
	Medicare preventive services				Spirometry, pre and post		94060		Pregnancy, blood		84703
	Pap		Q0091		Tympanometry		92567		Pregnancy, urine		81025
	Pelvic & breast		G0101		Vasectomy		55250		Renal panel		80069
	Prostate/PSA		G0103		**Skin procedures**		**Units**		Sedimentation rate		85651
	Tobacco counseling/3-10 min		99406		Burn care, initial	16000			Strep, rapid		86403
	Tobacco counseling/>10 min		99407		Foreign body, skin, simple	10120			Strep culture		87081
	Welcome to Medicare exam		G0344		Foreign body, skin, complex	10121			Strep A		87880
	ECG w/Welcome to Medicare exam		G0366		I&D, abscess	10060			TB		86580
	Flexible sigmoidoscopy		G0104		I&D, hematoma/seroma	10140		X	UA, complete, non-automated		81000
	Hemoccult, guaiac		G0107		Laceration repair, simple	120____			UA, w/o micro, non-automated		81002
	Flu shot		G0008		Site: _____ Size: ____				UA, w/ micro, non-automated		81003
	Pneumonia shot		G0009		Laceration repair, layered	120____			Urine colony count		87086
	Consultation/preop clearance				Site: _____ Size: ____				Urine culture, presumptive		87088
	Expanded problem focused		99242		Lesion, biopsy, one	11100			Wet mount/KOH		87210
	Detailed		99243		Lesion, biopsy, each add'l	11101			**Vaccines**		
	Comprehensive/mod complexity		99244		Lesion, destruct., benign, 1-14	17110			DT, <7 y		90702
	Comprehensive/high complexity		99245		Lesion, destruct., premal., single	17000			DTP		90701
	Other services				Lesion, destruct., premal., ea. add'l	17003			DtaP, <7 y		90700
	After posted hours		99050		Lesion, excision, benign	114____			Flu, 6-35 months		90657
	Evening/weekend appointment		99051		Site: _____ Size: ____			X	Flu, 3 y +		90658
	Home health certification		G0180		Lesion, excision, malignant	116____			Hep A, adult		90632
	Home health recertification		G0179		Site: _____ Size: ____				Hep A, ped/adol, 2 dose		90633
	Post-op follow-up		99024		Lesion, paring/cutting, one	11055			Hep B, adult		90746
	Prolonged/30-74 min		99354		Lesion, paring/cutting, 2-4	11056			Hep B, ped/adol 3 dose		90744
	Special reports/forms		99080		Lesion, shave	113____			Hep B-Hib		90748
	Disability/Workers comp		99455		Site: _____ Size: ____				Hib, 4 dose		90645
	Radiology				Nail removal, partial	11730			HPV		90649
					Nail removal, w/matrix	11750			IPV		90713
					Skin tag, 1-15	11200			MMR		90707
	Diagnoses				**Medications**		**Units**		Pneumonia, >2 y		90732
1	Z00.00				Ampicillin, up to 500mg	J0290			Pneumonia conjugate, <5 y		90669
2	Z23				B-12, up to 1,000 mcg	J3420			Td, >7 y		90718
3	E11.9				Epinephrine, up to 1ml	J0170			Varicella		90716
4					Kenalog, 10mg	J3301			**Immunizations & Injections**		**Units**
Next office visit					Lidocaine, 10mg	J2001			Allergen, one	95115	
Recheck Prev PRN _____ D W M Y					Normal saline, 1000cc	J7030			Allergen, multiple	95117	
Instructions:					Phenergan, up to 50mg	J2550		X	Imm admin, one	90471	
					Progesterone, 150mg	J1055			Imm admin, each add'l	90472	
					Rocephin, 250mg	J0696			Imm admin, intranasal, one	90473	
					Testosterone, 200mg	J1080			Imm admin, intranasal, each add'l	90474	
Referral					Tigan, up to 200 mg	J3250			Injection, joint, small	20600	
To:					Toradol, 15mg	J1885			Injection, joint, intermediate	20605	
					Miscellaneous services				Injection, joint, major	20610	
Instructions:									Injection, ther/proph/diag	90772	
					Glucose - 82947				Injection, trigger point	20552	
Physician signature									**Supplies**		
X _____											

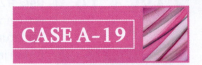

CASE A-19

Capital City Medical—123 Unknown Boulevard, Capital City, NY 12345-2222, (555) 555-1234

Phil Wells, M.D., Mannie Mends, M.D., Bette R. Soone, M.D.

Patient Information Form

Tax ID: 75-0246810

Group NPI: 1513171216

Patient Information:

Name: (Last, First) Fields, Chester   ☒ Male   ☐ Female   Birth Date: 08/31/1943

Address: 1902 Birch Ave, Capital City, NY 12345   Phone: (555) 555-1112

Social Security Number: 652-91-3046   Full-Time Student: ☐ Yes   ☒ No

Marital Status: ☐ Single   ☒ Married   ☐ Divorced   ☐ Other

Employment:

Employer: Retired   Phone: ( )

Address:

Condition Related to: ☐ Auto Accident   ☐ Employment   ☐ Other Accident

Date of Accident: _____ State _____

Emergency Contact: _____   Phone: ( ) _____

Primary Insurance: Medicare   Phone: ( ) _____

Address: P.O. Box 9834, Capital City, NY 12345

Insurance Policyholder's Name: Same   ☐ M   ☐ F   DOB:

Address:

Phone: _____   Relationship to Insured: ☒ Self   ☐ Spouse   ☐ Child   ☐ Other

Employer: _____   Phone: ( ) _____

Employer's Address:

Policy/I.D. No: 359560568A   Group No: ____   Percent Covered: 80 %, Copay Amt: $___

Secondary Insurance: Blue Cross Blue Shield Medigap   Phone: ( ) _____

Address: 379 Blue Plaza, Capital City, NY 12345

Insurance Policyholder's Name: Same   ☐ M   ☐ F   DOB:

Address:

Phone: _____   Relationship to Insured: ☒ Self   ☐ Spouse   ☐ Child   ☐ Other

Employer: _____   Phone: ( ) _____

Employer's Address:

Policy/I.D. No: YYZ65281623   Group No: ____   Percent Covered: ___%, Copay Amt: $___

Reason for Visit: Having chest pain

Known Allergies:

Were you referred here? If so, by whom?:

CASE A-19 SOAP

04/24/20XX
Assignment of Benefits: Y
Signature on File: Y
Referring Physician: N

S: Chester Fields presents with complaints of CP.

O: BP stable at 118/80, P 94. EKG reveals normal sinus rhythm with no ST-T changes. Holter ordered. Pt. does admit to palpitations × 2 days.

A: 1. Angina pectoris—ICD-10 (I20.8)

　　2. Palpitations—ICD-10 (R00.2)

　　3. HTN; benign—ICD-10 (I11.9)

P: 1. Refill BP med Norvasc.

　　2. Return tomorrow for Holter monitor disconnection.

　　3. Refer to Dr. Iva Hart, cardiology, for possible stress test.

_____

Phil Wells, M.D.

Family Practice

NPI: 1234567890

PIN: 657891

Date of service:	04/24/XX		Waiver? ☐		
Patient name:	Chester Fields		Insurance:		
			Subscriber name:		
Address:	1902 Birch Ave		Group #:		Previous balance:
	Capital City, NY 12345		Copay:		Today's charges:
Phone:	555-555-5678		Account #:		Today's payment: check#
DOB:	08/31/1943 Age: Sex:		Physician name:		Balance due:

RANK	Office visit	New	Est	RANK	Office procedures			RANK	Laboratory	
	Minimal		99211		Anoscopy		46600	X	Venipuncture	36415
	Problem focused	99201	99212		Audiometry		92551		Blood glucose, monitoring device	82962
X	Expanded problem focused	99202	99213		Cerumen removal		69210		Blood glucose, visual dipstick	82948
	Detailed	99203	99214		Colposcopy		57452	X	CBC, w/ auto differential	85025
	Comprehensive	99204	99215		Colposcopy w/biopsy		57455		CBC, w/o auto differential	85027
	Comprehensive (new patient)	99205			ECG, w/interpretation		93000		Cholesterol	82465
	Significant, separate service	-25	-25		ECG, rhythm strip		93040		Hemoccult, guaiac	82270
	Well visit	**New**	**Est**		Endometrial biopsy		58100		Hemoccult, immunoassay	82274
	< 1 y	99381	99391		Flexible sigmoidoscopy		45330		Hemoglobin A1C	85018
	1-4 y	99382	99392		Flexible sigmoidoscopy w/biopsy		45331		Lipid panel	80061
	5-11 y	99383	99393		Fracture care, cast/splint		29____		Liver panel	80076
	12-17 y	99384	99394		Site:				KOH prep (skin, hair, nails)	87220
	18-39 y	99385	99395		Nebulizer		94640		Metabolic panel, basic	80048
	40-64 y	99386	99396		Nebulizer demo		94664		Metabolic panel, comprehensive	80053
	65 y +	99387	99397		Spirometry		94010		Mononucleosis	86308
	Medicare preventive services				Spirometry, pre and post		94060		Pregnancy, blood	84703
	Pap		Q0091		Tympanometry		92567		Pregnancy, urine	81025
	Pelvic & breast		G0101		Vasectomy		55250		Renal panel	80069
	Prostate/PSA		G0103		**Skin procedures**		**Units**		Sedimentation rate	85651
	Tobacco counseling/3-10 min		99406		Burn care, initial	16000			Strep, rapid	86403
	Tobacco counseling/>10 min		99407		Foreign body, skin, simple	10120			Strep culture	87081
	Welcome to Medicare exam		G0344		Foreign body, skin, complex	10121			Strep A	87880
	ECG w/Welcome to Medicare exam		G0366		I&D, abscess	10060			TB	86580
	Flexible sigmoidoscopy		G0104		I&D, hematoma/seroma	10140			UA, complete, non-automated	81000
	Hemoccult, guaiac		G0107		Laceration repair, simple	120____			UA, w/o micro, non-automated	81002
	Flu shot		G0008		Site: _____ Size: ____				UA, w/ micro, non-automated	81003
	Pneumonia shot		G0009		Laceration repair, layered	120____			Urine colony count	87086
	Consultation/preop clearance				Site: _____ Size: ____				Urine culture, presumptive	87088
	Expanded problem focused		99242		Lesion, biopsy, one	11100			Wet mount/KOH	87210
	Detailed		99243		Lesion, biopsy, each add'l	11101			**Vaccines**	
	Comprehensive/mod complexity		99244		Lesion, destruct., benign 1-14	17110			DT, <7 y	90702
	Comprehensive/high complexity		99245		Lesion, destruct., premal., single	17000			DTP	90701
	Other services				Lesion, destruct., premal., ea. add'l	17003			DtaP, <7 y	90700
	After posted hours		99050		Lesion, excision, benign	114____			Flu, 6-35 months	90657
	Evening/weekend appointment		99051		Site: _____ Size: ____				Flu, 3 y +	90658
	Home health certification		G0180		Lesion, excision, malignant	116____			Hep A, adult	90632
	Home health recertification		G0179		Site: _____ Size: ____				Hep A, ped/adol, 2 dose	90633
	Post-op follow-up		99024		Lesion, paring/cutting, one	11055			Hep B, adult	90746
	Prolonged/30-74 min		99354		Lesion, paring/cutting, 2-4	11056			Hep B, ped/adol 3 dose	90744
	Special reports/forms		99080		Lesion, shave	113____			Hep B-Hib	90748
	Disability/Workers comp		99455		Site: _____ Size: ____				Hib, 4 dose	90645
	Radiology				Nail removal, partial	11730			HPV	90649
					Nail removal, w/matrix	11750			IPV	90713
					Skin tag, 1-15	11200			MMR	90707
	Diagnoses				**Medications**		**Units**		Pneumonia, >2 y	90732
1	I20.8				Ampicillin, up to 500mg	J0290			Pneumonia conjugate, <5 y	90669
2	R00.2				B-12, up to 1,000 mcg	J3420			Td, >7 y	90718
3	I11.9				Epinephrine, up to 1ml	J0170			Varicella	90716
4					Kenalog, 10mg	J3301			**Immunizations & Injections**	**Units**

Next office visit				
Recheck	Prev	PRN	_____	D W M Y

		Units
Lidocaine, 10mg	J2001	
Normal saline, 1000cc	J7030	
Phenergan, up to 50mg	J2550	
Progesterone, 150mg	J1055	
Rocephin, 250mg	J0696	
Testosterone, 200mg	J1080	
Tigan, up to 200 mg	J3250	
Toradol, 15mg	J1885	

		Units
Allergen, one	95115	
Allergen, multiple	95117	
Imm admin, one	90471	
Imm admin, each add'l	90472	
Imm admin, intranasal, one	90473	
Imm admin, intranasal, each add'l	90474	
Injection, joint, small	20600	
Injection, joint, intermediate	20605	
Injection, joint, major	20610	
Injection, ther/proph/diag	90772	
Injection, trigger point	20552	

Instructions:

Miscellaneous services

electrocardiograph recording - 93225
Routine ECG - 93000
Pulse oximetry - 94760

Supplies

Referral

To:

Instructions:

Physician signature

X _____

CASE A-19 ENCOUNTER FORM

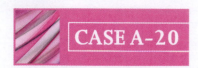

CASE A-20

Capital City Medical—123 Unknown Boulevard, Capital City, NY 12345-2222, (555) 555-1234
Phil Wells, M.D., Mannie Mends, M.D., Bette R. Soone, M.D.

Patient Information Form
Tax ID: 75-0246810
Group NPI: 1513171216

Patient Information:

Name: (Last, First) Huckle, Gertrude   ☐ Male   ☐ Female   Birth Date: 04/08/1939

Address: 901 Poplar Rd, Capital City, NY 12345   Phone: (555) 555-1213

Social Security Number: 309-18-0684   Full-Time Student: ☐ Yes   ☒ No

Marital Status: ☐ Single   ☒ Married   ☐ Divorced   ☐ Other

Employment:

Employer: Retired   Phone: ( ) _____

Address: _____

Condition Related to: ☐ Auto Accident   ☐ Employment   ☐ Other Accident

Date of Accident: _____   State _____

Emergency Contact: _____   **Phone: ( )** _____

Primary Insurance: Medicare   **Phone: ( )** _____

Address: P.O. Box 9834, Capital City, NY 12345

Insurance Policyholder's Name: Same   ☐ M ☐ F DOB: _____

Address: _____

Phone: _____ Relationship to Insured: ☒ Self ☐ Spouse ☐ Child ☐ Other

Employer: _____   Phone: ( ) _____

Employer's Address: _____

Policy/I.D. No: 238123565A Group No: _____ Percent Covered: 80 %, Copay Amt: $__

Secondary Insurance: Health America   **Phone: ( )** _____

Address: 2031 Healthica Center, Capital City, NY 12345

Insurance Policyholder's Name: Same   ☐ M ☐ F DOB: _____

Address: _____

Phone: _____ Relationship to Insured: ☒ Self ☐ Spouse ☐ Child ☐ Other

Employer: Retired   Phone: ( ) _____

Employer's Address: _____

Policy/I.D. No: 0004594 Group No: 9048000 Percent Covered: 80 %, Copay Amt: $__

Reason for Visit: Check up on pilonidal cyst and possible removal of it

Known Allergies: _____

Were you referred here? If so, by whom? _____

CASE A-20
SOAP

11/09/20XX
Assignment of Benefits: Y
Signature on File: Y
Referring Physician: N

S: Gertrude Huckle is here for a follow-up on her pilonidal cyst. She has had it × 3 weeks.

O: Pt. still complains of pain associated with sitting. She says that it is so bad, she can't even sit for 10 minutes. Upon exam, there is no change in the size of the cyst. Simple I&D will be necessary.

A: 1. Pilonidal cyst—ICD-10 (L05.91)

P: 1. Keep bandaged for 1 week.

   2. Do not take baths, only showers.

   3. Return in 7 days for suture removal.

_____

Mannie Mends, M.D.
General Surgeon
NPI: 012345689
PIN: 446213

Date of service:	11/09/XX		Waiver? ☐		
Patient name:	Gertrude Huckle		Insurance:		
			Subscriber name:		
Address:	901 Poplar Rd		Group #:		Previous balance:
	Capital City, NY 12345		Copay:		Today's charges:
Phone:	555-555-1213		Account #:		Today's payment: check#
DOB:	04/08/1939 Age: Sex:		Physician name:		Balance due:

RANK	Office visit	New	Est	RANK	Office procedures			RANK	Laboratory	
	Minimal		99211		Anoscopy		46600		Venipuncture	36415
	Problem focused	99201	99212		Audiometry		92551		Blood glucose, monitoring device	82962
	Expanded problem focused	99202	99213		Cerumen removal		69210		Blood glucose, visual dipstick	82948
	Detailed	99203	99214		Colposcopy		57452		CBC, w/ auto differential	85025
	Comprehensive	99204	99215		Colposcopy w/biopsy		57455		CBC, w/o auto differential	85027
	Comprehensive (new patient)	99205			ECG, w/interpretation		93000		Cholesterol	82465
	Significant, separate service	-25	-25		ECG, rhythm strip		93040		Hemoccult, guaiac	82270
	Well visit	**New**	**Est**		Endometrial biopsy		58100		Hemoccult, immunoassay	82274
	< 1 y	99381	99391		Flexible sigmoidoscopy		45330		Hemoglobin A1C	85018
	1-4 y	99382	99392		Flexible sigmoidoscopy w/biopsy		45331		Lipid panel	80061
	5-11 y	99383	99393		Fracture care, cast/splint		29____		Liver panel	80076
	12-17 y	99384	99394		Site: _____				KOH prep (skin, hair, nails)	87220
	18-39 y	99385	99395		Nebulizer		94640		Metabolic panel, basic	80048
	40-64 y	99386	99396		Nebulizer demo		94664		Metabolic panel, comprehensive	80053
	65 y +	99387	99397		Spirometry		94010		Mononucleosis	86308
	Medicare preventive services				Spirometry, pre and post		94060		Pregnancy, blood	84703
	Pap		Q0091		Tympanometry		92567		Pregnancy, urine	81025
	Pelvic & breast		G0101		Vasectomy		55250		Renal panel	80069
	Prostate/PSA		G0103		**Skin procedures**		**Units**		Sedimentation rate	85651
	Tobacco counseling/3-10 min		99406		Burn care, initial	16000			Strep, rapid	86403
	Tobacco counseling/>10 min		99407		Foreign body, skin, simple	10120			Strep culture	87081
	Welcome to Medicare exam		G0344		Foreign body, skin, complex	10121			Strep A	87880
	ECG w/Welcome to Medicare exam		G0366		I&D, abscess	10060			TB	86580
	Flexible sigmoidoscopy		G0104		I&D, hematoma/seroma	10140			UA, complete, non-automated	81000
	Hemoccult, guaiac		G0107		Laceration repair, simple	120____			UA, w/o micro, non-automated	81002
	Flu shot		G0008		Site: _____ Size: ____				UA, w/ micro, non-automated	81003
	Pneumonia shot		G0009		Laceration repair, layered	120____			Urine colony count	87086
	Consultation/preop clearance				Site: _____ Size: ____				Urine culture, presumptive	87088
	Expanded problem focused		99242		Lesion, biopsy, one	11100			Wet mount/KOH	87210
	Detailed		99243		Lesion, biopsy, each add'l	11101			**Vaccines**	
	Comprehensive/mod complexity		99244		Lesion, destruct., benign, 1-14	17110			DT, <7 y	90702
	Comprehensive/high complexity		99245		Lesion, destruct., premal., single	17000			DTP	90701
	Other services				Lesion, destruct., premal., ea. add'l	17003			DtaP, <7 y	90700
	After posted hours		99050		Lesion, excision, benign	114____			Flu, 6-35 months	90657
	Evening/weekend appointment		99051		Site: _____ Size: ____				Flu, 3 y +	90658
	Home health certification		G0180		Lesion, excision, malignant	116____			Hep A, adult	90632
	Home health recertification		G0179		Site: _____ Size: ____				Hep A, ped/adol, 2 dose	90633
	Post-op follow-up		99024		Lesion, paring/cutting, one	11055			Hep B, adult	90746
	Prolonged/30-74 min		99354		Lesion, paring/cutting, 2-4	11056			Hep B, ped/adol 3 dose	90744
	Special reports/forms		99080		Lesion, shave	113____			Hep B-Hib	90748
	Disability/Workers comp		99455		Site: _____ Size: ____				Hib, 4 dose	90645
	Radiology				Nail removal, partial	11730			HPV	90649
					Nail removal, w/matrix	11750			IPV	90713
					Skin tag, 1-15	11200			MMR	90707
	Diagnoses				**Medications**		**Units**		Pneumonia, >2 y	90732
1	L05.91				Ampicillin, up to 500mg	J0290			Pneumonia conjugate, <5 y	90669
2					B-12, up to 1,000 mcg	J3420			Td, >7 y	90718
3					Epinephrine, up to 1ml	J0170			Varicella	90716
4					Kenalog, 10mg	J3301			**Immunizations & Injections**	**Units**
Next office visit					Lidocaine, 10mg	J2001			Allergen, one	95115
Recheck	Prev	PRN	____ D W M Y		Normal saline, 1000cc	J7030			Allergen, multiple	95117
Instructions:					Phenergan, up to 50mg	J2550			Imm admin, one	90471
					Progesterone, 150mg	J1055			Imm admin, each add'l	90472
					Rocephin, 250mg	J0696			Imm admin, intranasal, one	90473
					Testosterone, 200mg	J1080			Imm admin, intranasal, each add'l	90474
Referral					Tigan, up to 200 mg	J3250			Injection, joint, small	20600
To:					Toradol, 15mg	J1885			Injection, joint, intermediate	20605
					Miscellaneous services				Injection, joint, major	20610
Instructions:									Injection, ther/proph/diag	90772
					I&D cyst - 10080				Injection, trigger point	20552
Physician signature									**Supplies**	
X _____										

Capital City Medical
Fee Schedule

New Patient OV		Punch Biopsy various codes	$80
Problem Focused 99201	$45	Nebulizer various codes	$45
Expanded Problem Focused 99202	$65	Cast Application 25600 various codes	$85
Detailed 99203	$85	Laryngoscopy 31505	$255
Comprehensive 99204	$105	Audiometry 92552	$85
Comprehensive/High Complex 99205	$115	Tympanometry 92567	$85
Well Exam Infant (less than 1 year) 99381	$45	Ear Irrigation 69210	$25
Well Exam 1–4 yrs. 99382	$50	Diaphragm Fitting 57170	$30
Well Exam 5–11 yrs. 99383	$55	IV Therapy (up to 1 hour) 96365	$65
Well Exam 12–17 yrs. 99384	$65	Each additional hour 96366	$50
Well Exam 18–39 yrs. 99385	$85	Oximetry 94760	$10
Well Exam 40–64 yrs. 99386	$105	ECG 93000	$75
Established Patient OV		Holter Monitor various codes	$170
Post-Op Follow-up Visit 99024	$0	Rhythm Strip 93040	$60
Minimum 99211	$35	Treadmill 93015	$375
Problem Focused 99212	$45	Cocci Skin Test 86490	$20
Expanded Problem Focused 99213	$55	X-ray, spine, chest, bone—any area various codes	$275
Detailed 99214	$65	Avulsion Nail 11730	$200
Comprehensive/High Complex 99215	$75	Laboratory	
Well Exam infant (less than 1 year) 99391	$35	Amylase 82150	$40
Well Exam 1–4 yrs. 99392	$40	B12 82607	$30
Well Exam 5–11 yrs. 99393	$45	CBC & Diff 85025	$95
Well Exam 12–17 yrs. 99394	$55	Comp Metabolic Panel 80053	$75
Well Exam 18–39 yrs. 99395	$65	Chlamydia Screen 87110	$70
Well Exam 40–64 yrs. 99396	$75	Cholestrerol 82465	$75
Obstetrics		Digoxin 80162	$40
Total OB Care 59400	$1700	Electrolytes 80051	$70
Injections		Estrogen, Total 82672	$50
Administration Through 18 Years 90460	$10	Ferritin 82728	$40
Allergy 95115	$35	Folate 82746	$30
DTP 90701	$50	GC Screen 87070	$60
Drug Various Codes	$35	Glucose 82947	$35
Influenza 90658	$25	Glycosylated HGB A1C 83036	$45
MMR 90707	$50	HCT 85014	$30
OPV 90712	$40	HDL 83718	$35
Pneumovax 90732	$35	HGB 85018	$30
TB Skin Test 86580	$15	Hep BSAG 83740	$40
TD 90718	$40	Hepatitis Panel, Acute 80074	$95
Tetanus Toxoid 90703	$40	HIV 86703	$100
		Iron & TIBC 83550	$45
		Kidney Profile 80069	$95
Vaccine/Toxoid Administration for Adult 90471	$10	Lead 83665	$55
Arthrocentesis/Aspiration/Injection		Lipase 83690	$40
Small Joint 20600	$50	Lipid Panel 80061	$95
Interm Joint 20605	$60	Liver Profile 80076	$95
Major Joint 20610	$70	Mono Test 86308	$30
Trigger Point/Tendon Sheath Inj. 20550	$90	Pap Smear 88155	$90
Other Invasive/Noninvasive Procedures		Pap Collection/Supervision 88142	$95
Catheterization 51701	$55	Pregnancy Test 84156	$90
Circumcision 54150	$150	Obstetric Panel 80055	$85
Colposcopy 57452	$225	Pro Time 85610	$50
Colposcopy w/Biopsy 57454	$250	PSA 84153	$50
Cryosurgery Premalignant Lesion various codes	$160	RPR 86592	$55
Endometrial Biopsy 58100	$190	Sed. Rate 85651	$50
Excision Lesion Malignant various codes	$145	Stool Culture 87045	$80
Excision Lesion Benign various codes	$125	Stool O & P 87177	$105
Curettement Lesion		Strep Screen 87880	$35
Single 11055	$70	Theophylline 80198	$40
2–4 11056	$80	Thyroid Uptake 84479	$75
> 4 11057	$90	TSH 84443	$50
Excision Skin Tags (1–15) 11200	$55	Urinalysis 81000	$35
Each Additional 10 11201	$30	Urine, bacterial culture 87086	$80
I & D Abscess Single/Simple 10060	$75	Drawing Fee 36415	$15
Multiple/Complex 10061	$95	Specimen Handling 99000	$10
I & D Pilonidal Cyst Simple 10080	$105		
I & D Pilonidal Cyst Complex 10081	$130		
Laceration Repair various codes	$60		

Completing the CMS-1500 Form for Physician Outpatient Billing Plus Determining the Correct Diagnostic and Procedure Codes

The case studies in this appendix are provided for additional practice in coding and in completing the CMS-1500 claim form for physician outpatient billing. By applying what you have learned in this text, your objective is to accurately code and complete each case study. In addition to completing the CMS-1500 form, you will be required to insert the correct diagnostic and procedure codes on the SOAP forms for each patient, for which you will need both the ICD and CPT manuals. Patient demographics and a brief case history are provided.

Complete the cases based on the following criteria:

- All patients have release of information and assignment of benefit signatures on file.
- All providers are participating and accept assignment.
- The group practice is the billing entity.
- 2017 ICD-10-CM and CPT codes are used.

For the cases in this appendix, the student should provide the ICD-10-CM code(s) on the claim forms. For other exercises in the textbook, when instructed, the student should provide the ICD-10-CM code(s).

When entering procedures, students should enter the E/M code first, followed by all other codes in descending cost order. The following history and exam levels should be used to determine E/M codes:

- Min = Minimal
- PF = Problem Focused
- EPF = Extended Problem Focused
- D = Detailed
- C = Comprehensive
- HC = Comprehensive with High Complexity Decision Making

CPT-4 codes in this appendix are from the CPT-4 2017 code set. CPT® is a registered trademark of the American Medical Association.

ICD-10-CM codes in this appendix are from the ICD-10-CM 2017 code set from the Department of Health and Human Services, Centers for Disease Control and Prevention.

Use eight-digit dates for birth dates. Use six-digit dates for all other dates. All street names should be entered using standard postal abbreviations, even if they are spelled out on the source documents. To complete each case study, copy the CMS-1500 form provided in Appendix D or download the form from MyHealthProfessionsKit or MyHealthProfessionsLab, which accompany this text. Refer to the Capital City Medical Fee Schedule on page 615 to determine the correct fees. For a list of abbreviations used in these case studies and their meanings, please refer to MyHealthProfessionsKit or MyHealthProfessionsLab, which accompany this text.

CASE STUDIES

Primary Payer

Case	Patient	Primary Payer
Case B-1	Roberto Muñoz	Medicaid
Case B-2	Aaron Abner	Blue Cross Blue Shield
Case B-3	Abbie Spencer	Blue Cross Blue Shield
Case B-4	Justin Leasure	Blue Cross Blue Shield
Case B-5	Shayla Robinson	Medicaid
Case B-6	Mia Lui	Health America
Case B-7	April O'Leary	Aetna
Case B-8	Abdul Qabiz	Aetna
Case B-9	Clyde Hedberg	TRICARE
Case B-10	Kelly Campbell	Accidents Happen (auto insurance)

Primary/Secondary Payers

Case	Patient	Primary Payer/Secondary Payer
Case B-11	Doree Marowski	Medicare/Medicaid
Case B-12	Joseph Hodreal	Medicare/Medicaid
Case B-13	Victoria Kozak	Medicare/Medicaid
Case B-14	Natasha Gubin	Medicare/Medicaid
Case B-15	Norma Casella	Medicare/Blue Cross Blue Shield (Medigap)
Case B-16	Earl Abbott	Blue Cross Blue Shield/Medicare (MSP)
Case B-17	Clifford McDavidson	Medicare/Aetna (Medigap)
Case B-18	Stewart Jenkins	Medicare/Medicaid
Case B-19	Adelphie Popazekus	Medicare/Aetna (Retiree)
Case B-20	Marsha Gambaro	Medicare/Health America (Retiree)

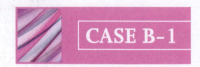

CASE B-1

Capital City Medical—123 Unknown Blvd, Capital City, NY 12345-2222, (555) 555-1234	Patient Information Form
Phil Wells, M.D., Mannie Mends, M.D., Bette R. Soone, M.D.	Tax ID: 75-0246810 Group NPI: 1513171216

Patient Information:

Name: (Last, First) Muñoz, Roberto   ☒ ☐ Male   ☐ Female   Birth Date: 11/27/1978

Address: 1210 Sunny Ave, Capital City, NY 12345   Phone: (555) 555-1541

Social Security Number: 794-58-3422   Full-Time Student: ☐ Yes   ☒ No

Marital Status: ☐ Single   ☒ Married   ☐ Divorced   ☐ Other

Employment:

Employer: 24-7 Mini Mart   Phone: (555) 555-8241

Address: 7472 W. Washington St, Capital City, NY 12345

Condition Related to: ☐ Auto Accident   ☐ Employment   ☐ Other Accident

Date of Accident: _____ State _____

Emergency Contact: _____   **Phone:** ( ) _____

Primary Insurance: Medicaid   **Phone:** ( ) _____

Address: 4875 Capital Blvd, Capital City, NY 12345

Insurance Policyholder's Name: _____   ☐ M   ☐ F   DOB: _____

Address: _____

Phone: _____ Relationship to Insured: ☒ Self   ☐ Spouse   ☐ Child   ☐ Other

Employer: _____   Phone: ( ) _____

Employer's Address: _____

Policy/I.D. No: 000174563256 Group No: ___ Percent Covered: ___ %, Copay Amt: $ 5.00

Secondary Insurance: _____   **Phone:** ( ) _____

Address: _____

Insurance Policyholder's Name: _____   ☐ M   ☐ F DOB: _____

Address: _____

Phone: _____ Relationship to Insured: ☐ Self ☐ Spouse ☐ Child ☐ Other

Employer: _____   Phone: ( ) _____

Employer's Address: _____

Policy/I.D. No: _____ Group No: ____ Percent Covered: _____%, Copay Amt: $ ___

Reason for Visit: Surgery follow-up for removal of a keloid scar _____

Known Allergies: _____

Were you referred here? If so, by whom? Dr. Eva N. Good, Internal Medicine, NPI: 8976453201

06/27/20XX
Assignment of Benefits: Y
Signature on File: Y
Referring Physician: N

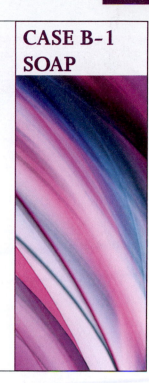

CASE B-1 SOAP

S: Roberto Muñoz presents for a follow-up on his keloid scar surgery.
O: Pt. had keloid scar on the abdomen removed 7 days ago. It has healed well. Skin intact.
No swelling, redness, drainage, or rash at site. Sutures to be removed today. The procedure has 10 global days for post-op follow-up. The payer requires reporting of the post-op visit (no charge).
A: 1. Surgical follow-up
2. Post-op follow-up
P: 1. Call office if any problems occur.

_____

Mannie Mends, M.D.
General Surgeon
NPI: 0123456789
Referral #35877562

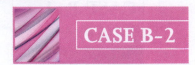

CASE B-2

| Capital City Medical—123 Unknown Blvd, Capital City, NY 12345-2222, (555) 555-1234 Phil Wells, M.D., Mannie Mends, M.D., Bette R. Soone, M.D. | Patient Information Form Tax ID: 75-0246810 Group NPI: 1513171216 |

Patient Information:

Name: (Last, First) Abner, Aaron   ☒ Male   ☐ Female   Birth Date: 01/28/1976

Address: 98 N. Rosewood Dr, Capital City, NY 12345   Phone: (555) 555-8852

Social Security Number: 367-77-1104   Full-Time Student: ☐ Yes   ☒ No

Marital Status: ☐ Single   ☒ Married   ☐ Divorced   ☐ Other

Employment:

Employer: M Mart   Phone: (555) 555-3200

Address: 1019 County Rd, Township, NY 12345

Condition Related to: ☐ Auto Accident   ☐ Employment   ☐ Other Accident

Date of Accident: _____ State _____

Emergency Contact: _____   **Phone: ( )** _____

Primary Insurance: Blue Cross Blue Shield   **Phone: ( )** _____

Address: 379 Blue Plz, Capital City, NY 12345

Insurance Policyholder's Name: Melissa Abner   ☐ M   ☒ F   DOB: 08/04/1974

Address: Same

Phone: _____ Relationship to Insured: ☐ Self   ☒ Spouse   ☐ Child   ☐ Other

Employer: Pasta USA   Phone: (555) 555-6213

Employer's Address: 421 Eight Ave, Township, NY 12345

Policy/I.D. No: YYJ744258013 Group No: 015386 Percent Covered: __%, Copay Amt: $ 10.00

Secondary Insurance: _____   **Phone: ( )** _____

Address: _____

Insurance Policyholder's Name: _____   ☐ M   ☐ F DOB: _____

Address: _____

Phone: _____ Relationship to Insured: ☐ Self   ☐ Spouse   ☐ Child   ☐ Other

Employer: _____   Phone: ( ) _____

Employer's Address: _____

Policy/I.D. No: _____ Group No: _____ Percent Covered: _____ %, Copay Amt: $ __

Reason for Visit: I am having feelings of anxiousness _____

Known Allergies: _____

Were you referred here? If so, by whom? _____

12/01/20XX
Assignment of Benefits: Y
Signature on File: Y
Referring Physician: N

S: New patient, Aaron Abner, is seen in the office for anxiousness, and a feeling of "dying."

O: ROS reveals no disease process. He has family history of CAD; father. Mother has asthma. He has no siblings. He says he gets these episodes more frequently since they started about a month ago. Pt. also complains of bloating, dizziness, palpitations, and a feeling of fainting during these episodes. He is a smoker, 1 pack a day, and he denies any alcohol use. EKG displays normal sinus rhythm. CBC and lytes are normal values. He has been experiencing a lot of stress lately at work and with his marriage. Medical decision making (MDM) is low complexity (LC).

A: 1. Panic disorder
2. Smoker
3. Family history of CAD
4. Family history of asthma
5. E/M (D)
6. Venipuncture
7. CBC with diff
8. Comprehensive Metabolic Panel (CMP)
9. EKG

P: 1. Start pt. on Paxil.
2. Refer pt. to psychiatrist.
3. Return after seeing the psychiatrist.
4. Xanax 1 p.o. t.i.d. #10.

Phil Wells, M.D.
Family Practice
NPI: 1234567890

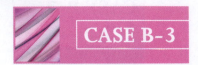

CASE B-3

Capital City Medical—123 Unknown Blvd, Capital City, NY 12345-2222, (555) 555-1234	Patient Information Form
Phil Wells, M.D., Mannie Mends, M.D., Bette R. Soone, M.D.	Tax ID: 75-0246810 Group NPI: 1513171216

Patient Information:

Name: (Last, First) Spencer, Abbie ☐ Male ☒ Female Birth Date: 03/21/2005

Address: 831 Crystal Dr, Capital City, NY 12345   Phone: (555) 555-7163

Social Security Number: 201-48-7302   Full-Time Student: ☐ Yes ☒ No

Marital Status: ☒ Single ☐ Married ☐ Divorced ☐ Other

Employment:

Employer: _____ Phone: ()_____

Address: _____

Condition Related to: ☐ Auto Accident ☐ Employment ☐ Other Accident

Date of Accident: _____ State _____

Emergency Contact: _____ **Phone: ( )** _____

Primary Insurance: Blue Cross Blue Shield   **Phone: ( )** _____

Address: 379 Blue Plz, Capital City, NY 12345

Insurance Policyholder's Name: Mila Spencer   ☐ M ☒ F DOB: 09/25/1987

Address: Same

Phone: _____ Relationship to Insured: ☐ Self ☐ Spouse ☒ Child ☐ Other

Employer: Travel Plus   Phone: (555) 555-0471

Employer's Address: 1632 Getaway Ln, Capital City, NY 12345

Policy/I.D. No: YYZ210529333 Group No: 521036 Percent Covered: __%, Copay Amt: $ 25.00

Secondary Insurance: _____ **Phone: ( )** _____

Address: _____

Insurance Policyholder's Name: _____ ☐ M ☐ F DOB: _____

Address: _____

Phone: _____ Relationship to Insured: ☐ Self ☐ Spouse ☐ Child ☐ Other

Employer: _____ Phone: ( ) _____

Employer's Address: _____

Policy/I.D. No: _____ Group No: ____ Percent Covered: ____%, Copay Amt: ____

Reason for Visit: Throat hurts really bad _____

Known Allergies: _____

Were you referred here? If so, by whom? _____

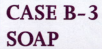
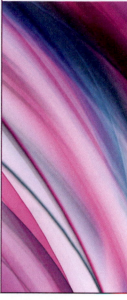

CASE B-3
SOAP

07/19/20XX
Assignment of Benefits: Y
Signature on File: Y
Referring Physician: N

S: Abbie Spencer, an established patient, presents in the office today with complaints of a
painful sore throat since this morning.

O: On exam, parotid glands swollen and the throat shows rubor. Eyes, ears, and nose clear.
Chest clear. Strep screen is positive.

A: 1. Strep throat
2. E/M (PF)
3. Strep screen

P: 1. Amox q.i.d.
2. Return as needed.

_____

Phil Wells, M.D.

Family Practice

NPI: 1234567890

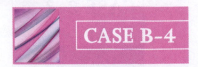

CASE B-4

Capital City Medical—123 Unknown Blvd, Capital City, NY 12345-2222, (555) 555-1234 Phil Wells, M.D., Mannie Mends, M.D., Bette R. Soone, M.D.	Patient Information Form Tax ID: 75-0246810 Group NPI: 1513171216

Patient Information:

Name: (Last, First) Leasure, Justin ☒ Male ☐ Female Birth Date: 12/07/1973

Address: 1820 Grandview Ave, Capital City, NY 12345 Phone: (555) 555-6043

Social Security Number: 329-81-7402 Full-Time Student: ☐ Yes ☒ No

Marital Status: ☐ Single ☒ Married ☐ Divorced ☐ Other

Employment:

Employer: _____ Phone: ( ) _____

Address: _____

Condition Related to: ☐ Auto Accident ☐ Employment ☐ Other Accident

Date of Accident: _____ State _____

Emergency Contact: _____ Phone: ( ) _____

Primary Insurance: Blue Cross Blue Shield **Phone: ( )** _____

Address: 379 Blue Plz, Capital City, NY 12345

Insurance Policyholder's Name: Tiffany Leasure ☐ M ☒ F DOB: 11/13/1977

Address: Same

Phone: _____ Relationship to Insured: ☐ Self ☒ Spouse ☐ Child ☐ Other

Employer: Capital Junior/Senior High School Phone: (555) 555-6986

Employer's Address: 1400 School House Rd, Capital City, NY 12345

Policy/I.D. No: YYJ426812684 Group No: 158386 Percent Covered: _%, Copay Amt: $ 10.00

Secondary Insurance: _____ **Phone: ( )** _____

Address: _____

Insurance Policyholder's Name: _____ ☐ M ☐ F DOB: _____

Address: _____

Phone: _____ Relationship to Insured: ☐ Self ☐ Spouse ☐ Child ☐ Other

Employer: _____ Phone: ( ) _____

Employer's Address: _____

Policy/I.D. No: _____ Group No: ____ Percent Covered: ____ %, Copay Amt: $ __

Reason for Visit: My blood pressure has been running higher than normal _____

Known Allergies: _____

Were you referred here? If so, by whom? _____

07/16/20XX
Assignment of Benefits: Y
Signature on File: Y
Referring Physician: N

CASE B-4 SOAP

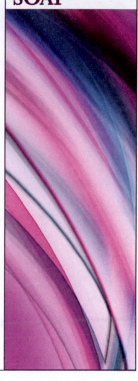

S: Justin Leasure, an established patient, presents today complaining that his BP has been running above normal × 1 week.

O: On exam, pt. denies any stress. Pt. does have family history of HTN. BP today 162/94. ROS unremarkable, except for his BP reading.

A: 1. Elevated BP
   2. Family history of HTN
   3. E/M (EPF)
   4. CBC with diff
   5. Comprehensive Metabolic Panel (CMP)

P: 1. CBC and CMP today.
   2. Return to the office for the next 3 days for BP check.
   3. If consistently above normal, start pt. on hypertensive medicine.
   4. Appointment on Monday.

_____

Phil Wells, M.D.

Family Practice

NPI: 1234567890

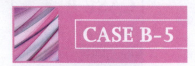

CASE B-5

Capital City Medical—123 Unknown Blvd, Capital City, NY 12345-2222, (555) 555-1234	Patient Information Form
Phil Wells, M.D., Mannie Mends, M.D., Bette R. Soone, M.D.	Tax ID: 75-0246810 Group NPI: 1513171216

Patient Information:

Name: (Last, First) Robinson, Shayla   ☐ Male   ☒ Female   Birth Date: 11/20/2012

Address: 621 Bluff St, Capital City, NY 12345   Phone: (555) 555-2080

Social Security Number: 553-680-0125   Full-Time Student: ☐ Yes   ☒ No

Marital Status: ☒ Single   ☐ Married   ☐ Divorced   ☐ Other

Employment:

Employer: _____ Phone: ( ) _____

Address: _____

Condition Related to: ☐ Auto Accident   ☐ Employment   ☐ Other Accident

Date of Accident: _____ State _____

Emergency Contact: _____ Phone: ( ) _____

Primary Insurance: Medicaid   Phone: ( ) _____

Address: 4875 Capital Blvd, Capital City, NY 12345

Insurance Policyholder's Name: Same   ☐ M   ☐ F   DOB: _____

Address: Same

Phone: _____ Relationship to Insured: ☒ Self   ☐ Spouse   ☐ Child   ☐ Other

Employer: _____ Phone: ( ) _____

Employer's Address: _____

Policy/I.D. No: 643566862 Group No: ____ Percent Covered: ____%, Copay Amt: $ 5.00

Secondary Insurance: _____ Phone: ( ) _____

Address: _____

Insurance Policyholder's Name: _____   ☐ M   ☐ F DOB: _____

Address: _____

Phone: _____ Relationship to Insured: ☐ Self   ☐ Spouse   ☐ Child   ☐ Other

Employer: _____ Phone: ( ) _____

Employer's Address: _____

Policy/I.D. No: _____ Group No: ____ Percent Covered: ____ %, Copay Amt: $ __

Reason for Visit: Here for 5-year well-child exam

Known Allergies: _____

Were you referred here? If so, by whom? _____

CASE B-5
SOAP

01/23/20XX
Assignment of Benefits: Y
Signature on File: Y
Referring Physician: N

S: Shayla Robinson returns for her 5-year well-child exam. Her mother has no complaints.
O: ROS: unremarkable. Ht. and Wt. appropriate for age and gender. There is no evidence
   of illness.
A: 1. Healthy child exam
   2. MMR vaccine
   3. Administration of vaccination (with counseling)
   4. Vaccine
P: 1. Return p.r.n.
   2. Make appointment for next well checkup.

Phil Wells, M.D.

Family Practice

NPI: 1234567890

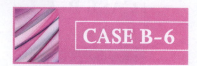

CASE B-6

Capital City Medical—123 Unknown Blvd, Capital City, NY 12345-2222, (555) 555-1234	Patient Information Form
Phil Wells, M.D., Mannie Mends, M.D., Bette R. Soone, M.D.	Tax ID: 75-0246810 Group NPI: 1513171216

Patient Information:

Name: (Last, First) Lui, Mia   ☐ Male   ☒ Female   Birth Date: 05/25/1967

Address: 51 Orchard Ln, Capital City, NY 12345   Phone: (555) 555-4798

Social Security Number: 660-89-5353   Full-Time Student: ☐ Yes   ☒ No

Marital Status: ☐ Single   ☒ Married   ☐ Divorced   ☐ Other

Employment:

Employer: Township County Court   Phone: (555) 555-7000

Address: 1 Court St, Suite 201, Township, NY 12345

Condition Related to: ☐ Auto Accident   ☐ Employment   ☐ Other Accident

Date of Accident: _____ State _____

Emergency Contact: _____ **Phone: ( )** _____

Primary Insurance: Health America   **Phone: ( )** _____

Address: 2031 Healthica Ctr, Capital City, NY 12345

Insurance Policyholder's Name: Same   ☐ M ☐ F DOB: _____

Address: _____

Phone: _____ Relationship to Insured: ☒ Self ☐ Spouse ☐ Child ☐ Other

Employer: _____ Phone: ( ) _____

Employer's Address: _____

Policy/I.D. No: YYJ062054621 Group No: 319521 Percent Covered: __%, Copay Amt: $ 20.00

Secondary Insurance: _____ **Phone: ( )** _____

Address: _____

Insurance Policyholder's Name: _____ ☐ M ☐ F DOB: _____

Address: _____

Phone: _____ Relationship to Insured: ☐ Self ☐ Spouse ☐ Child ☐ Other

Employer: _____ Phone: ( ) _____

Employer's Address: _____

Policy/I.D. No: _____ Group No: _____ Percent Covered: _____ %, Copay Amt: $ ___

Reason for Visit: I haven't been having a period

Known Allergies: _____

Were you referred here? If so, by whom? _____

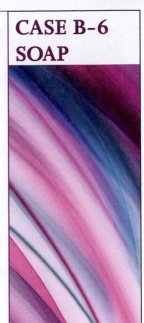

CASE B-6 SOAP

07/16/20XX
Assignment of Benefits: Y
Signature on File: Y
Referring Physician: N

S: Mia Lui is here for a follow-up on menopausal screen.
O: Pt. still experiencing absence of menstruation. Estrogen and progesterone levels have decreased since last visit. Pt. was informed of hormone replacement therapy, its risks, and benefits. Pt. has agreed to proceed.
A: 1. Menopausal
    2. E/M (PF)
    3. Total estrogen
    4. Venipuncture
P: 1. Premarin 1 p.o. daily.
    2. Follow up in 6 months.

Bette R. Soone, M.D.
Obstetrics/Gynecology
NPI: 0987654321

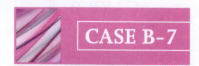

CASE B-7

Capital City Medical—123 Unknown Blvd, Capital City, NY 12345-2222, (555) 555-1234

Phil Wells, M.D., Mannie Mends, M.D., Bette R. Soone, M.D.

Patient Information Form

Tax ID: 75-0246810

Group NPI: 1513171216

Patient Information:

Name: (Last, First) O'Leary, April   ☐ Male   ☒ Female   Birth Date: 04/03/1980

Address: 872 Hickory Pl, Capital City, NY 12345   Phone: (555) 555-4289

Social Security Number: 102-84-2471   Full-Time Student: ☐ Yes   ☒ No

Marital Status: ☒ Single   ☐ Married   ☐ Divorced   ☐ Other

Employment:

Employer: _____ Phone: ( ) _____

Address: _____

Condition Related to: ☐ Auto Accident   ☐ Employment   ☐ Other Accident

Date of Accident: _____ State _____

Emergency Contact: _____ Phone: ( ) _____

Primary Insurance: Medicaid   Phone: ( ) _____

Address: 4875 Capital Blvd, Capital City, NY 12345

Insurance Policyholder's Name: Same   ☐ M   ☐ F   DOB: _____

Address: _____

Phone: _____ Relationship to Insured: ☒ Self   ☐ Spouse   ☐ Child   ☐ Other

Employer: _____ Phone: ( ) _____

Employer's Address: _____

Policy/I.D. No: 9839505   Group No: ___ Percent Covered: ____ %, Copay Amt: $ 35.00

Secondary Insurance: _____ Phone: ( ) _____

Address: _____

Insurance Policyholder's Name: _____   ☐ M   ☐ F   DOB: _____

Address: _____

Phone: _____ Relationship to Insured: ☐ Self   ☐ Spouse   ☐ Child   ☐ Other

Employer: _____ Phone: ( ) _____

Employer's Address: _____

Policy/I.D. No: _____ Group No: _____ Percent Covered: ____ %, Copay Amt: $ ____

Reason for Visit: Here for checkup on pregnancy

Known Allergies: _____

Were you referred here? If so, by whom? _____

10/07/20XX
Assignment of Benefits: Y
Signature on File: Y
Referring Physician: N

**CASE B-7
SOAP**

S: April O'Leary presents for her 8-week prenatal exam. (LMP 7/29/XX)
O: Pt. hasn't had any problems so far. Obstetric panel is normal. She is still considered high risk. (Medicaid pays separately for prenatal visits until patient has selected a participating OB)
A: 1. High-risk pregnancy
   2. E/M (PF)
   3. Venipuncture
   4. Obstetric panel
P: 1. Register with an OB on your Medicaid managed care plan so you can get on a regular program.

_____

Phil Wells, M.D.
Family Practice
NPI: 1234567890

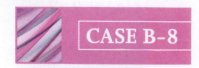

CASE B-8

Capital City Medical—123 Unknown Blvd, Capital City, NY 12345-2222, (555) 555-1234	Patient Information Form
Phil Wells, M.D., Mannie Mends, M.D., Bette R. Soone, M.D.	Tax ID: 75-0246810
	Group NPI: 1513171216

Patient Information:

Name: (Last, First) Qabiz, Abdul ☒ Male ☐ Female   Birth Date: 02/17/1985

Address: 278 Covert Rd, Capital City, NY 12345   Phone: (555) 555-8725

Social Security Number: 655-34-4385   Full-Time Student: ☐ Yes ☒ No

Marital Status: ☐ Single ☒ Married ☐ Divorced ☐ Other

Employment:

Employer: Goodhealth Unlimited, Inc   Phone: ( )

Address: 13 Mile Blvd, Capital City, NY 12345

Condition Related to: ☐ Auto Accident ☐ Employment ☐ Other Accident

Date of Accident: _____ State _____

Emergency Contact: _____ Phone: ( ) _____

Primary Insurance: Aetna   Phone: ( )

Address: 1625 Healthcare Bldg, Capital City, NY 12345

Insurance Policyholder's Name: Same ☐ M ☐ F DOB: _____

Address: _____

Phone: _____ Relationship to Insured: ☒ Self ☐ Spouse ☐ Child ☐ Other

Employer: _____ Phone: ( ) _____

Employer's Address: _____

Policy/I.D. No: 6523483 Group No: 85624 Percent Covered: 90 %, Copay Amt: $____

Secondary Insurance: _____ Phone: ( ) _____

Address: _____

Insurance Policyholder's Name: _____ ☐ M ☐ F DOB: _____

Address: _____

Phone: _____ Relationship to Insured: ☐ Self ☐ Spouse ☐ Child ☐ Other

Employer: _____ Phone: ( ) _____

Employer's Address: _____

Policy/I.D. No: _____ Group No: _____ Percent Covered: ____ %, Copay Amt: $ ____

Reason for Visit: Need a physical _____

Known Allergies: _____

Were you referred here? If so, by whom? _____

10/26/20XX
Assignment of Benefits: Y
Signature on File: Y
Referring Physician: N

S: New patient, Abdul Qabiz, is being seen today for an annual checkup. He is 32 years old and has no complaints at this time.

O: ROS: Unremarkable. Vitals: T 98.6°F, P 74, R 18, BP 114/70. Pt. has no complaints. U/A shows no evidence of WBCs, glucose, or any other abnormality. CBC, CMP, and lipid panels present unremarkable. MDM is SF.

A: 1. General health checkup
    2. E/M
    3. Venipuncture
    4. CBC with diff
    5. Comprehensive Metabolic Panel (CMP)
    6. Lipid panel
    7. U/A dipstick

P: 1. Return p.r.n.

_____

Phil Wells, M.D.
Family Practice
NPI: 1234567890

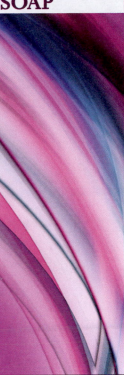

**CASE B-8
SOAP**

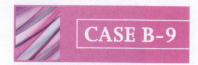

CASE B-9

Capital City Medical—123 Unknown Blvd, Capital City, NY 12345-2222, (555) 555-1234	Patient Information Form
Phil Wells, M.D., Mannie Mends, M.D., Bette R. Soone, M.D.	Tax ID: 75-0246810
	Group NPI: 1513171216

Patient Information:

Name: (Last, First) Hedberg, Clyde   ☒ Male   ☐ Female   Birth Date: 05/02/1969

Address: 939 Freedom Rd, Capital City, NY 12345   Phone: (555) 555-4546

Social Security Number: 897-51-7831   Full-Time Student: ☐ Yes   ☒ No

Marital Status: ☐ Single   ☒ Married   ☐ Divorced   ☐ Other

Employment:

Employer: _____ Phone: ( ) _____

Address: _____

Condition Related to: ☐ Auto Accident   ☐ Employment   ☐ Other Accident

Date of Accident: _____ State _____

Emergency Contact: _____ **Phone: ( )** _____

Primary Insurance: TRICARE   Phone: ( ) _____

Address: 7594 Forces-Run Rd, Militaryville, NY 12345

Insurance Policyholder's Name: Same   ☐ M   ☐ F   DOB: _____

Address: _____

Phone: _____ Relationship to Insured: ☒ Self   ☐ Spouse   ☐ Child   ☐ Other

Employer: United States Army Reserves   Phone: ( ) _____

Employer's Address: 43 S. Army Blvd, Militaryville, NY 12345

Policy/I.D. No: 897517831   Group No: ___   Percent Covered: 80 %, Copay Amt: _____

Secondary Insurance: _____ Phone: ( ) _____

Address: _____

Insurance Policyholder's Name: _____ ☐ M   ☐ F   DOB: _____

Address: _____

Phone: _____ Relationship to Insured: ☐ Self   ☐ Spouse   ☐ Child   ☐ Other

Employer: _____ Phone: ( ) _____

Employer's Address: _____

Policy/I.D. No: _____ Group No: _____ Percent Covered: ____ %, Copay Amt: $ _____

Reason for Visit: I have been having a burning sensation in my throat. _____

Known Allergies: _____

Were you referred here? If so, by whom? _____

12/30/20XX
Assignment of Benefits: Y
Signature on File: Y
Referring Physician: N

S: New patient, Clyde Hedberg, presents with complaints of a burning sensation in his esophagus.

O: ROS shows no visceromegaly; sounds are normal. Vitals normal. Pt. says that for about 2 months he has been experiencing a burning sensation in his throat, as if his esophagus were eroding. He says that it is worse after meals, especially fried foods.

A: 1. GERD
   2. E/M (EPF)

P: 1. Nexium daily.
   2. Schedule an upper GI and esophageal X-ray.
   3. Return in 1 week.
   4. Avoid fatty and fried foods.
   5. Avoid caffeine.
   6. Give pamphlet on GERD.

_____

Phil Wells, M.D.

Family Practice

NPI: 1234567890

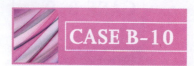

CASE B-10

Capital City Medical—123 Unknown Blvd, Capital City, NY 12345-2222, (555) 555-1234	Patient Information Form
Phil Wells, M.D., Mannie Mends, M.D., Bette R. Soone, M.D.	Tax ID: 75-0246810 Group NPI: 1513171216

Patient Information:

Name: (Last, First) Campbell, Kelly   ❑ Male   ☒ Female   Birth Date: 09/12/1985
Address: 565 Cottage Ln, Capital City, NY 12345   Phone: (555) 555-2631
Social Security Number: 598-77-5432   Full-Time Student: ❑ Yes   ☒ No
Marital Status: ☒ Single   ❑ Married   ❑ Divorced   ❑ Other

Employment:

Employer: Quick Fill Pharmacy   Phone: (555) 555-2683
Address: Brier Rd, Township, NY 12345
Condition Related to: ❑ Auto Accident   ❑ Employment   ❑ Other Accident
Date of Accident: 12/17/20XX   State NY
Emergency Contact: _____   Phone: ( ) _____

Primary Insurance: Accidents Happen Insurance Co.   **Phone: ( )** _____
Address: 8100 Crash Blvd, Capital City, NY 12345
Insurance Policyholder's Name: Same   ❑ M   ❑ F   DOB: _____
Address: _____
Phone: _____ Relationship to Insured: ☒ Self   ❑ Spouse   ❑ Child   ❑ Other
Employer: _____   Phone: ( ) _____
Employer's Address: _____
Policy/I.D. No: 658235476 Group No: ____ Percent Covered: ____ %, Copay Amt: $ ____

Secondary Insurance: Health America (if denied by auto) **Phone: ( )** _____
Address: 2031 Healthica Ctr, Capital City, NY 12345
Insurance Policyholder's Name: Same   ❑ M   ❑ F   DOB: _____
Address: _____
Phone: _____ Relationship to Insured: ☒ Self   ❑ Spouse   ❑ Child   ❑ Other
Employer: _____   Phone: ( ) _____
Employer's Address: _____
Policy/I.D. No: 658235476 Group No: QFP624 Percent Covered: ____ %, Copay Amt: $35.00

Reason for Visit: Here to get checked out for a car accident that happened yesterday

Known Allergies: _____

Were you referred here? If so, by whom? _____

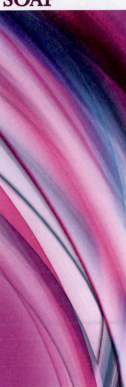

CASE B-10

SOAP

12/18/20XX
Assignment of Benefits: Y
Signature on File: Y
Referring Physician: N

S: Kelly Campbell, an established patient, presents in office today after a motor vehicle collision yesterday around 2:00 P.M. She was driving and slid on ice through a stop sign, hitting a tree on the opposite side of the road. She was at the ER yesterday afternoon following the accident.

O: Pt. complains of cervical vertebrae pain. She is not wearing the neck support because she says that it hurts more with it on. X-rays from the ER show cervical sprain at C-3 and C-4.

A: 1. Cervical sprain
   2. MVA
   3. E/M (EPF)

P: 1. Continue ibuprofen as ordered by the hospital.
   2. Vicodin 1 q 6 h p.r.n. #20.
   3. Refer to physical therapy 3 × week × 4 weeks.
   4. Return after therapy is completed.
   5. Off work until further notice:

Phil Wells, M.D.

Family Practice

NPI: 1234567890

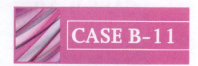

CASE B-11

Capital City Medical—123 Unknown Blvd, Capital City, NY 12345-2222, (555) 555-1234	Patient Information Form
Phil Wells, M.D., Mannie Mends, M.D., Bette R. Soone, M.D.	Tax ID: 75-0246810 Group NPI: 1513171216

Patient Information:

Name: (Last, First) Marowski, Doree   ☐ Male   ☒ Female   Birth Date: 11/02/1944

Address: 3940 Holiday Way, Capital City, NY 12345   Phone: (555) 555-2007

Social Security Number: 494-61-7105   Full-Time Student: ☐ Yes   ☒ No

Marital Status: ☐ Single   ☐ Married   ☒ Divorced   ☐ Other

Employment:

Employer: Retired   Phone: ( )

Address:

Condition Related to: ☐ Auto Accident   ☐ Employment   ☐ Other Accident

Date of Accident: _____ State _____

Emergency Contact: _____ **Phone: ( )** _____

Primary Insurance: Medicare   Phone: ( )

Address: P.O. Box 9834, Capital City, NY 12345

Insurance Policyholder's Name: Same   ☐ M   ☐ F   DOB:

Address:

Phone: _____ Relationship to Insured: ☐ Self   ☐ Spouse   ☐ Child   ☐ Other

Employer: _____ Phone: ( )

Employer's Address:

Policy/I.D. No: 953255475A   Group No: ___ Percent Covered: 80 %, Copay Amt: $ ___

Secondary Insurance: Medicaid   Phone: ( )

Address: 4875 Capital Blvd, Capital City, NY 12345

Insurance Policyholder's Name: Same   ☐ M   ☐ F   DOB:

Address:

Phone: _____ Relationship to Insured: ☒ Self   ☐ Spouse   ☐ Child   ☐ Other

Employer: _____ Phone: ( )

Employer's Address:

Policy/I.D. No: 00008776732   Group No: ___ Percent Covered: ___ %, Copay Amt: $ 5.00

Reason for Visit: Here to find out what my EMG results are for pain in both arms

Known Allergies:

Were you referred here? If so, by whom?

03/24/20XX
Assignment of Benefits: Y
Signature on File: Y
Referring Physician: N

S: Doree Marowski is being seen for a follow-up on an EMG of R/L arms.

O: On exam, edema is still present bilaterally. She still complains of pain, tingling, and weakness. EMG is consistent with CTS.

A: 1. Carpal tunnel syndrome; bilateral
    2. E/M (EPF)

P: 1. Continue ibuprofen.
    2. Set up surgery with Dr. Mends.

Phil Wells, M.D.

Family Practice

NPI: 1234567890

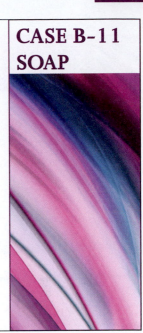

**CASE B-11
SOAP**

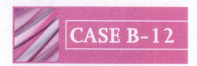

CASE B-12

Capital City Medical—123 Unknown Blvd, Capital City, NY 12345-2222, (555) 555-1234

Phil Wells, M.D., Mannie Mends, M.D., Bette R. Soone, M.D.

Patient Information Form
Tax ID: 75-0246810
Group NPI: 1513171216

Patient Information:

Name: (Last, First) Hodreal, Joseph   ☒ Male   ☐ Female   Birth Date: 09/06/1938

Address: 11 Round St, Capital City, NY 12345   Phone: (555) 555-9798

Social Security Number: 153-96-2004   Full-Time Student: ☐ Yes   ☒ No

Marital Status: ☐ Single   ☒ Married   ☐ Divorced   ☐ Other

Employment:

Employer: Retired   Phone: ( )

Address:

Condition Related to: ☐ Auto Accident   ☐ Employment   ☐ Other Accident

Date of Accident: _____ State _____

Emergency Contact: _____   **Phone: ( )** _____

Primary Insurance: Medicare   Phone: ( )

Address: P.O. Box 9834, Capital City, NY 12345

Insurance Policyholder's Name: Same   ☐ M   ☐ F   DOB:

Address:

Phone: _____ Relationship to Insured: ☒ Self   ☐ Spouse   ☐ Child   ☐ Other

Employer: _____   Phone: ( ) _____

Employer's Address:

Policy/I.D. No: 153521115A   Group No: ___ Percent Covered: 80 %, Copay Amt: $ ___

Secondary Insurance: Medicaid   **Phone: ( )** _____

Address: 4875 Capital Blvd, Capital City, NY 12345

Insurance Policyholder's Name: Same   ☐ M   ☐ F   DOB: _____

Address:

Phone: _____ Relationship to Insured: ☒ Self   ☐ Spouse   ☐ Child   ☐ Other

Employer: _____   Phone: ( ) _____

Employer's Address:

Policy/I.D. No: 00235883216   Group No: ___ Percent Covered: ___ %, Copay Amt: $ 5.00

Reason for Visit: To see how my prostate and blood pressure are doing

Known Allergies: _____

Were you referred here? If so, by whom? _____

05/05/20XX
Assignment of Benefits: Y
Signature on File: Y
Referring Physician: N

CASE B-12 SOAP

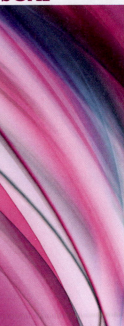

S: Joseph Hodreal, an established patient, is in the office for a checkup on his prostate and HTN.

O: ROS shows no bladder or colon incontinence at this time. BP 122/86. PSA has increased by 0.2.

A: 1. Benign prostatic hypertrophy
2. HTN
3. E/M (EPF)
4. Venipuncture
5. PSA

P: 1. Repeat PSA in 2 months.
2. Return in 2 months.

Phil Wells, M.D.
Family Practice
NPI: 1234567890

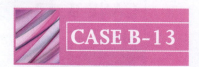

CASE B-13

Capital City Medical—123 Unknown Blvd, Capital City, NY 12345-2222, (555) 555-1234

Phil Wells, M.D., Mannie Mends, M.D., Bette R. Soone, M.D.

Patient Information Form
Tax ID: 75-0246810
Group NPI: 1513171216

Patient Information:

Name: (Last, First) Kozak, Victoria ☐ Male ☒ Female Birth Date: 09/03/1937

Address: 501 Locust St, Capital City, NY 12345 Phone: (555) 555-3374

Social Security Number: 156-73-0953 Full-Time Student: ☐ Yes ☒ No

Marital Status: ☐ Single ☐ Married ☒ Divorced ☐ Other

Employment:

Employer: Retired Phone: ( )

Address:

Condition Related to: ☐ Auto Accident ☐ Employment ☐ Other Accident

Date of Accident: State

Emergency Contact: Phone: ( )

Primary Insurance: Medicare Phone: ( )

Address: P.O. Box 9834, Capital City, NY 12345

Insurance Policyholder's Name: Same ☐ M ☐ F DOB:

Address:

Phone: Relationship to Insured: ☒ Self ☐ Spouse ☐ Child ☐ Other

Employer: Phone: ( )

Employer's Address:

Policy/I.D. No: 698334572A Group No: Percent Covered: 80 %, Copay Amt: $

Secondary Insurance: Medicaid Phone: ( )

Address: 4875 Capital Blvd, Capital City, NY 12345

Insurance Policyholder's Name: Same ☐ M ☐ F DOB:

Address:

Phone: Relationship to Insured: ☒ Self ☐ Spouse ☐ Child ☐ Other

Employer: Phone: ( )

Employer's Address:

Policy/I.D. No: 00060268359 Group No: Percent Covered: %, Copay Amt: $ 5.00

Reason for Visit: Follow-up on cancer of the pancreas

Known Allergies:

Were you referred here? If so, by whom?

08/11/20XX
Assignment of Benefits: Y
Signature on File: Y
Referring Physician: N

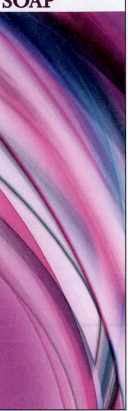

CASE B-13
SOAP

S: Victoria Kozak presents for a checkup on chronic pancreatitis and cancer of the pancreas that I have been following.

O: Pt. starts chemotherapy and radiation next week. Amylase and lipase unchanged. Abdomen reveals enlargement of the pancreas due to the cancer. Pt. still drinks excessively every day. Everything is clear to proceed with the chemo and radiation.

A: 1. Pancreatic cancer of islet cells (neoplasm)
    2. Chronic pancreatitis
    3. Continuing alchol abuse
    4. E/M (EPF)
    5. Venipuncture
    6. Amylase
    7. Lipase

P: 1. Clearance o.k. for chemo and radiation therapy.
    2. Return in 1 week.
    3. Stop drinking.

_____

Phil Wells, M.D.
Family Practice
NPI: 1234567890

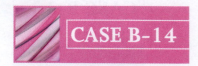

CASE B-14

Capital City Medical—123 Unknown Blvd, Capital City, NY 12345-2222, (555) 555-1234

Phil Wells, M.D., Mannie Mends, M.D., Bette R. Soone, M.D.

Patient Information Form

Tax ID: 75-0246810

Group NPI: 1513171216

Patient Information:

Name: (Last, First) Gubin, Natasha ☐ Male ☒ Female Birth Date: 04/18/1946

Address: 1589 Ridge Ave, Capital City, NY 12345 Phone: (555) 555-4142

Social Security Number: 253-00-6295 Full-Time Student: ☐ Yes ☒ No

Marital Status: ☐ Single ☒ Married ☐ Divorced ☐ Other

Employment:

Employer: Retired Phone: ( )

Address:

Condition Related to: ☐ Auto Accident ☐ Employment ☐ Other Accident

Date of Accident: State

Emergency Contact: Phone: ( )

Primary Insurance: Medicare Phone: ( )

Address: P.O. Box 9834, Capital City, NY 12345

Insurance Policyholder's Name: Same ☐ M ☐ F DOB:

Address:

Phone: Relationship to Insured: ☒ Self ☐ Spouse ☐ Child ☐ Other

Employer: Phone: ( )

Employer's Address:

Policy/I.D. No: 53168465A Group No: Percent Covered: 80 %, Copay Amt: $

Secondary Insurance: Medicaid Phone: ( )

Address: 4875 Capital Blvd, Capital City, NY 12345

Insurance Policyholder's Name: Same ☐ M ☐ F DOB:

Address:

Phone: Relationship to Insured: ☒ Self ☐ Spouse ☐ Child ☐ Other

Employer: Phone: ( )

Employer's Address:

Policy/I.D. No: 001544358706 Group No: Percent Covered: %, Copay Amt: $ 5.00

Reason for Visit: I think I have a sinus infection causing me shortness of breath

Known Allergies:

Were you referred here? If so, by whom?

09/09/20XX
Assignment of Benefits: Y
Signature on File: Y
Referring Physician: N

**CASE B-14
SOAP**

S: Natasha Gubin comes in today complaining of a sinus infection and SOB.

O: On exam, pt. has fever; T 99.9°F. Nares are patent, but there is mucosal drainage. Chest reveals wheezes. Pt. does have asthma. Pt. was here a month ago with same complaints. Inhaled treatment with albuterol given. CXR negative.

A: 1. Asthma, exacerbated
   2. Chronic sinusitis
   3. E/M (EPF)
   4. CXR
   5. Nebulizer

P: 1. Levaquin 1 daily for 7 days.
   2. Prednisone 2 sprays q 6 h.
   3. Return p.r.n.

_____

Phil Wells, M.D.
Family Practice
NPI: 1234567890

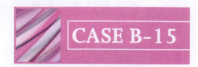

CASE B-15

| Capital City Medical—123 Unknown Blvd, Capital City, NY 12345-2222, (555) 555-1234 Phil Wells, M.D., Mannie Mends, M.D., Bette R. Soone, M.D. | Patient Information Form Tax ID: 75-0246810 Group NPI: 1513171216 |

Patient Information:

Name: (Last, First) Casella, Norma   ☐ Male   ☒ Female   Birth Date: 03/19/1945

Address: 200 Liberty Ave, Capital City, NY 12345   Phone: (555) 555-7183

Social Security Number: 8622-29-3546   Full-Time Student: ☐ Yes   ☒ No

Marital Status: ☒ Single   ☐ Married   ☐ Divorced   ☐ Other

Employment:

Employer: Retired   Phone: ( )

Address:

Condition Related to: ☐ Auto Accident   ☐ Employment   ☐ Other Accident

Date of Accident: _____ State _____

Emergency Contact: _____ Phone: ( )

Primary Insurance: Medicare   **Phone: ( )**

Address: P.O. Box 9834, Capital City, NY 12345

Insurance Policyholder's Name: Same   ☐ M   ☐ F   DOB:

Address:

Phone: _____ Relationship to Insured: ☒ Self   ☐ Spouse   ☐ Child   ☐ Other

Employer: _____ Phone: ( )

Employer's Address:

Policy/I.D. No: 216933650A   Group No: ___ Percent Covered: 80 %, Copay Amt: $ ___

Secondary Insurance: Blue Cross Blue Shield Medigap   **Phone: ( )**

Address: 379 Blue Plz, Capital City, NY 12345

Insurance Policyholder's Name: Same   ☐ M   ☐ F   DOB:

Address:

Phone: _____ Relationship to Insured: ☒ Self   ☐ Spouse   ☐ Child   ☐ Other

Employer: _____ Phone: ( )

Employer's Address:

Policy/I.D. No: YYZ007893521   Group No: ___ Percent Covered: ___ %, Copay Amt: $ ___

Reason for Visit: My left heel is hurting all the time

Known Allergies:

Were you referred here? If so, by whom?

04/24/20XX
Assignment of Benefits: Y
Signature on File: Y
Referring Physician: N

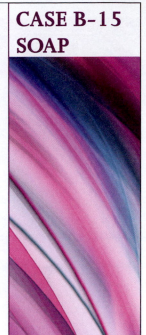

S: Norma Casella, an established patient, presents today for complaints of pain in her left heel.

O: Exam shows that pt. has pain when walking or standing. She says it is worse when she has been sitting, and then gets up. The first couple of steps feels like she's walking on a broken heel. X-ray reveals a spur on the heel bone. I would like to see if steroids will help before operating.

A: 1. Heel spur
   2. E/M (PF)
   3. X-ray; heel
   4. Administration of injection

P: 1. Cortisone injection at site.
   2. Return in 2 weeks to evaluate status.

Mannie Mends, M.D.
General Surgeon
NPI: 0123456789

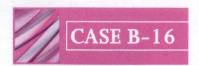

CASE B-16

Capital City Medical—123 Unknown Blvd, Capital City, NY 12345-2222, (555) 555-1234

Phil Wells, M.D., Mannie Mends, M.D., Bette R. Soone, M.D.

Patient Information Form
Tax ID: 75-0246810
Group NPI: 1513171216

Patient Information:

Name: (Last, First) Abbott, Earl   ☒ Male   ☐ Female   Birth Date: 08/30/1932

Address: 34 Diamond Ln, Capital City, NY 12345   Phone: (555) 555-4608

Social Security Number: 410-11-6293   Full-Time Student: ☐ Yes   ☒ No

Marital Status: ☐ Single   ☒ Married   ☐ Divorced   ☐ Other

Employment:

Employer: Retired   Phone: ( )

Address:

Condition Related to: ☐ Auto Accident   ☐ Employment   ☐ Other Accident

Date of Accident: _____ State _____

Emergency Contact: _____   **Phone: ( )** _____

Primary Insurance: Blue Cross Blue Shield   Phone: ( ) _____

Address: 379 Blue Plz, Capital City, NY 12345

Insurance Policyholder's Name: Sheila Abbott   ☐ M   ☒ F   DOB: 09/05/1944

Address: Same

Phone: _____ Relationship to Insured: ☐ Self   ☒ Spouse   ☐ Child   ☐ Other

Employer: Spotless Cleaning Co.   Phone: ( )

Employer's Address: 624 Dust Rd, Capital City, NY 12345

Policy/I.D. No: XYZ4427895235 Group No: 490003 Percent Covered: _ %, Copay Amt: $ 25.00

Secondary Insurance: Medicare   Phone: ( ) _____

Address: P.O. Box 9834, Capital City, NY 12345

Insurance Policyholder's Name: Same   ☐ M   ☐ F   DOB: _____

Address:

Phone: _____ Relationship to Insured: ☒ Self   ☐ Spouse   ☐ Child   ☐ Other

Employer: _____   Phone: ( ) _____

Employer's Address:

Policy/I.D. No: 800563798A Group No: ____ Percent Covered: 80 %, Copay Amt: $ ____

Reason for Visit: Heart checkup

Known Allergies: _____

Were you referred here? If so, by whom? _____

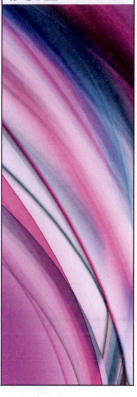

**CASE B-16
SOAP**

03/11/20XX
Assignment of Benefits: Y
Signature on File: Y
Referring Physician: N

S: Earl Abbott is in for a checkup on his heart. He is an established patient.

O: Pt. has old MI, s/p CABG for CAD, and HTN. BP: 136/78. Pt. denies angina, SOB, or any other symptoms. EKG shows old MI, otherwise normal. No carotid bruits. Lipid panel shows mild elevation.

A: 1. CAD
   2. HTN
   3. Old MI
   4. Status post CABG
   5. E/M (EPF)
   6. EKG
   7. Venipuncture
   8. Lipid panel

P: 1. Refill medications.
    2. Return in 2 months.

Phil Wells, M.D.
Family Practice
NPI: 1234567890

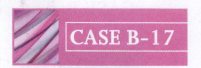

CASE B-17

Patient Information:

Name: (Last, First) McDavidson, Clifford   ☒ Male   ❑ Female   Birth Date: 05/23/1947

Address: 717 Hillcrest Dr, Capital City, NY 12345   Phone: (555) 555-7585

Social Security Number: 673-51-1149   Full-Time Student: ❑ Yes   ☒ No

Marital Status: ☒ Single   ❑ Married   ❑ Divorced   ❑ Other

Employment:

Employer: Retired   Phone: ( )

Address:

Condition Related to: ❑ Auto Accident   ❑ Employment   ❑ Other Accident

Date of Accident: State

Emergency Contact: Phone: ( )

Primary Insurance: Medicare   Phone: ( )

Address: P.O. Box 9834, Capital City, NY 12345

Insurance Policyholder's Name: Same   ❑ M   ❑ F   DOB:

Address:

Phone: Relationship to Insured: ☒ Self   ❑ Spouse   ❑ Child   ❑ Other

Employer: Phone: ( )

Employer's Address:

Policy/I.D. No: 468752139A   Group No: Percent Covered: 80 %, Copay Amt: $

Secondary Insurance: Aetna Medigap   Phone: ( )

Address: 1625 Healthcare Bldg, Capital City, NY 12345

Insurance Policyholder's Name: Same   ❑ M   ❑ F   DOB:

Address:

Phone: Relationship to Insured: ☒ Self   ❑ Spouse   ❑ Child   ❑ Other

Employer: Phone: ( )

Employer's Address:

Policy/I.D. No: 0321227 Group No: Percent Covered: %, Copay Amt: $

Reason for Visit: I have a cough and am really congested

Known Allergies:

Were you referred here? If so, by whom?

09/07/20XX
Assignment of Benefits: Y
Signature on File: Y
Referring Physician: N

CASE B-17 SOAP

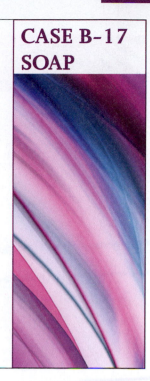

S: Clifford McDavidson is being seen today for cough and congestion.

O: Chest sounds are that of his COPD, but with congestion. CXR shows this disorder. He is on oxygen therapy, 2 L/min.

A: 1. Chronic bronchitis with acute exacerbation of COPD
   2. E/M (EPF)
   3. CXR

P: 1. Augmentin 1 b.i.d. for 10 days.
   2. Plenty of rest and fluids.
   3. Return for normal appointment scheduled in October.

_____

Phil Wells, M.D.

Family Practice

NPI: 1234567890

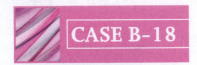
CASE B-18

Patient Information:

Name: (Last, First) Jenkins, Stewart   ☒ Male   ☐ Female   Birth Date: 07/29/1947

Address: 27 Highland Ave, Capital City, NY 12345   Phone: (555) 555-9475

Social Security Number: 429-66-0631   Full-Time Student: ☐ Yes   ☒ No

Marital Status: ☐ Single   ☒ Married   ☐ Divorced   ☐ Other

Employment:

Employer: Retired   Phone: ( )

Address:

Condition Related to: ☐ Auto Accident   ☐ Employment   ☐ Other Accident

Date of Accident: _____ State _____

Emergency Contact: _____   **Phone: ( )** _____

Primary Insurance: Medicare   **Phone: ( )** _____

Address: P.O. Box 9834, Capital City, NY 12345

Insurance Policyholder's Name: Same   ☐ M   ☐ F   DOB: _____

Address:

Phone: _____ Relationship to Insured: ☒ Self   ☐ Spouse   ☐ Child   ☐ Other

Employer: _____   Phone: ( ) _____

Employer's Address:

Policy/I.D. No: 238823364A Group No: ___ Percent Covered: 80 %, Copay Amt: $ ____

Secondary Insurance: Medicaid   **Phone: ( )** _____

Address: 4875 Capital Blvd, Capital City, NY 12345

Insurance Policyholder's Name: Same   ☐ M   ☐ F   DOB: _____

Address:

Phone: _____ Relationship to Insured: ☐ Self   ☐ Spouse   ☐ Child   ☐ Other

Employer: _____   Phone: ( ) _____

Employer's Address:

Policy/I.D. No: 00005733268 Group No: ___ Percent Covered: ___ %, Copay Amt: $ 5.00

Reason for Visit: I have a wart on my right index finger

Known Allergies: _____

Were you referred here? If so, by whom? _____

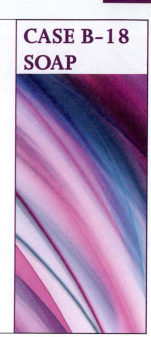

CASE B-18
SOAP

11/09/20XX
Assignment of Benefits: Y
Signature on File: Y
Referring Physician: N

S: Stewart Jenkins, an established patient, presents today with complaints of a wart on his right index finger.

O: Pt. says that he tried to "cut it out," but it only made it 2 times bigger. He would like it removed.

A: 1. Wart; right index finger
    2. Cryosurgery; wart

P: 1. Ibuprofen b.i.d.

_____

Mannie Mends, M.D.
General Surgeon
NPI: 0123456789

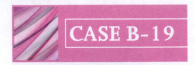

CASE B-19

Capital City Medical—123 Unknown Blvd, Capital City,
NY 12345-2222, (555) 555-1234
Phil Wells, M.D., Mannie Mends, M.D., Bette R. Soone, M.D.

Patient Information Form
Tax ID: 75-0246810
Group NPI: 1513171216

Patient Information:

Name: (Last, First) Popazekus, Adelphie   ☐ Male   ☒ Female   Birth Date: 09/08/1942

Address: 333 Violet Cir, Capital City, NY 12345   Phone: (555) 555-0853

Social Security Number: 729-04-6278   Full-Time Student: ☐ Yes   ☒ No

Marital Status: ☐ Single   ☒ Married   ☐ Divorced   ☐ Other

Employment:

Employer: Retired   Phone: ( )

Address:

Condition Related to: ☐ Auto Accident   ☐ Employment   ☐ Other Accident

Date of Accident: _____ State _____

Emergency Contact: _____   **Phone: ( )** _____

Primary Insurance: Medicare   **Phone: ( )** _____

Address: P.O. Box 9834, Capital City, NY 12345

Insurance Policyholder's Name: Same   ☐ M   ☐ F   DOB: _____

Address:

Phone: _____ Relationship to Insured: ☒ Self   ☐ Spouse   ☐ Child   ☐ Other

Employer: _____   Phone: ( ) _____

Employer's Address:

Policy/I.D. No: 653284563A   Group No: ____   Percent Covered: 80 %, Copay Amt: $ ____

Secondary Insurance: Aetna   **Phone: ( )** _____

Address: 1625 Healthcare Bldg, Capital City, NY 12345

Insurance Policyholder's Name: Samuel Popazekus   ☒ M   ☐ F   DOB: 10/14/1941

Address: Same

Phone: _____ Relationship to Insured: ☐ Self   ☒ Spouse   ☐ Child   ☐ Other

Employer: Retired   Phone: ( ) _____

Employer's Address:

Policy/I.D. No: 210805   Group No: 496000   Percent Covered: ___ %, Copay Amt: $ 30.00

Reason for Visit: Checkup on diabetes

Known Allergies: _____

Were you referred here? If so, by whom? _____

03/17/20XX
Assignment of Benefits: Y
Signature on File: Y
Referring Physician: N

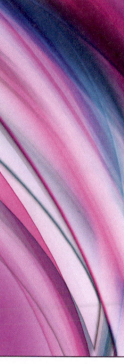

CASE B-19
SOAP

S: Adelphie Popazekus is being seen for evaluation of her DM II.
O: Pt. only complains of symptoms related to her diabetic neuropathy. Her pedal pulses are 2+. There is no evidence of wounds. Glucose 174. She says that she ate within the past hour. She has gained 7 lbs. since her last visit. Pt. instructed to lose weight.
A: 1. DM II
   2. Diabetic polyneuropathy
   3. Obesity
   4. E/M (EPF)
   5. Venipuncture
   6. Glucose
P: 1. Continue medications.
   2. Recheck in 1 month.
   3. Refer to hospital dietary services for weight loss.

_____

Phil Wells, M.D.
Family Practice
NPI: 1234567890

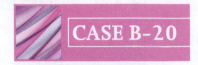

CASE B-20

Capital City Medical—123 Unknown Blvd, Capital City, NY 12345-2222, (555) 555-1234	Patient Information Form
Phil Wells, M.D., Mannie Mends, M.D., Bette R. Soone, M.D.	Tax ID: 75-0246810
	Group NPI: 1513171216

Patient Information:

Name: (Last, First) Gambaro, Marsha   ❑ Male   ☒ Female   Birth Date: 04/15/1932

Address: 19 Crestview Pl, Capital City, NY 12345   Phone: (555) 555-4737

Social Security Number: 873-12-9784   Full-Time Student: ❑ Yes   ☒ No

Marital Status: ❑ Single   ☒ Married   ❑ Divorced   ❑ Other

Employment:

Employer: Retired   Phone: ( )

Address:

Condition Related to: ❑ Auto Accident   ❑ Employment   ❑ Other Accident

Date of Accident: _____ State _____

Emergency Contact: _____   **Phone: ( )** _____

Primary Insurance: Medicare   **Phone: ( )** _____

Address: P.O. Box 9834, Capital City, NY 12345

Insurance Policyholder's Name: Same   ❑ M   ❑ F   DOB: _____

Address:

Phone: _____ Relationship to Insured: ☒ Self   ❑ Spouse   ❑ Child   ❑ Other

Employer: _____ Phone: ( ) _____

Employer's Address:

Policy/I.D. No: 231481483A Group No: ____ Percent Covered: 80 %, Copay Amt: $ ____

Secondary Insurance: Health America   **Phone: ( )** _____

Address: 2031 Healthica Ctr, Capital City, NY 12345

Insurance Policyholder's Name: Same   ❑ M   ❑ F   DOB: _____

Address:

Phone: _____ Relationship to Insured: ☒ Self   ❑ Spouse   ❑ Child   ❑ Other

Employer: Retired   Phone: ( ) _____

Employer's Address:

Policy/I.D. No: 0548726   Group No: 6843 Percent Covered: ____ %, Copay Amt: $ 15.00

Reason for Visit: Checkup on Alzheimer's and thyroid

Known Allergies: _____

Were you referred here? If so, by whom? _____

11/09/20XX
Assignment of Benefits: Y
Signature on File: Y
Referring Physician: N

S: Marsha Gambaro presents in the office for a regular checkup on Alzheimer's
   and hypothyroidism.
O: Pt. is brought in by daughter Ann, who says that her mother has been doing well.
   Pt. is in no acute distress. TSH shows stable functioning.
A: 1. Alzheimer's disease
   2. Hypothyroidism
   3. E/M (PF)
   4. TSH
   5. Venipuncture
P: 1. Refill Synthroid and Aricept.
   2. Return in 3 months.

_____

Phil Wells, M.D.
Family Practice
NPI: 1234567890

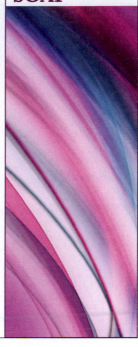

**CASE B-20
SOAP**

Completing the UB-04 Form for Hospital Billing

The case studies in this appendix are provided for additional practice in completing the UB-04 claim form for hospital billing. By applying what you have learned in this text, your objective is to accurately complete each case study. All of the information you need is provided, including patient demographics, diagnostic and procedure codes, and a brief case history of each patient's health problem.

Complete the cases based on the following criteria:

- All patients have release-of-information and assignment-of-benefit signatures on file.
- All physicians and hospitals participate in all of the health care plans listed, and all physicians and hospitals accept assignment for these plans.
- The hospital is the billing entity.
- 2017 ICD-10-CM and CPT codes are to be used to complete the exercises.

For the cases in this appendix the student should provide the ICD-10-CM code(s) on the claim forms. Use six-digit dates for ALL dates. All street names should be entered using standard postal abbreviations, even if they are spelled out on the source documents. Room charges reflect the daily rate and should be multiplied times the number of days to get the total room charge for the stay. All other services reflect the total charges for all units provided. To complete each case study, copy the UB-04 form provided in Appendix D or download the form from MyHealthProfessionsKit or MyHealthProfessionsLab, which accompany this text. For a list of abbreviations used in these case studies, also refer to the MyHealthProfessionsKit or MyHealthProfessionsLab.

CPT-4 codes in this appendix are from the CPT-4 2017 code set. CPT® is a registered trademark of the American Medical Association.
ICD-10-CM codes in this appendix are from the ICD-10-CM 2017 code set from the Department of Health and Human Services, Centers for Disease Control and Prevention.

CASE STUDIES

Inpatient Hospital

Case	Patient	Primary Payer
C-1	Nestor Willis	Medicaid
C-2	Melvin Lyles	Blue Cross Blue Shield
C-3	Emilio Mendez	Blue Cross Blue Shield
C-4	Harold Janovich	Aetna
C-5	Ramesh Kedar	Health America
C-6	Arthur Zbegan	Medicare
C-7	Rita Mangino	Aetna
C-8	Dorothy Greer	Medicare
C-9	Virginia Moore	Medicaid
C-10	Albert Kim	Medicare

Outpatient Hospital

Case	Patient	Primary Payer
C-11	Olivia Marselle	Medicaid
C-12	Antonio Rodriquez	Blue Cross Blue Shield
C-13	Randall Paul	Aetna
C-14	Megan Bishop	Blue Cross Blue Shield
C-15	Patricia Vlah	Aetna
C-16	Bryson Chung	Health America
C-17	Keith Lombardo	Medicare
C-18	Tyrone Clark	Medicaid
C-19	Dawn Hunt	Medicare
C-20	Jenna Masters	Medicare

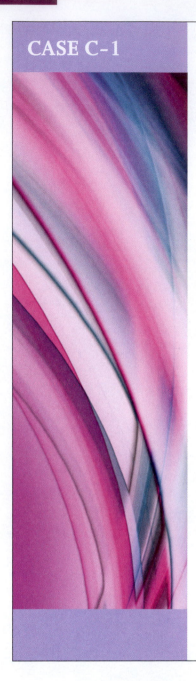

CASE C-1

Capital City Memorial Hospital
700 Shady Street
Capital City, NY 12345
(555) 555-0700

Patient Information:	Nestor Willis
	63 Park Avenue, Capital City, NY 12345
	(555) 555-2901
DOB:	09-29-1952
Gender:	Male
SSN:	873-02-6447
Status:	Married Student: No
Employer:	Retired
Responsible Party:	Nestor Willis
	Address—same as above

Insurance Information:	Medicaid
	4875 Capital Boulevard, Capital City, NY 12345
ID #:	322654921345 Group #:
Insured's Name:	Same Relationship to Patient: Self
Insured's Address:	

Insured's Employer:

Authorization:	3.2191321 Approved # of Days: 4
Attending Physician:	Phil Wells, M.D.
Federal Tax ID #:	75-1234567
NPI:	1234567890
Group NPI:	1513171216

Reason for visit: I'm having chest pain, and I'm short of breath.

HPI: This is an African American male admitted on July 28, 20XX, at 1:17 A.M. with CP and SOB. Pt. has emphysema, has smoked 2 packs a day for 34 years, and still smokes. Pt. denies N&V. Mouth breathing noted. CXR reveals pneumonia in the RLL of lung. Sputum cultures ordered. Pt. was discharged on August 1, 20XX, at 3:20 P.M.

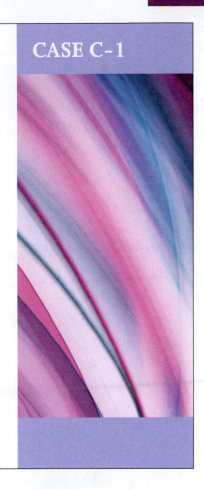

CASE C-1

Patient Control #:	56139844	Type of Admission:	1
MR #:	659431896	Source of Admission:	1
Hospital NPI:	3434343434	Discharge Status:	01
Hospital Tax ID:	75-0750750	Type of Bill Code:	111

Fees:

Revenue Codes	Units	Total Charges	Date of Service
120 Room/Board/Semi	4	$ 450.00/day	07/28/20XX–08/01/20XX
260 IV Therapy	4	$1,000.00	07/28/20XX–07/31/20XX
300 Lab	1	$ 235.00	07/28/20XX
320 Radiology	1	$ 250.00	07/28/20XX
900 Respiratory Services	4	$ 400.00	07/28/20XX–07/31/20XX
001 TOTAL		$3,685.00	

Principal DX:	ICD-10 (J18.9), ICD-10 (J43.9)
Admitting DX:	ICD-10 (R07.89)
Principal Procedure Code:	BW03ZZZ

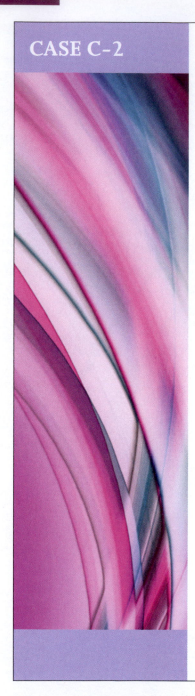

CASE C-2

Capital City General Hospital
1000 Cherry Street
Capital City, NY 12345
(555) 555-1000

Patient Information:	Melvin Lyles
	2001 Meadow Road, Capital City, NY 12345
	(555) 555-1342
DOB:	05-14-1972
Gender:	Male
SSN:	178-37-2456
Status:	Married **Student:** No
Employer:	None
Responsible Party:	Melvin Lyles
	Address—same as above

Insurance Information:	Blue Cross Blue Shield
	379 Blue Plaza, Capital City, NY 12345
ID #:	YYJ561319821 **Group #:** 025648
Insured's Name:	Shelby Lyles **Relationship to Patient:** Spouse
Insured DOB:	05/03/1971 **Insured Party's Gender:** Female
Insured's Address:	Same

Insured's Employer:	Green Landscaping Co.
	1315 Green Avenue, Capital City, NY 12345
	(555) 555-8503
Authorization:	846465315 **Approved # of Days:** 3
Attending Physician:	Elby Alright, M.D.
Federal Tax ID #:	75-7654321
NPI:	9876543210

Reason for visit: My sugar has been running high.

HPI: This is a Caucasian male admitted on October 10, 20XX, at 8:44 P.M. for uncontrolled DM II. Pt. has had a recent change in medicines, and these may be the contributor to his condition. Pt. does admit to noncompliance with diet. Pt. was discharged on October 13, 20XX, at 7:45 A.M.

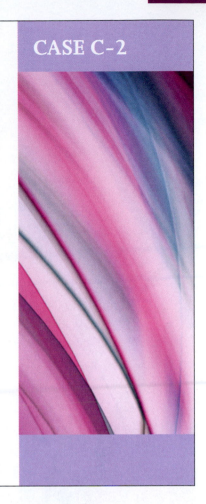

CASE C-2

Patient Control #:	6132198	Type of Admission:	1
MR #:	ML18913	Source of Admission:	1
Hospital NPI:	1212121212	Discharge Status:	01
Hospital Tax ID:	75-7575757	Type of Bill Code:	111

Fees:

Revenue Codes	Units	Total Charges	Date of Service
120 Room/Board/Semi	3	$ 400.00/day	10/10/20XX–10/13/20XX
250 Pharmacy	8	$ 375.00	10/10/20XX–10/13/20XX
260 IV Therapy	2	$ 850.00	10/10/20XX–10/12/20XX
300 Lab	5	$ 450.00	10/10/20XX–10/12/20XX
320 Radiology	1	$ 900.00	10/11/20XX
001 TOTAL		$3,775.00	

Principal DX:	ICD-10 (E11.65), ICD-10 (583.81), ICD-10 (E66.9), ICD-10 (Z71.3), ICD-10 (Z68.32)
Admitting DX:	ICD-10 (E11.65)
Principal Procedure Code:	B40FYZZ, B50BYZZ

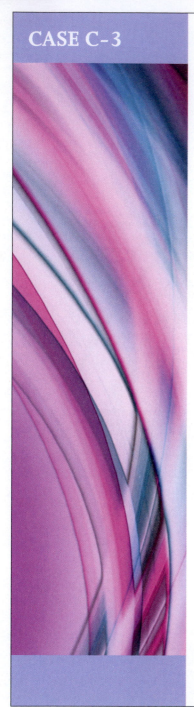

CASE C-3

Capital City General Hospital
1000 Cherry Street
Capital City, NY 12345
(555) 555-1000

Patient Information: Emilio Mendez
                                 3009 River Road, Capital City, NY 12345
                                 (555) 555-3839
DOB: 09-30-1984
Gender: Male
SSN: 548-37-0081
Status: Married   **Student:** Yes
Employer: Tough Guy's Gym
                                 79 W. Boron Avenue,
                                 Township, NY 12345
                                 (555) 555-4816
Responsible Party: Emilio Mendez
                                 Address—same as above

Insurance Information: Blue Cross Blue Shield
                                 379 Blue Plaza, Capital City, NY 12345
ID #:   YYZ156349873   **Group #:** 252354
Insured's Name: Same   **Relationship to Patient:** Self

Insured's Address:

Insured's Employer:

Authorization: 5168431313   **Approved # of Days:** 4
Attending Physician: Elby Alright, M.D.
Federal Tax ID #:   75-7654321
NPI: 9876543210

Reason for visit: I think that I have an infection from my wisdom tooth surgery.

HPI: This is a Latin American male admitted on June 7, 20XX, at 5:42 P.M. for an infected wisdom tooth. Pt. recently underwent wisdom tooth extraction and now has septicemia. He says that he stopped taking his antibiotic because he felt better. Pt. was discharged on June 10, 20XX, at 11:00 A.M.

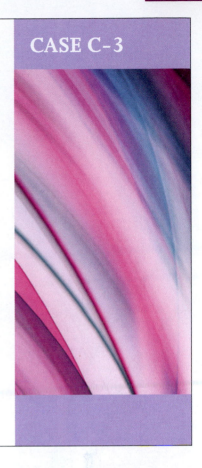

CASE C-3

Patient Control #:	646413	Type of Admission:	1
MR #:	84616489	Source of Admission:	7
Hospital NPI:	212121212	Discharge Status:	01
Hospital Tax ID:	75-7575757	Type of Bill Code:	111

Fees:

Revenue Codes	Units	Total Charges	Date of Service
120 Room/Board/Semi	3	$ 400.00/day	06/07/20XX–06/10/20XX
250 Pharmacy	7	$ 400.00	06/07/20XX–06/09/20XX
260 IV Therapy	3	$ 900.00	06/07/20XX–06/09/20XX
300 Lab	6	$ 700.00	06/07/20XX–06/09/20XX
001 TOTAL		$3,600.00	

Principal DX:	ICD-10 (A41.2), ICD-10 (M27.3)
Admitting DX:	ICD-10 (M27.3)
Principal Procedure Code:	

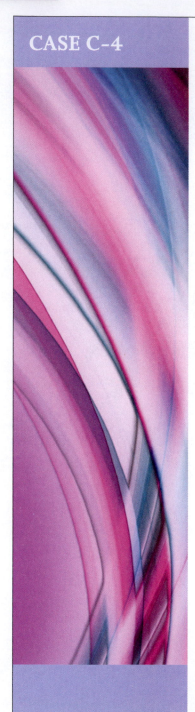

CASE C-4

Capital City Community Hospital
1600 Clover Street
Capital City, NY 12345
(555) 555-1600

Patient Information:	Harold Janovich
	532 Creek Street, Capital City, NY 12345
	(555) 555-8824
DOB:	12-12-1971
Gender:	Male
SSN:	401-64-7228
Status:	Single **Student:** No
Employer:	Buy 'N Save Grocers, Ltd.
	927 Interstate Plaza, Township, NY 12345
	(555) 555-8193
Responsible Party:	Harold Janovich
	Address—same as above
Insurance Information:	Aetna
	1625 Heath Care Building
	Capital City, NY 12345
ID #:	65321313 **Group #:** 97390
Insured's Name:	Same **Relationship to Patient:** Self
Insured's Address:	
Insured's Employer:	
Authorization:	10564598 **Approved # of Days:** 2
Attending Physician:	Mannie Mends, M.D.
Federal Tax ID #:	75-1234567
NPI:	0123456789
Group NPI:	1513171216

Reason for visit: My stomach hurts, I've been vomiting, and I have the chills.

HPI: Pt. presents in the ER on November 22, 20XX, at 6:19 P.M. He is complaining of N&V, chills, and RLQ pain. Pt. tolerated appendectomy well and was discharged on November 24, 20XX, at 5:15 P.M.

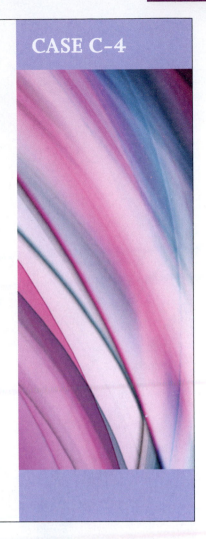

CASE C-4

Patient Control #:	564321	Type of Admission:	1
MR #:	005332496	Source of Admission:	7
Hospital NPI:	6767676767	Discharge Status:	01
Hospital Tax ID:	70-707070	Type of Bill Code:	111
Fees:	$ 950.00		

Revenue Codes	Units	Total Charges	Date of Service
120 Room/Board/Semi	2	$ 400.00/day	11/22/20XX–11/24/20XX
250 Pharmacy	5	$ 400.00	11/22/20XX–11/23/20XX
260 IV Therapy	2	$ 950.00	11/22/20XX–11/23/20XX
270 Med/Surg Supplies	1	$ 500.00	11/22/20XX
300 Lab	2	$ 300.00	11/22/20XX–11/23/20XX
320 Radiology	1	$ 650.00	11/22/20XX
360 OR Services	1	$1,200.00	11/22/20XX
370 Anesthesia	1	$ 600.00	11/22/20XX
001 TOTAL		$5,400.00	

Principal DX:	ICD-10 (K35.80)
Admitting DX:	ICD-10 (R10.31)
Principal Procedure Code:	0DTJ0ZZ, BW40ZZZ

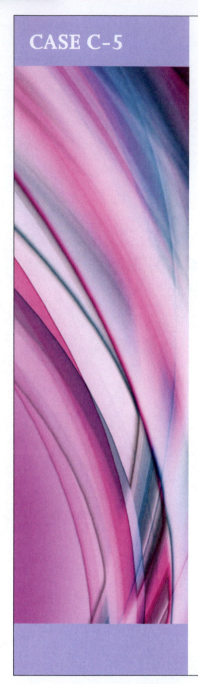

CASE C-5

Capital City Memorial Hospital
700 Shady Street
Capital City, NY 12345
(555) 555-0700

Patient Information:	Ramesh Kedar
	14 Berry Lane, Capital City, NY 12345
	(555) 555-2624
DOB:	03-07-1967
Gender:	Male
SSN:	534-69-7184
Status:	Divorced **Student:** No
Employer:	Wholsale Electronics, Inc.
	5634 Electric Boulevard, Capital City, NY 12345
	(555) 555-1476
Responsible Party:	Ramesh Kedar
	Address—same as above

Insurance Information:	Health America
	2031 Healthica Center, Capital City, NY 12345
ID #:	65432678 **Group #:** 6649
Insured's Name:	Same **Relationship to Patient:** Self
Insured's Address:	

Insured's Employer:

Authorization:	545777888 **Approved # of Days:** 2
Attending Physician:	Iva Hart, M.D.
Federal Tax ID #:	75-0246802
NPI:	0246802468

Reason for visit: I feel anxious and my chest hurts.

HPI: This is an Asian male admitted on December 12, 20XX, at 12:25 P.M. for CP and anxiousness. Pt. is hypertensive. CXR showed no abnormalities. Labs positive for clotting issues. VQ scan of lung reveals pulmonary embolism. Pt. was discharged on December 14, 20XX, at 10:30 A.M.

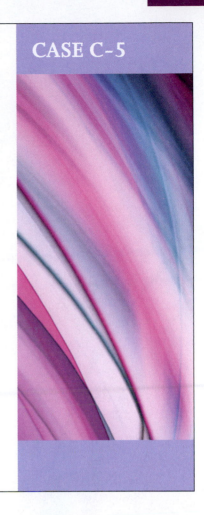

CASE C-5

Patient Control #:	594313		Type of Admission:	1
MR #:	RK654142		Source of Admission:	1
Hospital NPI:	3434343434		Discharge Status:	01
Hospital Tax ID:	75-0750750		Type of Bill Code:	111

Fees:

Revenue Codes	Units	Total Charges	Date of Service
120 Room/Board/Semi	2	$ 400.00/day	12/12/20XX–12/14/20XX
250 Pharmacy	3	$ 375.00	12/12/20XX–12/14/20XX
260 IV Therapy	3	$1,200.00	12/12/20XX–12/14/20XX
300 Lab	6	$ 450.00	12/12/20XX–12/14/20XX
320 Radiology	1	$1,000.00	12/12/20XX
730 EKG	1	$ 150.00	12/12/20XX
001 TOTAL		$3,975.00	

Principal DX:	ICD-10 (I26.99), ICD-10 (F41.9), ICD-10 (I10)
Admitting DX:	ICD-10 (R06.02)
Principal Procedure Code:	CB12TZZ, 4A02X4Z

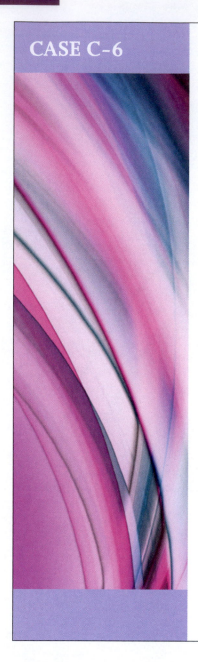

CASE C-6

Capital City General Hospital
1000 Cherry Street
Capital City, NY 12345-2222
(555) 555-1000

Patient Information:	Arthur Zbegan
	9832 Grass Road, Capital City, NY 12345
	(555) 555-6549
DOB:	04-11-1939
Gender:	Male
SSN:	457-67-2470
Status:	Married **Student:** No
Employer:	Retired
Responsible Party:	Arthur Zbegan
	Address—same as above

Insurance Information:	Medicare
	P.O. Box 9834, Capital City, NY 12345
ID #:	629417113A **Group #:**
Insured's Name:	Same **Relationship to Patient:** Self
Insured's Address:	

Insured's Employer:

Authorization:	5463664535 **Approved # of Days:** 4
Attending Physician:	Iva Hart, M.D.
Federal Tax ID #:	75-0246802
NPI:	0246802468

Reason for visit: I can't breathe. I feel winded very easily.

HPI: This is a Caucasian male admitted on September 1, 20XX, at 2:39 A.M. for coronary artery disease, HTN, and angina. Pt. had s/p CABG 12 years ago. Coronary artery blockage requires CABG. Pt. was discharged on September 5, 20XX, at 11:00 A.M.

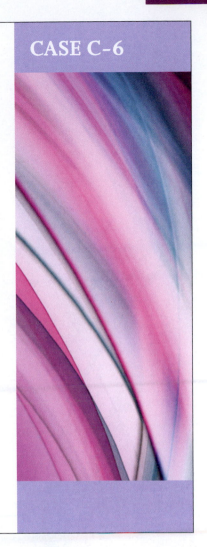

CASE C-6

Patient Control #:	4616549	Type of Admission:	1
MR #:	ZA16836401	Source of Admission:	7
Hospital NPI:	1212121212	Discharge Status:	01
Hospital Tax ID:	75-7575757	Type of Bill Code:	0111

Fees:

Revenue Codes	Units	Total Charges	Date of Service
0210 Coronary Care	4	$ 650.00/day	09/01/20XX–09/05/20XX
0250 Pharmacy	5	$ 425.00	09/01/20XX–09/05/20XX
0260 IV Therapy	4	$1,200.00	09/01/20XX–09/04/20XX
0270 Med/Surg Supplies	1	$ 800.00	09/02/20XX
0300 Lab	5	$ 450.00	09/01/20XX–09/05/20XX
0360 OR Services	1	$2,300.00	09/02/20XX
0370 Anesthesia	1	$ 675.00	09/02/20XX
0730 EKG	1	$ 175.00	09/01/20XX
0001 TOTAL		$8,625.00	

Principal DX:	ICD-10 (I24.0), ICD-10 (I25.10), ICD-10 (I11.9), ICD-10 (Z95.1)
Admitting DX:	ICD-10 (I20.8)
Principal Procedure Code:	021108W, 4A02X4Z

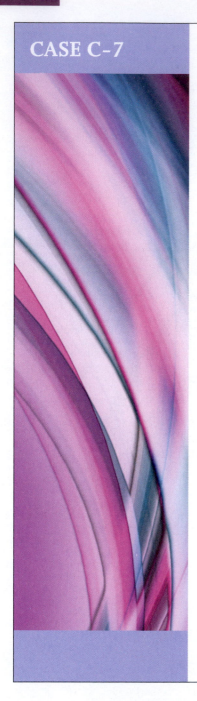

CASE C-7

Capital City General Hospital
1000 Cherry Street
Capital City, NY 12345
(555) 555-1000

Patient Information:	Rita Mangino	
	4 S. Orange Way, Capital City, NY 12345	
	(555) 555-5776	
DOB:	02-08-1957	
Gender:	Female	
SSN:	243-51-6328	
Status:	Married	**Student:** No
Employer:	Retired	
Responsible Party:	Rita Mangino	
	Address—same as above	

Insurance Information:	Aetna	
	1625 Healthcare Building, Capital City, NY 12345	
ID #:	4783900	**Group #:** 493
Insured's Name:	Bruce Mangino	**Relationship to Patient:** Husband
DOB:	11/06/1957	**Gender:** Male
Insured's Address:	Same	

Insured's Employer:	Critter's Campus	
	6291 Grove Boulevard, Township, NY 12345	
	(555) 555-3374	
Authorization:	5331648	**Approved # of Days:** 2
Attending Physician:	Phil Wells, M.D.	
Federal Tax ID #:	75-1234567	
NPI:	1234567890	

Reason for visit: I'm having an asthma attack.

CASE C-7

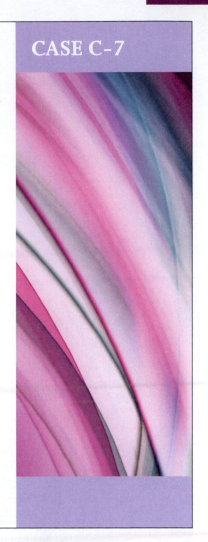

HPI: Caucasian female admitted on January 14, 20XX, at 6:05 A.M. for exacerbation of asthma. Chest auscultation and percussion show severe wheezes, and SpO_2 is 86%. CXR revealed atelectasis, and a thoracentesis was performed to expand the right lung. Thoracentesis was performed without complications. Pt. was discharged on January 16, 20XX, at 1:30 P.M.

Patient Control #:	0063259	Type of Admission:	1
MR #:	000233168	Source of Admission:	1
Hospital NPI:	1212121212	Discharge Status:	01
Hospital Tax ID:	75-7575757	Type of Bill Code:	111

Fees:

Revenue Codes	Units	Total Charges	Date of Service
120 Room/Board/Semi	2	$ 450.00/day	01/14/20XX–01/16/20XX
250 Pharmacy	3	$ 375.00	01/14/20XX–01/16/20XX
260 IV Therapy	2	$ 820.00	01/14/20XX–01/15/20XX
270 Med/Surg Supplies	1	$ 400.00	01/14/20XX
300 Lab	1	$ 105.00	01/14/20XX
320 Radiology	2	$ 500.00	01/14/20XX–01/15/20XX
900 Respiratory Services	3	$ 600.00	01/14/20XX–01/16/20XX
001 TOTAL		$3,700.00	

Principal DX:	ICD-10 (J45.901)
Admitting DX:	ICD-10 (J45.901)
Principal Procedure Code:	0W993ZZ, BW03ZZZ

CASE C-8

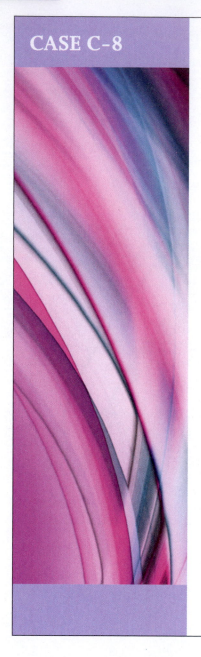

Capital City General Hospital
1000 Cherry Street
Capital City, NY 12345-2222
(555) 555-1000

Patient Information: Dorothy Greer
777 Sycamore Circle, Capital City, NY 12345
(555) 555-5682

DOB: 10-02-1949

Gender: Female

SSN: 738-53-2081

Status: Married   **Student:** No

Employer: Retired

Responsible Party: Dorothy Greer
Address—same as above

Insurance Information: Medicare
P.O. Box 9834, Capital City, NY 12345

ID #:   629417113A   **Group #:**

Insured's Name: Same   **Relationship to Patient:** Self

Insured's Address:

Insured's Employer:

Authorization: 198131332   **Approved # of Days:** 5

Attending Physician: Iva Hart, M.D.

Federal Tax ID #:   75-0246802

NPI: 0246802468

Reason for visit: I fainted this morning.

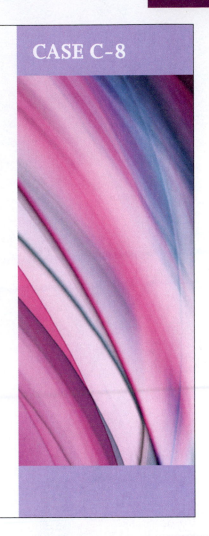

CASE C-8

HPI: This is an African American female admitted on August 14, 20XX, at 9:15 A.M. for syncope. Pt. has history of SSS and has a pacemaker. Pacemaker has failed, and a new one needs to be implanted. Pt. was discharged on August 18, 20XX, at 2:00 P.M.

Patient Control #:	198761	Type of Admission:	1
MR #:	00025643189	Source of Admission:	7
Hospital NPI:	1212121212	Discharge Status:	01
Hospital Tax ID:	75-7575757	Type of Bill Code:	0111

Fees:

Revenue Codes	Units	Total Charges	Date of Service
0210 Coronary Care	4	$ 600.00/day	08/14/20XX–08/18/20XX
0250 Pharmacy	5	$ 350.00	08/14/20XX–08/18/20XX
0260 IV Therapy	4	$1,000.00	08/14/20XX–08/17/20XX
0270 Med/Surg Supplies	1	$ 900.00	08/14/20XX
0300 Lab	4	$ 600.00	08/14/20XX–08/17/20XX
0360 OR Services	1	$1,950.00	08/14/20XX
0370 Anesthesia	1	$ 700.00	08/14/20XX
0730 EKG	1	$ 150.00	08/14/20XX
0001 TOTAL		$8,050.00	

Principal DX:	ICD-10 (T82.190A), ICD-10 (R55)
Admitting DX:	ICD-10 (R55)
Principal Procedure Code:	0JH607Z, 4A02XM4, B244YZZ, 4A02X4Z

CASE C-9

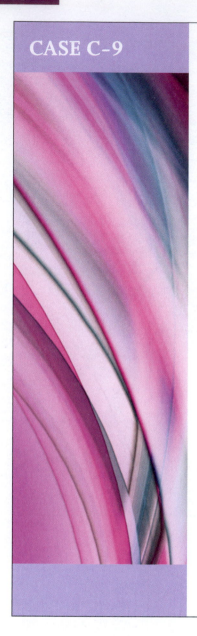

Capital City General Hospital
1000 Cherry Street
Capital City, NY 12345
(555) 555-1000

Patient Information: Virginia Moore
                             934 Smithfield Street, Capital City, NY 12345
DOB: 01-27-1944
Gender: Female
SSN: 237-02-3331
Status: Divorced   Student: No
Employer: Retired
Responsible Party: Virginia Moore
                             Address—same as above

Insurance Information: Medicaid
                             4875 Capital Boulevard, Capital City, NY 12345
ID #:   629417113972   Group #:
Insured's Name: Same   Relationship to Insured: Self
Insured's Address:

Insured's Employer:

Authorization: 519843131   Approved # of Days: 5
Attending Physician: Arthur I. Tiss, M.D.
Federal Tax ID #:   75-1135791
NPI: 1357613579

Reason for visit: I am having hip surgery.

HPI: This white female admitted on March 11, 20XX, at 5:30 P.M. for left hip replacement; total. Pt. has history of HTN, osteoporosis, and osteoarthritis. She tolerated the procedure well. Pt. was discharged on March 15, 20XX, at 2:00 P.M.

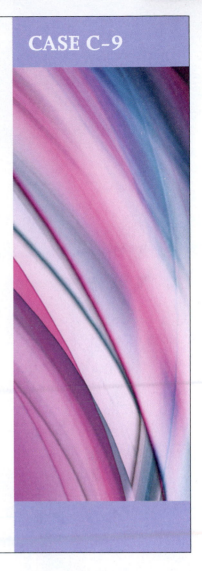

CASE C-9

Patient Control #:	578877	Type of Admission:	2
MR #:	654943233	Source of Admission:	1
Hospital NPI:	1212121212	Discharge Status:	62
Hospital Tax ID:	75-7575757	Type of Bill Code:	111

Fees:

Revenue Codes	Units	Total Charges	Date of Service
120 Room/Board/Semi	4	$ 650.00/day	03/11/20XX–03/15/20XX
250 Pharmacy	5	$ 400.00	03/11/20XX–03/15/20XX
260 IV Therapy	4	$1,200.00	03/11/20XX–03/14/20XX
270 Med/Surg Supplies	1	$1,200.00	03/12/20XX
300 Lab	2	$ 400.00	03/11/20XX–03/12/20XX
320 Radiology	1	$ 250.00	03/11/20XX
360 OR Services	1	$2,600.00	03/12/20XX
370 Anesthesia	1	$ 800.00	03/12/20XX
730 EKG	1	$ 175.00	03/11/20XX
001 TOTAL		$9,775.00	

Principal DX:	ICD-10 (S72.109A), ICD-10 (M84.40XA), ICD-10 (M15.0), ICD-10 (I10)
Admitting DX:	ICD-10 (S72.109A)
Principal Procedure Code:	0SR90J9, BQ000ZZ, 4A02XAZ

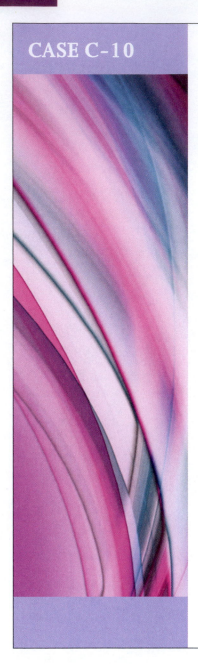

CASE C-10

Capital City General Hospital
1000 Cherry Street
Capital City, NY 12345-2222
(555) 555-1000

Patient Information:	Albert Kim	
	601 Sunflower Drive, Capital City, NY 12345	
	(555) 555-6843	
DOB:	06-02-1930	
Gender:	Male	
SSN:	563-56-7031	
Status:	Married	**Student:** No
Employer:	Retired	
Responsible Party:	Albert Kim	
	Address—same as above	

Insurance Information:	Medicare	
	P.O. Box 9834, Capital City, NY 12345	
ID #:	629417113A	**Group #:**
Insured's Name:	Same	**Relationship to Patient:** Self
Insured's Address:		

Insured's Employer:

Authorization:	646819900	**Approved # of Days:** 5
Attending Physician:	Iva Hart, M.D.	
Federal Tax ID #:	75-0246802	
NPI:	0246802468	

Reason for visit: I'm having trouble breathing, and I'm very tired.

HPI: This Asian male presents in the ER on April 3, 20XX, at 4:43 P.M. He is complaining of SOB and excessive tiredness. Exam revealed increased BP, respiration, and pulse rate. Pt. denies any CP. Says he just feels uncomfortably full. B/L pitting ankle edema 2+. Pt. does have a history of malignant HTN. Pt. was admitted for further workup. Over the course of the stay, CXR revealed pleural effusion. Thoracentesis was performed without complications. Pt. was discharged on April 7, 20XX, at 12:30 P.M.

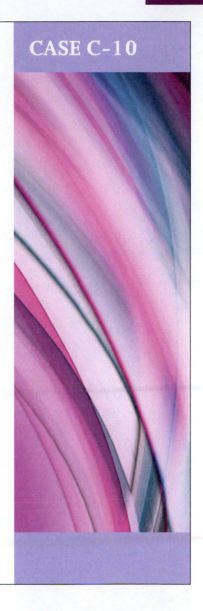

CASE C-10

Patient Control #:	015356	Type of Admission:	1
MR #:	AK45329	Source of Admission:	7
Hospital NPI:	1212121212	Discharge Status:	03
Hospital Tax ID:	75-5757575	Type of Bill Code:	0111

Fees:

Revenue Codes	Units	Total Charges	Date of Service
0210 Coronary Care	4	$ 650.00/day	04/03/20XX–04/07/20XX
0250 Pharmacy	5	$ 375.00	04/03/20XX–04/07/20XX
0260 IV Therapy	4	$1,000.00	04/03/20XX–04/06/20XX
0270 Med/Surg Supplies	1	$ 400.00	04/05/20XX
0300 Lab	2	$ 220.00	04/03/20XX; 04/06/20XX
0320 Radiology	2	$ 550.00	04/03/20XX; 04/05/20XX
0730 EKG	1	$ 150.00	04/03/20XX
0900 Respiratory Services	1	$ 400.00	04/05/20XX
0001 TOTAL		$5,695.00	

Principal DX:	ICD-10 (I11.0), ICD-10 (I50.9)
Admitting DX:	ICD-10 (R06.02)
Principal Procedure Code:	0W993ZZ, BW03ZZZ

CASE C-11

Capital City General Hospital Outpatient Services
1000 Cherry Street
Capital City, NY 12345
(555) 555-1000

Patient Name:	Olivia Marselle
	4142 Valley Road, Capital City, NY 12345
	(555) 555-1037
DOB:	10-29-1975
Gender:	Female
SSN:	993-92-7046
Status:	Married **Student:** No
Employer:	Sandwiches Plus
	26 Seneca Boulevard, Capital City, NY 12345
	(555) 555-3300
Responsible Party:	Olivia Marselle
	Address—same as above
Insurance Information:	Medicaid
	4875 Capital Boulevard, Capital City, NY 12345
ID #:	0564616665659 **Group #:**
Insured's Name:	Same **Relationship to Patient:** Self
Insured's Address:	
Insured's Employer:	
Authorization:	
Emergency Physician:	Karen A. Lotts, M.D.
Federal Tax ID #:	75-1471471
NPI:	1471471471

Reason for visit: Nausea & vomiting.

Capital City General Hospital Emergency Services

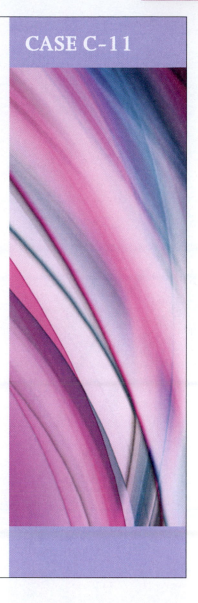

CASE C-11

Patient's Name: Olivia Marselle
Date of Procedure: 08/23/20XX
Emergency Physician: Karen A. Lotts, M.D.

DOB: 10/29/1975
PCP: Phil Wells, M.D.
MR#: OM 24965

This is a white female who presents to the ER on August 23, 20XX, at 6:32 P.M. with complaints of N&V. She is asthmatic and has recently started prednisone and tetracycline for exacerbation and bronchitis. She says that she has taken prednisone before without any problems. Patient denies any possibility of being pregnant. Lab values are negative. She is advised to stop the tetracycline. Augmentin given, and clear liquid diet ×2 days. Follow up with PCP.

Reason for Visit: ICD-10 (R11.2)
DX Code: ICD-10 (T36.4X1A), E930.4
    (this code does not convert to ICD-10),
    ICD-10 (J44.1)
CPT Procedure Code: 85025, 80053, 36415

Source of Admission: 7

Discharge Status: 01

Hospital NPI:	1212121212		Type of Bill Code:	131
Hospital Tax ID:	75-7575757		Patient Control #:	313652

Fees:

Revenue Codes	Units	Total Charges	Date of Service
300 Lab 36415	1	$ 20.00	08/23/20XX
301 Lab 80053	2	$230.00	08/23/20XX
305 Lab 85025	1	$ 25.00	08/23/20XX
450 ER	1	$350.00	08/23/20XX
001 TOTAL		$625.00	

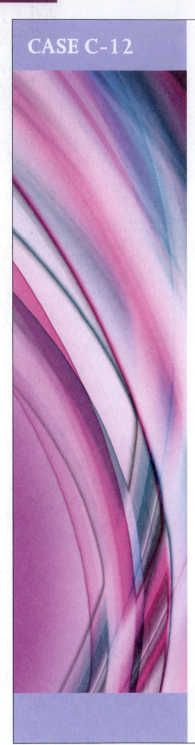

CASE C-12

Capital City General Hospital Outpatient Services
1000 Cherry Street
Capital City, NY 12345
(555) 555-1000

Patient Name:	Antonio Rodriguez
	32 Plank Circle, Capital City, NY 12345
	(555) 555-2015
DOB:	04-28-1954
Gender:	Male
SSN:	259-70-0732
Status:	Married **Student:** No
Employer:	The Builder's Outlet
	6391 Graceland Highway, Capital City, NY 12345
	(555) 555-7439
Responsible Party:	Antonio Rodriguez
	Address—same as above

Insurance Information:	Blue Cross Blue Shield
	379 Blue Plaza, Capital City, NY 12345
ID #:	YYZ94004954 **Group #:** 727524

Insured's Name:	Cassandra Rodriguez **Relationship to Patient:** Spouse
DOB:	07/30/1959 **Gender:** Female
Insured's Address:	Same

Insured's Employer:	Richie Rich Bank of USA
	7384 Dollar Avenue, Capital City, NY 12345
	(555) 555-0195
Operating Physician:	Mannie Mends, M.D.
Federal Tax ID #:	75-0123456
NPI:	0123456789
Group NPI:	1513171216

Reason for visit: I am scheduled for a colonoscopy.

Capital City General Hospital Outpatient Surgery

CASE C-12

Patient Name: Antonio Rodriguez   DOB: 04/28/1954
Date of Procedure: 05/18/20XX
Surgeon: Mannie Mends, M.D.   PCP: Elby Alright, M.D.
Anesthesia: Twilight   MR#: AR 3461
Preoperative Diagnosis: Melena
Postoperative Diagnosis: Carcinoma of the Colon; In Situ
PROCEDURE: COLONOSCOPY

Patient is prepped and draped in the usual sterile fashion. The scope is entered up and through the rectum for visualization. There are 3 polyps noted. They were excised by and sent to pathology for further evaluation. Patient tolerated the procedure well with minimal blood loss.
Exam is consistent with carcinoma.

Source of Admission: 1
Discharge Status: 01
DX Code: ICD-10 (D01.0)   Type of Bill Code: 131
CPT Procedure Code: 45384   Patient Control #: 869244

Hospital NPI:	1212121212
Hospital Tax ID: 75-7575757	
Fees:	

Revenue Codes	Units	Total Charges	Date of Service
260 IV Therapy	1	$ 400.00	05/18/20XX
270 Med/Surg Supplies	1	$ 500.00	05/18/20XX
500 Ambul Surg	1	$2,200.00	05/18/20XX
001 TOTAL		$3,100.00	

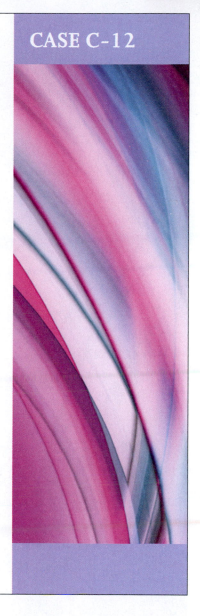

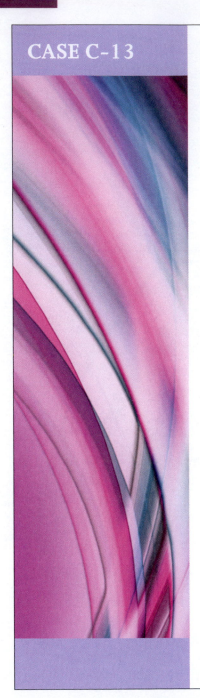

CASE C-13

Capital City Community Hospital Outpatient Services
1600 Clover Street
Capital City, NY 12345
(555) 555-1600

Patient Name:	Randall Paul
	231 Boston Avenue, Apt. 5, Capital City, NY 12345
	(555) 555-3644
DOB:	12-09-1959
Gender:	Male
SSN:	468-37-9631
Status:	Divorced **Student:** No
Employer:	Randy's Gaming Stop
	118 Swellsville Square, Capital City, NY 12345
	(555) 555-1941
Responsible Party:	Randall Paul
	Address—same as above

Insurance Information: Aetna
1625 Healthcare Building, Capital City, NY 12345

ID #: YYZ204753589   **Group #:** 200754

Insured's Name: Same   **Relationship to Patient:** Self

Insured's Address:

Insured's Employer:

Authorization:
Ordering Physician: Elby Alright, M.D.
Federal Tax ID #: 75-7654321
NPI: 9876543210

Reason for visit: Abdominal pain.

Capital City Community Hospital Outpatient Radiology

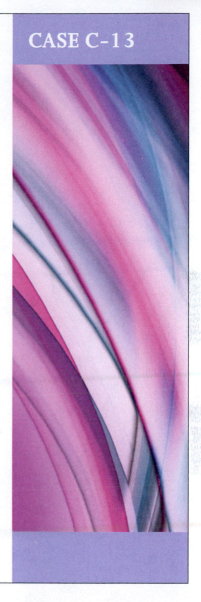

CASE C-13

Patient's Name: Randall Paul

Date of Procedure: 11/25/20XX

Ordering Physician: Elby Alright, M.D.

Report #: RP-0251

Diagnosis: Mass, kidney

Procedure: CT OF THE ABDOMEN

DOB: 12/09/1959

PCP: Elby Alright, M.D.

MR #: MR 1297

Exam is performed with the administration of oral and IV contrast. Noncontrast studies are performed of the kidneys and liver before the contrast introduction.

Liver presents normal in size and mass. There is, however, a 5 × 5.2-cm mass noted in the caudad lobe of the left kidney. The gallbladder presents as normal. Kidneys, spleen, and abdominal aorta are negative of any findings.

	Source of Admission: 1
	Discharge Status: 01
DX Code: ICD-10 (R19.00)	**Type of Bill Code:** 131
CPT Procedure Code: 74170	**Patient Control #:** 04698

Hospital NPI:	6767676767
Hospital Tax ID:	70-7070707

Fees:

Revenue Codes	Units	Total Charges	Date of Service
250 Pharmacy	1	$ 90.00	11/25/20XX
260 IV Therapy	1	$ 575.00	11/25/20XX
320 Radiology	1	$ 850.00	11/25/20XX
001 TOTAL		$1,515.00	

CASE C-14

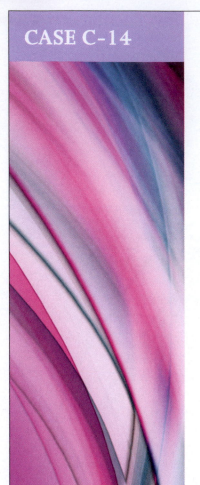

Capital City General Hospital Outpatient Services
1000 Cherry Street
Capital City, NY 12345
(555) 555-1000

Patient Name:	Megan Bishop
	5834 Cliff Street, Capital City, NY 12345
	(555) 555-1107
DOB:	10-31-1962
Gender:	Female
SSN:	501-18-6349
Status:	Single **Student:** No
Employer:	Videos Plus
	800 Mead Boulevard, Capital City, NY 12345
	(555) 555-3275
Responsible Party:	Megan Bishop
	Address—same as above
Insurance Information:	Blue Cross Blue Shield
	379 Blue Plaza, Capital City, NY 12345
ID #:	YYJ846168930 **Group #:** 688112
Insured's Name:	Same **Relationship to Patient:** Self
Insured's Address:	
Insured's Employer:	
Authorization:	
Ordering Physician:	Bette R. Soone, M.D.
Federal Tax ID #:	75-7654321
NPI:	0987654321

Reason for visit: Routine annual mammogram.

Capital City General Hospital Outpatient Radiology

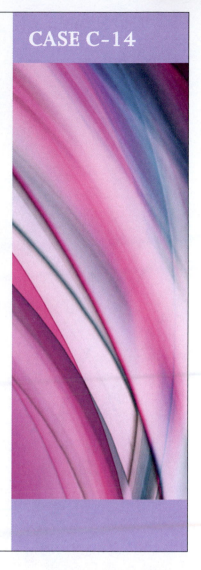

CASE C-14

Patient's Name: Megan Bishop
Date of Procedure: 09/16/20XX
Ordering Physician: Bette R. Soone, M.D.
Report #: MG-82206
Diagnosis: Routine yearly exam
Procedure: BILATERAL MAMMOGRAM

DOB: 10/31/1962
PCP: Elby Alright, M.D.
MR #: MB 8020

Comparison is made using patient's mammogram films from last year's exam. The mammary glands are primarily fatty. Margins are well defined, and there is no evidence of any suspicious masses.

Both breasts present unremarkable.

Source of Admission: 1
Discharge Status: 01
Type of Bill Code: 131
Patient Control #: 462013

DX Code: ICD-10 (Z12.31)
CPT Procedure Code: 77057

Hospital NPI:	1212121212
Hospital Tax ID:	75-7575757

Fees:

Revenue Codes	Units	Total Charges	Date of Service
320 Radiology	1	$775.00	09/16/20XX
972 Radiologist	1	$100.00	09/16/20XX
001 TOTAL		$875.00	

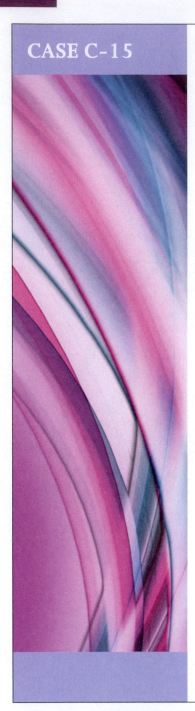

CASE C-15

Capital City Community Hospital Outpatient Surgery
1600 Clover Street
Capital City, NY 12345
(555) 555-1600

Patient Name:	Patricia Vlah
	988 Mill Run Road, Capital City, NY 12345
	(555) 555-2015
DOB:	02-11-2000
Gender:	Female
SSN:	747-03-6473
Status:	Single **Student:** Yes
Employer:	None
Responsible Party:	Patricia Vlah
	Address—same as above

Insurance Information:	Aetna
	1625 Health Care Building, Capital City, NY 12345
ID #:	6561946
Group #:	649104
Insured's Name:	Suzanne Vlah **Relationship to Patient:** Mother
DOB:	10/18/1982 **Gender:** Female
Insured's Address:	Same

Insured's Employer:	Cut-'N Curls Salon
	53 Second Avenue, Township, NY 12345
Authorization:	
Operating Physician:	Mannie Mends, M.D.
Federal Tax ID #:	75-0123456
NPI:	0123456789
Group NPI:	1513171216

Reason for visit: Tonsillectomy with adenoidectomy.

Capital City Community Hospital Outpatient Surgery

CASE C-15

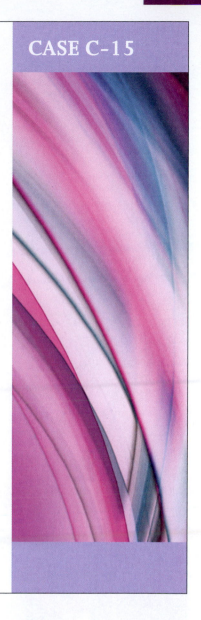

Patient Name: Patricia Vlah

Date of Procedure: 06/19/20XX

Surgeon: Mannie Mends, M.D.

Anesthesia: General

Preoperative Diagnosis: Adenotonsillitis; chronic

Postoperative Diagnosis: Adenotonsillitis; chronic

PROCEDURE: TONSILLECTOMY WITH ADENOIDECTOMY

DOB: 02/11/2000

PCP: Elby Alright, M.D.

MR #: PV 7539

Patient is prepped and draped in the usual sterile fashion. There is severe swelling of the tonsils and adenoidal tissue. This area is grasped and excised. Patient tolerated the procedure well.

Source of Admission: 1
Discharge Status: 01
Type of Bill Code: 131
Patient Control #:   665090

DX Code: ICD-10 (J35.03)

CPT Procedure Code: 42820

Hospital NPI:	6767676767
Hospital Tax ID:	70-7070707

Fees:

Revenue Codes	Units	Total Charges	Date of Service
250 Pharmacy	1	$ 150.00	06/19/20XX
260 IV Therapy	1	$ 750.00	06/19/20XX
270 Med/Surg Supplies	1	$ 400.00	06/19/20XX
370 Anesthesia	1	$ 700.00	06/19/20XX
500 Ambul Surg	1	$1,500.00	06/19/20XX
001 TOTAL		$3,500.00	

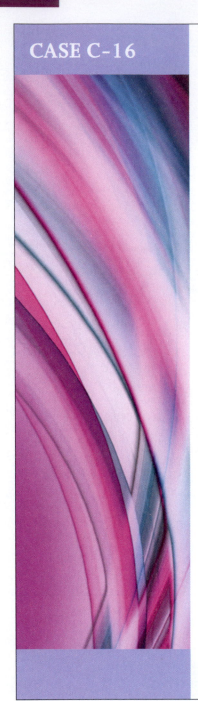

CASE C-16

Capital City General Hospital Outpatient Services
1000 Cherry Street
Capital City, NY 12345
(555) 555-1000

Patient Name:	Bryson Chung
	205 Glass Road, Capital City, NY 12345
	(555) 555-3749
DOB:	01-21-2010
Gender:	Male
SSN:	115-84-5974
Status:	Single Student: Yes
Employer:	None
Responsible Party:	Melissa Chung
	Address—same as above

Insurance Information:	Health America
	2031 Healthica Center, Capital City, NY 12345
ID #:	4684646 **Group #:** 5215
Insured's Name:	Michael Chung **Relationship to Patient:** Father, not financially responsible
DOB:	04/28/1978 **Gender:** Male
Insured's Address:	Same

Insured's Employer:	Best Furniture
	8999 Wood Road, Capital City, NY 12345
	(555) 555-0012
Authorization:	
Emergency Physician:	Karen A. Lotts, M.D.
Federal Tax ID #:	75-1471471
NPI:	1471471471

Reason for visit: Having diarrhea all morning.

Capital City General Hospital Emergency Services

CASE C-16

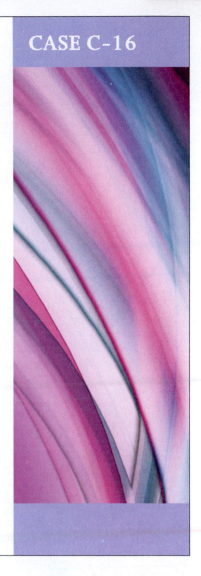

Patient's Name: Bryson Chung
Date of Procedure: 11/01/20XX
Emergency Physician: Karen A. Lotts, M.D.

DOB: 01/21/1997
PCP: Phil Wells, M.D.
MR #: BC 69281

This is an Asian American male presenting to the ER on November 1, 20XX, at 10:18 A.M. with complaints of diarrhea all morning. He has a fever of 101°F. Lab values are negative for dehydration or any other processes. Patient is to rest, drink clear liquids, take children's Tylenol, and follow up with his pediatrician for abdominal flu.

Source of Admission: 7
Discharge Status: 01
DX Code: ICD-10 (J11.2)
Type of Bill Code: 131
CPT Procedure Code: 36415, 85025, 80053
Patient Control #: 925259

Hospital NPI:	1212121212
Hospital Tax ID:	75-7575757

Fees:

Revenue Codes	Units	Total Charges	Date of Service
250 Pharmacy	1	$ 75.00	11/01/20XX
300 Lab 36415	1	$ 20.00	11/01/20XX
301 Lab 80053	1	$250.00	11/01/20XX
305 Lab 85025	1	$ 30.00	11/01/20XX
450 ER	1	$350.00	11/01/20XX
001 TOTAL		$725.00	

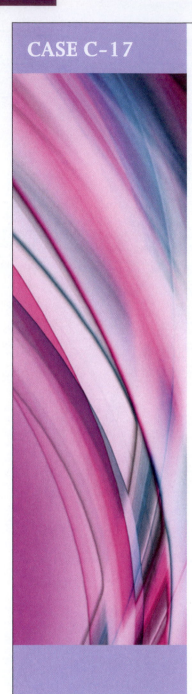

CASE C-17

Capital City Memorial Hospital Outpatient Services
700 Shady Street
Capital City, NY 12345-2222
(555) 555-0700

Patient Name:	Keith Lombardo
	174 Jefferson Street, Capital City, NY 12345
	(555) 555-8413
DOB:	05-13-1933
Gender:	Male
SSN:	165-40-3199
Status:	Married **Student:** No
Employer:	Retired
Responsible Party:	Keith Lombardo
	Address—same as above

Insurance Information:	Medicare
	P.O. Box 9834, Capital City, NY 12345
ID #:	649331304A **Group #:**
Insured's Name:	Same **Relationship to Patient:** Self
Insured's Address:	

Insured's Employer:

Authorization:

Ordering Physician:	Phil Wells, M.D.
Federal Tax ID #:	75-1234567
NPI:	1234567890
Group NPI:	1513171216

Reason for visit: Patient has a continuing high diastolic number. Dr. Wells has recommended a renal ultrasound to rule out any underlying kidney function problems.

Capital City Memorial Hospital Outpatient Radiology

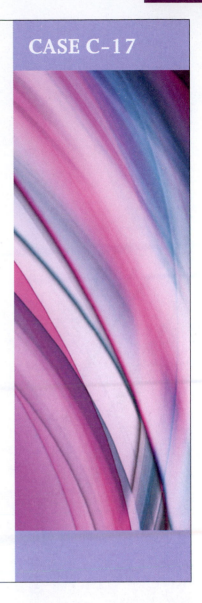

CASE C-17

Patient's Name: Keith Lombardo

Date of Procedure: 01/06/20XX

Ordering Physician: Phil Wells, M.D.

Report #: KL-56460

Diagnosis: Renal calculi

Procedure: RENAL ULTRASOUND

DOB: 05/13/1933

PCP: Phil Wells, M.D.

MR #: KL 693321

Ultrasound reveals a small area of echogenicity with some shadowing in the midportion of the right kidney that is consistent with renal calculus diagnosis. Otherwise, both kidneys are unremarkable.

There is no visualization of the urinary bladder.

Source of Admission:	1
Discharge Status:	01
Type of Bill Code:	0131
Patient Control #:	728438

DX Code: ICD-10 (N20.0)

CPT Procedure Code: 76770

Hospital NPI:	3434343434
Hospital Tax ID:	75-0750750

Fees:

Revenue Codes	Units	Total Charges	Date of Service
0320 Radiology	1	$300.00	01/06/20XX
0972 Radiologist	1	$125.00	01/06/20XX
0001 TOTAL		$425.00	

Information on File

CASE C-18

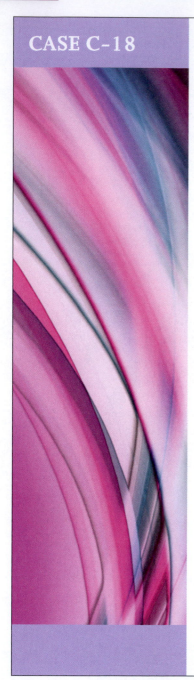

Capital City Memorial Hospital Outpatient Services
700 Shady Street
Capital City, NY 12345
(555) 555-0700

Patient Name:	Tyrone Clark
	55 Lockwood Drive, Capital City, NY 12345
	(555) 555-7578
DOB:	06-15-1980
Gender:	Male
SSN:	817-39-6220
Status:	Single Student: No
Employer:	Suzie's Styles
	42 West Deer Road, Capital City, NY 12345
	(555) 555-6776
Responsible Party:	Tyrone Clark
	Address—same as above
Insurance Information:	Medicaid
	4875 Capital Boulevard, Capital City, NY 12345
ID #:	498481614 Group #:
Insured's Name:	Same Relationship to Patient: Self
Insured's Address:	
Insured's Employer:	
Authorization:	
Emergency Physician:	Karen A. Lotts, M.D.
Federal Tax ID #:	75-1471471
NPI:	1471471471

Reason for visit: I have poison ivy really bad near my eye.

Capital City Memorial Hospital Emergency Services

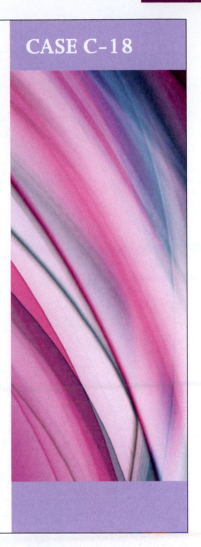

CASE C-18

Patient's Name: Tyrone Clark
Date of Procedure: 08/21/20XX
Emergency Physician: Karen A. Lotts, M.D.

DOB: 06/15/1980
PCP: Phil Wells, M.D.
MR #: TC 11720

This is an African American male presenting to the ER on August 21, 20XX, at 7:55 P.M. for poison ivy. He thinks that he had gotten it when he took his grandson for a walk in the woods 2 days ago. Since then, it has "gotten out of hand." He says that he used OTC medicine on it without any relief. It has now spread to the outer aspects of his right eyelid.

Depo-Medrol injection given for systemic reaction.

Source of Admission: 1
Discharge Status: 01
DX Code: ICD-10 (N20.0)
CPT Procedure Code: None

Type of Bill Code: 131
Patient Control #:   210158

Hospital NPI:	3434343434		
Hospital Tax ID:	75-0750750		
Fees:			

Revenue Codes	Units	Total Charges	Date of Service
250 Pharmacy	1	$ 50.00	08/21/20XX
450 ER	1	$275.00	08/21/20XX
001 TOTAL		$325.00	

CASE C-19

Capital City General Hospital Outpatient Services
1000 Cherry Street
Capital City, NY 12345-2222
(555) 555-1000

Patient Name:	Dawn Hunt
	46 Harley Drive, Capital City, NY 12345
	(555) 555-8852
DOB:	09-21-1943
Gender:	Female
SSN:	341-67-5051
Status:	Married **Student:** No
Employer:	Retired
Responsible Party:	Dawn Hunt
	Address—same as above

Insurance Information:	Medicare
	P.O. Box 9834, Capital City, NY 12345
ID #:	532865149A **Group #:**
Insured's Name:	Same **Relationship to Patient:** Self
Insured's Address:	

Insured's Employer:

Authorization:

Emergency Physician:	Karen A. Lotts, M.D.
Federal Tax ID #:	75-1471471
NPI:	1471471471

Reason for visit: Fell down my stairs and hurt my left arm.

Capital City General Hospital Emergency Services

CASE C-19

Patient's Name: Dawn Hunt

Date of Procedure: 11/25/20XX

Emergency Physician: Karen A. Lotts, M.D.

DOB: 09/21/1943

PCP: Phil Wells, M.D.

MR #: DH 40195

This is a white female presenting to the ER on November 25, 20XX, at 3:30 P.M. with complaints of falling down her basement stairs about an hour ago. She has since experienced pain and swelling in her left arm and wrist. On exam she has limited ROM. X-ray of the left arm and wrist are consistent with fracture with ulnar and radial involvement toward the distal aspect of the arm. Casting was applied. Ibuprofen and Tylenol #3 given. Follow up with orthopedist ASAP.

Source of Admission: 7

Discharge Status: 01

DX Code: ICD-10 (S52.609A),
　　　　　ICD-10 (W10.8XXA)

Type of Bill Code: 0131

CPT Procedure Code: 73090, 73100, 29075

Patient Control #: 319654

Hospital NPI:	1212121212
Hospital Tax ID:	75-7575757

Fees:

Revenue Codes	Units	Total Charges	Date of Service
0320 Radiology 73090	1	$200.00	11/25/20XX
0320 Radiology 73100	1	$200.00	11/25/20XX
0450 ER	1	$300.00	11/25/20XX
0700 Casting 29075	1	$ 95.00	11/25/20XX
0001 TOTAL		$795.00	

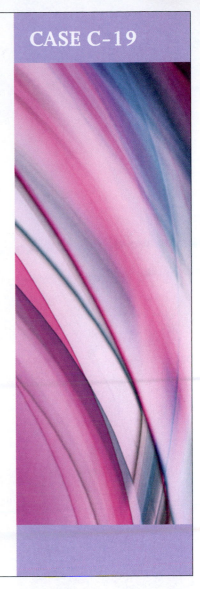

CASE C-20

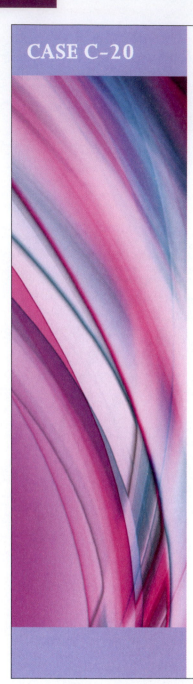

Capital City Memorial Hospital Outpatient Services
700 Shady Street
Capital City, NY 12345-2222
(555) 555-0700

Patient Name:	Jenna Masters
	388 Atlantic Avenue, Capital City, NY 12345
	(555) 555-9751
DOB:	03-12-1950
Gender:	Female
SSN:	485-72-3982
Status:	Divorced **Student:** No
Employer:	Retired
Responsible Party:	Jenna Masters
	Address—same as above

Insurance Information: Medicare
P.O. Box 9834, Capital City, NY 12345
ID #:   853614253A   **Group #:**
Insured's Name: Same   **Relationship to Patient:** Self
Insured's Address:

Insured's Employer:

Authorization:
Operating Physician: Mannie Mends, M.D.
Federal Tax ID #:   75-0123456
NPI: 0123456789
Group NPI: 1513171216

Reason for visit: Due to enlargement of cervical lymph nodes, a biopsy has been ordered to rule out infection or malignancies.

Capital City Memorial Hospital Outpatient Surgery

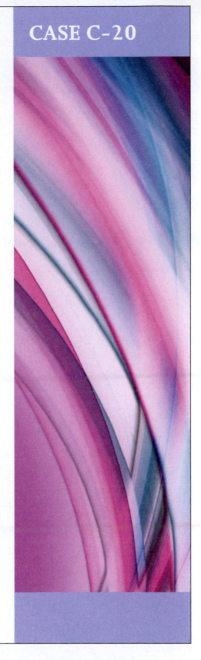

CASE C-20

Patient Name: Jenna Masters   **DOB:** 03/12/1950
Date of Procedure: 07/20/20XX
Surgeon: Mannie Mends, M.D.   **PCP:** Phil Wells, M.D.
Anesthesia: General   **MR #:** JM 820135
Preoperative Diagnosis: Lymph node enlargement; cervical
Postoperative Diagnosis: Left cervical lymphadenopathy
PROCEDURE: CERVICAL LYMPH NODE EXCISION FOR BIOPSY

Patient is prepped and draped in the usual sterile fashion. Incision is made into the left region of the left cervical nodes. The node is grasped and excised and sent to pathology for examination.

Source of Admission:	I
Discharge Status:	01
Type of Bill Code:	131
Patient Control #:	751259

DX Code: ICD-10 (R59.9)
CPT Procedure Code: 38510

Hospital NPI:	3434343434
Hospital Tax ID:	75-0750750

Fees:

Revenue Codes	Units	Total Charges	Date of Service
0250 Pharmacy	I	$ 175.00	07/20/20XX
0260 IV Therapy	I	$ 825.00	07/20/20XX
0270 Med/Surg Supplies	I	$ 450.00	07/20/20XX
0300 Lab	I	$ 375.00	07/20/20XX
0310 Lab/Path	I	$ 300.00	07/20/20XX
0370 Anesthesia	I	$ 750.00	07/20/20XX
0500 Ambul Surg	I	$1,700.00	07/20/20XX
0001 TOTAL		$4,575.00	

Medical Forms

The forms included in this appendix are documents that medical office specialists use. The format may vary from one facility to another; however, the information is universal. Exercises in the textbook will require students to utilize the following forms:

Advance Beneficiary Notice (ABN), p. 701

Assignment of Benefits (Sample), p. 702

Lifetime Assignment of Benefits (Sample), p. 703

CMS-1500 Claim Form, p. 704

E/M Audit Tool, pp. 705 and 706

Explanation of Benefits (Sample), p. 707

Financial Agreement (Sample), pp. 708–710

Insurance Verification Worksheet (Sample), p. 711

Medical Record Release Form (Sample), p. 712

Medicare Limiting Charge Form, p. 713

Medicare Secondary Payer (MSP) Form, pp. 714–717

Medicare Redetermination Request Form, p. 718

Patient Information/Registration Form (Samples), pp. 719 and 720

Precertification Form (Sample), p. 721

Preoperative Verification Form (Hospital Outpatient Benefits Form) (Sample), p. 722

Privacy Policy/HIPAA Form (Sample), pp. 723–729

Superbill/Encounter Form (Samples), p. 730

Tool to Choose the Correct CPT® Code, pp. 731–733

UB-04 (CMS-1450) Form, p. 734

CPT-4 codes in this appendix are from the CPT-4 2017 code set. CPT® is a registered trademark of the American Medical Association.

Patient's Name: _____   Medicare # (HICN): _____

ADVANCE BENEFICIARY NOTICE (ABN)

NOTE: You need to make a choice about receiving these healthcare items or services.

We expect that Medicare will not pay for the item(s) or service(s) that are described below. Medicare does not pay for all of your healthcare costs. Medicare only pays for covered items and services when Medicare rules are met. The fact that Medicare may not pay for a particular item or service does not mean that you should not receive it. There may be a good reason your doctor recommended it. Right now, in your case, **Medicare probably will not pay for—**

Items or Services:
Because:

The purpose of this form is to help you make an informed choice about whether or not you want to receive these items or services, knowing that you might have to pay for them yourself. Before you make a decision about your options, you should **read this entire Notice carefully**.

- Ask us to explain, if you do not understand why Medicare probably will not pay.
- Ask us how much these items or services will cost you (**Estimated Cost: $_____**), in case you have to pay for them yourself or through other insurance.

PLEASE CHOOSE **ONE** OPTION. CHECK **ONE** BOX. **SIGN** and **DATE** YOUR CHOICE.

☐ **Option 1. YES. I want to receive these items or services.**

I understand that Medicare will not decide whether to pay unless I receive these items or services. Please submit my claim to Medicare. I understand that you may bill me for items or services and that I may have to pay the bill while Medicare is making its decision. If Medicare does pay, you will refund to me any payments I made to you that are due to me. If Medicare denies payment, I agree to be personally and fully responsible for payment—that is, I will pay personally, either out of pocket or through any other insurance that I have. I understand I can appeal Medicare's decision.

☐ **Option 2. NO. I have decided not to receive these items or services.**

I will not receive these items or services. I understand that you will not be able to submit a claim to Medicare and that I will not be able to appeal your opinion that Medicare will not pay.

_____   _____
          Date   Signature of patient or person acting on patient's behalf

NOTE: Your health information will be kept confidential. Any information that we collect about you on this form will be kept confidential in our offices. If a claim is submitted to Medicare, your health information on this form may be shared with Medicare. Your health information, which Medicare sees, will be kept confidential by Medicare.

OMB Approval No. 0938-0566 Form No. CMS-R-131-G (March 2011)

ASSIGNMENT OF BENEFITS (SAMPLE)

I authorize payment of medical benefits to Allied Medical Center or the physician specified below.

Elizabeth S. Braceland, M.D.   Samson Westheimer, M.D.

_____   _____

Patient/Guarantor's Signature   **Date**

LIFETIME ASSIGNMENT OF BENEFITS (SAMPLE)

Financial Responsibility

All professional services rendered are charged to the patient and are due at the time of service, unless other arrangements have been made in advance with our business office. Necessary forms will be completed to file for insurance carrier payments.

Assignment of Benefits

I hereby assign all medical and surgical benefits, to include major medical benefits to which I am entitled. I hereby authorize and direct my insurance carrier(s), including Medicare, private insurance, and any other health/medical plan, to issue payment check(s) directly to Dr. Sean Robin Kirk for medical services rendered to myself and/or my dependents regardless of my insurance benefits, if any. I understand that I am responsible for any amount not covered by insurance.

Authorization to Release Information

I hereby authorize Dr. Sean Robin Kirk to (1) release any information necessary to insurance carriers regarding my illness and treatments; (2) process insurance claims generated in the course of examination or treatment; and (3) allow a photocopy of my signature to be used to process insurance claims for the period of the policy lifetime. This order will remain in effect until revoked by me in writing.

I have requested medical services from Dr. Sean Robin Kirk on behalf of myself and/or my dependents, and I understand that by making this request I become fully financially responsible for any and all charges incurred in the course of the treatment authorized.

I further understand that fees are due and payable on the date that services are rendered, and I agree to pay all such charges incurred in full immediately upon presentation of the appropriate statement. A photocopy of this assignment is to be considered as valid as the original.

_____   _____

Patient/Responsible Party Signature   Date

_____   _____

Witness   Date

CMS-1500 CLAIM FORM

HEALTH INSURANCE CLAIM FORM

APPROVED BY NATIONAL UNIFORM CLAIM COMMITTEE (NUCC) 02/12

☐☐ PICA | PICA ☐☐

1. MEDICARE ☒ (Medicare#) MEDICAID ☐ (Medicaid#) TRICARE ☐ (ID#/DoD#) CHAMPVA ☐ (Member ID#) GROUP HEALTH PLAN ☐ (ID#) FECA BLK LUNG ☐ (ID#) OTHER ☐ (ID#) | 1a. INSURED'S I.D. NUMBER (For Program in Item 1)

2. PATIENT'S NAME (Last Name, First Name, Middle Initial) | 3. PATIENT'S BIRTH DATE MM DD YY SEX M☐ F☐ | 4. INSURED'S NAME (Last Name, First Name, Middle Initial)

5. PATIENT'S ADDRESS (No., Street) | 6. PATIENT RELATIONSHIP TO INSURED Self☐ Spouse☐ Child☐ Other☐ | 7. INSURED'S ADDRESS (No., Street)

CITY | STATE | 8. RESERVED FOR NUCC USE | CITY | STATE

ZIP CODE | TELEPHONE (Include Area Code) ( ) | ZIP CODE | TELEPHONE (Include Area Code) ( )

9. OTHER INSURED'S NAME (Last Name, First Name, Middle Initial) | 10. IS PATIENT'S CONDITION RELATED TO: | 11. INSURED'S POLICY GROUP OR FECA NUMBER

a. OTHER INSURED'S POLICY OR GROUP NUMBER | a. EMPLOYMENT? (Current or Previous) YES☐ NO☐ | a. INSURED'S DATE OF BIRTH MM DD YY SEX M☐ F☐

b. RESERVED FOR NUCC USE | b. AUTO ACCIDENT? YES☐ NO☐ PLACE (State) | b. OTHER CLAIM ID (Designated by NUCC)

c. RESERVED FOR NUCC USE | c. OTHER ACCIDENT? YES☐ NO☐ | c. INSURANCE PLAN NAME OR PROGRAM NAME

d. INSURANCE PLAN NAME OR PROGRAM NAME | 10d. CLAIM CODES (Designated by NUCC) | d. IS THERE ANOTHER HEALTH BENEFIT PLAN? YES☐ NO☐ If yes, complete items 9, 9a, and 9d.

READ BACK OF FORM BEFORE COMPLETING & SIGNING THIS FORM.

12. PATIENT'S OR AUTHORIZED PERSON'S SIGNATURE I authorize the release of any medical or other information necessary to process this claim. I also request payment of government benefits either to myself or to the party who accepts assignment below.

SIGNED _____ DATE _____

13. INSURED'S OR AUTHORIZED PERSON'S SIGNATURE I authorize payment of medical benefits to the undersigned physician or supplier for services described below.

SIGNED _____

14. DATE OF CURRENT ILLNESS, INJURY, or PREGNANCY (LMP) MM DD YY QUAL | 15. OTHER DATE QUAL MM DD YY | 16. DATES PATIENT UNABLE TO WORK IN CURRENT OCCUPATION FROM MM DD YY TO MM DD YY

17. NAME OF REFERRING PROVIDER OR OTHER SOURCE | 17a. | 17b. NPI | 18. HOSPITALIZATION DATES RELATED TO CURRENT SERVICES FROM MM DD YY TO MM DD YY

19. ADDITIONAL CLAIM INFORMATION (Designated by NUCC) | 20. OUTSIDE LAB? YES☐ NO☐ $ CHARGES

21. DIAGNOSIS OR NATURE OF ILLNESS OR INJURY Relate A-L to service line below (24E) ICD Ind. | 22. RESUBMISSION CODE ORIGINAL REF. NO.

A. ___ B. ___ C. ___ D. ___
E. ___ F. ___ G. ___ H. ___
I. ___ J. ___ K. ___ L. ___

23. PRIOR AUTHORIZATION NUMBER

24. A. DATE(S) OF SERVICE From MM DD YY	To MM DD YY	B. PLACE OF SERVICE	C. EMG	D. PROCEDURES, SERVICES, OR SUPPLIES (Explain Unusual Circumstances) CPT/HCPCS MODIFIER	E. DIAGNOSIS POINTER	F. $ CHARGES	G. DAYS OR UNITS	H. EPSDT Family Plan	I. ID. QUAL	J. RENDERING PROVIDER ID. #
1										NPI
2										NPI
3										NPI
4										NPI
5										NPI
6										NPI

25. FEDERAL TAX I.D. NUMBER SSN☐ EIN☐ | 26. PATIENT'S ACCOUNT NO. | 27. ACCEPT ASSIGNMENT? (For govt. claims, see back) YES☐ NO☐ | 28. TOTAL CHARGE $ | 29. AMOUNT PAID $ | 30. Rsvd. for NUCC Use

31. SIGNATURE OF PHYSICIAN OR SUPPLIER INCLUDING DEGREES OR CREDENTIALS (I certify that the statements on the reverse apply to this bill and are made a part thereof.)

SIGNED _____ DATE _____

32. SERVICE FACILITY LOCATION INFORMATION
a. NPI b.

33. BILLING PROVIDER INFO & PH # ( )
a. NPI b.

NUCC Instruction Manual available at: www.nucc.org | PLEASE PRINT OR TYPE | APPROVED OMB-0938-1197 FORM 1500 (02-12)

Clear Form

E/M Audit Tool

Patient Information

Patient:	Visit Date:	History Level
Examined By:		Exam Level
Patient Status:	DOB:	Decision Making
Service Type:	Sex:	Insurance Carrier

CPT® Code(s) Billed   DOCUMENTED   DIAGNOSIS CODE(S) BILLED   DOCUMENTED

History

History of Present Illness
- ❏ location
- ❏ quality
- ❏ severity
- ❏ duration
- ❏ timing
- ❏ context
- ❏ modifying factors
- ❏ associated signs and symptoms
- ❏ No. of chronic diseases

History _____

Review of Systems
- ❏ Constitutional symptoms
- ❏ Eyes
- ❏ Ears, nose, mouth, throat
- ❏ Cardiovascular
- ❏ Respiratory
- ❏ Gastrointestinal
- ❏ Genitourinary
- ❏ Integumentary
- ❏ Musculoskeletal
- ❏ Neurologic
- ❏ Psychiatric
- ❏ Endocrine
- ❏ Hematologic/lymphatic
- ❏ Allergic/immunologic

Past, Family & Social History

PAST
- ❏ current medication
- ❏ prior illnesses and injuries
- ❏ operations and hospitalizations
- ❏ age-appropriate immunizations
- ❏ allergies   ❏ dietary status

FAMILY
- ❏ health status or cause of death of parents siblings, and children
- ❏ hereditary or high-risk diseases
- ❏ diseases related to CC, HPI, ROS

SOCIAL
- ❏ living arrangements
- ❏ marital status   ❏ sexual history
- ❏ occupational history
- ❏ use of drugs, alcohol, or tobacco
- ❏ extent of education
- ❏ current employment   ❏ other

❏ PFSH form reviewed no change   ❏ PFSH form reviewed, updated   ❏ PFSH form new

General Multi-System Examination

Constitutional
- ❏ 3 of 7 (2 BP, pulse, respir, tmp, hgt, wgt)
- ❏ General Appearance

Eyes
- ❏ Conjunctivac, Lids
- ❏ Eyes: Pupils, Irises
- ❏ Opthal exam-Optic discs, Pos Seg

ENT
- ❏ Ears Nose
- ❏ Oto exam-Aud canals, Tymp membr
- ❏ Hearing
- ❏ Nasal mucosa, Septum, Turbinates
- ❏ ENTM: Lips, Teeth, Gums
- ❏ Oropharynx-oral mucosa, palates

Neck
- ❏ Neck
- ❏ Thyroid

Respiratory
- ❏ Respiratory effort
- ❏ Percussion of chest
- ❏ Palpation of chest
- ❏ Auscultation of lungs

Cardiovascular
- ❏ Palpation of heart
- ❏ Auscultation of heart (& sounds)
- ❏ Carotid arteries Abdominal aorta
- ❏ Femoral arteries
- ❏ Pedal pulses
- ❏ Extrem for periph edema/varicosities

Chest
- ❏ Inspect Breasts
- ❏ Palpation of Breasts & Axillae

Gastrointestinal
- ❏ Abd (+/− masses or tenderness)
- ❏ Liver, Spleen
- ❏ Hernia (+/−)
- ❏ Anus, Perineum, Rectum
- ❏ Stool for occult blood

GU/Female
- ❏ Female: Genitalia, Vagina
- ❏ Female Urethra
- ❏ Bladder
- ❏ Cervix
- ❏ Uterus
- ❏ Adnexa/parametria

GU/Male
- ❏ Scrotal Contents
- ❏ Penis
- ❏ Digital Rectal of Prostate

Lymphatic
- ❏ Lymph: Neck
- ❏ Lymph: Axillae
- ❏ Lymph: Groin
- ❏ Lymph: Other

Musculoskeletal
- ❏ Gait (… ability to exercise)
- ❏ Palpation Digits, Nails
- ❏ Head/Neck: Inspect, Percuss, Palp
- ❏ Head/Neck: Motion (+/− pain, crepit)
- ❏ Head/Neck: Stability (+/− lux, sublux)
- ❏ Head/Neck: Muscle strength & tone
- ❏ Spine/Rib/Pelv: Inspect, Percuss, Palp
- ❏ Spine/Rib/Pelv: Motion
- ❏ Spine/Rib/Pelv: Stability
- ❏ Spine/Rib/Pelv: Strength and tone

- ❏ R. Up Extrem: Inspect, Percuss, Palp
- ❏ R. Up Extrem: Motion (+/− pain, crepit)
- ❏ R. Up Extrem: Stability (+/− lux, sublux)
- ❏ R. Up Extrem: Muscle strength & tone
- ❏ L. Up Extrem: Inspect, Percuss, Palp
- ❏ L. Up Extrem: Motion (+/− pain, crepit)
- ❏ L. Up Extrem: Muscle strength & tone
- ❏ R. Low Extrem: Inspect, Percuss, Palp
- ❏ R. Low Extrem: Motion (+/− pain, crepit)
- ❏ R. Low Extrem: Stability (+/− lux, laxity)
- ❏ R. Low Extrem: Muscle strength & tone
- ❏ L. Low Extrem: Inspect, Percuss, Palp
- ❏ L. Low Extrem: Motion (+/− pain, crepit)
- ❏ L. Low Extrem: Sability (+/− lux, sublux)
- ❏ L. Low Extrem: Muscle strength & tone

Skin
- ❏ Skin: Inspect Skin & Subcut tissues
- ❏ Skin: Palpation Skin & Subcut tissues

Neuro
- ❏ Neuro: Cranial nerves (+/− deficits)
- ❏ Neuro: DTRs (+/− pathological reflexes)
- ❏ Neuro: Sensations

Psychiatry
- ❏ Psych: Judgment, Insight
- ❏ Psych: Mood, Affect (depression, anxiety)

Exam Documented _____

(continued)

Number of Diagnoses/ Management Options	Points
Self-limited or minor (Stable, improved, or worsened)—Maximum 2 points in this category.	1
Established problem (to examining MD); stable or improved	1
Established problem (to examining MD); worsening	2
New problem (to examining MD); no additional workup planned— Maximum 1 point in this category.	3
New problem (to examining MD); additional workup (eg., admit/ transfer)	4
Total	

Amount and/or complexity of Data Reviewed	Points
Lab ordered and/or reviewed (regardless of # ordered)	1
X-ray ordered and/or reviewed (regardless of # ordered)	1
Medicine section (90701-99199) ordered and/or reviewed	1
Discussion of test results with performing physician	1
Decision to obtain old record and/or obtain hx from someone other than patient	1
Review and summary of old records and/or obtaining hx from someone other than patient and/or discussion with other health provider	2
Independent visualization of image, tracing, of specimen (not simply review of report)	2
Total	

Table of Risk

Level of Risk	Presenting Problem(s)	Diagnostic Procedure(s) Ordered	Management Options Selected
Minimal	• One self-limited or minor problem, e.g., cold, insect bite, tinea corporis	• Laboratory tests requiring venipuncture • Chest x-rays • EKG/EEG • Urinalysis • Ultrasound, eg, echocardi-ography • KOH prep	• Rest • Gargles • Elastic bandages • Superficial dressings
Low	• Two or more self-limited or minor problem • One stable chronic illness, e.g., well-controlled hyper-tension, non-insulindepend-ent diabetes, cataract, BPH • Acute uncomplicated illness or injury, e.g., cystitis allergic rhinitis, simple sprain	• Physiologic tests not under stress, e.g., pulmonary functions tests • Noncardiovascular imaging studies with contrast, e.g., barium enema • Superficial needle biopsies • Clinical laboratory tests requiring arterial puncture • Skin biopsies	• Over-the-counter drugs • Minor surgery with no identified risk factors • Physical therapy • Occupational therapy • IV fluids without addi-tives
Moderate	• One or more chronic ill-nesses with mild exacerba-tion, progression, or side effects of treatment • Two or more stable chronic illness • Undiagnosed new problem with uncertain prognosis, e.g., lump in breast • Acute illness with systemic symptoms, e.g., pyelone-phritis, pneumonitis, colitis • Acute complicated injury, e.g., head injury with brief loss of consciousness	• Physiologic tests under stress, e.g., cardiac stress tests, fetal contraction stress test • Diagnostic endoscopies with no identified risk fac-tors • Deep needle or incisional biopsy • Cardiovascular imaging studies with contrast and no identified risk factors, eg, arteriogram, cardiac catheterization • Obtain fluid from body cavity, e.g., lumbar punc-ture, thoracentesis, culdo-centesis	• Minor surgery with identified risk factors • Elective major surgery (open, percutaneous, or endoscopic) with no identified risk factors • Prescription drug man-agement • Therapeutic nuclear medicine • IV fluids with additives • Closed treatment of fracture or dislocation without manipulation
High	• One or more chronic ill-nesses with severe exacer-bation, progression, or side effects of treatment • Acute or chronic illnesses or injuries that pose a threat to life or bodily function, eg, multiple trauma, acute MI, pulmo-nary embolus, severe res-piratory distress, progressive severe rheu-matoid arthritis, psychiatric illness with potential threat to self or others, peritoni-tis, acute renal failure • An abrupt change in neuro-logic status, e.g., seizure, TIA, weakness, sensory loss	• Cardiovascular imaging studies with contrast with identified risk factors • Cardiac electrophysiologi-cal tests • Diagnostic endoscopies with identified risk factors • Discography	• Elective major surgery (open, percutaneous, or endoscopic) with identi-fied risk factors • Emergency major sur-gery (open, percutane-ous, or endoscopic) • Parenteral controlled substances • Drug therapy requiring intensive monitoring for toxicity • Decision not to resusci-tate or to deescalate care because of poor prognosis

Medical Decision Making	SF	LOW	MOD	HIGH
Number of Diagnoses or Treatment Options	1	2	3	4
Amount and/or Complexity of Data to be Reviewed	1	2	3	4
Risk of Complications, Morbidity, Mortality	Minimal	Low	Moderate	High
E/M Level= 2 out of 3				

MDM _____

Chart Note
❏ Dictated   ❏ Handwritten
❏ Form   ❏ Illegible
❏ Note signed
❏ Signature missing

Other Services or Modalities:

Auditor:

EXPLANATION OF BENEFITS (SAMPLE)

For Students Use Only.

Payer's Name and Address

Today's Date:

Provider's Name and Address

This statement covers payments for the following patient(s):

Claim Detail Section (if there are number in the "SEE REMARKS" column, see the Remarks Section for explanation)

Patient Name	Patient Account Number:
Patient ID Number:	Insured's Name:
Group Number:	
Provider Name:	Inventory Number: Claim Control Number:

Service Date(s)	Procedure	Charges	Adjustment	Allowed	Copay	Deduct/Not Covered	Coins	Paid Amt.	Provider Paid/ Remarks
TOTALS									

BALANCE DUE FROM PATIENT: PT'S DED/NOT COV $_____

PT'S COINSURANCE $_____

PAYMENT SUMMARY SECTION (Totals)

Charges	Adjustment	Allowed	Copay	Deduct/Not Covered	Coins	Total Paid

Financial Agreement (Sample)
Allied Medical Center
1933 E. Frankford Road, Suite 110

Carrollton, TX 12345

Phone: (910) 555-1716

FAX: (910) 555-1717

Please read the following carefully and sign below that you understand and accept Allied Medical Center's basic operating policies and agree to the financial terms:

<u>Payment is expected at time of service</u>:

Unless insurance is verified by the office or a treatment payment plan is arranged, clients are responsible for making full payment at the time of service.

<u>Schedule of Fees</u>:

Clients will be provided a schedule of fees regarding their treatment and payment options.

<u>Health Insurance</u>:

Allied Medical Center participates (in-network) with several major insurers, and the practice will make every reasonable effort to work with your insurance plan to file for all covered services.

If coverage cannot be verified, full payment at time of service is required. After the office receives payment with an Explanation of Benefits from your insurer, any surplus payment for services will be credited to your account or refunded promptly.

Once insurance coverage is verified, clients are responsible for payment of all copays, coinsurance, deductibles, and uncovered balances at time of service.

If insurance is used, please understand that it is the client's (or client's legal guardian's) responsibility to notify Allied Medical Center of any changes in insurance coverage. You are responsible for prompt and full payment of services not covered by insurance. When insurance is used to pay for services, the client agrees to assign any insurance benefit payments to Allied Medical Center for services rendered.

<u>Limitations of Insurance</u>:

Not all insurance plans cover all services, and Allied Medical Center does not participate in all plans. Some plans require preauthorization, referrals, or justification of medical necessity, which limit or deny reimbursement. Also, some insurance companies regard therapy, including biofeedback, for medical conditions to be reimbursed under mental health coverage, which frequently has less coverage than medical benefits. Please check with your carrier to determine specifics of your policy and your mental health coverage for this type of treatment.

If you participate in an insurance plan in which Allied Medical Center is not in-network, it is strongly recommended that you provide a physician referral letter so the practice can better assist you in advocating for payment by your insurance company. Allied Medical Center will submit your claim to the insurance carrier for consideration of out-of-network reimbursement, but full payment at time of service is your responsibility.

Prompt Payment:

The practice provides the most cost-effective, high-quality care possible. To do this, costs related to billing overhead are kept to a minimum. Therefore clients are obliged to make prompt payment for all fees due. Charges for late payment, collections, or missed appointments will be assessed as needed to recover these costs.

Late Charges:

All outstanding balances are due within 30 days of services rendered or by the date due for prearranged payment plans. A 5% per month fee is assessed for overdue balances. Balances that exceed 90 days are considered delinquent and will be assigned to collections. Clients are responsible for payment of all fees related to collecting the unpaid balance.

Returned Checks:

There is a $50.00 fee for returned checks.

Missed Appointments:

Scheduled appointments are time that is blocked out for you, and the practice does not overbook appointments that might limit or delay your appointment. Therefore, clients are responsible for payment for their reserved time.

Late Cancellations:

Appointments must be cancelled or rescheduled by 5:00 P.M. of the prior day, or the client will be charged the full appointment charge (even if the client does not show for the appointment). Allied Medical Center will make every reasonable effort to forgive missed appointments due to an unforeseen emergency, but all missed or late cancelled appointments need to be discussed and approved. After two missed appointments without adequate notification or explanation, Allied Medical Center reserves the right to terminate treatment.

Appointment Notification:

Allied Medical Center will remind you of your scheduled appointment by telephone or e-mail. (Please state your preference of e-mail or telephone or neither.) However, it is your responsibility to keep your appointment as scheduled or notify the practice as outlined above if you need to cancel or reschedule.

Telephone Consults:

The services that Allied Medical Center offers are elective in nature. Allied Medical Center does not offer emergency medical or psychiatric care. Therefore, emergency telephone calls are generally not accepted. Clients should contact their medical providers for any medically oriented emergencies. Telephone calls outside of prearranged consultations or as a medical consultation scheduled by the client will be billed at the hourly rate in 15-minute increments. Telephone consults are typically not reimbursable by insurance.

Ancillary Services:

Legal and disability support is offered through the practice, with advance arrangement and approval only. Court appearances, correspondence, report writing, and other

(continued)

efforts for legal action or disability work are not reimbursable by health insurance and will be billed on a time and materials basis.

Questions about Payment or Insurance:

For payment or insurance questions or concerns, contact the practice administrator via e-mail at billing@alliedmedcenter.com or phone: (910) 555-1717.

I received a copy of the current Allied Medical Center fee schedule.
I have read, understand, and agree to the policies outlined in this agreement.

_____

Patient's Name

_____   _____

Patient/Guardian Signature   Date

Financial Agreement (Sample) (continued)

INSURANCE VERIFICATION WORKSHEET (SAMPLE)

Patient's Name: _____ Chart Number: _____ Appt. Date: _____

DOB: _____ Policy ID Number: _____ Group Number: _____

Policyholder: _____ DOB: _____

Insurance Co. Name: _____ Referral Number Required: ❑ No ❑ Yes

Telephone Number: _____ Referral Number: _____

Mailing Address: _____

Employer's Name: _____

Employer's Phone Number: _____

Effective Date: _____ Lifetime Maximum: _____

Pre-Cert Required: ❑ Yes ❑ No

Deductible Met:

Copay: _____ Deductible _____ ❑ No ❑ Yes

Pays @ _____%

Exclusion/Preexisting: _____

Chief Complaint/Diagnosis: _____

Insurance Rep's Name: _____ Ext Number: _____

Voice Tracking Number: _____ Date: _____ Time: _____

Verified by: _____ Date: _____

MEDICAL RECORD RELEASE FORM (SAMPLE)

I, _____ ACTING ON
BEHALF OF: (Print Name of Patient or Legally Authorized Representative)

_____ HEREBY AUTHORIZE THE RELEASE
(Print Name of Patient)
OF INFORMATION AS INDICATED:

My Healthcare Information

_____ I authorize disclosure of healthcare information (related to my medical history, diagnosis, treatment, or prognosis) to all inquiries or only to the following people or entities (for example, family friends, employer, insurance companies, clergy):

List Names:

_____

_____

Limited Healthcare Information:

_____ I wish to limit disclosure of only certain kinds of healthcare information (related to my medical history, diagnosis, treatment, or prognosis) to the following people or entities:

List Names   **List information that may be released**

_____   _____

_____   _____

No Information:

_____ I do not authorize release of any information regarding my admission or treatment. I wish to be a "no information" patient, and I realize that flowers, telephone calls, and visitors will be refused on my behalf.

_____   _____
(Signature of Patient or Legally Authorized Representative)   (Date)

MEDICARE LIMITING CHARGE FORM

Limiting Charge
Overview

Note: This form will only be sent if the beneficiary requests it.

We were advised by TrailBlazer Health Enterprises, LLC, on (insert date), that the services described below were billed with charges that exceeded the amounts permitted under Medicare rules. In accordance with their instructions, we are refunding the excess amount or posting a credit to your account.

TODAY'S DATE: _____

BENEFICIARY (PATIENT) NAME: _____

BENEFICIARY HICN: _____

DATE(S) OF SERVICE: _____

PROCEDURE CODE(S): _____

DESCRIPTION OF THE PROCEDURE(S): _____

_____

AMOUNT OF REFUND: _____

NAME AND ADDRESS OF PHYSICIAN OR NON-PHYSICIAN PRACTITIONER:

_____

_____

_____

_____

Medicare Secondary Payer Questionnaire Form

1. Are you receiving Black Lung (BL) Benefits?
   ♦ The Black Lung Benefits Act of 1981 provides benefits to miners totally disabled due to pneumoconiosis arising out of coal mine employment. Black Lung IS PRIMARY ONLY FOR CLAIMS RELATED TO Black Lung diagnosis.
   _____ If no, write "N" and go to the next question.
   _____ If yes, write "Y" and document the date benefits began: CCYY/MM/DD.
   Black Lung is primary, only for claims related to Black Lung.

2. Will this be paid by a government program (e.g., research grant)?
   ♦ If the services provided are part of any government **program**, they may be paid by a source other than Medicare. Your patient will know whether it is a research grant or another program that is paying for their services.
   _____ If no, write "N" and go to the next question.
   _____ If yes, write "Y" and determine who the primary payer is. Government programs will be primary for these services.

3. Has Department of Veterans Affairs (DVA) authorized and agreed to pay?
   ♦ If the DVA has authorized and agreed to pay, ask the patient for the authorization.
   _____ If no, write "N" and go to the next question.
   _____ If yes, write "Y" and enter as the primary insurance. DVA is primary for these services.

4. Was the illness/injury due to a work-related accident/condition?
   ♦ If the illness/injury is due to a work-related accident, MEDICARE IS NOT PRIMARY, WORKERS' COMPENSATION IS THE PRIMARY PAYER ONLY FOR CLAIMS RELATED TO WORK-RELATED INJURIES OR ILLNESS. GO TO PART III.
   _____ If no, this is not a work-related illness/accident. GO TO PART II.
   _____ If yes, write "Y" and enter the date of injury/illness: CCYY/MM/DD. Workers' compensation is primary payer only for claims related to work-related injury or illness. STOP.

   _____
   Date of injury/illness: _____
   _____
   _____
   Record the policy or identification number: _____
   Document the name and address of the patient's employer: _____
   _____
   _____
   _____
   _____

Part II

1. Was the illness/injury due to a non-work-related accident
   ♦ (e.g., automobile, fall in the home, fall in business)?
   _____ If no, GO TO PART III.
   _____ If yes, record the date of accident: CCYY/MM/DD.

2. Was the accident automobile related?
   _____ If no, GO TO PART III.
   _____ If yes, record the name and address of nofault or liability insurer.
   _____
   _____
   Insurance Claim Number: _____

3. Was another party responsible for this accident?
   _____ If no, GO TO PART III.

_____ If yes, record the name and address of the liability insurer. LIABILITY INSURER IS PRIMARY ONLY FOR THOSE RELATED TO THE ACCIDENT. GO TO PART III.

Name and address of any liability insurer:

_____

_____

_____

_____

Insurance claim number: _____

Part III

1. Are you entitled to Medicare based on any of the following?
   - ◆ Age (people 65 years of age and older). GO TO PART IV.
   - ◆ Disability (some people with disabilities under 65 years of age). GO TO PART V.
   - ◆ End-stage renal disease (ESRD)—permanent kidney failure treated with dialysis or a transplant. GO TO PART VI.

Part IV

If you are entitled to Medicare based on age:

1. Are you currently employed?

   _____ If no, record the date of retirement: CCYY/MM/DD.

   _____ If yes, record the name and address of your employer.

   _____

   _____

2. Is your spouse currently employed?

   _____ If no, record the date of his or her retirement: CCYY/MM/DD.

   _____ If yes, record the name and address of your spouse's employer:

   _____

   _____

   _____

   _____

   IF THE PATIENT ANSWERED NO TO BOTH QUESTIONS 1 AND 2, MEDICARE IS PRIMARY. DO NOT PROCEED ANY FURTHER. IF YES TO QUESTIONS 1 AND 2, GO TO QUESTIONS 3 AND 4.

3. If either you or your spouse is employed, do you have group health plan (GHP) coverage?

   _____ If no, STOP. MEDICARE IS PRIMARY.

   _____ If yes, does the employer that sponsors your GHP employ 20 or more employees?

   _____ If no, STOP. MEDICARE IS PRIMARY.

   _____ If yes, the GROUP HEALTH PLAN IS PRIMARY. RECORD THE FOLLOWING INFORMATION.

   Name and address of GHP:

   _____

   _____

   _____

   _____

   Policy ID Number: _____

   Group ID Number: _____

   Name of Policyholder: _____

   Relationship to Patient: _____

Part V

If you are entitled to Medicare based on a disability:

1. Are you currently employed?

   _____ If no, record the date of retirement: CCYY/MM/DD.

   _____ If yes, record the name and address of your employer:

   _____

   _____

   _____

2. Is a family member currently employed?
_____ IF THE PATIENT ANSWERS NO TO BOTH QUESTIONS 1 AND 2, MEDICARE IS PRIMARY, DO NOT PROCEED ANY FURTHER.
_____ If yes, record the name and address of employer:
_____
_____
_____
_____

3. Do you have group health plan (GHP) coverage based on your own or a family member's current employment?
_____ If no, STOP. MEDICARE IS PRIMARY.
_____ If yes, does the employer that sponsors your GHP employ 100 or more employees?
_____ If no, STOP. MEDICARE IS PRIMARY.
_____ If yes, the Group Health Plan is PRIMARY. OBTAIN THE FOLLOWING INFORMATION:

Name and address of GHP:
_____
_____
_____
_____

Policy ID Number: _____
Group ID Number: _____
Name of Policyholder: _____
Relationship to Patient: _____

Part VI
Are you entitled to Medicare based on ESRD?
1. Do you have group health plan (GHP) coverage?
_____ If no, STOP. MEDICARE IS PRIMARY.
_____ If yes, record the name and address of GHP:
_____
_____
_____
_____

Policy ID Number: _____
Group ID Number: _____
Name of Policyholder: _____
Relationship to Patient: _____
Name and address of employer, if any, from which you receive GHP coverage: _____

2. Have you received a kidney transplant?
_____ If no, continue to the next question.
_____ If yes, record the date of transplant: CCYY/MM/DD. GO TO QUESTION 3.

3. Have you received maintenance dialysis treatments? (These are dialysis treatments relating to transplant and should be billed as part of the transplant cost.)
_____ If no, continue to the next question.
_____ If yes, record the date dialysis began: CCYY/MM/DD. GO TO QUESTION 4.
If you participated in a self-dialysis program, provide date training started: CCYY/MM/DD.

4. Are you within the 30-month coordination period?

When a patient is diagnosed with ESRD, the patient's group health plan (GHP) must pay claims for the first 30 months after diagnosis.
_____ If no, STOP. MEDICARE IS PRIMARY.
_____ If yes, GO TO QUESTION 5.

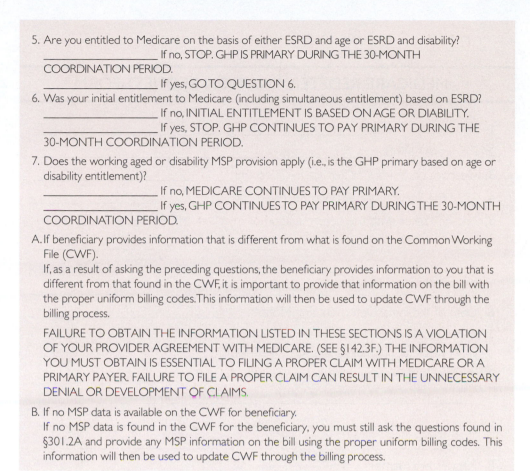

5. Are you entitled to Medicare on the basis of either ESRD and age or ESRD and disability?

_____ If no, STOP. GHP IS PRIMARY DURING THE 30-MONTH COORDINATION PERIOD.

_____ If yes, GO TO QUESTION 6.

6. Was your initial entitlement to Medicare (including simultaneous entitlement) based on ESRD?

_____ If no, INITIAL ENTITLEMENT IS BASED ON AGE OR DIABILITY.

_____ If yes, STOP. GHP CONTINUES TO PAY PRIMARY DURING THE 30-MONTH COORDINATION PERIOD.

7. Does the working aged or disability MSP provision apply (i.e., is the GHP primary based on age or disability entitlement)?

_____ If no, MEDICARE CONTINUES TO PAY PRIMARY.

_____ If yes, GHP CONTINUES TO PAY PRIMARY DURING THE 30-MONTH COORDINATION PERIOD.

A. If beneficiary provides information that is different from what is found on the Common Working File (CWF).

If, as a result of asking the preceding questions, the beneficiary provides information to you that is different from that found in the CWF, it is important to provide that information on the bill with the proper uniform billing codes. This information will then be used to update CWF through the billing process.

FAILURE TO OBTAIN THE INFORMATION LISTED IN THESE SECTIONS IS A VIOLATION OF YOUR PROVIDER AGREEMENT WITH MEDICARE. (SEE §142.3F.) THE INFORMATION YOU MUST OBTAIN IS ESSENTIAL TO FILING A PROPER CLAIM WITH MEDICARE OR A PRIMARY PAYER. FAILURE TO FILE A PROPER CLAIM CAN RESULT IN THE UNNECESSARY DENIAL OR DEVELOPMENT OF CLAIMS.

B. If no MSP data is available on the CWF for beneficiary.

If no MSP data is found in the CWF for the beneficiary, you must still ask the questions found in §301.2A and provide any MSP information on the bill using the proper uniform billing codes. This information will then be used to update CWF through the billing process.

DEPARTMENT OF HEALTH AND HUMAN SERVICES
CENTERS FOR MEDICARE & MEDICAID SERVICES

MEDICARE REDETERMINATION REQUEST FORM

1. Beneficiary's Name: _____

2. Medicare Number: _____

3. Description of Item or Service in Question: _____

4. Date the Service or Item Was Received: _____

5. I do not agree with the determination of my claim. MY REASONS ARE:

   _____

   _____

   _____

6. Date of the Initial Determination Notice: _____

   (If you received your Initial Determination Notice more than 120 days ago, include your reason for not making this request earlier.)

7. Additional Information Medicare Should Consider:

   _____

   _____

   _____

8. Requester's Name: _____

9. Requester's Relationship to the Beneficiary: _____

10. Requester's Address: _____

    _____

    _____

    _____

11. Requester's Telephone Number: _____

12. Requester's Signature: _____

13. Date Signed: _____

14. ❑ I have evidence to submit. (Attach such evidence to this form.)
    ❑ I do not have evidence to submit.

NOTICE: Anyone who misrepresents or falsifies essential information requested by this form may upon conviction be subject to fine or imprisonment under Federal Law.

Form CMS-20027 (05/05) EF 05/2005

PATIENT INFORMATION/REGISTRATION FORM (SAMPLE)

Allied Medical Center
REGISTRATION FORM

(Please Print)

Today's date: _____   PCP: _____

PATIENT INFORMATION

Patient's last name:	First:	Middle:	❑ Mr. ❑ Miss ❑ Mrs. ❑ Ms.	Marital status (circle one) Single / Mar / Div / Sep / Wid

Is this your legal name? ❑ Yes ❑ No	If not, what is your legal name?	(Former name):	Birth date:	Age:	Sex: ❑ M ❑ F

Street address:	Social Security no.:	Home phone no.:

P.O. box:	City:	State:	ZIP Code:

Occupation:	Employer:	Employer phone no.: ( )

Chose clinic because/Referred to clinic by (please choose one):	❑ Dr.	❑ Insurance Plan	❑ Hospital

❑ Family	❑ Friend	❑ Close to home/work	❑ Yellow Pages	❑ Other

Other family members seen here: _____   **REASON FOR THIS VISIT:**

INSURANCE INFORMATION

(Please give your insurance card to the receptionist.)

Person responsible for bill:	Birth date: / /	Address (if different):	Home phone no.: ( )

Is this person a patient here?   ❑ Yes   ❑ No

Occupation:	Employer:	Employer address:	Employer phone no.: ( )

Is this patient covered by insurance? ❑ Yes   ❑ No

Please indicate primary insurance	Claims Mailing Address:		
	PHONE:		

Subscriber's name:	Subscriber's S.S. no.:	Birth date:	❑ M ❑ F	Group no.:	Policy no.:	Copayment:

Patient's relationship to subscriber: ❑ Self ❑ Spouse ❑ Child ❑ Other

Name of secondary insurance (if applicable):	Subscriber's name and DOB:	❑ M ❑ F	Group no.:	Policy no.:

Patient's relationship to subscriber: ❑ Self ❑ Spouse ❑ Child ❑ Other Claims Address:

IN CASE OF EMERGENCY

Name of local friend or relative (not living at same address):	Relationship to patient:	Home phone no.:	Work phone no.:

The above information is true to the best of my knowledge. I authorize my insurance benefits be paid directly to the physician. I understand that I am financially responsible for any balance. I also authorize ALLIED MEDICAL CENTER or insurance company to release any information required to process my claims.

_____   _____
Patient/Guardian signature   *Date*

PATIENT INFORMATION/REGISTRATION FORM (SAMPLE)

Capital City Medical—123 Unknown Blvd, Capital City, NY 12345–2222 (555)555–1234

Phil Wells, M.D., Mannie Mends, M.D., Bette R. Soone, M.D.

Patient Information Form

Tax ID: 75–0246810

Group NPI: 1513171216

Patient Information:

Name: (Last, First) _____ ❑ Male ❑ Female   Birth Date: _____

Address: _____ Phone: ( ) _____

Social Security Number: _____ FullTime Student: ❑ Yes   ❑ No

Marital Status: ❑ Single   ❑ Married   ❑ Divorced   ❑ Other

Employment:

Employer: _____ Phone: ( ) _____

Address: _____

Condition Related to: ❑ Auto Accident   ❑ Employment   ❑ Other Accident

Date of Accident: _____ State _____

Emergency Contact: _____ Phone: ( ) _____

Primary Insurance: _____ Phone: ( ) _____

Address: _____

Insurance Policyholder's Name: _____ ❑ M   ❑ F   DOB: _____

Address: _____

Phone: _____ Relationship to Insured: ❑ Self ❑ Spouse ❑ Child ❑ Other

Employer: _____ Phone: ( ) _____

Employer's Address: _____

Policy/ID No: _____ Group No: ___ Percent Covered: ___%, Copay Amt: $___

Secondary Insurance: _____ Phone: ( ) _____

Address: _____

Insurance Policyholder's Name: _____ ❑ M   ❑ F   DOB: _____

Address: _____

Phone: _____ Relationship to Insured: ❑ Self ❑ Spouse ❑ Child ❑ Other

Employer: _____ Phone: ( ) _____

Employer's Address: _____

Policy/ID No: _____ Group No: ___ Percent Covered: ___%, Copay Amt: $___

Reason for Visit: _____

Known Allergies: _____

Were you referred here? If so, by whom? _____

Precertification Form (Sample)

Name: _____   DOB: _____

Chart: _____   DOS: _____

Policyholder: _____   Policy ID: _____

Group Number: _____

PTS DX: _____   Procedure to Be Done: _____

Insurance Co: _____   Phone: _____

Precert Rep's Name: _____   Phone: _____

Authorization Number: _____   Time: _____

OPS or IP: _____

Global Period (# of days): _____

Other Comments: _____

Voice Tracking Number: _____

Verified by: _____   Date: _____

Requested verification in writing to fax number or e-mail: _____

Preoperative Verification Form (Hospital Outpatient Benefits Form) (Sample)

PATIENT NAME _____   ACCT NUMBER _____

POLICY ID NUMBER _____   GROUP NUMBER _____

POLICY HOLDER _____   RELATION _____

SERVICE DATE _____   PROCEDURE _____

CONTRACTED WITH _____ PLAN

PLAN TYPE: HMO _____ PPO _____ POS _____ EPO _____ MC _____ INDEM _____

　　　　　　　　　WORKERS' COMP _____ SUBSCRIBER/NON-SUBSCRIBER _____

COVERAGE EFFECTIVE DATE _____   LIFETIME MAXIMUM _____

COPAY _____ DOES PREEXISTING APPLY? ❑YES ❑NO WHAT _____

DEDUCTIBLE: _____ MET ❑YES ❑NO HOW MUCH? _____

INS PAYS _____%   PATIENT PAYS _____%

OOP _____ MET: ❑YES ❑NO HOW MUCH? _____ THEN PAYS _____

BENEFITS REP. NAME _____   TELEPHONE # _____

DATE YOU SPOKE TO REP: _____   TIME: _____

SUBMIT CLAIMS TO: _____

VOICE TRACKING NUMBER _____

REFERAL NEEDED? ❑YES ❑NO   REFFERAL NUMBER: _____

PCP NAME _____   PHONE NUMBER _____

ADDITIONAL
COMMENTS _____

PRE CERT REP NAME _____   PHONE NUMBER _____

AUTHORIZATION NUMBER _____ IS THIS OPS (outpatient surgery) _____
or CLI (clinical admission inpatient) _____?

If this is for a surgery, is 23-hour observation included?   ❑YES ❑NO

Exclusions: ❑Y ❑N WHAT _____

VERIFIED BY: _____ DATE: _____

Privacy Policy/HIPAA Form (Sample)

ALLIED MEDICAL CENTER
Notice of Privacy Policies and Practices

This Notice of Privacy and Practices (the "Notice") tells you about the ways we may use and disclose medical information about you and your rights and our obligations regarding the use and disclosure of your medical information. This Notice applies to Allied Medical Center and its employees, and it is effective beginning April 14, 20XX.

I. <u>OUR OBLIGATIONS.</u>

We are required by law to:

- Make sure that the medical information we have about you is kept private, to the extent required by state and federal law;

- Give you this Notice explaining our legal duties and privacy practices with respect to medical information about you; and

- Follow the terms of the version of the Notice that is currently in effect at the time we acquire medical information about you.

II. <u>HOW WE MAY USE AND DISCLOSE MEDICAL INFORMATION ABOUT YOU.</u>

The following categories describe the different reasons that we typically use and disclose medical information. These categories are intended to be generic descriptions only, and not a list of every instance in which we may use or disclose medical information. Please understand that for these categories, the law generally does not require us to get your consent in order for us to release your medical information.

A. <u>For Treatment</u>. We may use medical information about you to provide you with medical treatment and services, and we may disclose medical information about you to doctors, nurses, technicians, medical students, or hospital personnel who are providing or involved in providing medical care to you. For example, we will provide information about the results of your test to your physicians and his or her office staff.

B. <u>For Payment</u>. We may use and disclose medical information about you so that we may bill and collect from you, an insurance company, or a third party for the services we provided. This may also include the disclosure of medical information to obtain prior authorization for treatment and procedures from your insurance plan. For example, we may send a claim for payment to your insurance company, and that claim may have a code on it that describes your diagnosis.

C. <u>For Healthcare Operations</u>. We may use and disclose medical information about you for our healthcare operations. These uses and disclosures are necessary to operate our practice appropriately and ensure that all of our patients receive quality care. For example, we may need to use or disclose your medical information in order to conduct certain cost-management practices, or to provide information to our insurance carriers.

(continued)

D. <u>Quality Assurance.</u> We may need to use or disclose your medical information for our internal processes to determine that we are providing appropriate care to our patients.

E. <u>Utilization Review.</u> We may need to use or disclose your medical information about you in order for us to review the credentials and actions of physicians to ensure they meet our qualifications and standards.

F. <u>Peer Review.</u> We may need to use or disclose your medical information about you in order for us to review the credentials and actions of physicians to ensure they meet our qualifications and standards.

G. <u>Treatment Alternatives.</u> We may use and disclose medical information to tell you about or recommend possible treatment options or alternatives that we believe may be of interest to you.

H. <u>Health-Related Benefits and Services.</u> We may use and disclose medical information to tell you about health-related benefits or services that we believe may be of interest to you.

I. <u>Individuals Involved in Your Care or Payment for Your Care.</u> We may release medical information about you to a friend or family member who is involved in your medical care, as well as to someone who helps pay for your care, but we will do so only as allowed by state or federal law, or in accordance with your prior authorization.

J. <u>As Required by Law.</u> We will disclose medical information about you when required to do so by federal, state, or local law.

K. <u>To Avert a Serious Threat to Health or Safety.</u> We may use and disclose medical information about you when necessary to prevent or decrease a serious and imminent threat to your health or safety or the health and safety of the public or another person. Such disclosure would only be to someone able to help prevent the threat, or to appropriate law enforcement officials.

L. <u>Organ and Tissue Donation.</u> If you are an organ donor, we may release medical information to organizations that handle organ procurement or organ, eye, or tissue transplantation or to an organ donation bank as necessary to facilitate organ or tissue donation and transplantation.

M. <u>Research.</u> We may use or disclose your medical information to an Institutional Review Board or other authorized research body if it has obtained your consent as required by law, or if the information we provide them is "de-identified."

N. <u>Military and Veterans.</u> If you are or were a member of the armed forces, we may release medical information about you as required by the appropriate military authorities.

O. <u>Workers' Compensation.</u> We may release medical information about you for your employer's workers' compensation or similar program. These programs provide benefits for work-related injuries. For example, if your injuries result from your employment, workers' compensation insurance or a state workers' compensation program may be responsible for payment for your care, in which case we might be required to provide information to the insurer or program.

Privacy Policy/HIPAA Form (Sample) (continued)

P. Public Health Risks. We may disclose medical information about you to public health authorities for public health activities. As a general rule, we are required by law to disclose the following types of information to public health authorities, such as the Texas Department of Health. These types of information generally include the following:

- To prevent or control disease, injury, or disability (including the reporting of a particular disease or injury)

- To report births and deaths

- To report suspected child abuse or neglect

- To report reactions to medications or problems with medical devices and supplies

- To notify people of recalls or products they may be using

- To notify people who may have been exposed to a disease or may be at risk for contracting or spreading a disease or condition

- To notify the appropriate government authority if we believe a patient has been the victim of abuse, neglect, or domestic violence (We will only make this disclosure if you agree or when required or authorized by law.)

- To provide information on certain medical devices

- To assist in public health investigations, surveillance, or interventions

Q. Health Oversight Activities. We may disclose medical information to a health oversight agency for activities authorized by law. These oversight activities include audits, civil, administrative, or criminal investigations and proceedings, inspections, licensure and disciplinary actions, and other activities necessary for the government to monitor the healthcare system, certain governmental benefit programs, certain entities subject to government regulation that relates to health information, and compliance with civil rights laws.

R. Lawsuits and Legal Proceedings. If you are involved in a lawsuit or a legal dispute, we may disclose medical information about you in response to a court or administrative order, subpoena, discovery request, or other lawful process. In addition to lawsuits, there may be other legal proceedings for which we may be required or authorized to use or disclose your medical information, such as investigations of healthcare providers, competency hearings on individuals, or claims over the payment of fees for medical services.

S. Law Enforcement. We may disclose your medical information if we are asked to do so by law enforcement officials, or if we are required by law to do so. Examples of these situations are:

- In response to a court order, subpoena, warrant, summons, or similar process

- To identify or locate a suspect, fugitive, material witness, or missing person

- About the victim of a crime

- About a death we believe may be the result of criminal conduct

- About criminal conduct in our office

(continued)

- In emergency circumstances to report a crime, the location of the crime of victims, or the identity, description, or location of the person who committed the crime

- To report certain types of wounds or physical injuries (e.g., gunshot wounds)

T. <u>Coroners, Medical Examiners, and Funeral Home Directors.</u> We may disclose your medical information to a coroner or medical examiner. This may be necessary, for example, to identify a deceased person or determine the cause of death. We may also release medical information about our patients to funeral home directors as necessary to carry out their duties.

U. <u>National Security and Intelligence Activities.</u> We may disclose medical information about you to authorized federal officials for intelligence, counterintelligence, and other national security activities authorized by law.

V. <u>Inmates.</u> If you are an inmate of a correctional institution or under custody of a law enforcement official, we may disclose medical information about you to the correctional institution or the law enforcement official. This would be necessary for the institution to provide you with health care, to protect your health and safety and the health and safety of others, or for the safety and security of the correctional institution or law enforcement official.

III. <u>OTHER USES OF MEDICAL INFORMATION.</u>

At times we may need or want to use or disclose your medical information other than for the reasons listed above, but to do so we will need your prior permission. If you provide us permission to use or disclose medical information about you for such other purposes, you may revoke that permission in writing at any time. If you revoke your permission, we will no longer use or disclose medical information about you for the reasons covered by your written authorization. You understand that we are unable to take back any disclosures we have already made with your permission, and that we are required to retain our records of the care that we provided to you.

IV. <u>YOUR RIGHTS REGARDING MEDICAL INFORMATION ABOUT YOU.</u>

Federal and state laws provide you with certain rights regarding the medical information we have about you. The following is a summary of those rights.

A. <u>Right to Inspect and Copy.</u> Under most circumstances, you have the right to inspect and/or copy your medical information that we have in our possession, which generally includes your medical and billing records. To inspect or copy your medical information, you must submit your request to do so in writing to the Allied Medical Center's Compliance Officer at the address listed in Section VI below.

If you request a copy of your information, we may charge a fee for the costs of copying, mailing, or other supplies associated with your request. The fee we may charge will be the amount allowed by state law.

In certain very limited circumstances allowed by law, we may deny your request to review or copy your medical information. Under federal law, you may not inspect or copy psychotherapy notes. We will give you any such denial in writing. If you are denied access to medical information, you may request that the denial be reviewed. Another licensed healthcare professional chosen by the Allied

Medical Center will review your request and the denial. The person conducting the review will not be the person who denied your request. We will abide by the outcome of the review.

B. <u>Right to Amend</u>. If you feel the medical information we have about you is incorrect or incomplete, you may ask us to amend the information. You have the right to request an amendment for as long as the information is kept by Allied Medical Center. To request an amendment, your request must be in writing and submitted to the Compliance Officer at the address listed in Section VI below. In your request, you must provide a reason as to why you want this amendment. If we accept your request, we will notify you of that in writing.

We may deny your request for an amendment if it is not in writing or does not include a reason to support the request. In addition, we may deny your request if you ask us to amend information that (i) was not created by us, (ii) is not part of the information kept by Allied Medical Center, (iii) is not part of the information that you would be permitted to inspect and copy, or (iv) is accurate and complete. If we deny your request, we will notify you of that denial in writing.

C. <u>Right to an Accounting of Disclosures.</u> You have the right to request an "accounting of disclosures" of your medical information. This is a list of the disclosures we have made for up to 6 years prior to the date of your request for your medical information, but it does not include disclosures for treatment, payment, or healthcare operations (as described in Sections II A, B, and C of this Notice), or certain other disclosures. To request this list of accounting, you must submit your request in writing to the Allied Medical Center's Compliance Officer at the address set forth in Section VI below. Your request must state a time period, which may not be longer than 6 years and may not include dates before April 14, 2003. Your request should indicate in what form you want the list (e.g., on paper or electronically). The first list you request within a 12-month period will be free. For additional lists, we may charge you a reasonable fee for the costs of providing the list. We will notify you of the cost involved, and you may choose to withdraw or modify your request at that time before any costs are incurred.

D. <u>Right to Request Restrictions</u>. You have the right to request a restriction or limitation on the medical information we use or disclose about you in various situations. You also have the right to request a limit on the medical information we disclose about you to someone who is involved in your care or the payment for your care, like a family member or friend. We are not required to agree to your request. If we do agree, we will comply with your request unless the information is needed to provide you with emergency treatment. In addition, there are certain situations where we will not be able to agree to your request, such as when we are required by law to use or disclose your medical information. To request restrictions, you must make your request in writing to Allied Medical Center's Compliance Officer at the address listed in Section VI below. In your request, you must specifically tell us what information you want to limit; whether you want us to limit our use, disclosure, or both; and to whom you want the limits to apply.

E. <u>Right to Request Confidential Communications.</u> You have the right to request that we communicate with you about medical matters in a certain way or at a certain location. For example, you can ask that we only contact you at home, not

(continued)

at work or conversely, or only at work and not at home. To request such confidential communications, you must make your request in writing to Allied Medical Center's Compliance Officer at the address listed in Section VI below.

We will not ask the reason for your request, and we will use our best efforts to accommodate all reasonable requests, but there are some requests with which we will not be able to comply. Your request must specify how and where you wish to be contacted.

F. <u>Business Associates.</u> Some services are provided in our organization through contracts with business associates. When these services are contracted, we may disclose your medical information to our business associates so that they can perform the job we have asked them to do. To protect your medical information, however, we require the business associate to appropriately safeguard your information.

G. <u>Right to a Paper Copy of This Notice.</u> You have the right to a paper copy of this Notice. You may ask us to give you a copy of this Notice at any time. To obtain a copy of this Notice, you must make your request in writing to Allied Medical Center's Compliance Officer at the address set forth in Section VI below.

V. <u>CHANGES TO THIS NOTICE.</u>

We reserve the right to change this Notice at any time, along with our privacy policies and practices. We reserve the right to make the revised or changed Notice effective for medical information we already have about you as well as any information we receive in the future. We will post a copy of the current Notice, along with an announcement that changes have been made, as applicable, in our offices. When changes have been made to the Notice, you may obtain a revised copy by sending a letter to Allied Medical Center's Compliance Officer at the address listed in Section VI below or by asking the office receptionist for a current copy of the Notice.

VI. <u>COMPLAINTS.</u>

If you believe that your privacy rights as described in this Notice have been violated, you may file a complaint with Allied Medical Center at the following address or phone number:

Allied Medical Center
Attn: Compliance Officer
1933 E. Frankford Road, Suite 110
Carrollton, TX 12345
(972) 555-5482

To file a complaint, you may either call or send a written letter. Allied Medical Center will not retaliate against any individual who files a complaint. If you do not want to file a complaint with Allied Medical Center, you may file one with the Secretary of the Department of Health and Human Services.

In addition, if you have any questions about this Notice, please contact Allied Medical Center's Compliance Officer at the address or phone number listed above.

Privacy Policy/HIPAA Form (Sample) (continued)

I hereby certify and state that I have read, and that I fully and completely understand the HIPAA policy above.

_____   _____
Signature (Patient)   Date
_____

_____   _____   _____
Signature (Patient Representative)   (Relationship to Patient)   Date
_____

_____   _____
Signature (Witness)   Date

SUPERBILL/ENCOUNTER FORM (SAMPLE)

Date of service:		Waiver? ☐		
Patient name:		Insurance:		
		Subscriber name:		
Address:		Group #:		Previous balance:
		Copay:		Today's charges:
Phone:		Account #:		Today's payment: check#
DOB: Age: Sex:		Physician name:		Balance due:

RANK	Office visit	New	Est
	Minimal		99211
	Problem focused	99201	99212
	Expanded problem focused	99202	99213
	Detailed	99203	99214
	Comprehensive	99204	99215
	Comprehensive (new patient)	99205	
	Significant, separate service	-25	-25
	Well visit	**New**	**Est**
	< 1 y	99381	99391
	1-4 y	99382	99392
	5-11 y	99383	99393
	12-17 y	99384	99394
	18-39 y	99385	99395
	40-64 y	99386	99396
	65 y +	99387	99397
	Medicare preventive services		
	Pap		Q0091
	Pelvic & breast		G0101
	Prostate/PSA		G0103
	Tobacco counseling/3-10 min		99406
	Tobacco counseling/>10 min		99407
	Welcome to Medicare exam		G0344
	ECG w/Welcome to Medicare exam		G0366
	Flexible sigmoidoscopy		G0104
	Hemoccult, guaiac		G0107
	Flu shot		G0008
	Pneumonia shot		G0009
	Consultation/preop clearance		
	Expanded problem focused		99242
	Detailed		99243
	Comprehensive/mod complexity		99244
	Comprehensive/high complexity		99245
	Other services		
	After posted hours		99050
	Evening/weekend appointment		99051
	Home health certification		G0180
	Home health recertification		G0179
	Post-op follow-up		99024
	Prolonged/30-74 min		99354
	Special reports/forms		99080
	Disability/Workers comp		99455
	Radiology		

Diagnoses
1
2
3
4

Next office visit

Recheck	Prev	PRN	_____ D W M Y

Instructions:

Referral

To:

Instructions:

Physician signature

X _____

RANK	Office procedures		
	Anoscopy		46600
	Audiometry		92551
	Cerumen removal		69210
	Colposcopy		57452
	Colposcopy w/biopsy		57455
	ECG, w/interpretation		93000
	ECG, rhythm strip		93040
	Endometrial biopsy		58100
	Flexible sigmoidoscopy		45330
	Flexible sigmoidoscopy w/biopsy		45331
	Fracture care, cast/splint		29____
	Site: _____		
	Nebulizer		94640
	Nebulizer demo		94664
	Spirometry		94010
	Spirometry, pre and post		94060
	Tympanometry		92567
	Vasectomy		55250
	Skin procedures		**Units**
	Burn care, initial	16000	
	Foreign body, skin, simple	10120	
	Foreign body, skin, complex	10121	
	I&D, abscess	10060	
	I&D, hematoma/seroma	10140	
	Laceration repair, simple	120___	
	Site: _____ Size: _____		
	Laceration repair, layered	120___	
	Site: _____ Size: _____		
	Lesion, biopsy, one	11100	
	Lesion, biopsy, each add'l	11101	
	Lesion, destruct., benign, 1-14	17110	
	Lesion, destruct., premal., single	17000	
	Lesion, destruct., premal., ea. add'l	17003	
	Lesion, excision, benign	114___	
	Site: _____ Size: _____		
	Lesion, excision, malignant	116___	
	Site: _____ Size: _____		
	Lesion, paring/cutting, one	11055	
	Lesion, paring/cutting, 2-4	11056	
	Lesion, shave	113___	
	Site: _____ Size: _____		
	Nail removal, partial	11730	
	Nail removal, w/matrix	11750	
	Skin tag, 1-15	11200	

Medications		Units
Ampicillin, up to 500mg	J0290	
B-12, up to 1,000 mcg	J3420	
Epinephrine, up to 1ml	J0170	
Kenalog, 10mg	J3301	
Lidocaine, 10mg	J2001	
Normal saline, 1000cc	J7030	
Phenergan, up to 50mg	J2550	
Progesterone, 150mg	J1055	
Rocephin, 250mg	J0696	
Testosterone, 200mg	J1080	
Tigan, up to 200 mg	J3250	
Toradol, 15mg	J1885	
Miscellaneous services		

RANK	Laboratory	
	Venipuncture	36415
	Blood glucose, monitoring device	82962
	Blood glucose, visual dipstick	82948
	CBC, w/ auto differential	85025
	CBC, w/o auto differential	85027
	Cholesterol	82465
	Hemoccult, guaiac	82270
	Hemoccult, immunoassay	82274
	Hemoglobin A1C	85018
	Lipid panel	80061
	Liver panel	80076
	KOH prep (skin, hair, nails)	87220
	Metabolic panel, basic	80048
	Metabolic panel, comprehensive	80053
	Mononucleosis	86308
	Pregnancy, blood	84703
	Pregnancy, urine	81025
	Renal panel	80069
	Sedimentation rate	85651
	Strep, rapid	86403
	Strep culture	87081
	Strep A	87880
	TB	86580
	UA, complete, non-automated	81000
	UA, w/o micro, non-automated	81002
	UA, w/ micro, non-automated	81003
	Urine colony count	87086
	Urine culture, presumptive	87088
	Wet mount/KOH	87210
	Vaccines	
	DT, <7 y	90702
	DTP	90701
	DtaP, <7 y	90700
	Flu, 6-35 months	90657
	Flu, 3 y +	90658
	Hep A, adult	90632
	Hep A, ped/adol, 2 dose	90633
	Hep B, adult	90746
	Hep B, ped/adol 3 dose	90744
	Hep B-Hib	90748
	Hib, 4 dose	90645
	HPV	90649
	IPV	90713
	MMR	90707
	Pneumonia, >2 y	90732
	Pneumonia conjugate, <5 y	90669
	Td, >7 y	90718
	Varicella	90716

Immunizations & Injections		Units
Allergen, one	95115	
Allergen, multiple	95117	
Imm admin, one	90471	
Imm admin, each add'l	90472	
Imm admin, intranasal, one	90473	
Imm admin, intranasal, each add'l	90474	
Injection, joint, small	20600	
Injection, joint, intermediate	20605	
Injection, joint, major	20610	
Injection, ther/proph/diag	90772	
Injection, trigger point	20552	
Supplies		

I acknowledge receipt of medical services and authorize the release of
any medical information necessary to process this claim for healthcare
payment only. I do authorize payment to the provider.

Patient Signature: _____

Total Estimated Charges: _____

Payment Amount: _____

Next Appointment: _____

Tool to Determine Correct CPT® Code

1) HISTORY

HPI (History of Present Illness): Characterize HPI by considering either the Status of chronic conditions or the number of elements recorded.	☐ Status of 1-2 chronic conditions	☐ Status of 1-2 chronic conditions	☐ Status of 3 chronic conditions	☐ Status of 3 chronic conditions
☐ 1 condition ☐ 2 conditions ☐ 3 conditions **OR** ☐ Location ☐ Severity ☐ Timing ☐ Modifying factors ☐ Quality ☐ Duration ☐ Context ☐ Associated signs and symptoms	☐ Brief (1-3)	☐ Brief (1-3)	☐ Extended (4 or more)	☐ Extended (4 or more)
ROS (Review of Systems): ☐ Constitutional (wt loss, etc.) ☐ Ears, nose, mouth, throat ☐ GI ☐ Integumentary (skin, breast) ☐ Endo ☐ Eyes ☐ Card/vasc ☐ GU ☐ Hem/lymph ☐ Musculo ☐ Neuro ☐ All/immuno ☐ Resp ☐ Psych	N/A	☐ Pertinent to problem (1 system)	☐ Extended (Pert and others) (2-9 systems)	☐ Complete (Pert and all others) (10 systems)
PFSH (Past medical, Family, Social History) areas: ☐ Past history (the patient's past experiences with illnesses, operation, injuries and treatments) ☐ Family history (a review of medical events in the patient's family, including diseases that may be hereditary or place the patient at risk) ☐ Social history (an age-appropriate review of past and current activities)	N/A	N/A	☐ Pertinent (1 history area)	☐ *Complete (2 or 3 history areas)

*Complete PFSH: 2 history areas: a) established patients - office (outpatient) care, domiciliary care, home care; b) emergency department; c) subsequent nursing facility care; d) subsequent hospital care; and, e) follow-up consultations.

3 history areas: a) new patients - office (outpatient) care, domiciliary care, home care; b) initial consultations; c) initial hospital care; d) hospital observation; and, e) comprehensive nursing facility assessments.

PROBLEM-FOCUSED	EXP. PROBLEM-FOCUSED	DETAILED	COMPREHENSIVE

Final History requires all 3 components above met or exceeded

2) EXAMINATION

CPT Exam Description	95 Guideline Requirements	97 Guideline Requirements	CPT Type of Exam
Limited to affected body area or organ system	One body area or organ system	1-5 bulleted elements	**PROBLEM-FOCUSED EXAM**
Affected body area or organ system and other symptomatic or related organ systems	2-7 body areas and/or organ systems	6-11 bulleted elements	**EXPANDED PROBLEM-FOCUSED EXAM**
Extended exam of affected body area or organ system and other symptomatic or related organ systems	2-7 body areas and/or organ systems	12-17 bulleted elements for 2 or more systems	**DETAILED EXAM**
General multi-system	8 or more body areas and/or organ systems	18 or more bulleted elements for 9 or more systems	**COMPREHENSIVE EXAM**
Complete single organ system exam	Not defined	See requirements for individual single system exams	

3) MEDICAL DECISION-MAKING

Final Result of Complexity for Medical Decision-Making Level				
A. Number of diagnoses and/or management options	≤ 2 Minimal	3-4 Limited	5-6 Multiple	≥ 7 Extensive
B. Amount and complexity of data reviewed/ordered	≤ 1 None/Minimal	2 Limited	3 Multiple	≥ 4 Extensive
C. Risk	Minimal	Low	Moderate	High
Type of medical decision-making	**Straightforward**	**Low Complexity**	**Moderate Complexity**	**High Complexity**

Final Medical Decision-Making requires 2 of 3 components above met or exceeded

A. Number of Diagnoses and/or Management Options (see Table A.1)	#DX	#TX	#DX + #TX
New or est problem(s), no evaluation/management mentioned and problem **is not** clearly co-morbid condition.	0	0	0
New or est problem(s), no evaluation/management mentioned and problem **is** a co-morbid condition.		0	
New or established problem(s), evaluation/management mentioned.			
		TOTAL	

(continued)

3 **MEDICAL DECISION-MAKING** (continued)

A.1 Treatments and Therapeutic Options	
DO NOT COUNT AS TREATMENT OPTIONS NOTATIONS SUCH AS Continue "same" therapy or "no change" in therapy (including drug management) without further description (record does not document what the current therapy plan is nor that the physician reviewed it)	0
Continue "same" therapy or "no change" in therapy without further description (record clearly documents what the current therapy plan is and that the physician reviewed it); or scheduled monitoring without specific therapy	1
Drug management, new prescriptions, or changes in dosing for current medications	1
Complex drug management (more than 3 medications/prescriptions and/or over-the-counter) new prescriptions or changes in dosing for current medications	2
Open or percutaneous therapeutic cardiac, surgical or radiological procedure – minor or major	1
Physical, occupational or speech therapy or other manipulation	1
Closed treatment for fracture or dislocation	1
IV fluids	1
Complex insulin prescription (SC or combo of SC/IV), hyperalimentation, insulin drip or other complex IV admix prescription	2
Conservative measures such as rest, ice, bandages, dietary	1
Radiation therapy	1
IM injection/aspiration or other pain management procedure	1
Patient educated on self or home care topics/techniques	1
Hospital admit	1
Hospital admit – other physician(s) contacted	2
Referral to another physician, consultation	1
Other – specify	
TOTAL	

B. Amount and/or Complexity of Data Reviewed or Ordered	
Order and/or review results of clinical lab tests	1
Order and/or review results of tests in Radiology section of CPT	1
Order and/or review results of tests in Medical section of CPT	1
Discuss case with consultant or order consultation or discuss case with other physician also managing the patient	1
Discuss test results with performing physician	1
Order (identify specific source of records ordered) and/or summarize old or other health care records (simple statements to the effect that other or old outside records were reviewed is insufficient to count)	1
Physiologic monitoring	1
Independently visualize and report findings from images, tracings, pathological specimens themselves (not the reports) for procedures and tests for which interpretation not separately billed by the provider	1
TOTAL	

C. Risk of Complication and/or Mortality (see Table C.1)				
Nature of the presenting illness	Minimal	Low	Moderate	High
Risk conferred by diagnostic options	Minimal	Low	Moderate	High
Risk conferred by therapeutic options	Minimal	Low	Moderate	High

Final Risk determined by highest of 3 components above

C.1 Risk of Complications and/or Morbitity or Mortality			
LEVEL OF RISK	PRESENTING PROBLEM(S)	DIAGNOSTIC PROCEDURE(S) ORDERED	MANAGEMENT OPTIONS SELECTED
Minimal	• One self-limited or minor problem, e.g., cold, insect bite, tinea corporis	• Laboratory tests requiring venipuncture • Chest x-rays • EKG/EEG • Urinalysis • Ultrasound, e.g., echo • KOH prep	• Rest • Gargles • Elastic bandages • Superficial dressings
Low	• Two or more self-limited or minor problems • One stable chronic illness, e.g., well-controlled hypertension or non-insulin-dependent diabetes, cataract, BPH • Acute uncomplicated illness or injury, e.g., cystitis, allergic rhinitis, simple sprain	• Physiologic tests not under stress, e.g., pulmonary function tests • Non-cardiovascular imaging studies with contrast, e.g., barium enema • Superficial needle biopsies • Clinical laboratory tests requiring arterial puncture • Skin biopsies	• Over-the-counter drugs • Minor surgery with no identified risk factors • Physical therapy • Occupational therapy • IV fluids without additives

C.1 Risk of Complications and/or Morbidity or Mortality			
LEVEL OF RISK	PRESENTING PROBLEM(S)	DIAGNOSTIC PROCEDURE(S) ORDERED	MANAGEMENT OPTIONS SELECTED
Moderate	• One or more chronic illnesses with mild exacerbation, progression or side effects of treatment • Two or more stable chronic illnesses • Undiagnosed new problem with uncertain prognosis, e.g., lump in breast • Acute illness with systemic symptoms, e.g., pyelonephritis, pneumonitis, colitis • Acute complicated injury, e.g., head injury with brief loss of consciousness	• Physiologic tests under stress, e.g., cardiac stress test, fetal contraction stress test • Diagnostic endoscopies with no identified risk factors • Deep needle or incisional biopsy • Cardiovascular imaging studies with contrast and no identified risk factors, e.g., arteriogram cardiac cath • Obtain fluid from body cavity, e.g., lumbar procedure, thoracentesis, culdocentesis	• Minor surgery with identified risk factors • Elective major surgery (open, percutaneous or endoscopic) with no identified risk factors • Prescription drug management • Therapeutic nuclear medicine • IV fluids with additives • Closed treatment of fracture or dislocation without manipulation
High	• One or more chronic illnesses with severe exacerbation, progression, or side effects of treatment • Acute or chronic illnesses or injuries that may pose a threat to life or bodily function, e.g., multiple trauma, acute MI, pulmonary embolus, severe respiratory distress, progressive severe rheumatoid arthritis, psychiatric illness with potential threat to self or others, peritonitis, acute renal failure • An abrupt change in neurologic status, e.g., seizure, TIA, weakness or sensory loss	• Cardiovascular imaging studies with contrast with identified risk factors • Cardiac electrophysiological tests • Diagnostic endoscopies with identified risk factors • Discography	• Elective major surgery (open, percutaneous or endoscopic with identified risk factors) • Emergency major surgery (open, percutaneous or endoscopic) • Parenteral controlled substances • Drug therapy requiring intensive monitoring for toxicity • Decision not to resuscitate or to de-escalate care because of poor prognosis

Tool to Determine Correct CPT® Code (continued)

4 LEVEL OF SERVICE

OUTPATIENT, CONSULTS (OUTPATIENT AND INPATIENT) AND ER

	New Office/Consults/ER						Established Office			
	Requires 3 components within shaded area						Requires 2 components within shaded area			
History	PF ER: PF	EPF ER: EPF	D ER: EPF	C ER: D	C ER: C	*Minimal problem that may not require presence of physician*	PF	EPF	D	C
Examination	PF ER: PF	EPF ER: EPF	D ER: EPF	C ER: D	C ER: C		PF	EPF	D	C
Complexity of Medical Decision	SF ER: SF	SF ER: L	L ER: M	M ER: M	H ER: H		SF	L	M	H
Average Time (minutes) (ER have no average time)	10 New (99201) 15 Outpt cons (99241) 20 Inpat cons (99251) ER (99281)	20 New (99202) 30 Outpt cons (99242) 40 Inpat cons (99252) ER (99282)	30 New (99203) 40 Outpt cons (99243) 55 Inpat cons (99253) ER (99283)	45 New (99204) 60 Outpt cons (99244) 80 Inpat cons (99254) ER (99284)	60 New (99205) 80 Outpt cons (99245) 100 Inpat cons (99255) ER (99285)	5 (99211)	10 (99212)	15 (99213)	25 (99214)	40 (99215)
Level	I	II	III	IV	V	I	II	III	IV	V

INPATIENT

	Initial Hospital/Observation			Subsequent Inpatient/Follow-up		
	Requires 3 components within shaded area			Requires 2 components within shaded area		
History	D or C	C	C	PF interval	EPF interval	D interval
Examination	D or C	C	C	PF	EPF	D
Complexity of Medical Decision	SF/L	M	H	SF/L	M	H
Average Time (minutes) (Observation care has no average time)	30 Init hosp (99221) Observ care (99218)	50 Init hosp (99222) Observ care (99219)	70 Init hosp (99223) Observ care (99220)	15 Subsequent (99231)	25 Subsequent (99232)	35 Subsequent (99233)
Level	I	II	III	I	II	III

NURSING FACILITY

	Annual Assessment/Admission			Subsequent Nursing Facility			
	Old Plan Review	New Plan	Admission	Requires 2 components within shaded area			
History	D/C	C	C	PF interval	EPF interval	D interval	C interval
Examination	D/C	C	C	PF	EPF	D	C
Complexity of Medical Decision	SF	M	M	SF	L	M	H
No Average Time Established (Confirmatory consults and ER have no average time)	(99304)	(99305)	(99306)	(99307)	(99308)	(99309)	(99310)
Level	I	II	III	I	II	III	IV

DOMICILIARY (REST HOME, CUSTODIAL CARE) AND HOME CARE

	New					Established			
	Requires 3 components within shaded area					Requires 2 components within shaded area			
History	PF	EPF	D	C	C	PF interval	EPF interval	D interval	C
Examination	PF	EPF	D	C	C	PF	EPF	D	C
Complexity of Medical Decision	SF	L	M	M	H	SF	L	M	H
Average Time (minutes)	20 Domiciliary (99324) 20 Home care (99341)	30 Domiciliary (99325) 30 Home care (99342)	45 Domiciliary (99326) 45 Home care (99343)	60 Domiciliary (99327) 60 Home care (99344)	75 Domiciliary (99328) 75 Home care (99345)	15 Domiciliary (99334) 15 Home care (99347)	25 Domiciliary (99335) 25 Home care (99348)	40 Domiciliary (99336) 40 Home care (99349)	60 Domiciliary (99337) 60 Home care (99350)
Level	I	II	III	IV	V	I	II	III	IV

PF = Problem focused   EPF = Expanded problem focused   D = Detailed   C = Comprehensive   SF = Straightforward   L = Low   M = Moderate   H = High

UB04 (CMS1450) FORM

1		2		3a PAT. CNTL #			4 TYPE OF BILL
				b. MED. REC. #			
				5 FED. TAX NO.	6 STATEMENT COVERS PERIOD FROM THROUGH	7	

8 PATIENT NAME	a		9 PATIENT ADDRESS	a			
b			b		c	d	e

10 BIRTHDATE	11 SEX	12 DATE	ADMISSION 13 HR	14 TYPE	15 SRC	16 DHR	17 STAT	18	19	20	21	CONDITION CODES 22	23	24	25	26	27	28	29 ACDT STATE	30

31 OCCURRENCE CODE DATE	32 OCCURRENCE CODE DATE	33 OCCURRENCE CODE DATE	34 OCCURRENCE CODE DATE	35 OCCURRENCE SPAN CODE FROM THROUGH	36 OCCURRENCE SPAN CODE FROM THROUGH	37
a						a
b						b

38			39 VALUE CODES CODE AMOUNT	40 VALUE CODES CODE AMOUNT	41 VALUE CODES CODE AMOUNT
		a			
		b			
		c			
		d			

42 REV. CD.	43 DESCRIPTION	44 HCPCS / RATE / HIPPS CODE	45 SERV. DATE	46 SERV. UNITS	47 TOTAL CHARGES	48 NON-COVERED CHARGES	49
1							1
2							2
3							3
4							4
5							5
6							6
7							7
8							8
9							9
10							10
11							11
12							12
13							13
14							14
15							15
16							16
17							17
18							18
19							19
20							20
21							21
22							22
23	*PAGE ___ OF ___*	*CREATION DATE*		**TOTALS ➡**			23

50 PAYER NAME	51 HEALTH PLAN ID	52 REL INFO	53 ASG. BEN.	54 PRIOR PAYMENTS	55 EST. AMOUNT DUE	56 NPI	
A							57 OTHER PRV ID
B							
C							

58 INSURED'S NAME	59 P.REL	60 INSURED'S UNIQUE ID	61 GROUP NAME	62 INSURANCE GROUP NO.
A				
B				
C				

63 TREATMENT AUTHORIZATION CODES	64 DOCUMENT CONTROL NUMBER	65 EMPLOYER NAME
A		
B		
C		

66 DX	67 A B C D E F G H I J K L M N O P Q	68

69 ADMIT DX	70 PATIENT REASON DX a b c	71 PPS CODE	72 ECI a b c	73

74 PRINCIPAL PROCEDURE CODE DATE	a. OTHER PROCEDURE CODE DATE	b. OTHER PROCEDURE CODE DATE	75	76 ATTENDING NPI QUAL
				LAST FIRST
c. OTHER PROCEDURE CODE DATE	d. OTHER PROCEDURE CODE DATE	e. OTHER PROCEDURE CODE DATE		77 OPERATING NPI QUAL
				LAST FIRST
80 REMARKS	81CC a			78 OTHER NPI QUAL
	b			LAST FIRST
	c			79 OTHER NPI QUAL
	d			LAST FIRST

UB-04 CMS-1450   APPROVED OMB NO. 0938-0997   **NUBC** National Uniform Billing Committee   THE CERTIFICATIONS ON THE REVERSE APPLY TO THIS BILL AND ARE MADE A PART HEREOF.

Appendix E

Acronyms and Abbreviations

ABN	Advance Beneficiary Notice
AFDC	Aid to Families with Dependent Children
AHA	American Hospital Association
ALJ	administrative law judge
AMA	American Medical Association; against medical advice
ANSI	American National Standards Institute
APC	Ambulatory Payment Classification
ASC	ambulatory surgical center
ASU	ambulatory surgical unit
BCBSA	Blue Cross Blue Shield Association
C&M	Coordination and Maintenance Committee
CBO	centralized billing office
CC	chief complaint; comorbidities and complications
CDM	charge description master
CE	covered entities
CHAMPUS	Civilian Health and Medical Program of the Uniformed Services
CHAMPVA	Civilian Health and Medical Program of the Department of Veterans Affairs
CHIP	Children's Health Insurance Program
CLIA	Clinical Laboratory Improvement Amendments
CMN	certificate of medical necessity
CMP	civil money penalty
CMS	Centers for Medicare and Medicaid Services
COB	coordination of benefits
COBRA	Consolidated Omnibus Budget Reconciliation Act of 1985
CPOE	computerized provider order entry
CPT	Current Procedural Terminology
CPU	central processing unit
CSRS	Civil Service Retirement System
DEERS	Defense Enrollment Eligibility Reporting System
DHHS	Department of Health and Human Services
DME	durable medical equipment
DMERC	durable medical equipment resource center
DOB	date of birth

DOJ	Department of Justice
DRG	diagnosis-related group
EDI	electronic data interchange
EEOICP	Energy Employees Occupational Illness Compensation Program Act
EHR	electronic health record
EIN	employer identification number
EMR	electronic medical record
EOB	Explanation of Benefits
EPHI	electronic protected health information
EPO	exclusive provider organization
EPSDT	early and periodic screening, diagnosis, and treatment
ER	emergency department
ERA	electronic remittance advice
ERISA	Employee Retirement Income Security Act of 1974
ESRD	end-stage renal disease
FDA	Food and Drug Administration
FECA	Federal Employees' Compensation Act
FFS	fee for service
FICA	Federal Insurance Contribution Act
FMAP	Federal Medical Assistance Percentage Program
FPN	facility provider number
g, gm	gram
GEM	General Equivalence Mappings (for ICD-9 to ICD-10 codes)
GHP	group health plan
GPCI	Geographic Practice Cost Index
GPN	group provider number
GTIN	global trade item number
HCFA	Health Care Financing Administration
HCPCS	Healthcare Common Procedure Coding System
HHS	Health and Human Services
HIAA	Health Insurance Association of America
HIBCC	Health Industry Business Communications Council
HIC	health insurance claim
HIM	health information management

HIPAA	Health Insurance Portability and Accountability Act of 1996
HITECH	Health Information Technology for Economic and Clinical Health Act
HMO	health maintenance organization
HPI	history of present illness
ICD-9	*International Classification of Diseases and Related Health Problems, Ninth Revision*
ICD-9-CM	*International Classification of Diseases, Ninth Revision, Clinical Modification*
ICD-9-PCS	*International Classification of Diseases, Ninth Revision, Procedure Classification System*
ICD-10	*International Classification of Diseases and Related Health Problems, Tenth Revision*
ICD-10-CM	*International Classification of Diseases, Tenth Revision, Clinical Modification*
ICD-10-PCS	*International Classification of Diseases, Tenth Revision, Procedure Classification System*
IDDM	insulin-dependent diabetes mellitus
IRO	independent review organization
LCD	Local Coverage Determination
LHWCA	Longshore and Harbor Workers' Compensation Act
LMRP	local Medicare review policy
LTR	lifetime reserve days
MA	Medicare Advantage
MCF	Medicare conversion factor
MCO	managed care organization
MDC	Major Diagnostic Categories
MDM	medical decision making
MFS	Medicare Fee Schedule
mL	milliliter
MOS	medical office specialist
MPM	medical practice management (software)
MQGE	Medicare-qualified government employment
MRN	Medicare Remittance Notice
MSA	medical savings account
MS-DRG	Medicare Diagnosis-Related Group
MSN	Medicare Summary Notice
MSP	Medicare secondary payer
MTF	military treatment facility
NAS	nonavailability statement
NCCI	National Correct Coding Initiative
NCHS	National Center for Health Statistics
NCQA	National Committee for Quality Assurance
NDC	National Drug Code
NEC	not elsewhere classified
NIDDM	non-insulin-dependent diabetes mellitus
NOC	not otherwise classified
NON-PAR	nonparticipating provider
NOS	not otherwise specified

NPI	National Provider Identifier
NUCC	National Uniform Claim Committee
OCR	Office of Civil Rights; optical character recognition
OIG	Office of Inspector General
ONC	Office of the National Coordinator for Health Information
OPPS	Outpatient Prospective Payment System
OTAF	obligated to accept as payment in full
OWCP	Office of Workers' Compensation Program
PACE	Programs for All-Inclusive Care for the Elderly
PAR	participating provider
PAS	patient account services
PCM	primary care manager
PCN	patient control number
PCP	primary care physician
PFSH	past family social history
PHI	protected health information
PIN	provider identification number
PMPM	per member per month
POA	present on admission
POS	point of service; place of service
PPACA	Patient Protection and Affordable Care Act
PPIN	preferred provider identification number
PPO	preferred provider organization
PQRI	Physicians Quality Reporting Initiative
PSO	provider-sponsored organization
QIC	qualified independent contractor
RBRVS	resource-based relative value scale
RHIT	registered health information technician
ROS	review of systems
RVU	relative value unit
SMI	supplemental medical insurance
SNF	skilled nursing facility
SOF	signature on file
SSA	Social Security Administration
SSDI	Social Security Disability Insurance
SSI	Supplemental Security Income
SSN	Social Security number
TANF	Temporary Assistance for Needy Families
TEFRA	Tax Equity Fiscal Responsibility Act
TIN	tax identification number
TFL	TRICARE for Life
TRHCA	Tax Relief and Healthcare Act of 2006
TRR	TRICARE Reserve Retired
TRS	TRICARE Reserve Select
TYA	TRICARE Young Adult
UCR	usual, customary, and reasonable
UPC	Universal Product Code
VOB	verification of benefits
WHO	World Health Organization

Medical Terminology Word Parts

Medical terms are like individual jigsaw puzzles. Once you divide the terms into their component parts and learn the meaning of the individual parts, you can use that knowledge to understand many other new terms. Four basic component parts are used to create medical terms:

Root
: The basic, or core, part that makes up the essential meaning of the term. The root usually, but not always, denotes a body part. Root words usually come from the Greek or Latin languages. For example, *bronch* is a root word that means "the air passages in the lungs" or "bronchial tubes." *Cephal* means "head." An extensive list of root words is given on pages 744–747.

Prefix
: One or more letters placed before the root to change its meaning. Prefixes usually, but not always, indicate location, time, number, or status. For example, the prefix *bi-* means "two" or "twice." When *bi* is placed before the root *lateral* ("side") to form *bilateral*, the meaning is "having two sides." An extensive list of prefixes is given on page 744.

Suffix
: One or more letters placed after the root to change its meaning. Suffixes usually, but not always, indicate the procedure, condition, disorder, or disease. For example, the suffix *-itis* means "inflammation"—that is, damaged tissue that is red and painful. The medical term *bronchitis* means "inflammation of the bronchial tubes." Another example is the suffix *-ectomy*, which means "removal." Hence, *appendectomy* means "removal of the appendix." An extensive list of suffixes is given on pages 747–749.

Combining vowel
: A letter used to combine roots with other word parts. The vowel is usually an *o*, but sometimes it is an *a* or *i*. When a combining vowel is added to a root, the result is called a combining form. For example, in the word *encephalogram*, the root is *cephal* ("head"), the prefix is *en-* ("inside"), and the suffix is *-gram* ("something recorded"). These word parts are joined by the combining vowel *o* to make a word easier to pronounce. *Cephal/o* is the combining form. An *encephalogram* is an X-ray of the inside of the head.

Analyzing a Medical Term

The meaning of a medical term can often by deciphered by breaking it down into its separate parts. Consider the following examples:

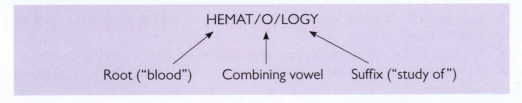

HEMAT/O/LOGY

Root ("blood")   Combining vowel   Suffix ("study of")

737

The term *hematology* is divided into three parts. To analyze a medical term, begin at the end of the word. The ending is called the suffix. Almost all medical terms contain suffixes. The suffix in *hematology* is *-logy*, which means "study of." Now look at the beginning of the word: *Hemat* is the root word, which means "blood." The root word gives the essential meaning of the term.

The third part of this term, which is the letter *o*, has no meaning of its own, but it is an important connector between the root (*hemat*) and the suffix (*logy*). It is the combining vowel. The letter *o* is the combining vowel usually found in medical terms.

Putting together the meanings of the suffix and the root, the term *hematology* means "the study of blood."

The combining vowel plus the root is called the combining form. A medical term can have more than one root word; therefore, there can be two combining forms. For example:

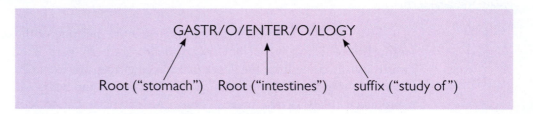

GASTR/O/ENTER/O/LOGY

Root ("stomach")   Root ("intestines")   suffix ("study of")

The two combining forms in the example are *gastr/o* and *enter/o*. The entire term (reading from the suffix, back to the beginning of the term, and across) means "the study of the stomach and the intestines."

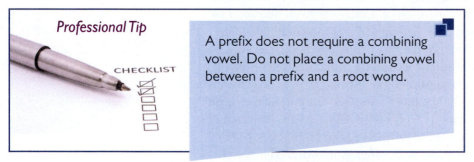

Professional Tip

CHECKLIST

A prefix does not require a combining vowel. Do not place a combining vowel between a prefix and a root word.

Rules for Using Combining Vowels

1. A combining vowel is not used when the suffix begins with a vowel (*a-e-i-o-u*). For example, when *neur/o* (nerve) is joined with the suffix *-itis* (inflammation), the combining vowel is not used because *-itis* begins with a vowel. *Neuritis* (new-RYE-tis) is an inflammation of a nerve or nerves.

2. A combining vowel is used when the suffix begins with a consonant. For example, when *neur/o* (nerve) is joined with the suffix *-plasty* (surgical repair), the combining vowel *o* is used because *-plasty* begins with a consonant. *Neuroplasty* (NEW-roh-plas-tee) is the surgical repair of a nerve.

3. A combining vowel is always used when two or more root words are joined. For example, when *gastr/o* (stomach) is joined with *enter/o* (small intestine), the combining vowel is used with *gastr/o*. *Gastroenteritis* (gas-troh-en-ter-EYE-tis) is an inflammation of the stomach and small intestine.

Word Part Guidelines

1. A single root word with a combining form cannot stand alone. A suffix must be added to complete the term.

2. The rules for the use of combining vowels apply when adding a suffix.

3. When a suffix begins with a consonant, a combining vowel such as O, is placed before the suffix.

Suffixes and Medical Terms Related to Pathology

Pathology is the study of disease and the following suffixes describe specific disease conditions. (A more complete list of suffixes appears on pages 747–749.)

Suffix	Meaning
-algia	pain and suffering
-dynia	pain
-ectomy	surgical removal
-graphy	process of recording a picture or record
-gram	record or picture
-necr/osis	death (tissue death)
-scler/osis	abnormal hardening
-sten/osis	abnormal narrowing
-centesis	surgical puncture to remove fluid for diagnostic purposes or to remove excess fluid
-plasty	surgical repair
-scopy	visual examination with an instrument

The Double RRs Suffixes

The following suffixes are often referred to as the "double RRs":

-rrhage and -rrhagia	Bursting form; an abnormal excessive discharge or bleeding. *Note: -rrhage* and *-rhagia* refer to the flow of blood.
-rrhaphy	To suture or stitch.
-rrhea	Abnormal flow or discharge; refers to the abnormal flow of most bodily fluids. *Note:* Although *-rrhea* and *-rrhage* both refer to abnormal flow, they are not used interchangeably.
-rrhexis	Rupture.

Contrasting and Confusing Prefixes

The following contrasting prefixes can be confusing. Study this list to make sure you know the differences between the contrasting terms. (A more complete list of prefixes begins on page 744.)

Ab- "away from." *Abnormal* means "not normal" or "away from normal."

Ad- "toward" or "in the direction." *Addiction* means "drawn toward" or "a strong dependence on a drug or substance."

Dys- "bad," "difficult," "painful." *Dysfunctional* means "an organ or body that is not working properly."

Eu- "good," normal, well, or easy. *Euthyroid* (you-THIGH-roid) means "a normally functioning thyroid gland."

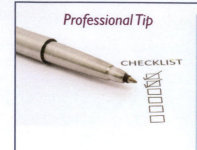

Learning to use a medical dictionary is an important part of mastering the correct use of medical terms. Some dictionaries use categories such as "Diseases and Syndromes" to group disorders with these terms in the titles. For example:

■ Venereal disease would be found under "disease, venereal."
■ Fetal alcohol syndrome would be found under "syndrome, fetal alcohol."

When you come across a term and cannot find it listed by the first word, the next step is to look under the appropriate category.

Hyper- "excessive" or "increased." *Hypertension* (high-per-TEN-shun) means "higher than normal blood pressure."

Hypo- "deficient" or "decreased." *Hypotension* (high-poh-TEN-shun) means "lower than normal blood pressure."

Inter- "between" or "among." *Interstitial* (in-ter-STISH-al) means "between, but not within, the parts of a tissue."

Intra- "within" "into." *Intramuscular* (in-trah-MUS-kyou-lar) means "within the muscle."

Sub- "under," "less," or "below." *Subcostal* (sub-KOS-tal) means "below a rib or ribs."

Supra- "above." *Supracostal* (sue-prah-KOS-tal) means "above or outside the ribs."

Singular and Plural Endings

Many medical terms have Greek or Latin origins. As a result of these different origins, the rules for changing a singular word into a plural form are unusual. In addition, English endings have been adopted for some commonly used terms.

Guidelines to Unusual Plural Forms

Guideline	Singular	Plural
1. If the term ends in an *a*, the plural is usually formed by adding an *e*.	bursa vertebra	bursae vertebrae
2. If the term ends in *ex* or *ix*, the plural is usually formed by changing the *ex* or *ix* to *ices*.	appendix index	appendices indices
3. If the term ends in *is*, the plural is usually formed by changing the *is* to *es*.	diagnosis metastasis	diagnoses metastases
4. If the term ends in *itis*, the plural is usually formed by changing the *is* to *ides*.	arthritis meningitis	arthritides meningitides
5. If the term ends in *nx*, the plural is usually formed by changes the *x* to *ges*.	phalanx meninx	phalanges meninges
6. If the term ends in *on*, the plural is usually formed by changing the *on* to *a*.	criterion ganglion	criteria ganglia

7. If the term ends in *um*, the plural is usually
   formed by changing the *um* to *a*.

   diverticulum   diverticula
   ovum   ova

8. If the term ends in *us*, the plural is usually
   formed by changing the *us* to i.

   alveolus   alveoli
   malleolus   malleoli

Basic Medical Terms

The following subsections discuss basic medical terms that are used to describe diseases and disease conditions, major body systems, and body direction.

Terms Used to Describe Diseases and Disease Conditions

The basic medical terms used to describe diseases and disease conditions are listed here:

- A *sign* is evidence of disease, such as fever, that can be observed by the patient and others. A sign is objective because it can be evaluated or measured by others.
- A *symptom*, such as pain or a headache, can only be experienced or defined by the patient. A symptom is subjective because it can be evaluated or measured only by the patient.
- A *syndrome* is a set of signs and symptoms that occur together as part of a specific disease process.
- *Diagnosis* is the identification of disease. To diagnose is the process of reaching a diagnosis.
- A *differential diagnosis* attempts to determine which of several diseases may be producing the symptoms.
- A *prognosis* is a forecast or prediction of the probable course and outcome of a disorder.
- An *acute* disease or symptom has a rapid onset, a severe course, and relatively short duration.
- A *chronic* symptom or disease has a long duration. Although chronic symptoms or diseases may be controlled, they are rarely cured.
- A *remission* is the partial or complete disappearance of the symptoms of a disease without having achieved a cure. A remission is usually temporary.
- Some diseases are named for the condition described. For example, *chronic fatigue syndrome* (CFS) describes a persistent overwhelming fatigue that does not resolve with bed rest.
- An *eponym* is a disease, structure, operation, or procedure that is named for the person who discovered or described it first. For example, Alzheimer's disease is named for Alois Alzheimer, a German neurologist who lived from 1864 to 1915.
- An *acronym* is a word formed from the initial letter or letters of the major parts of a compound term. For example, the acronym *AMA* stands for American Medical Association.

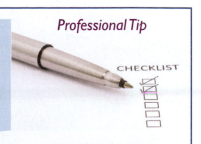

Professional Tip

Accuracy in spelling medical terms is extremely important. Changing just one or two letters can completely change the meaning of the word—and this difference could literally be a matter of life or death for the patient.

CHECKLIST

Terms Used to Describe Major Body Systems

The following is a list of the major body systems and some common related combining forms used with each:

Major Structures and Body System	Related Roots with Combining Forms

Cardiovascular system	heart (card/o, cardi/o)
	   arteries (arteri/o)
	   veins (phleb/o, ven/o)
	   blood (hem/o, hemat/o)

Digestive system	mouth (or/o)
	   esophagus (esophag/o)
	   stomach (gastr/o)
	   small intestines (enter/o)
	   large intestines (col/o)
	   liver (hepat/o)
	   pancreas (pancreat/o)

Endocrine system	adrenals (adren/o)
	   pancreas (pancreat/o)
	   pituitary (pituit/o)
	   thyroid (thyr/o, thyroid/o)
	   parathyroids (parathyroid/o)
	   thymus (thym/o)

Integumentary system	glands (aden/o)
	   skin (cutane/o, dermat/o, derm/o)
	   sebaceous glands (seb/o)
	   sweat glands (hidraden/o)

Lymphatic and immune systems	lymph, lymph vessels, and lymph
	   nodes (lymph/o), (lymphangi/o)
	   tonsils (tonsill/o)
	   spleen (splen/o)
	   thymus (thym/o)

Muscular system	muscles(my/o)
	   ligaments (syndesm/o)
	   tendons (ten/o, tend/o, tendin/o)

Nervous system	nerves (neur/o)
	   brain (encephal/o)
	   spinal cord (myel/o)
	   eyes (ocul/o, ophthalm/o)
	   ears (acoust/o, ot/o)

Respiratory system	nose (nas/o, rhin/o)
	   pharynx (pharyng/o)
	   trachea (trache/o)
	   larynx (laryng/o)
	   lungs (pneum/o, pneumon/o)

Skeletal system	bones (oste/o)
	   joints (arthr/o)
	   cartilage (chondr/o)

Urinary system	kidneys (nephr/o, ren/o) ureters (ureter/o)

urinary bladder (cyst/o, vesic/o)

urethra (urethr/o)

Reproductive system   *Male:*

testicles (orch/o, orchid/o)

Female:

ovaries (oophor/o, ovari/o)

uterus (hyster/o, metr/o, metri/o, uter/o)

Terms Used to Describe Body Direction

Certain terms are used to describe the location of body parts relative to the trunk or other parts of the anatomy:

Ventral (VEN-tral) refers to the front or belly side of the body or organ (*ventr* means "belly side" of the body, and *al* means "pertaining to").

Dorsal (DOR-sal) refers to the back of the body or organ (*dors* means "back of body," and *al* means "pertaining to").

Anterior (an-TEER-ee-or) means situated in the front. It also means on the forward part of an organ (*anter* means "front" or "before," and *ior* means "pertaining to"). For example, the stomach is located anterior to (in front of) the pancreas. *Anterior* is also used in reference to the ventral surface of the body.

Posterior (pos-TEER-ee-or) means situated in the back. It also means on the back portion of an organ (*poster* means "back" or "after," and *ior* means "pertaining to"). For example, the pancreas is located posterior to (behind) the stomach. *Posterior* is also used in reference to the dorsal surface of the body.

Superior means uppermost, above, or toward the head. For example, the lungs are superior to (above) the diaphragm.

Inferior means lowermost, below, or toward the feet. For example, the stomach is located inferior to (below) the diaphragm.

Cephalic (seh-FAL-ick) means toward the head (*cephal* means "head," and *ic* means "pertaining to").

Caudal (KAW-dal) means toward the lower part of the body (*caud* means "tail" or "lower part," of the body and *al* means "pertaining to").

Proximal (PROCK-sih-mal) means situated nearest the midline or beginning of a body structure. For example, the proximal end of the humerus (the bone of the upper arm) forms part of the shoulder. It may be easier to think of *proximal* as "closer to the origin of the body part or the point of attachment of a limb to the body trunk."

Distal (DIS-tal) means situated farthest from the midline or beginning of a body structure. For example, the distal end of the humerus forms part of the elbow.

Medial means the direction toward or nearer the midline. For example, the medial ligament of the knee is near the inner surface of the leg.

Lateral means the direction toward or nearer the side and away from the midline. For example, the lateral ligament of the knee is near the outside surface of the leg.

Bilateral means relating to, or having, two sides.

Prefixes, Root Words, and Suffixes

The most common medical prefixes, root words, and suffixes are listed here. Knowing these common prefixes, roots, and suffixes will help you decipher medical terms.

Prefixes

a	without or absence of	inter	between
ab	from; away from	intra	within
ad	to; toward	mal	bad
an	without or absence of	meso	middle
ante	before	meta	after; beyond; change
anti	against	micro	small
bi	two	multi	many
bin	two	neo	new
brady	slow	nulli	none
con	together	pan	all; total
contra	against	para	outside; beyond; around
de	from; down from; lack of	per	through
dia	through; complete; between; apart	peri	surrounding (outer)
		poly	many; much
dis	to undo; free from	post	after
dys	difficult; labored; painful; abnormal	pre	before; in front of
		pro	before
ec	out	quadri	four
ecto	outside	re	back
endo	within	retro	back; behind
epi	on; upon; over	semi	half
eso	inward	sub	under; below
eu	normal; good	super	over; above
ex	outside; outward	supra	above; beyond; on top
exo	outside; outward	sym	together; joined
extra	outside of; beyond	syn	together; joined
hemi	half	tachy	fast; rapid
hyper	above; excessive	tetra	four
hypo	below; incomplete; deficient	trans	through; across; beyond
		tri	three
in	in; into; not	ultra	beyond; excess
infra	under; below	uni	one

Root Words

abdomin	abdomen	aut	self
aden	gland	bil	bile
adren	adrenal gland	bio	life
adrenal	adrenal gland	blephar	eyelid
aer	air; oxygen; gas	bronch	airway; bronchus
alveol	alveolus	bronchiol	bronchiole
angi	blood or lymph vessel	burs	bursa
ankyl	crooked; stiff; bent	carcin	cancer
appendic	appendix	cardi	heart
arteri, arter	artery	caud	tail; toward lower part of the body
arteriol	arteriole (small artery)		
arthr	joint	cephal	head
ather	yellowish; fatty plaque	cerebell	cerebellum
aur	ear	cerebr	cerebrum; brain

cervic	neck; cervix	glauc	gray
cheil	lip	gloss	tongue
chiro	hand	gluc	sweetness; sugar
cholangi	bile duct	glyc	sugar; glucose
chole	gall; bile	glycos	sugar; glucose
chondr	cartilage	gnos	knowledge; a knowing
coccyg	coccyx; tailbone	gonad	gonad; sex glands
col	colon; large intestine	gyn	woman
conjunctiv	conjunctiva	gynec	woman
corne	cornea	gyr	turning; folding
coron	heart; crown of the head	hem	blood
cost	rib	hemat	blood
crani	cranium; skull	hepat	liver
cutane	skin	hidr	sweat
cyan	blue	hist	tissue
cyst	bladder; sac	hom	same
cyt, cyte	cell	home	sameness; unchanging
dacry	tears; tear duct	hydr	water
dactyl	fingers or toes	hyster	uterus
dent	tooth	ile	ileum
derm	skin	ili	ilium
dermat	skin	immun	immune
dipl	two; double	irid	iris
diverticul	diverticulum	kerat	horny tissue; hard
dors	back (of the body)	kin	movement
duoden	duodenum	kinesi	movement; motion
ectop	located away from usual place	labi	lips
		lacrim	tear duct; tear
edema	swelling	lact	milk
electr	electricity; electrical activity	lapar	abdomen
		laryng	larynx
encephal	brain	later	side
endocrin	endocrine	lei	smooth
enter	intestines (usually small intestine)	leuk	white
		lingu	tongue
epiglott	epiglottis	lip	fat
epitheli	epithelium	lith	stone; calculus
erythr	red	lob	lobe
esophag	esophagus	lymph	lymph
esthesi	sensation; feeling; sensitivity	macr	abnormal largeness
		mamm	breast
eti	cause (of disease)	mast	breast
exocrin	secrete out of	meat	opening or passageway
faci	face	melan	black
fasci	fascia; fibrous band	men	menstruation
fract	break; broken	mening	meninges
galact	milk	ment	mind
gastr	stomach	mes, meso	middle
ger	old age; aged	metr	uterus
geront	old age; aged	mon	one
gingiv	gums	morbid	disease; sickness

muc	mucus	pneumon	lung; air
my, myos	muscle	pod	foot
myc	fungus	poli	gray matter
myel	bone marrow; spinal cord	polyp	polyp; small growth
myelon	bone marrow	poster	back (of body)
myring	eardrum	prim	first
narc	stupor; numbness	proct	rectum
nas	nose	pseud	fake; false
nat	birth	psych	mind
necr	death (cells; body)	pulmon	lung
nephr	kidney	py	pus
neur	nerve	pyel	renal pelvis
noct	night	pylor	pylorus
nyct	night	pyr	fever; heat
nyctal	night	quadr	four
ocul	eye	rect	rectum
onc	tumor	ren	kidney
onych	nail	retin	retina
oophor	ovary	rhin	nose
ophthalm	eye	sacr	sacrum fallopian (uterine)
or	mouth	salping	tube
orth	straight	sanit	soundness; health
oste	bone	sarc	flesh; connective tissue
ot	ear	scler	sclera; white of eye; hard
ox	oxygen	scoli	crooked; curved
palpat	touch; feel; stroke	seb	sebum; oil
pancreat	pancreas	seps	infection
par, part	bear; give birth to; labor	sept	infection; partition; septum
parathyroid	parathyroid	sial	saliva
path	disease; suffering	sinus	inus
pector	chest; muscle	somat	body
ped	child; foot	somn	sleep
pelv	pelvis; pelvic bone	son	sound
pen	penis	sopor	sleep
perine	perineum	sperm	sperm, spermatazoa; seed
peritone	peritoneum	spermat	sperm, spermatazoa; seed
petr	stone; portion of temporal bone	spher	round; sphere; ball
		sphygm	pulse
phac	lens of the eye	spin	spine; backbone to
phag	eat; swallow	spir	breathe
phak	lens of the eye	splen	spleen
phalang	finger or toe bone	spondyl	vertebra; spinal or vertebral column
pharyng	pharynx, throat		
phas	speech	staphyl	grapelike clusters
phleb	vein	stern	breastbone
phot	light	steth	chest (muscles)
phren	mind	stoma	mouth; opening
physi	nature	stomat	mouth; opening
pleur	pleura	strab	squint; squint-eyed
pneum	lung; air	synovi	synovia; synovial membrane
pneumat	lung; air		

system	system	valv	valve
ten, tend	tendon	valvul	valve
tendin	tendon	vas	vessel; duct
test	testis; testicle	vascul	blood vessel; little vessel
therm	heat	ven	vein
thorac	thorax; chest	versicul	seminal vesicles; blister
thromb	clot	vertebr	vertebra; backbone
thym	thymus gland; soul	vesic	urinary bladder
thyr	thyroid gland	vir	poison; virus
thyroid	thyroid gland	viril	masculine; manly
tom	cut; section	vis	seeing; sight
ton	tension; pressure	visc	sticky
tone	to stretch	viscer	viscera; internal organs; sternum
tonsill	tonsils		
top	place; position; location	viscos	sticky
tox, toxic	poison; poisonous	vit	life
trach, trache	trachea; windpipe	xanth	yellow
trachel	neck; necklike	xen	strange; foreign
trich	hair	xer	dry
tubercul	little knot; swelling	zygot	joined together
tympan	eardrum; middle ear		

Additional Root Words

ulcer	sore; ulcer
ungu	nail
ur	urine; urinary tract
ureter	ureter
urethr	urethra
uria	urination; urine
urin	urine or urinary organs
uter	uterus
uvul	vula; little grape
vagin	vagina

caus	burning sensation; capable of burning
cusp	point; cusp
flexion	bending
genital	pertaining to birth
lumb	lumbar; loin region
mediastin	mediastinum
tens, tensi	pressure, force, stretching

Suffixes

Suffixes Meaning "Pertaining to"

ac			eal	ous
al	ine		ial	
ar	ior		ic	
ary	ory		ical	tic

Suffixes about "Conditions"

ago	abnormal condition, disease
esis	abnormal condition, disease
ia	abnormal condition, disease
iasis	abnormal condition, disease
ion	condition
ism	condition; abnormal condition
osis	disease

Other Common Suffixes Used in Medical Terminology

algia	pain, suffering	meter	instrument used to measure
asthenia	weakness		
cele	hernia, protrusion	metry	measurement
centesis	surgical puncture to remove fluid	morph	form; shape
		oid, ode	resembling
cidal	killing	oma	tumor; mass
clasia	break	opia	vision (condition)
clasis	break	opsy	to view
clast	break	oxia	oxygen
clysis	irrigating; washing	paresis	slight paralysis
coccus	berry shaped (a form of bacterium)	pathy	disease
		penia	abnormal reduction in number; lack of
crine	separate; secrete		
crit	to separate	peps, pepsia	digestion
cyte	cell	pexy	surgical fixation; suspension
desis	fusion; to bind; to tie together		
		phagia	eating; swallowing
drome	run; running	philia	love
ductor	to lead or pull	phily	love
dynia	pain	phobia	abnormal fear of or adversion to specific objects or things
ectasis	stretching out; dilation; expansion		
ectomy	excision or surgical removal		
		phonia	sound or voice
ectopia	displacement	phoria	feeling
emesis	vomiting	physis	growth
emia	blood; blood condition	plasia	formation; development; a growth
gen	producing, forming		
genesis	producing; forming	plasm	growth; formation; substance
genic	producing, forming		
gnosis	a knowing	plasty	plastic or surgical repair
gram	record; X-ray		
graph	instrument used to record	plegia	paralysis; stroke
		pnea	breathing
graphy	process of recording; X-ray filming	porosis	lessening in density; porous condition
ictal	seizure; attack	praxia	in front of; before
ism	state of	ptosis	drooping; sagging; prolapse
itis	inflammation		
lepsy	seizure	ptysis	spitting
logist	specialist	rrhage	bursting forth; an abnormal excessive discharge or bleeding
logy	study of		
lysis	destruction; reduce; separation		
		rrhagia	bursting forth; an abnormal excessive discharge or bleeding
malacia	softening		
mania	madness; insane desire		
megaly	enlargement		

rrhaphy	to suture or stitch	stasis	control; stop; standing still
rrhea	abnormal flow or discharge	stat	to stop
rrhexis	rupture	stenosis	narrowing; constriction
schisis	split; fissure		
sclerosis	hardening	stomy	new artificial opening
scope	instrument used for visual exam	therapy	treatment
scopic	visual exam	tome	instrument used to cut
scopy	visual exam with an instrument	tomy	cutting into; surgical incision
sepsis	infection		
sis	state of	tripsy	crushing
spasm	sudden involuntary muscle contraction	trophy	nourishment
		ule	little
stalsis	contraction; constriction	uria	urine; urination

Glossary

abuse: Improper billing practices that result in financial benefit to the provider but are not fraudulent.

Accountable Care Organization (ACO): A contract between a health insurance company and group of healthcare providers that adopt alternative payment models (e.g., capitation) and agree to take on a shared responsibility for the managed care of a defined population of patients (e.g., Medicare).

addendum: An addition made to a book or publication, normally at the end, to document a change or revision. Plural is addenda.

add-on codes: CPT codes with a + symbol in front, used to specify procedures in addition to the primary procedure. An add-on code cannot be used alone.

adjudication: The insurance carrier's process of evaluating a claim for payment, which includes investigating the details of the claim to determine which items should be paid and how much should be paid on each.

adjustment: A positive or negative change to a patient's account balance. This is done to make changes, corrections, or discount write-offs.

administrative law judge (ALJ) hearing: The third level of appeal for physician claims with Medicare. Physicians have 60 days to file an appeal. Medicare must make a decision within 90 days.

administrative services only (ASO): Administrative services only is an arrangement in which an organization funds its own employee benefit plan, such as a pension plan or health insurance program, but hires an outside firm to perform specific administrative services.

Admission of Liability: Acknowledgment to an employee that the workers' compensation claim has been accepted or approved.

admitting clerk: Clerk who enters patient's demographic information into a computer and obtains signed statement(s) from patients to protect hospitals' interests. Responsibilities of the admitting clerk may also include general filing of patient charts.

admitting physician: The doctor responsible for admitting a patient to a hospital or other inpatient health facility.

advance beneficiary notice (ABN): A written notification that must be signed by the patient or guardian prior to the provider rendering a service to a Medicare beneficiary that could be potentially denied or deemed "not medically necessary" and will be the patient's financial responsibility.

adverse affect: An undesired condition that results from use of a medication or drug given in the correct dosage.

advisory opinion: An opinion issued by legal counsel that advises a healthcare professional on the legal rights of the facility.

Affordable Care Act (ACA): The law known as "Patient Protection and Affordable Care Act." Also known as "Obamacare."

Aid to Families with Dependent Children (AFDC): A cash assistance program of Medicaid that was repealed in 1996 with the implementation of Temporary Assistance to Needy Families (TANF), which limited the amount and duration of cash assistance.

allowed charges: Maximum amount an insurance payer considers reasonable for a medical service. Participating providers agree by contract to accept the allowed charge for services they provide.

Ambulatory Payment Classification (APC) system: Prospective payment system patterned after that of ambulatory patient groups. APCs are used for outpatient services, certain Medicare Part B services, and partial hospitalization. This payment method is based on procedures rather than diagnoses.

ambulatory surgical center (ASC): Facility designed for patients receiving minor surgical procedures who are expected to be discharged the same day.

ambulatory surgical unit (ASU): Facility within a hospital designed for patients receiving minor surgical procedures who are expected to be discharged the same day.

American Medical Association (AMA): Professional society that assists patients and physicians by creating a sense of unity in the medical industry. It implemented the first standard terms and descriptors to document procedures in the medical record.

appeal: The process used by a provider to ask an insurance carrier to reconsider a denied claim. The provider bases an appeal on documentation that backs up the medical necessity of the medical treatment.

assignment of benefits: Request made by a patient to allow the insurance carrier to pay the healthcare professional directly rather than issuing monies to the patient.

assumption coding: Billing for reasonable undocumented services presumably performed by the healthcare professional as part of the documented procedure.

attending physician: Physician primarily responsible for the medical care of a patient; supervises medical students and residents.

audit: A formal examination of patients' medical records and accounts.

audit/edit report: Feedback from the insurance company documenting the progress of individual claims that have been submitted. This report documents changes to be made or additional information to be submitted on a claim.

balance billing: Billing patients for the dollar amount left over after the insurance carrier has paid. If the provider has a contract with the third-party payer, balance billing may be prohibited.

batching out: The process used by a medical office specialist to calculate all monies received, tally all cash on hand, and compare the totals with the Patient Day Sheet report.

beneficiary: A person eligible to receive benefits under an insurance policy.

benefit period: A period of time during which medical benefits are available to an insurance beneficiary.

billing services: A third-party agency outside of the hospital or physician's practice that is responsible for submitting claims for the hospital or physician's practice.

birthday rule: Determines which insurance is primary when two policies are valid for a child. The plan of the parent whose birthday comes first in the calendar year is usually primary.

Body Mass Index (BMI): A weight-to-height ratio used as an indicator of obesity and underweight.

bundled code: A group of related procedures covered by a single code.

burial benefits: Benefits paid to the person who pays a deceased worker's funeral expenses.

business associate (BA): Any organization or person working in with or providing services to a covered entity who handles or discloses health information or health records.

capitation plan: Contract that a provider signs with a carrier agreeing to treat a certain number of members in the carrier's plan. The carrier then pays the provider based on a designated fee each month for each member in that plan.

carriers: Parties responsible for issuing insurance policies.

case manager: A person who coordinates patient care by assessing, monitoring, and evaluating options of cost-effective care.

catastrophic cap: Limits the amount of out-of-pocket expenses a family will have to pay for TRICARE-covered medical services.

categorically needy: The Medicaid eligibility group that includes cash recipients of Aid to Families with Dependent Children (AFDC)—now known as Temporary Assistance to Needy Families (TANF), most cash recipients of Social Security Income (SSI), and certain other groups of low-income, aged, and disabled persons.

Centers for Medicare and Medicaid Services (CMS): The department of the federal government responsible for administering Medicare and Medicaid. Formerly the Health Care Financing Administration (HCFA).

centralized billing office (CBO): Specializes in maintaining patient accounting records, filing health insurance claims, working with insurance carriers to receive reimbursement on insurance claims filed, and appealing denied claims.

certifications: Training received in particular fields that acknowledges a medical office specialist's expertise.

CHAMPVA: *See* Civilian Health and Medical Program of the Department of Veterans Affairs.

charge-based fees: Fees providers routinely charge for medical procedures performed. Providers reference the nationwide fee database to determine if their fees will be at the high, midpoint, or low range to be competitive with other providers of their specialty.

charges: Amounts a practice charges for medical services rendered.

charge description master (CDM): A database that contains a detailed narrative of each procedure, service, dollar amount, and revenue code that is used in inpatient facilities. This information is transferred to the patient bill or UB-04 after the patient is discharged.

chief complaint (CC): A concise statement describing the symptom, problem, condition, diagnosis, or other factor that is the reason for the patient encounter.

Children's Health Insurance Program (CHIP): A program that provides health insurance to all uninsured children and teens who are not eligible for or enrolled in Medical Assistance.

Children's Health Insurance Program Reauthorization Act (CHIPRA): A program administered by the U.S. Department of Health and Human Services that provides matching funds to states for health insurance to families with children. It is designed to cover uninsured children in families with low to modest incomes.

Civilian Health and Medical Program of the Uniformed Services (CHAMPUS): Comprehensive health benefit program designed by Congress for military personnel and their families. Now called TRICARE.

Civilian Health and Medical Program of the Department of Veterans Affairs (CHAMPVA): Healthcare for veterans with 100% service-related disabilities and their families.

civil money penalty (CMP): A punitive fine imposed by a civil court on a covered entity that has profited from illegal or unethical activity.

claim attachment: Additional documentation or information necessary when submitting a claim.

clean claims: Claims that have no data errors when submitted to an insurance carrier.

clearinghouse: A company that receives claims from multiple providers, evaluates them, and batches them for electronic submission to multiple insurance carriers.

Clinical Laboratory Improvement Amendment (CLIA): An act passed by Congress establishing quality standards for all laboratory testing to ensure the accuracy, reliability, and timeliness of patient test results regardless of where the test was performed.

CMS-1500 claim form: Standard claim form used by physicians and other healthcare professionals to bill for services rendered.

code edits: Computer program function that screens for improperly or incorrectly reported procedure codes.

code linkage: The process of joining a diagnosis code and a procedure code for the purpose of justifying medical necessity.

coinsurance: Percentage of the allowed amount that is the patient's responsibility.

combination code: A single code that classifies more than one condition, such as both the etiology and the manifestation of an illness or injury.

commercial health insurance (CHI): Any type of health insurance not paid for by a government agency. The policy can be based on fee for service or managed care. Also known as private health insurance.

comorbidity: One or more diseases or disorders that presents in addition to the primary disease or disorder.

compliance officer: Individual responsible for reviewing office policies and procedures to ensure that all applicable HIPAA laws, rules, and regulations are being followed.

complication: The disease or condition that arises during the course of treatment or during a medical procedure.

complication code: A diagnostic code that defines a complication that occurs when a patient suffers a problem resulting directly from a procedure that was performed by a physician.

computerized provider order entry (CPOE): A process of electronic entry of medical practitioner instructions for the treatment of patients under the provider's care. These orders are communicated over a computer network to the medical staff or to the departments responsible for fulfilling the order.

concierge medicine: A small, personalized medical practice that takes care of a limited number of patients. This allows each patient to receive the time they need with the physician. Urgent visits are seen the same or next day. It also offers home visits and follows its patients at hospitals, nursing homes, and assisted living residences.

Consolidated Omnibus Budget Reconciliation Act of 1985 (COBRA): Contains provisions giving former employees, retirees, spouses, and dependent children the right to temporary continuation of health coverage for 18 months after employment has ended. Group health coverage for COBRA participants is usually more expensive than health coverage for active employees because the COBRA participant usually has to pay the part of the premium that was formerly paid by the employer.

consultation: Service by a physician whose opinion or advice regarding a patient's condition and/or treatment is requested by another physician. The consulting physician must communicate the findings, results, and recommendations in a written report to the requesting physician.

consumer-driven health care (CDHC): Consumer-driven plans are subject to the provisions of the Affordable Care Act, which mandates that routine and/or health maintenance claims must be covered with no cost-sharing (copays, co-insurance, or deductibles) to the patient.

contractual adjustment: The difference between the provider's standard or customary fee and the allowed payment from the carrier.

conventions: Formatting used in coding books that is exclusive to each volume and publisher.

conversion factor: A dollar amount used to multiply relative value units (RVU) in order to arrive at the price for a service.

Coordination and Maintenance (C&M) Committee: A committee that reviews proposals regarding diagnostic codes and determines if a code is modified, added, or deleted. Suggestions for modifications come from both the public and private sectors.

coordination of benefits (COB): When a patient has more than one insurance policy, insurance carriers work together to coordinate the insurance benefit so that the maximum payment does not exceed 100% of the charge.

copayment: A fixed dollar amount the patient pays at each office visit or hospital encounter, as specified in the patient's insurance policy.

cost outlier: Medical services rendered for extenuating circumstances that cannot be assigned to a Diagnosis Related Group (DRG). Reimbursement is based on the DRG rate, plus an additional payment for services rendered.

cost share: The amount of healthcare charges that are the responsibility of the sponsor or family member.

counseling: A method of a healthcare professional providing advice and guidance to a patient. This could include physician discussion with a patient and/or family regarding the diagnosis, diagnostic testing results, prognosis, and treatment options.

covered entities (CE): Healthcare providers who transmit any health information in electronic form.

crossover: Reassignment of gaps in coverage that eliminates the need for a beneficiary to file a separate claim with his or her Medigap insurer. It usually requires the beneficiary to sign release-of-information and assignment-of-benefit forms with their providers.

cross-references: A coding and documentation guide that assist a medical coder to select the correct diagnosis code.

crosswalk: A reference aid that compares information in one system to information in another system. A crosswalk between the ICD-9 and ICD-10 will allow a coder to look up an ICD-9 code and see what the corresponding code is in the new ICD-10 system.

Current Procedural Terminology (CPT): A system of five-digit codes used to describe what procedures were performed.

death benefits: Benefits that can replace a portion of lost family income for eligible family members of workers killed on the job.

deductible: Amount a beneficiary is responsible for before the insurance company pays as stated in the insurance policy.

Defense Enrollment Eligibility Reporting System (DEERS): A support office for TRICARE. Sponsors and family members can contact DEERS to check the status of enrollment or inquire about plan benefits.

default code: In medical coding, the code next to the main term is called the default code.

descriptor: All Current Procedural Terminology codes are five digits followed by a descriptor, which is a brief description of the procedure.

designated doctor: 1. Treating physician chosen by the employer for initial treatment of injured employees. 2. An independent physician who has not seen the patient chosen by the Workers' Compensation Insurance Board to examine the patient for an independent medical review.

diagnosis: The process of determining by examination the nature and circumstances of a diseased condition.

Diagnosis-Related Group (DRG): A patient classification method that categorizes patients, for reimbursement purposes, who are medically related with respect to diagnosis and treatment and who are statistically similar in terms of their length of hospital stay.

diagnostic statement: The main reason for the patient encounter along with the descriptions of additional conditions or symptoms that have been treated or related to the patient's current illness.

dirty claim: A claim that is incorrect or is missing information when submitted.

disability: A physical or mental handicap, especially one that prevents a person from holding a gainful job.

disability compensation programs: Programs that reimburse a covered individual for wages lost due to a disability that prevents the individual from working.

discounted fee: A financial reimbursement system whereby a provider agrees to supply services on an FFS basis, but with the fees discounted by a certain percentage from the physician's usual and customary charges. An agreed upon rate for service between the provider and payer that is usually less than the provider's full fee.

District of Columbia Workers' Compensation Act: Provides benefits for any employee performing work on a regular basis in the District of Columbia.

documentation: A consistent medical record format, often in chronological order, that records facts and observations regarding a patient's health status.

downcode: Occurs when the procedure code billed is for a procedure that is less involved than the procedure actually documented in the chart. Carriers will downcode or deny payment when the documentation fails to justify the level of service billed.

durable medical equipment (DME): Any medical device, equipment, or instrument used in the care of a patient.

durable medical equipment number (DMEN): A number assigned to a medical device or piece of equipment or instrument for billing purposes.

Early and Periodic Screening, Diagnostic, and Treatment (EPSDT): Medicaid's comprehensive and preventive child health program for individuals under the age of 21; includes periodic screening, vision, dental, and hearing services.

electronic claims: The process of submitting medical claims electronically versus on paper.

electronic data interchange (EDI): Standardized transmission of data between covered entities by electronic means. It is used to transfer electronic documents or business data from one computer system to another computer system.

electronic health records (EHR): Electronic records of patient health information that originate in a delivery setting such as a hospital, physician's practice, multispecialty outpatient facility, or clinic. All records of patient care are retained in the EHR, including information from other systems such as X-rays, consultations, and so on. All providers that have a relationship with the patient can view the EHR. An EHR creates and gathers cumulatively across more than one healthcare organization.

electronic media claims (EMC): Insurance claims submitted to the carrier in a flat file format via electronic means, such as tape, diskette, direct wire, direct data entry, or telephone lines.

electronic medical records (EMR): Contain health-related information on a patient that is created, gathered, managed, and consulted by licensed clinicians and staff from a single organization who are involved in an individual's health and care. Electronic medical records are not integrated with other providers' systems.

electronic protected health information (EPHI): Refers to protected health information of an individual that is transmitted by electronic media or transmitted or maintained in any other form or medium.

Electronic Remittance Advice (ERA): An electronic notification sent to the provider who accepts assignment. The ERA lists the dates of service, type of service, and charges filed on the claim.

E/M codes: CPT code numbers 99201 to 99499. These codes are used to report encounters in which the physician evaluates the patient's problem or complaint, considers treatment options, and recommends a plan of treatment. The most common E/M visits are "office visits" and "hospital visits." Codes are categorized by place of service and subdivided based on the complexity of the problem and treatment options. Three to five levels of codes are available for reporting purposes. The number of levels in a category varies and is dependent on the types of services that might be provided.

emergency care: Urgent care necessary to sustain life and limbs.

Employee Retirement Income Security Act (ERISA) of 1974: Act that set standards for administering health insurance plans. It protects the interests of beneficiaries who depend on benefits from private employee benefit plans.

employer identification number (EIN): A number issued by the Internal Revenue Service to any medical facility, provider, or business for tax purposes.

Employer's First Report of Injury or Illness: Form filled out by the employer and sent to the insurance company in workers' compensation cases. A case number will not be assigned to workers' compensation injury or illness until this form has been filled out and received by the insurance carrier.

encrypted: Describes information that is "scrambled" during the time it is being transmitted by rotating letters in the alphabet and/or numbers.

encryption: Process of "scrambling" information during the time it is being transmitted by rotating letters in the alphabet and/or numbers.

end-stage renal disease (ESRD): Total or nearly complete failure of the kidneys.

Energy Employees Occupational Illness Compensation Program Act (EEOICP): Act that provides benefits to eligible and former employees of the U.S. Department of Energy, its contractors and subcontractors, and certain survivors of such individuals.

enforcement rule: Provisions relating to compliance and investigations, the imposition of civil money penalties for violations of the HIPAA Administrative Simplification Rules, and procedures for hearings.

enrollee: An individual who takes out an insurance policy in his or her name.

eponym: A procedure or diagnosis name derived from the name of a person.

established patient: One who has received professional services from a physician or another physician of the same specialty who belongs to the same group practice within the past 3 years.

etiology: The cause or origin of a disease.

evaluation and management (E&M) codes: *See* E/M codes.

examination: An evaluation performed by a physician who is involved in a patient's care for the purpose of establishing a medical diagnosis and treatment.

excluded services: Services not covered by an insurance payer as stated in the insurance policy.

Explanation of Benefits (EOB): Hard-copy notification sent by an insurance carrier to a patient and provider (if provider accepts assignment) to indicate the disposition of a claim. It shows the dates of service, type of service, and charges filed on the claim, as well as what was paid and the reason(s) for any denials.

external audit: An investigation performed by an external party to review patient documentation and records.

facility provider number (FPN): Number issued to a facility and used by a physician to report services provided at a particular location.

Federal Coal Mine Health and Safety Act (Black Lung Benefits Reform Act): Act that provides benefits to current coal mine employees as well as monthly payments to surviving dependents of deceased workers.

Federal Employees' Compensation Act (FECA): Provides benefits to millions of civilian employees of the United States, members of the Peace Corps, and Vista volunteers.

Federal Medical Assistance Percentages (FMAP): Program that specifies the formula for calculating federal medical assistance percentages. This program is available to certain children who qualify for medical assistance.

final report: Report filed by the treating physician in a state's workers' compensation case when the patient is released from medical care and is fit to return to work.

flexible spending accounts (FSA): A tax-advantaged financial account that can be set up through an employer in the United States. An FSA allows an employee to set aside a portion of earnings to pay for qualified expenses as established in the plan, most commonly for medical expenses but often for dependent care or other expenses. Money deducted from an employee's pay into an FSA is not subject to taxes; therefore it is a payroll tax savings.

follow-up: Refers to checking on the status of a claim by a variety of methods, such as calling the insurance carrier, checking the status of the claim online, or writing an appeal letter.

Food and Drug Administration (FDA): A federal agency responsible for monitoring trading and safety standards in the food and drug industries.

form locators: The boxes located on the UB-04 and CMS-1500 claim forms. Each form locator is assigned a number and requires designated information to be entered into that field.

fragmented billing: Occurs when procedures are reported separately that should have been included under a bundled code.

fraud: An intentional deception or misrepresentation that an individual knows, or should know, to be false, or does not believe to be true, and makes, knowing the deception could result in some unauthorized benefit to himself or some other person(s).

fraud indicators: With regard to workers' compensation, unusual events or circumstances that sometimes mean an employer, employee, or attorney is attempting to falsify facts for financial gain.

General Equivalence Mappings (GEM) files: Tool to assist with the conversion of *International Classification of Diseases*, Ninth Revision, Clinical Modification (ICD-9-CM) codes to *International Classification of Diseases*, Tenth Revision (ICD-10-CM), and the conversion of ICD-10-CM codes back to ICD-9-CM.

Geographic Practice Cost Index (GPCI): An adjustment that accounts for geographic variations in the costs of practicing medicine in different areas of the country. This adjustment factor is applied to each component (work, practice expense, and malpractice) used in calculating a physician payment.

global period: The number of days surrounding a surgical procedure during which all services relating to the procedure—preoperative, during the surgery, and postoperative—are considered part of the surgical package.

global surgical concept: A surgical package that includes specific services in addition to the operation.

group insurance: An insurance policy offered to groups of employees and often their dependents covered under a single policy and issued by an employer or other group.

group provider number (GPN): A number assigned to a group for billing purposes.

grouper: A computer software program that abstracts data from a medical record and assigns the DRG payment group.

guarantor: The person who is ultimately responsible for paying for the healthcare services rendered.

HCPCS: *See* Health Care Common Procedure Coding System.

Health and Human Services (HHS): The United States federal department that administers all federal programs dealing with health and welfare. HIPAA requires the HHS to adopt standards that covered entities (CE), health plans, healthcare clearinghouses, certain healthcare providers, employer-sponsored health plans, and health insurers must use when electronically conducting certain healthcare administrative transactions.

Healthcare Common Procedure Coding System (HCPCS): Standard code set for reporting professional services, procedures, and supplies.

health information clerk: These professionals organize and maintain health data in electronic and paper systems within various healthcare settings. They are responsible for reviewing patient records, organizing databases, tracking patient outcomes, and protecting patients' health information.

health information management (HIM): A department in a healthcare facility that maintains patients' medical records.

health information system (HIS): Refers to any technical system used to enter, store, manage, or transmit information related to the patient demographics, health insurance, billing, and care of patient.

Health Information Technology for Economic and Clinical Health (HITECH) Act: Act contained in the American Recovery and Reinvestment Act of 2009 to strengthen HIPAA privacy and security protections, enhance enforcement efforts, and provide public education about privacy protections.

Health Insurance Portability and Accountability Act (HIPAA): Act that required the Department of Health and Human Services to establish national standards for electronic healthcare transactions and national identifiers for providers, health plans, and employers. It also addressed the security and privacy of health data.

health maintenance organization (HMO): A medical center or designated group of medical professionals that provide medical services to subscribers for a fixed monthly or annual rate of pay.

health reimbursement accounts (HRA): Employer-funded plans that reimburse employees for incurred medical expenses that are not covered by the company's standard insurance plan.

health savings accounts (HSA): Tax savings account that helps cover additional costs not covered by a health insurance plan.

high-deductible health plans (HDHP): Health insurance plan with lower premiums and higher deductibles than a traditional health plan. Being covered by an HDHP is also a requirement for having a health savings account.

history: Information gained by a healthcare professional by asking the patient specific questions with the aim of obtaining information useful in formulating a diagnosis and providing medical care to the patient.

history of present illness (HPI): A chronological description of the development of the patient's present illness from the first sign or symptom to the present.

hospice: Palliative care for a person who is dying that is given at home, in day care, or in a hospice facility. Services may include pain control, symptom relief, skilled nursing care, and counseling but not active treatment of the terminal condition.

hospital acquired conditions (HAC): Serious conditions that patients may get during an inpatient hospital stay. Medicare does not pay for any of these conditions, and patients cannot be billed for them if they got them while in the hospital. Medicare will only pay for these conditions if patients already had them when they were admitted to the hospital.

ICD-10-CM: *See International Classification of Diseases*, Tenth Revision (ICD-10-CM). A coding system used to code signs, symptoms, injuries, diseases, and conditions.

ICD-10 Procedure Coding System (ICD-10-PCS): A system of medical classification used for procedural codes that track various health interventions taken by medical professionals. It is referred to as Volume 3 in a coding manual. It applies to hospital inpatient use only.

impairment: With regard to workers' compensation claims, permanent physical damage to a worker's body from a work-related injury or illness.

impairment income benefits: Benefits paid to an injured worker if the injured worker is found to have permanent impairment from a work-related injury or illness.

impairment rating: With regard to workers' compensation claims, describes the degree, in percentages, of permanent damage done to a worker's body as a whole.

income benefits: With regard to workers' compensation claims, benefits that replace a portion of any wages a worker loses because of a work-related injury or illness.

independent review organization (IRO): A company that provides a third-party assessment of a treatment plan and patient's status when the insurance carrier has denied treatment or considers the services medically unnecessary or inappropriate. The injured worker must request an appeal process before an IRO is called in.

inpatient: A patient who has been admitted to the hospital and is expected to stay 24 hours or more.

inpatient care: Care provided to a patient whose hospital stay is expected to be for 24 hours or more; usually requires approval by a patient's insurance carrier to prove medical necessity.

insurance commissioner: An elected official in each state charged with consumer protection and regulation of the state's insurance industry.

insurance verification representative: Coordinates all financial aspects of patient visits and admissions, including insurance verification, precertification information, follow-up of third-party payment denials, and financial counseling.

insured: An individual who is covered under an insurance agreement.

intermediaries: Private companies that have a contract with Medicare to pay Part A and some Part B bills.

internal audit: A review of claims that is performed by a facility to protect against submitting fraudulent or upcoded claims.

International Classification of Diseases, Tenth Revision (ICD-10-CM): Provided by the Centers for Medicare and Medicaid Services (CMS) and the National Center for Health Statistics (NCHS) for medical coding and reporting in the United States, the ICD-10-CM is based on the ICD-10, the statistical classification of diseases published by the World Health Organization (WHO). ICD-10 replaces ICD-9.

International Classification of Function (ICF): Framework for describing and organizing information on functioning and disability. Provides a standard language and a conceptual basis for the definition and measurement of health and disability.

late effect: A condition that remains after a patient's acute illness or injury.

Level I (HCPCS): CPT coding levels published by the American Medical Association that are made up of five numeric digits. These codes are used to report services and procedures when billing insurance carriers.

Level II (HCPCS): Alphanumeric CPT coding levels published by CMS that consist of one letter followed by four numbers. These codes are used to report certain medical services not included in the CPT manual, services by nonphysician providers and ambulances, and durable medical equipment and supplies when billing insurance carriers.

Level III (HCPCS): Local CPT coding levels used to electronically process claims for services where a Level I or Level II code has not yet been established. These codes were originally developed by Medicaid and Medicare state contractors and were discontinued in 2004.

lifetime income benefits: Benefits that an injured worker becomes eligible for from the date of disability if the injury is the loss of both feet at or above the ankle; the loss of both hands at or above the wrist; the loss of one foot at or above the ankle; the loss of one hand at or above the wrist; and other injuries of permanent damage.

lifetime maximum: As stated in the insurance policy, the maximum amount of money a plan will pay toward healthcare services over the lifetime of the insured. Once this amount has been met, no more benefits will be paid.

limiting charge: The maximum amount a nonparticipating physician can charge a Medicare patient on a nonassigned claim.

Local Coverage Determination (LCD): A decision by a Medicare fiscal intermediary or carrier on whether to cover a particular service on an intermediary-wide or carrier-wide basis in accordance with Section 1862(a)(1)(A) of the Social Security Act (i.e., a determination as to whether the service is reasonable and necessary).

Longshore and Harbor Workers' Compensation Act (LHWCA): Act that covers maritime workers injured or killed on navigable waters of the United States and those working on or adjoining piers, docks, and terminals.

main term: The term used when searching for a specific diagnosis code. Usually the chief complaint (CC).

managed care: A system of healthcare delivery aimed at controlling costs by shifting utilization risk to the provider.

managed care organization (MCO): Organization designed to provide quality healthcare that is cost effective. Through supervision, monitoring, and advising, managed care plans seek to ensure a certain standard of care, measure performance, and control costs. In addition, some managed care plans seek to assist members in staying healthy through prevention.

manifestation: A symptom related to the patient's condition.

manual review: Occurs when a claim is removed from an automated claims processing system and sent to a claims examiner to request additional information in order to complete the processing of the claim.

mapping: Reflects the complexity of the code sets rather than oversimplifying. It demonstrates the hierarchical relationships, taking into consideration the 68,000 diagnostic codes in ICD-10, compared to 13,000 in ICD-9.

master patient index: Identifies all patients who have been treated in a facility or hospital and lists the medical record or identification number associated with each patient.

maximum medical improvement: With regard to workers' compensation claims, the point in time at which an injured worker's injury or illness has improved as much as it is likely to improve.

meaningful use: A set of requirements that is designed to move the healthcare industry toward the implementation of standardized, certified, interoperable electronic health records and related technologies.

medical benefits: In the context of workers' compensation, medical care that is reasonable and necessary to treat a work-related injury or illness.

medical biller: Individual who submits and tracks all insurance claims and ensures that insurance companies correctly reimburse the healthcare provider.

medical coder: Individual who assigns numerical codes to diagnoses and procedures using the ICD-10 manuals, CPT manuals, and other such resources.

medical decision making (MDM): The process of establishing a diagnosis and selecting a management option as measured by the number of diagnoses or treatment options, the amount and complexity of data (medical records, test result, or other information) to be reviewed, and the risk of complications, morbidity, or mortality.

medical and health services manager: Plans and directs the health services in facilities, medical practices, or specific clinical departments.

medical practice management (MPM) software: Medical software database used in medical practices that stores physician's charges, patient data, adjustment information, and demographic and other information within a medical practice.

medically needy: An optional Medicaid program that allows states to extend Medicaid eligibility to additional qualified persons who may have too much income to qualify under the mandatory or optional categorically needy groups. Generally, those qualifying under the medically needy program receive medical services, but not cash assistance.

Medicare abuse: Includes improper payments for items or services when there was no legal entitlement to that payment; may directly or indirectly result in costs to the Medicare or Medicaid programs.

Medicare Administrative Contractor (MAC): Previously referred to as fiscal intermediaries and carriers; entities awarded contracts by CMS to adjudicate and pay Medicare claims.

Medicare Advantage (MA): Option that offers expanded benefits for a fee through private health insurance programs such as health maintenance organizations and preferred provider organizations that have contracts with Medicare. Also known as Medicare Part C.

Medicare conversion factor (MCF): Determined by Centers for Medicare and Medicaid Services, the MCF is a national value that converts the total relative value units into a payment amount to reimburse providers for medical services.

Medicare Development Letter: A letter sent to a provider by Medicare requesting additional information or documentation to process a claim.

Medicare DRG (CMS-DRG & MS-DRG): A DRG system that implements hospital acquired conditions (HAC). These are certain conditions that are no longer considered complications if they were not present on admission.

Medicare Fee Schedule (MFS): Based on the resource-based relative value scale (RBRVS) fees. This amount is the most Medicare will allow to be paid for a procedure.

Medicare fraud: Knowingly and intentionally executing a plan to scheme or defraud healthcare claims in order to obtain, by means of false or fraudulent pretenses, any money or property.

Medicare Part A: The U.S. government's health insurance program for the elderly, individuals with disabilities, and individuals with qualifying end-stage renal disease. This portion covers hospital fees.

Medicare Part B: Medical insurance that helps pay for physicians' services, outpatient hospital care, durable medical equipment, and some medical services that are not covered by Medicare Part A.

Medicare Part C: Offers expanded benefits for a fee through private health insurance programs such as health maintenance organizations and preferred provider organizations that have contracts with Medicare. Also called Medicare Advantage.

Medicare Part D: Medicare prescription drug coverage program.

Medicare Remittance Notice (MRN): Notice sent to providers by Medicare contractors on assigned claims; details how a claim was processed.

Medicare Secondary Payer (MSP): Any situation in which a payer is required by federal law to pay before Medicare pays. In several instances another payer could be primary to Medicare.

Medicare Summary Notice (MSN): An easy-to-read document that clearly lists the health insurance claim information. The MSN lists the details of the services rendered by a provider and shows amounts paid and beneficiaries' responsibilities.

Medigap: A privately offered, Medicare-supplemental health insurance policy designed to provide additional coverage for services that Medicare does not pay for and for noncovered services.

Medi-Medi: Term used to refer to a beneficiary who is covered under the Medicare program but is also eligible for coverage through the Medicaid program.

military treatment facility (MTF): A clinic, hospital, or provider within the military or armed forces. Some TRICARE plans require that sponsors and their families go to an MTF.

modifiers: Two-digit numbers placed after the five-digit CPT code to indicate that the description of the service or procedure has been altered.

morbidity: The condition of being diseased.

morphology: The study of the structure of words.

National Center for Health Statistics (NCHS): An organization component of the Centers for Disease Control and Prevention charged with providing statistical information to guide actions and policies to improve the health of the American people.

National Committee for Quality Assurance (NCQA): Promotes quality in the delivery of healthcare in managed care organizations by rating their performance from information obtained from the Healthcare Effectiveness Data and Information Set (HEDIS). NCQA works with managed care organizations to help them in their efforts to improve the delivery of quality healthcare to their members.

National Correct Coding Initiative (NCCI): Coding policies to standardize bundled codes and control improper coding that would lead to inappropriate payment for Medicare claims for physician services.

National Center for Health Statistics (NCHS): A division of the Centers for Disease Control and Prevention (CDC), a federal agency. As such, NCHS is under the U.S. Department of Health and Human Services (HHS).

National Provider Identifier (NPI): A unique 10-digit number for HIPAA-covered healthcare providers to be used in the administrative and financial transactions adopted under HIPAA.

nationally uniform relative value: A standardized scale, based on three cost elements: the physician's effort or amount of work to account for each service, the practice cost associated with delivering the service, and the professional liability insurance to cover the procedure being performed. Used as a basis for establishing Medicare fees for physicians.

nature of the presenting problem: Determines the medical necessity for history, exam, and medical decision-making. It justifies the level of care of evaluation and management during the encounter.

NEC (not elsewhere classified): A designation used in the ICD-10-CM coding manual that indicates a more specific code is not available to describe the condition, even though there is more detailed information in the medical record.

network: An organization of members contracted with a managed care organization.

new patient: A person who has not received any professional services within the past 3 years from the physician or another physician of the same specialty who belongs to the same group practice.

nomenclature: A listing of descriptive terms, guidelines, and identifying codes for reporting medical services and procedures.

nonavailability statement (NAS): Document that must be obtained through the DEERS office in order for a sponsor or family member to see a civilian provider or be treated in a nonmilitary facility.

non-PAR MFS: Amount that applies to unassigned services performed by physicians and suppliers who choose not to participate in the Medicare program, which is 5% less than the MFS for participating providers. Providers who are non-PAR and not accepting assignment may charge a limiting charge of 115% of the nonparticipating fee amount.

nonparticipating provider (non-PAR): A provider who does not have a contract with a designated insurance carrier and is not obligated to offer discounted rates.

NOS (not otherwise specified): A designation used in the ICD-10-CM coding manual that indicates there is lack of sufficient details in the medical record to assign a more specific code.

Notice of Contest: With regard to workers' compensation claims, notice issued to an employee if his or her employer denies a workers' compensation claim.

Obamacare: The law known as "Patient Protection and Affordable Care Act."

occupational diseases and illnesses: Health problems that are the direct result of a workplace health hazard, such as dust, gas, and radiation. These can come on rapidly or develop over time.

Occupational Safety and Health Act: Act that gave the federal government the authority to set and enforce safety and health standards for most employees in the United States; administered by the Occupational Safety and Health Administration.

Occupational Safety and Health Administration (OSHA): A federal agency that oversees the federal laws requiring employers to provide employees with a workplace free from hazardous conditions.

Office for Civil Rights (OCR): The Office for Civil Rights enforces the HIPAA Privacy Rule, which protects the privacy of individually identifiable health information; the HIPAA Security Rule, which sets national standards for the security of electronic protected health information; and the confidentiality provisions of the Patient Safety Rule, which protect identifiable information being used to analyze patient safety events and improve patient safety.

Office of Inspector General (OIG): The largest inspector general's office in the federal government, it is dedicated to combating fraud, waste, and abuse, and to improving the efficiency of HHS programs. The majority of OIG's resources goes toward overseeing Medicare and Medicaid programs.

Office of the National Coordinator for Health Information (ONC): A staff division of the Office of the Secretary, within the U.S. Department of Health and Human Services. It is primarily focused on coordination of nationwide efforts to implement and use health information technology and the electronic exchange of health information.

Office of Workers' Compensation Programs (OWCP): U.S. Department of Labor office that administers compensation programs for work-related injuries and illness for civilian employees of federal agencies.

OIG Fraud Alerts: Alerts that are periodically issued and posted on the Centers for Medicare and Medicaid Services website to advise providers of problematic actions that have come to the Office of Inspector General's attention.

OIG Work Plan: Office of Inspector General plan that lists the year's planned projects for sampling types of billing to determine if there are any problems.

ombudsman: A representative of workers' compensation insurance plans who can assist the injured worker with the workers' compensation claim at no charge. The ombudsman is not a lawyer but knows the law as it pertains to workers' compensation claims.

operating physician: A physician who performed the surgical procedure being billed on a specific claim.

optical character recognition (OCR): The mechanical or electronic translation of images of typewritten text into machine-editable text. Software used with a scanner allows for the transfer of printed or typed text and bar codes to an insurance company's computer memory.

out-of-pocket expenses: Amount of healthcare expenses for which a policyholder or patient is responsible. The amount is determined by the payer and is listed in the insured's policy. The payer reimburses services at 100% once the out-of-pocket expenses are met in a calendar year.

outpatient: A patient who is treated at a hospital or other medical facility during a stay of less than 24 hours.

outpatient care: Does not require the patient to stay overnight.

Outpatient Prospective Payment System (OPPS): The method that Medicare uses to pay for most outpatient services at hospitals or community mental health centers under Medicare Part B.

panel: A group of tests ordered together to detect particular diseases or malfunctioning organs.

participating provider (PAR): A provider who signs a contract with an insurance carrier to see patients at a discounted rate. PARs are usually listed in a provider book given to beneficiaries at enrollment.

past, family, and social history (PFSH): A review of the past medical experiences of the patient and the patient's family as well as an age-appropriate review of past and current social activities such as marital status, employment, sexual history, and use of drugs, alcohol, and tobacco.

patient account services (PAS): A facility that centralizes the process of billing patients and carriers for treatment received at an inpatient facility.

patient control number (PCN): Unique alphanumeric identifier assigned by a provider to facilitate retrieval of individual case records and posting of payments. Found on the UB-04.

patient financial services (PFS): The departments responsible for processing claims that include billing, revenue integrity, collections, support services, and others.

patient information form: Form that contains demographic, employment, and insurance information about a patient. The form varies from one practice to another.

Patient Protection and Affordable Care Act (PPACA): A U.S. federal statute signed into law by President Barack Obama on March 23, 2010. PPACA reforms certain aspects of the private health insurance industry and public health insurance programs, increases insurance coverage of preexisting conditions, expands access to insurance to over 30 million Americans, and increases projected national medical spending while lowering projected Medicare spending.

payer(or): Generally refers to entities other than the patient that finance or reimburse the cost of health services.

payer of last resort: Under the Medicaid program, if an insured person has any insurance in addition to Medicaid, then those insurance carriers will be approached first for payment and Medicaid will be approached as payer of last resort.

payment: Money received in a physician's practice. Includes insurance payments attached to an Explanation of Benefits or patient payments by check, money order, or cash.

peer review: An objective, unbiased review by a group of physicians employed by an insurance carrier to determine what payment is adequate for the services provided. This review is used by a physician as a last attempt to resolve an appeal dispute when all other efforts at resolution have failed.

pending claim: A claim that has been received by the carrier but has not yet been processed. Usually additional information is requested from the provider to continue processing of the claim.

per member per month (PMPM): Refers to the fees paid on a capitation plan. The rate is based on a list with a number of members sent to the provider at the beginning of the month. The provider is paid up front for medical services rendered whether the patients are treated or not.

physical status modifier: A two-character code beginning with "P," required after a CPT code for anesthesia to indicate the patient's health status at the time anesthesia is administered. Established by the American Society of Anesthesiologists.

physician of record: With regard to workers' compensation claims, physician who treats a patient's injury or illness; also known as the treating doctor.

point-of-service (POS): A type of managed healthcare plan that allows the member to choose between an HMO, PPO, or indemnity plan at the time of service.

policyholder: Owner of an insurance policy.

preauthorization: Authorization from an insurance company that allows a patient to receive treatment using their benefits. Some insurance companies require this prior to admission for a hospital stay or outpatient surgery.

pre-existing condition: A diagnosis or condition for which a beneficiary has already received medical advice or treatment prior to the effective date of coverage with his or her insurance carrier. Anything for which symptoms were present and a prudent person would have sought treatment.

preferred provider organization (PPO): Organization that contracts with physicians and facilities to perform services for preferred provider members for specified rates.

premiums: Dollar amounts a person pays for an insurance policy. Often deducted from an employee's paycheck.

present on admission (POA): POA indicators apply to all diagnosis codes and clarify if the diagnosis was present at the time of admission.

presenting problem: *See* nature of the presenting problem.

primary care manager (PCM): Physician who coordinates and manages a TRICARE Prime patient's care. This can be a civilian or military provider.

primary care physician (PCP): A provider who coordinates a patient's care.

primary diagnosis: The condition that requires the most resources and care. Many times the primary and principal diagnosis (the conditions that cause the patient to be admitted) are the same.

primary procedure: The most resource-intensive CPT procedure done during a patient encounter.

principal diagnosis: The condition established, after all tests and procedures are completed, to be chiefly responsible for the admission of a patient to a hospital for care.

privacy compliance officer: A contact person, usually a staff member, responsible for receiving and responding to requests of medical records and receiving complaints.

Privacy Rule: Regulates the use and disclosure of protected health information.

professional component: The part of the relative value associated with a procedure that represents a physician's skill, time, and expertise used in performing the procedure.

Program of All-Inclusive Care for the Elderly (PACE): Features a comprehensive service delivery system and integrated Medicare and Medicaid financing. The PACE program was developed to address the needs of long-term care clients, providers, and payers. For most participants, the comprehensive service package permits them to continue living at home while receiving services rather than be institutionalized.

prospective audit: Completed before the claim is submitted for payment.

prospective payment system: A method of reimbursement in which third-party payment is made based on a predetermined, fixed amount, based on the classification of type of service. Medicare DRGs are a major example.

protected health information (PHI): Individually identifiable health information, held or maintained by a covered entity or its business associates acting for the covered entity, that is transmitted or maintained in any form or medium.

provider identification number (PIN): Unique identification number given to providers for billing purposes.

providers: Individuals or facilities providing medical care.

qualified independent contractors (QICs): Companies that contract with Medicare to conduct all second-level appeals (reconsiderations) for Medicare, Medicaid, and SCHIP (State Children's Health Insurance Plan).

reason codes: Numeric or alphabetic digits that indicate the reason why a claim was not paid in full, how the claim was calculated, or why the claim was denied. Also known as remark codes.

recovery audit contractor (RAC): Audits the processed claims by MAC and recovers improper paid claims.

redetermination: The first level of appeal for physician claims with Medicare. The provider has 120 days to file this request from the date of denial. Medicare carriers must process these requests with 30 days.

referral: The transfer of total care or a specific portion of care of a patient from one physician to another.

registered health information administrator (RHIA): An expert in managing patient health information and medical records, administering computer information systems, collecting and analyzing patient data, and using classification systems.

registered health information technician (RHIT): Coordinates services related to inpatient medical coding, medical documentation, abstracting, data collection, and reimbursement requirements; supervises inpatient medical coding.

registration: The process of collecting a patient's personal information, including insurance information, and entering it into the hospital's computer system. Includes scheduling the hospital stay, completing preadmission testing, receiving and following all of the appropriate preadmission instructions, completing all consent forms, and verifying insurance benefits.

relative value unit (RVU): Unit of measure assigned to a medical procedure based on the time required to perform it. This system is composed of three elements: work, practice expense, and liability insurance.

release of information form: Specifies which information from a patient's medical chart may be released and to whom it may be released.

remark codes: *See* reason codes.

rendering physician: A provider who renders a service—for example, a radiologist.

residual effect: A condition that remains after a patient's acute injury or illness.

resource-based fees: Fees based on resource-based relative value scale (RBRVS).

resource-based relative value scale (RBRVS): A payment schedule system that represents the resources used to perform a procedure or service by assigning a relative value for each procedure.

restricted status: Status that requires a beneficiary to see a designated physician or pharmacy for eligible persons covered under the Medicaid program.

retention schedule: Determines how long patient records must be stored. This determination is based on state regulations and federal laws.

retrospective audit: Audit completed after payment has been received from a carrier.

review of systems (ROS): An inventory of body systems obtained through a series of questions asked by the physician, who seeks to identify signs or symptoms that the patient may be experiencing.

rule out (R/O): A designation for an uncertain diagnosis for which the provider orders tests or studies in an attempt to eliminate it as the cause of the patient's complaint. When coding outpatient services, R/O diagnoses are not to be coded; rather, the presenting signs and symptoms should be coded.

schedule of benefits (SOB): A list of medical services covered under an insurance policy and the amount paid for each treatment.

scrubbing: Intricate cleaning of a claim by a clearinghouse before submission. "Cleaning" refers to making sure all required data has been entered accurately.

secondary insurance: Any insurance a patient may have in addition to his or her primary insurance. Claims can be submitted to secondary insurance carriers for the balance of a medical claim not paid by the primary insurer.

secondary procedure: A procedure performed in addition to the primary procedure.

Security Rule: Specifies that safeguards be implemented to protect electronic protected health information (EPHI).

separate procedure: A descriptor used in coding for a procedure that is sometimes part of a surgical package but can be performed separately and billed separately.

sequela: A late effect, also referred to as a residual effect.

sign: An indication of a particular disorder that can be observed or measured by a physician.

skilled nursing facility (SNF): A nursing facility with the staff and equipment to provide skilled nursing care or skilled rehabilitation services and other related health services.

SOAP format: A documentation method that records the patient's Subjective complaint, the provider's Objective evaluation and examination, the Assessment or diagnosis, and the Plan for treatment.

Social Security Disability Insurance (SSDI): Federal disability compensation program that pays benefits to employed or self-employed individuals with disabilities who are under age 65 and have paid Social Security taxes for a minimum number of calendar year quarters. The number of quarters worked varies depending on the age of the individual. Pays benefits to people who cannot work because they have a medical condition that is expected to last at least 1 year or result in death.

special report: A report to detail the reason for a new, variable, or unlisted procedure or service; it explains the patient's condition and justifies the procedure's medical necessity.

special risk insurance: Insurance that an individual can purchase to protect against a certain type of accident or illness.

spend-down program: Program that allows patients to pay a portion of their medical expenses each month with Medicaid available to assist with the remaining medical expenses. This program is for persons who are at or below the state income level. Medicaid eligibility is then determined month to month.

sponsor: The beneficiary or policyholder of a TRICARE plan.

State Children's Health Insurance Program (SCHIP): Health insurance for children through the Medicaid program. SCHIP is jointly financed by the state and federal governments and administered by the states. Each state determines the guidelines for its own program, eligibility groups, benefit packages, payment levels for coverage, and administrative and operating procedures.

state license number (SLN): Unique identification number issued by the state for billing purposes.

subscribers: Persons responsible for payment of insurance premiums or persons whose employment or group affiliation is the basis for membership in a health plan.

subterms: Coding terms that provide more specific information than the main term. They also provide the anatomic site affected by the disease or injury.

superbill: Document that contains ICD-10 and CPT codes for the diagnoses and services that the office routinely uses. Also referred to as an encounter form, charge slip, or routing slip.

supplemental income benefits: With regard to workers' compensation claims, benefits that may be issued to an injured worker due to the percent of impairment rating, or if the worker has not been able to find employment that matches his or her ability to work.

supplemental insurance: Provides coverage for medical services not covered by the primary plan. An example of supplemental insurance would be a Medigap policy that pays the insured's coinsurance and items not covered by Medicare.

Supplemental Security Income (SSI): Government program funded by general taxes that helps pay living expenses for low-income older people and those who are blind or have disabilities. May be issued to an injured worker due to the percent of impairment rating, or if the worker has not been able to find employment that matches his or her ability to work.

supplementary terms: Nonessential words or phrases that help to define a code in the ICD-10-CM; usually enclosed in parentheses or brackets.

surgical package: The services before and after a surgical procedure that are considered to be part of the CPT code billed and should not be billed separately. The CPT manual defines the "CPT surgical package," but payers may vary this to suit their needs. Also called a global package.

symbols: Used in the CPT book to show changes and alert the reader to new codes, deletions, or alterations to a code. The symbol is located before the code number for 1 year, after which it becomes part of the next annual printing.

symptom: An indication of a disorder or disease that the patient reports to the physician, but that the physician cannot observe or measure.

tax identification number (TIN): Identification number used by the Internal Revenue Service in the administration of tax laws.

Tax Relief and Health Care Act (TRHCA): Act that helps to maintain key tax reforms, expand the U.S. commitment to renewable energy resources, make it easier for Americans to afford health insurance, and open markets overseas for farmers and small businesses.

technical component: Part of the relative value associated with a procedure that reflects the technologist, equipment, and processing including pre-injection and post-injection services.

telemedicine (telehealth): The remote diagnosis and treatment of patients via telecommunications technology (telephone, computer, etc.).

Temporary Assistance for Needy Families (TANF): A time-limited (5 years) cash assistance benefit for families that qualify based on the state income or poverty level. TANF replaced Aid to Families with Dependent Children (AFDC) in 1996.

temporary income benefits: With regard to workers' compensation claims, benefits a worker may receive if an injury or illness caused the worker to lose some or all income for 7 days.

third-party administrator: Organization that processes insurance claims for a separate entity. In the case of insurance claims, it handles the claims processing for an employer that self-insures its employees.

transactions: The task of entering a charge, payment, or adjustment on a patient's account.

transactions and code set rule: Rule to standardize the electronic exchange of patient-identifiable, health-related information.

treating doctor: With regard to workers' compensation claims, doctor who treats the injured worker; also known as the physician of record.

TRICARE: The civilian health and medical program of the uniformed services for qualified family members of military personnel. (Note: The name changed from CHAMPUS to TRICARE in January 1994, but it continues to be listed as CHAMPUS on the CMS-1500 form.)

TRICARE Extra: A PPO type of managed care plan that allows TRICARE beneficiaries who do not have priority at a military treatment facility to receive services primarily from a civilian provider at a reduced fee.

TRICARE for Life (TFL): Medicare-wraparound coverage available to all Medicare-eligible TRICARE beneficiaries, regardless of age or place of residence, provided they have Medicare Parts A and B.

TRICARE Prime: A voluntary HMO-style plan for TRICARE beneficiaries that offers preventive care and routine physical examinations. Each individual on this plan is assigned a primary care manager.

TRICARE Prime Remote (TPR): A healthcare plan that is available to active-duty members who are stationed more than 50 miles from a military treatment facility, enabling them to receive treatment from a civilian provider.

TRICARE Reserve Retired (TRR): A premium-based, worldwide health plan that qualified retired Reserve members and survivors may purchase

TRICARE Reserve Select (TRS): Healthcare program serving active-duty service members, National Guard and Reserve members, retirees, their families, survivors, and certain former spouses worldwide.

TRICARE Senior Prime: Healthcare coverage for Medicare-eligible beneficiaries ages 65 and older.

TRICARE Standard: A fee-for-service health plan for families of active-duty personnel and retirees that goes into effect when treated by a civilian provider. Most enrollees pay an annual deductible.

TRICARE Young Adult (TYA): A premium-based healthcare plan that qualified dependents may purchase. TRICARE Young Adult provides medical and pharmacy benefits, but dental coverage is excluded.

turnaround time: Length of time an insurance carrier takes to process a claim from the time it is received in the carrier's office.

UB-04 claim form: Standard health insurance claim form used by institutional providers, such as hospital, skilled nursing facility, and rehabilitation centers, to file insurance claims with Medicare Part A and other health insurance companies. The UB-04 replaced the UB-92 and was mandatory beginning in 2007.

unbundling: Occurs when separate procedures are reported that should have been included under a bundled code.

unique identifier rule: Unique identification number for all HIPAA administrative and financial transactions, covered healthcare providers, and all health plans and healthcare clearinghouses.

Unique Provider Identification Number (UPIN): A number assigned by Medicare to physicians, doctors of osteopathy, limited licensed practitioners, and some nonphysician practitioners who are enrolled in the Medicare program. In 2007 the UPIN was replaced with the NPI.

unlisted procedure: A service or procedure that does not have a unique code listed in the CPT codebook. Each section's guidelines have codes for unlisted procedures.

upcode: Occurs when the procedure code stated is for a procedure that is more involved than the one actually documented in the chart.

urgent care: Immediate medical care for a condition that requires prompt attention but does not pose an immediate, serious health threat.

usual, customary, and reasonable (UCR): A fee determined by third-party payers to reimburse providers based on the provider's normal fee, the range of fees charged by providers of the same specialty in the same geographic area, and other factors to determine appropriate fees in unusual situations.

utilization guidelines: A review process that compares requests for medical services to treatment guidelines that are deemed appropriate for such services and includes the preparation of a recommendation based on that comparison.

verification of benefits (VOB) form: Form used to identify and record the benefits a patient has with the insurance company, before service is rendered, to ensure that the patient is eligible.

Veteran's Disability Compensation: Benefits paid to a veteran because of injury or disease that happened while on active duty, or were made worse because of active military service.

Veteran's Disability Pension Benefits: Benefits paid to wartime veterans with limited income who are no longer able to work.

vocational rehabilitation: The retraining of an employee so he or she can return to the workforce.

walkout receipt: A printed statement, given to the patient at the end of a visit, that lists the patient's charges for that day.

Welfare Reform Bill: Term used for a policy change in state-administered social welfare systems that reduced dependence on welfare, as demanded by political conservatives. It made restrictive changes regarding eligibility for SSI benefits.

Wisconsin Physicians Services (WPS): Claims processor for all TRICARE Senior Prime claims.

withhold: Under a capitation plan, this is a percentage of the provider's payment that is deducted from the check to offset any additional costs. At the end of the year, any withhold not used is distributed as a bonus.

Work Status Report: Form issued by the state for transmission of information between the employee and the employer's insurance carrier and the treating physician. Also known as progress report or supplemental report.

World Health Organization (WHO): A specialized agency of the United Nations (UN) that is concerned with international public health. The WHO supports the development and distribution of safe and effective vaccines, pharmaceutical diagnostics, and drugs.

write-offs: Negative adjustments to patient accounts. Usually when the provider has a contract with a carrier, the difference between the billed amount and the allowed amount is written off.

Credits

Text Credits

Chapter 1   Page 5: Deborah Vines.

Chapter 3   Page 63: U.S. Department of Justice; page 65: From U.S. Advisory Commission on Consumer Protection and Quality in the Health Care Industry. Published by Agency for Healthcare Research and Quality; page 67: From *A New Patient's Bill of Rights*. Published by The White House.

Chapter 4   Page 83: Office of Inspector General.

Chapter 6   Page 144: "Elements for Each Level of Medical Decision Making" from Evaluation and Management Services. Published by Centers for Medicare and Medicaid Services (CMS).

Chapter 8   Page 187: From HCPCS Level II Coding. Published by U. S. Department of Health and Human Services; page 191: Office of Inspector General; pages 192–193: United States Department of Justice.

Chapter 9   Pages 210–211: E/M Audit Checklist Tool. Copyright by American Academy of Professional Coders (AAPC); page 213: "Elements Required for Each Type of History" from Evaluation and Management Services. Published by Centers for Medicare & Medicaid Services; page 217: From Evaluation and Management Services. Published by Centers for Medicare & Medicaid Services; pages 217–218: From 1997 Documentation Guidelines for Evaluation and Management Services. Published by Centers for Medicare & Medicaid Services; page 218: Cardiovascular Examination from Evaluation and Management Services. Published by Centers for Medicare & Medicaid Services; pages 219–220: From Evaluation and Management Services. Published by Centers for Medicare & Medicaid Services; page 223: Table of Risk from Evaluation and Management Services. Published by Centers for Medicare & Medicaid Services.

Chapter 10   Page 265: From Health Insurance Claim Form-1500. Published by Centers for Medicare and Medicaid Services.

Chapter 11   Pages 313–314: Centers for Medicare and Medicaid Services; page 324: https://www.thehealthplan.com/documents/providers/ub04_instructions.pdf; pages 324–331: Geisinger Health Plan site, https://www.geisinger.org, https://www.thehealthplan.com/documents/providers/ub04_instructions.pdf.

Chapter 12   Page 376: From Medicare Fraud & Abuse: Prevention, Detection and Reporting. Published by Centers for Medicare and Medicaid Services; page 377: From Health Care Fraud and Program Integrity: An Overview for Providers. Published by Centers for Medicare and Medicaid Services.

Chapter 14   Page 420: From Showing Your ID to Providers. Published by Tricare; page 422: Deborah Vines-Allen, Ann Braceland, Elizabeth Rollins, Susan H. Miller, Comprehensive Health Insurance: Billing, Coding & Reimbursement, 3e, © 2018. Pearson Education, Inc., New York, NY.; page 423: CMS-1500 Claim Form. Published by Centers for Medicare and Medicaid Services.

Chapter 15   Page 435: CMS-1500 Claim Form, Centers for Medicare and Medicaid Services; page 435: UB-04 Claim Form, Centers for Medicare and Medicaid Services; page 436: Deborah Vines-Allen, Ann Braceland, Elizabeth Rollins, Susan H. Miller, *Comprehensive Health Insurance: Billing, Coding & Reimbursement*, 3e, © 2018. Pearson Education, Inc., New York, NY; page 439: From Report 4 of the Council on Medical Service (I-14). Published by American Medical Association, © 2014.

Chapter 16   Page 505: Quote by Karl Menninger.

Chapter 17   Page 529: From Disability Evaluation Under Social Security. Published by Social Security Administration.

Appendix D   Page 701: From Form No. CMS-R-131-G (June 2002). Published by Centers for Medicare and Medicaid Services; Page 704: From Health Insurance Claim Form-1500. Published by Centers for Medicare and Medicaid Services; page 718: From Form CMS-20027 (05/05) EF 05/2005. Published by Centers for Medicare and Medicaid Services; page 734: From UB-04 (CMS-1450) Form. Published by Centers for Medicare and Medicaid Services.

Image Credits

Chapter 2   Page 29: Iodrakon/Fotolia; page 33: "…Make me a bigger offer?" by Larry Wright

Chapter 3   Page 65: Robert Englehart, *Hartford Courant*

Chapter 12   Page 366: Medicare.gov

Index

Index note: Page numbers with an f indicate a figure. Page numbers with a t indicate a table.

A

A-1 case study, 555–557
A-2 case study, 558–560
A-3 case study, 561–563
A-4 case study, 564–566
A-5 case study, 567–569
A-6 case study, 570–572
A-7 case study, 573–575
A-8 case study, 576–578
A-9 case study, 579–581
A-10 case study, 582–584
A-11 case study, 585–587
A-12 case study, 588–590
A-13 case study, 591–593
A-14 case study, 594–596
A-15 case study, 597–599
A-16 case study, 600–602
A-17 case study, 603–605
A-18 case study, 606–608
A-19 case study, 609–611
A-20 case study, 612–615
abuse
    fraud and, 194–195
    Medicare fraud and abuse, 376f,
      377–380
ACA. *See* Affordable Care Act
accountable care organizations
    (ACOs), 61
accounts receivable, 432–479
    funds remittance, 478–479
    patient account adjustments,
      464–477, 464f
accreditation audits, 208–209
acknowledgment report, 245–246,
    245f
acronyms and abbreviations table,
    735–736
acute conditions, ICD-10-CM coding
    for, 120
add-on codes, CPT coding, 163–164
adjudication
    allowed charges, 443–444, 444f
    fee determination, 439
    insurance claims, 437–438, 438f
    Medicare conversion factor, 441
    Medicare fee determination,
      441–443, 442f
    patient account adjustments,
      464–477
    payers' policies, 444–450
    resource-based relative value scale,
      439–441

adjustment, patient accounts,
    464–477, 464f
Administration Simplification Compli-
    ance Act (ASCA), 78, 372–373
administrative law, fraud in healthcare
    and, 194
administrative law judge (ALJ)
    hearing, 500
Admission of Liability, 526
admitting clerk, 8
admitting physician, 309–310
Advance Beneficiary Notice (ABN),
    360–361
    documentation, 371
    HCPCS, 186
    Medicaid, 392–393
    Medicare treatment caps, 188
    sample form, 701–702
adverse effects, 105
advisory opinion, fraudulent actions,
    198–199
Affordable Care Act (ACA), 45–46
    audits, 206
    contracts for, 68, 71f–72f
    diagnoses coding, 102–103
    fraudulent claims and, 190
    healthcare delivery under, 60–61
    Medicaid projections, 394–396
    Omnibus Rule, 79–80
allowed charges
    claims adjudication, 443–444,
      444f
    managed care, 30
Alphabetic Index (ICD-10-CM),
    103–104
    abbreviations, 114–115
    acute and chronic conditions, 120
    code verification, 111
    hyphen usage, 106
    instructional terms, 113–114
    main term entries, 111–112
    manifestation, 111
    punctuation, 115
Ambulatory Payment Classification
    (APC), 308–309
ambulatory surgical center (ASC), 312
ambulatory surgical unit (ASU), 312
American Health Information Manage-
    ment Association (AHIMA), 11
American Medical Association
    (AMA), 528
    Current Procedural Terminology
      coding and, 130–131

American Medical Billing Association
    (AMBA), 13
American Recovery and Reinvestment
    Act (ARRA), 88
appeals
    claims process, 437–438,
      490–491, 491f, 492f, 493f
    customer service and, 503–506
    "denial upheld" and, 505–506
    ERISA appeals, 498–499
    formal registration, 496
    letters, guidelines for, 500–502,
      501f–503f
    for medical necessity, 501, 504f
    Medicare appeals, 499–500
    necessity of, 495–496
    process for, 496–498, 498t
assignment of benefits, 49, 238,
    240–241
    form, 238, 240f
assumption coding, 196
attending physician, 310
attitude, appeal of denied claims and,
    505–506
audits
    carrier audits, 494
    coding error prevention, 227–228
    dirty claims, 245
    evaluation and management (E/M)
      audit tool, 210f–211f, 212,
      705–706
    evaluation and management (E/M)
      codes, 210f–211f, 212
    history of present illness, 213–214,
      213f
    key elements of service, 212–227,
      213–214, 213f
    purpose of, 206–207
    rebilling abuse, 487–488, 488t
    types, 207–209
automobile insurance, 369

B

B-1 case study, 618–619
B-2 case study, 620–621
B-3 case study, 622–623
B-4 case study, 624–625
B-5 case study, 626–627
B-6 case study, 628–629
B-7 case study, 630–631
B-8 case study, 632–633
B-9 case study, 634–635
B-10 case study, 636–637

B-11 case study, 638–639
B-12 case study, 640–641
B-13 case study, 642–643
B-14 case study, 644–645
B-15 case study, 646–647
B-16 case study, 648–649
B-17 case study, 650–651
B-18 case study, 652–653
B-19 case study, 654–655
B-20 case study, 656–657
balance billing, 453
Balanced Budget Act of 1997, 391
Bankulla, Renuka, 91
basic days (inpatient care), 353
beneficiary eligibility
    TRICARE, 414
    workmens' compensation, 535
benefit period, 351–354
benefit plan, 64
benefits
    assignment of, 49
    comparison of common benefits,
      451–452, 452t
    coordination of, 64
    schedule of, 58–59
    termination, 535
    verification of, 241, 242f
    workers' compensation, 533–535
benefits period (Medicare Part A), 351
billing guidelines
    accounts receivable, 432–479
    balance billing, 453
    CMS-1500 provider billing claim
      form, 248–250
    diagnostic and procedure coding,
      case studies, 616–657
    errors relating to, 196
    fraud in healthcare and, 194–196
    hospital medical billing, 306–338,
      658–699
    inpatient billing process, 306–307
    insurance billing, 372–373
    managed care organizations, 57–59
    Medicaid, 387–406
    Medicare billing, 346–380
    physician medical billing, 236–298
    physician outpatient billing, case
      studies, 553–615
    rebilling, 487–488, 488t
    TRICARE billing, 413–425
billing services, 246–248
birthday rule, secondary insurance,
    285–286

Black Lung Benefits Reform Act, 525
blood banks, 352
Blue Cross Blue Shield, provider billing claim form, 249–250
bundled codes, CPT coding, 165
Bureau of Labor Statistics (BLS), 11
burial benefits, 535
business associates (BAs), 78

C

C-1 case study, 660–661
C-2 case study, 662–663
C-3 case study, 664–665
C-4 case study, 666–667
C-5 case study, 668–669
C-6 case study, 670–671
C-7 case study, 672–673
C-8 case study, 674–675
C-9 case study, 676–677
C-10 case study, 678–679
C-11 case study, 680–681
C-12 case study, 682–683
C-13 case study, 684–685
C-14 case study, 686–687
C-15 case study, 688–689
C-16 case study, 690–691
C-17 case study, 692–693
C-18 case study, 694–695
C-19 case study, 696–697
C-20 case study, 698–699
capitation plan, 449–450
capitation rate, 449–450
carriers (insurance), 26
    audits of, 494
case manager, medically necessary patient care, 32
case mix index (CMI), 310
case studies. *See also* A-1 through A-20 case studies; B-1 through B-20 case studies; C-1 through C-20 case studies
    diagnostic and procedural coding, outpatient billing, 616–657
    physician outpatient billing, 553–615
    UB-04 claim forms, 658–699
catastrophic health insurance, 43
    TRICARE catastrophic cap, 417–418, 420
categorically needy, Medicaid eligibility, 387–388
CDHC. *See* consumer-driven health care
Centers for Medicare and Medicaid Services (CMS)
    Children's Health Insurance Program, 390
    Current Procedural Terminology coding and, 130–131
    incentive payments, 195–196
    Medicare administration, 348–349
    privacy and security protections, 91
centralized billing office (CBO) contracts, 56

professional billing and coding careers, 5–6
certifications
    laboratory testing, 174–175
    listing, 12–14
    medical coding, 11
    professional billing and coding careers, 8–10
certified coding associate (CCA)
    certification, 13
    examination, 11
certified coding specialist (CCS)
    certification, 14
    examination, 11
certified coding specialist-physician (CCS-P), 14
certified medical administrative assistant (CMAA), 13
Certified Medical Billing Specialist (CMBS), 13
certified medical reimbursement specialist (CMRS), 13
certified professional coder (CPC), 13
certified professional coder-hospital (CPC-H), 13–14
Certifying Board of the American Medical Billing Association (CBAMBA), 13
charge-based fee structure, 439
charge description master (CDM), 307–308, 307f
checks, mailing of, 478
chief complaint (CC)
    audits, 213
    CPT coding, 141
Children's Health Insurance Program Reauthorization Act (CHIPRA), 389–390
chiropractic services, 361
chronic conditions, ICD-10-CM coding for, 120
Civil False Claims Act, 189–190, 194–196
Civilian Health and Medical Program of the Department of Veterans Affairs (CHAMPVA), 415, 420–421
Civilian Health and Medical Program of the Uniformed Services (CHAMPUS), 414. *See also* TRICARE
civil law, fraud in healthcare and, 194
Civil Monetary Penalties Law (CMPL), 88
civil money penalties (CMPs), 88
Civil Practice and Remedies Code 16.004, 509
claims
    accepted claims sample, 246f
    accounts receivable guidelines, 432–479
    appeal of denial, 437–438, 490–491, 491f, 492f, 493f
    attachment, 244
    electronic filing of, 486
    electronic health record (OCR), 248

filing guidelines, 434–437
    insurance claims, 244–248
    Medicaid claims, 396–406
    Medicare Part B claims process, 372–374
    paper *vs.* electronic, 244–248
    patient questions concerning, 489–490
    pending claims, 454
    physician medical billing, 236–298
    physician's identification numbers, 263–264
    processing of, 437–438, 438f
    rejected claims sample, 246f, 456f–457f
    rejection follow-up, 486–487
    review of information, 463
    scrubbing of, 373–374
    secondary claims, 284–299
    settlement report sample, 246, 247f
    TRICARE submission guidelines, 421–424, 421f, 422f
    TRICARE timely filing requirements, 415
    workers' compensation claims, 538–539
clean claims, 245
clearinghouse, electronic claims, 244–245, 486
Clinical Laboratory Improvement Act (CLIA), 174–175
CMAA. *See* certified medical administrative assistant
CMBS. *See* certified medical billing specialist
CMRS. *See* certified medical reimbursement specialist
CMS. *See* Centers for Medicare and Medicaid Services (CMS)
CMS-1500 claim form, 244
    A-1 case study, 555–557
    A-2 case study, 559
    A-3 case study, 561
    A-4 case study, 564
    A-5 case study, 567
    A-6 case study, 570
    A-7 case study, 573
    A-8 case study, 576
    A-9 case study, 579
    A-13 case study, 591
    A-14 case study, 594
    A-15 case study, 597
    A-16 case study, 600
    A-17 case study, 603
    A-18 case study, 606
    A-19 case study, 609
    A-20 case study, 612
    abbreviations, 250t
    B-1 case study, 618
    B-2 case study, 620
    B-3 case study, 622
    B-4 case study, 624
    B-5 case study, 626
    B-6 case study, 628

B-7 case study, 630
    B-8 case study, 632
    B-9 case study, 634
    B-10 case study, 636
    B-11 case study, 638
    B-12 case study, 640
    B-13 case study, 642
    B-14 case study, 644
    B-15 case study, 646
    B-16 case study, 648
    B-17 case study, 650
    B-18 case study, 652
    B-19 case study, 654
    B-20 case study, 656
    completion guidelines, 250–262
    delayed or rejected forms, reasons for, 280, 281f–284f
    diagnostic and procedure coding, billing using, 616–657
    form locators (*See* Form locators (CMS-1500 claim form))
    HIPPA compliance, 284
    Medicaid claims, 397–406
    patient registration locators, 435, 435f, 436f
    physician outpatient billing case studies, 553–615
    practice exercises, 264–280
    provider billing, 248–250
    sample form, 251f, 704
    TRICARE claims, 421–424, 423f
    workers' compensation claims, 538–539, 540f
CMS Claim Forms
    A-10 case study, 582
    A-11 case study, 585
    A-12 case study, 588
CMS-DRG, 311–312
COBRA insurance, 43–44
code edits, 209
code linkage, 188–189, 196–197
coding. *See also* Current Procedural Terminology (CPT) coding; *International Classification of Diseases, Tenth Revision, Clinical Modification* (ICD-10-CM)
    case studies, 616–657
    certification, 13–14
    combination or multiple coding, 120–122
    diagnosis coding, 102–103
    error prevention guidelines, 227–228
    federal compliance, 199–200
    hospital billing systems, 308–309
    National Correct Coding Initiative, 196–198
    procedures and services, 152–176
    reason codes, 454
    remark codes, 454
    on UB-04 claim form, 322–338
Cohen, Lawrence, 91
coinsurance
    days, inpatient care, 353
    defined, 30
    Medicare coverage, 351

collection of payments
    insurance payments, 49
    medical collector, 7
combination codes, ICD-10-CM,
    120–122
commercial health insurance, 41–42
comorbidity, 311, 311f
compensation guidelines
    managed care organizations, 57–59
    for services, 65, 66f–68f
compliance, coding requirements,
    199–200
*Compliance Program Guidance for Individual and
    Small Group Physicians*, 199–200
complication codes
    audits, 221–222
    ICD-10-CM, 103
computerized provider order entry
    (CPOE), 89–91
concierge contract, 68, 69f
conditional payment, Medicare,
    370–371
confidential information, TRICARE
    claims, 424–425
Consolidated Omnibus Budget
    Reconciliation Act of 1985
    (COBRA), 369
consultation, CPT coding, 139
consumer-driven health care
    (CDHC), 44
contracted services, 64
contracts
    compensation and billing guide-
        lines, 57–59
    concierge contract, 68, 69f
    covered medical expenses in,
        58–59
    definitions, 64–65
    as legal agreement, 57
    managed care organizations, 56
    payment in, 59
    purpose, 56
    for specialists, 68, 69f–70f
contractual adjustment. *See* write-off
conversion factor, 441
coordination of benefits (COB), 64
    information review, 463
    Medicare, 369–370
    secondary claims and, 285–286
coordination of care, documentation,
    222, 224f–226f, 227
copayment
    calculation of, 451
    coordination of benefits and, 64
    defined, 30
    Medicare coverage, 351
    overpayments, 508–513
cost outliers, hospital billing systems,
    310–312
counseling
    CPT coding, 145
    documentation, 222,
        224f–226f, 227
covered entities (CE), in HIPPA, 78
covered medical expenses, managed
    care contracts, 58–59

covered persons, 64
covered services, 64
CPT. *See* Current Procedural Terminol-
    ogy (CPT) coding
criminal law, fraud in healthcare
    and, 194
crossover coverage, 358
cross-references, CPT coding, 157
Current Procedural Terminology (CPT)
    coding, 10–11
    add-on codes, 163–164
    anesthesia coding, 164–166,
        165f, 166f
    assignment of code, 148
    billing codes, 189–196
    categories, 131–133, 133f
    charge description master,
        307–308, 307f
    code ranges, 155, 156f
    coding steps, 164
    correct code determination tool,
        731–733
    counseling, 145
    cross-references, 157
    development of, 130–131
    errors, 195–196
    evaluation and management modi-
        fiers, 135–138
    extent of examination, 143
    formatting, 155–156, 156f
    guidelines, 134
    HCPCS Level 1 codes and, 179
    index organization, 154–157
    level of E/M service, 139, 141–148
    medicine codes, 175–176
    modifiers, 134–136, 158–163
    nature of the presenting problem,
        146–148
    nomenclature, 133–134
    office vs. hospital services, 137–138
    pathology and laboratory codes,
        174–175
    to place of service, 136–137
    private payer regulations, 209
    radiology codes, 172–174
    section guidelines, 157–158
    separate procedures, 169–170
    superbills, 241–242, 243f
    supplies and services, 172
    surgical coding, 166–169, 167f
    surgical package/global surgery
        concept, 170–172
    symbols, 134
    type of patient, 138–139
customary fee, managed care, 30
customer service, appeals and,
    503–506

D

data complexity, audits, 221
date of service (DOS), Medicaid
    claims, 396
death, injury resulting in, 528
death benefits, 535
deductibles
    in managed care, 26

patient charge calculations,
    450–451
default code (ICD-10-CM), 115
Defense Enrollment Eligibility Report-
    ing System (DEERS), 415
delivery of healthcare, changes to,
    60–61
denial of claims, 437–438, 490–491.
    See also appeals
    customer service for management
        of, 503–506
    follow-up procedures, 486–487
descriptor, in CPT coding,
    155–156, 173
designated doctor, workmens' com-
    pensation claims, 529–531
diagnosis related group (DRG) system,
    309–312
    Medicaid claims, 396
diagnostic coding, 102–103
    case studies, 616–657
diagnostic statement (ICD-10-CM),
    115
dirty claims, 245
disability
    compensation programs, 535–536
    defined, 528
    Medicare coverage, 369
    permanent disability, 528
    temporary disability, 527–528
    work-related injuries, 527–528
discounted fee, 29
District of Columbia Workers' Com-
    pensation Act, 525
documentation
    in audits, 222, 224f–226f, 227
    of claims process, 494–495
downcoding, 206, 212, 438
driver's license, copy of patient's, 367
durable medical equipment (DME)
    HCPCS coding, 185
    number for, 264
    protected health information and,
        82–84

E

Early and Periodic Screening,
    Diagnosis, and Treatment
    (EPSDT) program (Medicaid),
    260, 391–392
edit report, dirty claims, 245
electronic claims (electronic media
    claims), 244–248, 486
electronic data interchange (EDI),
    Transactions and Code Set Rule
    (HIPPA), 84–85
electronic funds transfer (EFT), 478
electronic health record (EHR), 85–87
    conversion, 238
    meaningful use principle, 89–91
electronic health record (OCR), opti-
    cal character recognition, 248
electronic medical records (EMR),
    85–87
electronic protected health
    information (EPHI), 85

Electronic Remittance Advice (ERA),
    208, 374–376, 434, 454–462,
    456f–458f, 463
    necessity of appeal, 495–496
    overpayments and, 506–513
    workers' compensation claims,
        538–539
emergency services, 64
    CPT coding, 138
    UB-04 claim, 312
emerging technologies, CPT Category
    III codes, 132–133
Employee Retirement Income Security
    Act (ERISA), 40, 498–499,
    508
employer identification number (EIN),
    physician, 263
Employer's First Report of Injury or
    Illness, 537
encounter form, 241–242,
    243f, 730
Encounter forms
    A-1 case study, 557
    A-2 case study, 560
    A-3 case study, 563
    A-4 case study, 566
    A-5 case study, 569
    A-6 case study, 572
    A-7 case study, 575
    A-8 case study, 578
    A-9 case study, 581
    A-10 case study, 584
    A-11 case study, 587
    A-12 case study, 590
    A-13 case study, 593
    A-14 case study, 596
    A-15 case study, 599
    A-16 case study, 602
    A-17 case study, 605
    A-18 case study, 608
    A-19 case study, 611
    A-20 case study, 614–615
encounter record. *See* claims
encryption
    electronic claims, 248
    patient records, 84
end-stage renal disease (ESRD),
    348, 369
Energy Employees occupational Illness
    Compensation Program Act
    (EEOICP), 525
Enforcement Rule (HIPPA), 88
enrollee, 32
EOB. *See* Explanation of Benefits
EPO. *See* exclusive provider
    organization
eponyms, ICD-10-CM coding, 118
ERA. *See* Electronic Remittance
    Advice
errors
    billing errors, 196
    in coding, 195–197
    prevention, in E/M coding,
        227–228
established patient, CPT coding,
    138–139

ethics
managed care, 60–63
medical coder, 200
medical office specialist,
62–64, 63f
etiology, in ICD-10-CM coding,
112, 117
evaluation and management
(E/M) codes
audits, 208
audit tool, 210f–211f, 212,
705–706
CPT coding, 135–148
error prevention, 227–228
medical necessity, 209, 212
*Evaluation and Management: Coding and
Documentation Pocket Reference* (Trailblazer Health Enterprises), 212
examination
audits, 216–218, 217t, 218t, 219t
CPT coding, extent of, 143
excluded services, 451–453
exclusive provider organization, 37
Explanation of Benefits (EOB), 208
account adjustments, 464–477,
464f
accounts receivable, 434
adjudication process, 437–438,
438f
claim filing guidelines, 434–437
denied claims, 490, 491f,
492f, 493f
fee determination, 439
Medicaid claims, 397
necessity of appeal, 495–496
overpayments and, 506–513
practice exercises, 459–463
processing, 453–463
remittance of funds, 478–479
review of information, 463
sample form, 707
secondary claims, 286
workers' compensation claims,
538–539
external audit, 207
External Causes Index
(ICD-10-CM), 105

F

facilities operations
in managed care, 47
professional careers in, 4–6, 9t–10t
facility provider number (FPN), 264
False Claims Act Legal Center, 191f
family deductibles, 451
Federal Coal Mine Health and Safety
Act, 525
federal compliance, 199–200
federal criminal penalties, HIPPA
violations, 88
Federal Employees' Compensation Act
(FECA), 525
Federal Insurance Contribution Act
(FICA), 536
Federal Medical Assistance Percentage
(FMAP), 386

Federal Poverty Level (FPL), 386
fee determination, claims adjudication
process, 439
fee for service
hospital billing systems, 308–309
managed care, 30
Medicare, 359
payment, 59
plans including, 42
final report, workmens' compensation
claims, 529
financial agreement form, 708–710
flexible spending accounts (FSAs), 45
follow-up procedures, claims
rejection, 486–487
Food and Drug Administration (FDA)
CPT Category III codes, 132–133
privacy requirements and, 82
Form locators (CMS-1500 claim form)
additional information (NUCC
designation) (19), 256–257
amount paid (29), 261
assignment acceptance by physician
(27), 261
billing provider information (33),
262
charges (24f), 259
condition related to visit
(10a-c), 253
date of current illness/injury/
pregnancy (14), 255
dates of service (locators 24 and
24a), 258
dates patient unable to work (16),
255–256
days or units of service (24g),
259–260
diagnosis or nature of illness/
injury (21), 257
diagnosis pointer (24e), 259
EMG (Emergency) (24c), 259
EPSDT Family Plan (24h), 260
facility name and address where
services were rendered (32), 262
hospitalization dates related to
current services (18), 256
insurance plan name/program
name (9d), 253
insured's address (7), 253
insured's/authorized person's
signature (13), 255
insured's date of birth/gender
(11a), 254
insured's ID number (1a), 252
insured's name (4), 252
insured's policy group/FECA number (11), 254
Medicaid claims, 397
Medicaid resubmission code/
original number (22),
257–258, 397
non-NPI qualifier identification
(24i), 260–261
non-NPI qualifier identification
(32b, 33b), 262
NPI number (17b), 256

NPI number (32a, 33a), 262
NUCC claim codes (10d), 254
other benefit plans (11d), 254
other claim ID (NUCC) (11b), 254
other date of current illness/
injury/pregnancy (15), 255
other insured's name (9), 253
other insured's policy or group
number (9a), 253
outside lab (20), 257
patient account number (26), 261
patient address (5), 252–253
patient's/authorized person's
signature (12), 254
patient's date of birth/
gender (3), 252
patient's name (2), 252
patient's relationship to insured
(6), 253, 397
physician or supplier signatures
(31), 262
place of service (24b), 258–259
prior authorization number (23),
258
procedures, services, supplies
(24d), 259
referring physician ID# (17a),
256
referring provider or other source,
name of (17), 255–256
Rendering Provider (24j),
260–261
tax ID number (25), 261
total charges (28), 261
type of insurance (1), 252
workers' compensation claims,
538–539
Form locators (UB-04 claim form),
322–338
admission/discharge hour codes
(13, 16), 324, 324t–325t
admission source code (15),
325, 326t
admission type codes (14), 324,
325t
bill codes (4), 322–324, 323t
condition codes (18-28), 326,
327t–328t
discharge status codes (17),
325, 327t
occurrence codes, 326, 329t
patient relationship (59), 330, 331t
revenue codes (42), 328, 330t
sex codes (11), 324, 324t
value codes (39-41), 328, 330t
fragmented billing, CPT coding,
170–172
fraud indicators, 542–543
fraud in healthcare, 63
billing codes, 189–196, 189f, 191f,
192f–193f
false claims, 189–196
fragmented billing, 170–172
fraudulent actions, 198–199
government investigation, 194–196
HIPPA penalties for, 88

Medicare fraud and abuse,
376–380, 376f
rebilling abuse, 487–488, 488t
workers' compensation fraud,
542–544
front desk representative, 8
FSA. *See* flexible spending accounts

G

GA modifier, HCPCS system, 186
Geographic Practice Cost Index
(GPCI), 440–441
global period, 170–171
global surgical concept, CPT coding,
170–172
glossary of terms, 770–782
government disability policies, 536
government medical billing, Medicare
billing, 346–380
grouper program, diagnosis related
group systems, 310
group HMO, 35
group insurance, 42
group provider number (GPN), 263
guarantor, 238
*Guides to the Evaluation of Permanent
Impairment* (AMA), 528

H

HCPCS. *See* Healthcare Common
Procedure Coding System
(HCPCS)
Health and Human Services (HHS),
78, 80
fraud settlements, 192f–193f
healthcare
cost control and management,
29–33
delivery systems, 60–61
fraud, 63
history in America of, 26–28
reform, 28–29, 91
Healthcare Common Procedure
Coding System (HCPCS), 13,
130, 172
billing CPT/ICD-10-PCS codes,
189–196
charge description master,
307–308, 307f
code linkage, 188–189, 196–197
coding compliance, 188
errors, 196–197
fraudulent claims, 189–196
history, 184
Index, 186
levels of codes, 185, 186t
Medicare insurance billing
requirements, 372–373
modifiers, 185–186, 187t
Health Care Financing Administration.
See Centers for Medicare and
Medicaid Services
healthcare finder (HCF), TRICARE
preauthorization, 416–417
Health Care Fraud and Abuse Control
(HCFAC) Program, 190

Health Care Fraud Prevention and
    Enforcement Action Team
    (HEAT), 190
healthcare information, defined, 241
health information clerk, 12
health information system (HIS), 306
Health Information Technology for
    Economic and Clinical Health
    (HITECH) Act, 79–80, 88–91
    electronic medical records, 242, 244
Health Insurance Portability and
    Accountability Act (HIPPA)
    Administrative Simplification
        Subsection, 249–250
    compliance alert, 284
    Current Procedural Terminology
        coding and, 131–133
    diagnoses coding, 102–103
    Enforcement Rule, 88
    HCPCS coding and, 184
    passage of, 78
    privacy compliance requirements,
        11, 78–82, 723–729
    Privacy Rule, 78–84, 83f
    records management
        requirements, 12
    Security Rule, 85–86
    Transactions and Code Set Rule,
        84–87, 372
    Version 5010 standards, 245
Health Maintenance Organization Act
    of 1973, 28–29
health maintenance organizations
    (HMOs)
    characteristics of, 34–35, 35f
    Medicaid and, 395
    Medicare, 359–360
health reimbursement accounts
    (HRAs), 44–45
health savings accounts (HSAs), 44–45
HealthSouth case, 194
high-deductible health plans
    (HDHP), 44
HIPPA. See Health Insurance Portability
    and Accountability Act
history of present illness (HPI)
    CPT coding, 141
    documentation, 222, 224f–226f,
        227
    key elements of service,
        213–214, 213f
HITECH. See Health Information
    Technology for Economic and
    Clinical Health Act
HMO. See health maintenance
    organizations
home- and community-based services
    (HCBS), 92
home healthcare, Medicare coverage, 351
hospice care, 312
    Medicare coverage, 351–352
hospital billing systems, 306–338
    charge description master,
        307–308, 307f
    coding and reimbursement
        methods, 308–309

cost outliers, 310–312
diagnosis related group system,
    309–312
inpatient billing process, 306–307
payer types, 308
UB-04 claim form, 312, 313f,
    314f, 315, 315f–321f,
    322–338, 658–699
hospital indemnity insurance, 42
hospital insurance, 42. See also
    Medicare, Part A
hospital services
    CPT coding, 137–138
    professional billing and coding
        careers, 5
HRA. See health reimbursement
    accounts
HSA. See health savings account

I

ICD-10-CM. See International Classifica-
    tion of Diseases, Tenth Revision,
    Clinical Modification
IDS. See integrated healthcare delivery
    systems
immigrants, Medicaid eligibility, 389
immunization, CPT coding for, 176f
immunoglobulins, CPT coding for,
    175–176
impairment income benefits, 534
impairment rating, 528, 531
incentive payments, 195
income benefits, workers' compensa-
    tion, 534
indemnity plan, 42
independent physician association
    (IPA), 40
independent review organizations
    (IROs), 539, 541
individual deductibles, 451
individual practice association (IPA)
    HMO, 35
injuries, worker rights and responsi-
    bilities, 528–529
injury classifications, 527–528
inpatient benefit days, 352–354, 353t
inpatient care
    billing process, 306–307
    hospital insurance, 42
    Medicare coverage, 351
    UB-04 claim forms, 312, 659
insurance
    carriers, 26, 436f, 443, 494
    claims, paper vs. electronic,
        244–248
    coverage, 42–44
    denied or delayed payments by,
        488–489
    Medicare insurance billing
        requirements, 372–373
    plans, 41–42
    secondary insurance, 284–286
    supplemental insurance, 44,
        285–286
    verification, 7–8, 47–48,
        436f, 711

insurance verification representative,
    7–8
integrated healthcare delivery systems
    (IDS), 39–40
intermediaries, 349–350
internal audit, 208
International Classification of Diseases, Tenth
    Revision, Clinical Modification
    (ICD-10-CM), 10
    abbreviations, 114–115
    acute and chronic conditions, 120
    additional characters and
        brackets, 115
    additional terms, 118
    Alphabetic Index, 103–104
    body mass index, 110
    carryover/turnover lines, 113
    checkmark, 106
    CMS-1500 claim form, codes on,
        257
    code assignment and sequencing,
        118
    coding condition, 110
    coding guidelines, 103
    coding procedure, 110–114
    cross references, 113, 115
    default codes, 115
    diagnosis related group (DRG)
        system, 309–312
    diagnostic statement, 115
    errors in coding, 195–196
    etiology, 112, 117
    External Causes Index, 105
    hyphen usage, 106
    instructional terms, 113–114
    late effects coding, 119–120
    laterality, 108–110
    manifestation in, 110–111, 117
    medical coding case study,
        101–102
    Medicare claims and coding from,
        373–374
    multiple coding, 120–122
    Neoplasm Table, 104
    placeholder, 108
    private payer regulations, 209
    punctuation, 115
    structure, 105
    superbills and coding from,
        241–242, 243f
    supplementary terms, 112
    surgical coding, 118–119
    Table of Drugs and Chemicals,
        104–105
    Tabular List, 103, 106–107, 107f
International Classification of Diseases, Tenth
    Revision, Procedure Cod-
    ing System (ICD-10-PCS),
    102–103
    billing codes, 189–196
IPA. See independent physician as-
    sociation

K

kickbacks, HIPPA penalties for, 88

L

laboratory testing, CPT coding,
    174–175
language barrier, protected health
    information, 82–83
large-group practice, professional bill-
    ing and coding in, 5
late effects coding, ICD-10-CM,
    119–120
legal agreement, contract as, 57
letters of appeal, 500–502, 501f–503f
liability insurance, 369
Lifetime Assignment of Benefits, 703
lifetime income benefit, 534
lifetime maximum benefit, 451
lifetime reserve days (LTR), inpatient
    care, 353–354
limiting charge (Medicare), 362, 713
Local Coverage Determination (LCD),
    Medicare claims, 374
lockbox services, 478–479
Longshore and Harbor Workers' Com-
    pensation Act (LHWCA), 525
long-term care insurance, 44

M

main term, ICD-10-CM coding,
    111–112
major medical insurance, 43
managed care
    appropriate providers in, 32–33
    cost control and management,
        29–33
    defined, 4
    ethics, 60–63
    fees for services, 30
    history of, 26–28
    Medicaid projections and, 394–396
    provider's view of, 46–47
    timeline, 27t–28t
managed care organizations (MCOs), 29
    advantages/disadvantages, 38t–39t
    classification of, 41t
    compensation and billing guide-
        lines, 57–59
    compensation for services, 65, 66f
    contracts, 56–57
    criticism of, 37–38
    least restrictive setting principle, 33
    medically necessary patient care, 32
    provider credentialing, 62
    types of, 34–39
    withholding programs, 33–34
manifestation, in ICD-10-CM coding,
    110–111, 117
manual review, insurance claims,
    437–438
master patient index, 306
maximum allowable fees (MAFs), 496
maximum medical improvement
    (MMI), 528, 531
MCO. See managed care organization
meaningful use principle, 89–91
    electronic claims, 244
    electronic medical records, 242, 244

Medicaid, 358
   amount and duration of services, 391–392
   appeals, time limits for, 396–397
   claims filing, 396–406
   eligibility groups, 387–389
   growth trends, 393–394
   guidelines, 387
   history of, 386
   managed care and, 394–396
   overpayments, 508
   payment for services, 392–393
   scope of services, 390–391
   special group eligibility, 389
   time limits on claims submission, 396–397
   verification, 395–396
medical and health services manager, 12
Medical Association of Billers (MAB), 13
medical benefits, workers' compensation, 533–534
medical biller, 6–7
medical billing specialist, certification, 13
medical claims. See claims
medical coder
   ethics for, 200
   job classification, 10–11
medical coding. See coding
medical collector, 7
medical decision making (MDM)
   audits, 219–221, 220t
   CPT coding, 144–145, 144f
medical director, 64
medical forms. See also specific forms, e.g. CMS-1500 claim form
   samples of, 700–734
medical insurance, 42–43
medically necessary patient care, 32
medically needy, Medicaid eligibility, 388
medically unlikely edits (MUEs), 197
medical necessity
   appeals based on, 501, 504f
   coding errors, 195–196
   defined, 64
   Medicare requirements for, 359
medical office assistant, 6
   certification, 12–13
medical office specialist
   assignment of benefits, 49
   CMS-1500 form, entry responsibilities, 252
   ethics, 62–64, 63f
medical records
   certification, 14
   electronic medical records, 85–87
   healthcare information in, 241
   HIPPA privacy requirements, 12, 78–82
   hospital records, 306–307
   notes, 215, 215f, 217f
   patient access and corrections, 84
   release form, 712
   RHIA/ RHIT classifications, 11–12
   workers' compensation, 541–542
medical terminology guidelines, 737–749

Medicare
   administration, 348–349
   appeals process, 499–500
   benefits period, 351
   billing guidelines, 346–380
   card for, 366–367, 366f
   claims process, Part B claims, 372–374
   coordination, 369–370
   coverage and eligibility requirements, 350–355
   coverage plans, 359–360
   deductibles, 353t
   documentation, 371
   electronic records, 78
   fee and limiting charge determination, 362–365, 441–443, 442f
   filing guidelines for claims, 374
   fraud and abuse, 376–380, 376f
   history, 348–349
   insurance billing requirements, 372–373
   limiting charge, 362–365
   local coverage determination, 374
   medical necessity requirements, 359
   overpayments, 508
   Part A, 348, 350–354, 360
   Part B, 348, 354–355, 360–362, 372–374
   Part C, 348, 356, 359
   Part D, 348, 356–357
   participating vs. nonparticipating Part B providers, 361–362
   patient registration, 366–371
   patient's financial responsibility, 362
   Physician Quality Reporting System, 360
   primary payers, 367–368
   providers, 360–362
   redetermination process, 499, 718
   remittance notice, 374–376
   secondary payers, 367–370, 714–717
   services not covered by, 357–358
   treatment caps, 188
   TRICARE eligibility, 414–415
   value-based payment modifier program, 360
Medicare Administrative Contractor (MAC), 349, 544
Medicare Advantage, 348, 356, 359
Medicare conversion factor (MCF), 441
Medicare Development Letter, 371–372
Medicare DRG, 311–312
Medicare Fee Schedule (MFS), 362
   workers' compensation claims, 538, 544–547
Medicare Limiting Charge, 362, 713
Medicare Remittance Notice (MRN), 374–376, 458f–459f
Medicare Secondary Payer (MSP), 369–370
Medicare Summary Notice (MSN), 374–376, 476f
Medicare Telehealth Parity Act of 2015, 355

Medicare Trust Funds, 190
medicine, CPT coding for, 175–176
Medigap, 358
Medi-Medi coverage, 358, 394
MFS. See Medicare Fee Schedule
military treatment facility (MTF), 414, 416, 419
modifier indicators, 197
morbidity, 102
   audits, 221–222
morphology, 105
mortality, audits, 221–222
MS-DRG, 311–312
multispecialty clinic, professional billing and coding careers, 5
mutually exclusive edits, medical coding, 197

N

National Certified Medical Office Assistant (NCMOA), 12–13
National Committee for Quality Assurance (NCQA), 62
National Correct Coding Initiative (NCCI), 196–198
nationally uniform relative scale, 440
National Provider Identifier (NPI), 87–88, 256, 262–263
National Uniform Claim Committee (NUCC), CMS-1500 claim form and, 250, 252–262
national uniform conversion factor, 441
nature of the presenting problem, CPT coding, 146–148
NCCI. See National Correct Coding Initiative
NCMOA. See National Certified Medical Office Assistant
Neoplasm Table (ICD-10-CM), 104
network
   HMO network, 35
   managed care contract, 57
newborn claim limits, Medicaid, 397
new patient, CPT coding, 138, 140f
no-fault insurance, 369
nonavailability statement (NAS), 416–417
non-par MFS, 362
nonparticipating provider (non-PAR), 57, 444–449, 445f
nonphysician practitioners, 361
not-elsewhere classified codes, 110–111, 114–115
Notice of Contest, 526
not-otherwise specified codes, 113, 115

O

Obamacare. See Affordable Care Act
occupational diseases and illnesses, 527
Occupational Safety and Health Administration (OSHA), 525
occurrence codes/occurrence span codes, 326, 329t
Office for Civil Rights (OCR), 84

Office of Inspector General (OIG)
   Compliance Program Guidance, 199
   fraud alerts, 195–196
   fraudulent claims and, 189–191, 192f–193f
   incentive payments and, 195
   Medicare fraud and abuse, 379–380
   OIG Work Plan, 194–195
Office of the National Coordinator for Health Information, 89
Office of Workers' Compensation Programs (OWCP), 525
office services, CPT coding, 137–138
OIG. See Office of Inspector General (OIG)
Oklahoma Option, 524
ombudsmen, workmens' compensation, 531–532
Omnibus Rule (ACA), 79–80
open access HMO, 35
operating physician, 310
opt out provisions, workers' compensation, 524
organ transplants, Medicare coverage, 352
out-of-pocket expenses, 451
outpatient care
   diagnostic and procedure coding, case studies, 616–657
   hospital billing, UB-04 claim forms, 659
   medical insurance for, 42–43
   physician outpatient billing, case studies, 553–615
   preoperative verification form, 722
Outpatient Prospective Payment System (OPPS), 309
overpayments, guidelines for, 506–513

P

Palmetto Government Benefits Administrators (PGBA), 424–425
panel test group, CPT coding, 174–175
paper claims, 244–248
PAR. See participating provider (PAR)
participating hospitals, defined, 65
participating provider (PAR), 57, 65
   allowed charges, 443–444, 444f–445f
   claims process and, 437–438
   TRICARE, 415–416
past, family, and social history (PFSH)
   audits, 213, 215–216, 217f
   CPT coding, 142–143
pathology, CPT coding, 174–175
patient care
   CPT type of patient coding, 138–139, 140f
   in managed care, 47
patient control number (PCN), 306
patient financial responsibilities
   account adjustments, 464–477, 464f
   calculation of patient charges, 450–451
   Medicare, 362

questions concerning claims, 489–490

TRICARE, 415

patient financial services (PFS), defined, 5

patient history
audits, 213
CPT coding for extent of, 141–143
documentation, 222, 224f–226f, 227

patient information form, 238, 239f, 719–720

Patient Protection and Affordable Care Act. See Affordable Care Act

Patient's Bill of Rights, 65

patient signatures, on Medicare forms, 367

payer (payor)
adjudication process and policies of, 444–449
defined, 4, 65
hospital billing systems, 308
payer ID, 373–374
primary and secondary payers, 367–368
private payer regulations, 209

pay for performance, managed care organizations, 33–34

payment. See also patient financial responsibilities
denied or delayed payments, 488–489
managed care contracts, 59
Medicaid services, 392–393

payment poster, 7

peer review, 492

penalties, workers' compensation fraud, 543

pending claims, 454

per diem payments, hospital billing systems, 308–309

performance measurement, CPT Category II codes, 132

per member per month (PMPM) fee, 449–450

per-member-per-month (PMPM) payments, 58–59

perseverance, in appeals, 505–506

pharmacies, protected health information and, 82–84

PHO. See physician-hospital organization

physical status modifier, CPT coding, 165, 165f

physician-hospital organization (PHO), 40

physician of record, workers' compensation claims, 528–531

Physician Quality Reporting System (PQRS), 360–361

physicians
admitting physicians, 309–310
attending physician, 310
billing guidelines, 236–298, 553–615
diagnostic and procedure coding, CMS-1500 form billing, 616–657

Medicare services, 361
operating physician, 310
rendering physician, 310
treating doctor/physician of record, 528–531

physician self-referral, 190–191, 193–194

physician's identification numbers, 263–264

physician's practice, professional billing and coding in, 4–5

physician standby services, CPT coding, 137

place of service, CPT coding to, 136–137

point-of-service (POS) options, 36–37

policyholders. See subscribers

POS. See point-of-service

PPO. See preferred provider organization

practice expense, RBRVS system, 440

preauthorization, 34, 36–37, 39, 47
overpayments, 509
workers' compensation, 537–538

precertification form, 721

pre-existing condition, 45–46

preferred provider organization (PPO), 36, 36f
Medicare, 359–360

premiums, 26–27, 35, 42, 46

preoperative verification form, 722

prescription drugs, Medicare Part D coverage, 348, 356–357

present on admission (POA) complications, 311–312

preventive medicine services, CPT coding, 138

primary care case management, Medicaid and, 395

primary care manager (PCM), 418

primary care physician (PCP)
managed care organizations, 32–33
Medicare coverage for, 359–360

primary diagnosis, 103

primary payers, 367–368
CMS-1500 case studies, 554–615, 616–657

primary procedure, add-on codes, 163–164

principal diagnosis, 103, 310

privacy
electronic health and medical records, 85–87
HIPPAA rules concerning, 78–82, 723–729
legal request guidelines, 80–81
release of medical information, designation for, 81f
security protection and, 91

privacy compliance officer, 11
legal requests and, 80–81

private payer regulations, 209

procedures, CPT Category I codes, 131–132, 133f
case studies, 616–657

procedure-to-procedure (PTP) code pairing, 196–198

professional billing and coding careers
certifications, 8, 9t–10t
employment demand, 4
facilities for, 4–6, 9t–10t
job titles and responsibilities, 5–6, 9t–10t
professional memberships, 14–15

professional component, CPT coding, 173

professional liability insurance, 440

professional memberships, 14–15

Program of All-Inclusive Care for the Elderly (PACE), 357, 391

prolonged services, CPT coding, 137

prospective audit, 208

prospective payment system (PPS), 308–309

protected health information (PHI). See also protected health information
electronic protected health information, 85–87
HIPAA privacy rule, 78–82
HITECH guidelines for, 88–91
language barriers and, 82–83
meaningful use principle and, 89–91
patient access and corrections, 84
pharmacies and durable medical equipment, 82–84

provider identification number (PIN), 263, 416

provider liability
Medicare fraud and abuse, 378–380
workers' compensation fraud, 543–544

providers
credentialing of, 62
history of, 26–28
identifying numbers, CMS-1500 claim form, 260–261
in managed care, 46–47
numbers on claims for, 255–256, 260–261, 263

provider's work, RBRVS system, 440

Q

qualified independent contractors (QICs), 500

R

radiology codes, CPT coding, 172–174

reason codes, 454, 498, 498t

rebilling procedures, 487–488, 488t

Recovery Audits Contractor (RAC) program, 349
Medicaid and, 394

redetermination, Medicare appeals process, 499, 718

referrals, 34–39
TRICARE preauthorization requirements, 416–417

refunds, guidelines for, 506–513

refund specialist, 7–8

registered health information administrator (RHIA)

certification, 14
classification, 11

registered health information technician (RHIT)
certification, 14
classification, 12

registration information, hospital billing, 306

reimbursement procedures
diagnosis related group (DRG) system, 309–312
hospital billing systems, 308–309
information processing, 464
workers' compensation, 544–547

reimbursement specialist, certification, 13

relative value unit (RVU), 440–441

release of information form, 238, 240–241, 240f

remark codes, 454

remittance of funds, 478–479

remote patient monitoring services (RPM), 355

rendering physician, 310

residual effect, 119

resource-based fee structure, 439

resource-based relative value scale (RBRVS), 59, 439–441

retention schedule, 463
wrongful retention, 509

retrospective audit, 208

review of systems (ROS)
audits, 213–214, 217t, 218t
CPT coding, 141–142

RHIA. See Registered Health Information Administrator

RHIT. See Registered Health Information Technician

risk assessment, audits, 221–222, 223t

Rivers, Joan, 91

S

schedule of benefits, 58–59

scrubbing of claims, 373–374

secondary claims, guidelines for, 284–299, 476f

secondary payers (Medicare), 367–368, 714–717
case studies, 554–615, 616–657

secondary procedure, CPT coding, 160

security, privacy and protection of, 91

Security Rule (HIPPA), 85–86

self-insured plans, 40, 508

separate procedure, CPT coding, 170–171

sequela, 119

service/military retiree, as TRICARE beneficiary, 414–415

services
CPT Category I codes, 131–132, 133f, 172–174
CPT surgical coding, 172
key elements of, 212–227

short-term health insurance, 43

signature on file (SOF), 367

skilled nursing facility (SNF), 312
Medicare coverage, 351

small-group practices, professional billing and coding in, 5
SOAP forms
A-1 case study, 556
A-2 case study, 559
A-3 case study, 562
A-4 case study, 565
A-5 case study, 568
A-6 case study, 571
A-7 case study, 574
A-8 case study, 577
A-9 case study, 580
A-10 case study, 583
A-11 case study, 586
A-12 case study, 589
A-13 case study, 592
A-14 case study, 595
A-15 case study, 598
A-16 case study, 601
A-17 case study, 604
A-18 case study, 607
A-19 case study, 610
A-20 case study, 613
B-1 case study, 618
B-2 case study, 621
B-3 case study, 623
B-4 case study, 625
B-5 case study, 627
B-6 case study, 629
B-7 case study, 631
B-8 case study, 633
B-9 case study, 635
B-10 case study, 637
B-11 case study, 639
B-12 case study, 641
B-13 case study, 643
B-14 case study, 645
B-15 case study, 647
B-16 case study, 649
B-17 case study, 651
B-18 case study, 653
B-19 case study, 655
B-20 case study, 657
record-keeping format, 495
Social Security Act, Title XIX, 386
Social Security Administration (SSA), 349
Social Security Disability Insurance (SSDI), 536
solo/private practice, professional billing and coding in, 4
specialists, contracts for, 68, 69f–70f
special risk insurance, 43
spend-down programs, 388
sponsor, TRICARE, 414, 421
staff model HMO, 35
Stark Law, 190–191, 193–194
State Children's Health Insurance Program (SCHIP), 389–390
state healthcare programs
Medicaid and, 391–392
workers' compensation plans, 524–526
State Insurance Commissioner, 492, 494
state license number (physician), 263

subscribers, in managed care, 26
superbills, 241–242, 243f, 730
supplemental insurance, 44, 285–286, 358, 476f
Supplemental Security Income (SSI), 388, 537
supplies
CPT coding, 172
Medicare coverage, 361
surgical coding
CPT codes, 166–169, 167f
ICD-10-CM codes, 118–119
surgical insurance, 43
surgical package, CPT coding, 170–172
symptom manifestation, in ICD-10-CM coding, 110–111
syndrome, ICD-10-CM coding, 118

T

Table of Drugs and Chemicals (ICD-10-CM), 104–105
Tabular List (ICD-10-CM), 103
checkmark, 106
code location in, 117
code verification, 111
punctuation, 115
structure, 106–107, 107f
Tax Equity and Fiscal Responsibility Act (TEFRA), 396
tax identification number (TIN)
patient, 261
physician, 263
Tax Relief and Health Care Act of 2006 (TRHCA), 349, 361
technical component, radiology coding, 172–173
telemedicine/telehealth, 354–355
Temporary Assistance for Needy Families (TANF), 389
third party payers, 209
tracking codes, CPT Category II codes, 132
Trailblazer Health Enterprises, 212
Transactions and Code Set Rule (HIPPA), 84–87
treating doctor, workers' compensation claims, 528–531
TRICARE
authorized providers, 415–416
billing guidelines for, 413–425
claims submission, 421–424, 421f, 422f
confidential and sensitive information in, 424–425
eligibility guidelines, 414–415
penalties and interest charges, 415
preauthorization requirements, 416–417
Prime plans, 417–420, 419f–420f
Prime Remote, 418–420
reform, 420
Senior Prime/TRICARE for Life, 420
Standard and Extra programs, 417–418

timely filing requirements, 415
turnaround time, claim filing, 434

U

UB-04 (CMS-1450) claim form, 244. *See also* Form locators (UB-04 claim form)
C-1 case study, 660–661
C-2 case study, 662–663
C-3 case study, 664–665
C-4 case study, 666–667
C-5 case study, 668–669
C-6 case study, 670–671
C-7 case study, 672–673
C-8 case study, 674–675
C-9 case study, 676–677
C-10 case study, 678–679
C-11 case study, 680–681
C-12 case study, 682–683
C-13 case study, 684–685
C-14 case study, 686–687
C-15 case study, 688–689
C-16 case study, 690–691
C-17 case study, 692–693
C-18 case study, 694–695
C-19 case study, 696–697
C-20 case study, 698–699
codes used on, 322–388
hospital billing, 312, 313f, 314f, 315, 658–699
instructions for completing, 315, 315t–321t
patient registration locators, 434, 435f
practice exercises, 330–338
sample forms, 313f, 314f, 734
TRICARE claims submissions, 421–424
unbundling, CPT procedures, 170–171
uniform code sets, 85
unique identifier rule (HIPPA), 87
United States ex rel. Bakid-Kunz v. Halifax Hospital Medical Center and Halifax Staffing, Inc., 193
upcode, 206
urgent care, 65, 312
usual, customary, and reasonable (UCR) fee, 439
usual fees, managed care, 30
utilization guidelines, 32

V

value-based payment (VBP), 360
value-based reimbursement, 450
verification
of benefits (VOB) form, 241, 242f
insurance coverage, 7–8, 47–48, 436f, 711
Medicaid, 395–396
preoperative verification form, 722
workers' compensation benefits, 537–538
veteran benefits, 369, 536. *See also* TRICARE

Veteran's Disability Compensation, 536
Veteran's Disability Pension Benefits, 536
vocational rehabilitation, injury requiring, 528

W

Welfare Reform Bill, 389
whistleblowers, health care fraud, 190
Wisconsin Physicians Service (WPS), 421
withholding of payment, 449–450
worker rights and responsibilities, 528–529
workers' compensation, 369
claims filing guidelines, 538–539
CMS-1500 claim form guidelines, 538–539, 540f
denied or delayed payment, 489
disputed maximum medical improvement/impairment rating, 531
eligibility requirements, 535
federal programs, 525
fraud, 542–544
history, 524–525
independent review organizations, 539, 541
injured worker rights and responsibilities, 528–529
injuries, illnesses and benefits covered by, 526–528
medical records, 541–542
ombudsmen, 531–532
physician's responsibilities, 529–531
practice exercise, 532–533
preauthorization, 537–538
reimbursements calculation, 544–547
state programs, 525–526
termination of benefits and compensation, 535–537
types of benefits, 533–535
verification of insurance benefits, 537
Workers' Compensation Commission Office of Investigations, 542
work-related injury classifications, 527–528
Work Status Report, 528–529
World Health Organization (WHO), 102
write-off, 30
filing guidelines, 434
wrongful retention, 509

X

XPress Claim, 422

Z

zero paid claims, 397, 457f–458f